C0-ATL-550

Biological Applications of Electron Spin Resonance

BIOLOGICAL APPLICATIONS OF ELECTRON SPIN RESONANCE

HAROLD M. SWARTZ

Departments of Radiology and Biochemistry
The Medical College of Wisconsin
Milwaukee, Wisconsin

JAMES R. BOLTON

Department of Chemistry
University of Western Ontario
London, Canada

DONALD C. BORG

Medical Research Center
Brookhaven National Laboratory
Upton, New York

WILEY-INTERSCIENCE, a Division of John Wiley & Sons, Inc.

New York · London · Sydney · Toronto

Library of Congress Cataloging in Publication Data

Swartz, Harold M

Biological applications of electron spin resonance.

Includes bibliographical references.

1. Electron paramagnetic resonance—Addresses, essays, lectures. 2. Biology—Technique—Addresses, essays, lectures. I. Bolton, James R., 1937– joint author. II. Borg, Donald C., joint author. III. Title.

QH324.9.E36S8 574′.028 72-39768

ISBN 0-471-83870-5

Printed in the United States of America.

10 9 8 7 6 5 4 3 2 1

Preface

The purpose of this book is to indicate the possibilities and problems in the use of electron spin resonance techniques in the biological sciences and to illustrate them with some of the current accomplishments. This book originated from discussions held during a symposium on Biological Applications of Electron Spin Resonance (ESR) held in Washington, D.C. The participants agreed that the full potential of ESR techniques in biology was not being realized, principally because biologists did not have an adequate understanding of this method. As a consequence it was not being applied in many situations in which it might be useful, and in many other instances it was being applied in a manner that could not produce meaningful results. It was generally agreed that a principal obstacle to its proper application was the lack of a good text on the technique, directed at the background and interests of the biologically oriented investigator.

Although many texts on ESR are available, they often assume a background in the physical sciences in excess of that usually possessed by biological scientists and, in addition, do not address themselves to many of the problems critical to biological applications. We felt, however, that an adequate understanding of ESR could be achieved by most biological scientists if the material were presented in a manner consistent with their backgrounds. Therefore we undertook to produce such a book, with the assistance and active collaboration of many colleagues, some of whom have contributed specific chapters.

Although we started at an elementary level, every attempt has been made to remain strictly accurate and to build up to material of a more advanced level. In the introduction and the first chapter, in which the theory of ESR is presented in some detail, a three-level approach has been used in recognition of the unfamiliarity to many readers of some of the concepts involved in ESR. In the introduction and the first chapter, in which the theory of ESR is presented in some detail, a three-level approach has been used in recognition of the unfamiliarity to many readers of some of the concepts involved in ESR. In the introduction a purely descriptive phenomenological approach is used to orient the inexperienced reader to general concepts. Within the body of the first chapter a more extensive (but still minimally mathematical) exposition is made. In addition, some aspects of the full mathematical quantum mechanical derivations of the theory are presented. The latter are set off in smaller type to emphasize the fact that although this presentation provides the fullest explanation of ESR the material need not be mastered to utilize this technique effectively. Smaller type also indicates theoretical or other aspects not essential to the main discussion of ESR.

The second chapter is a combined effort of the editors in which we have attempted to indicate the experimental aspects of ESR that we have found to be important in our own work. Within this chapter we have also made cross references to chapters that provide more extensive examples of the principles discussed.

The balance of the book is made up of contributed chapters. In each instance we believe that the authors are leaders in the field who provide authoritative overviews of their subjects with detailed considerations of only certain aspects. Each contributor was asked to tailor his chapter to the purposes of this book and not simply to provide a review. We are grateful for the splendid cooperation we have received in this respect. Our goal has been a unified book that will provide an introduction into biological applications of ESR rather than just a compilation of the current status in certain fields. It was inevitable that many topics would be omitted. We chose those subjects that we felt best exemplified the potentialities and problems of ESR studies in biology. We regret that space limitations prevented us from including other topics. One omitted subject, heme proteins, was planned for inclusion in the book, but the contributing author was unable to complete his chapter in time.

Frequently several terms are in common use in ESR spectroscope to denote the same concepts; we have attempted to cross reference them in the index. In general, we have attempted to use a single, "best" term within the text. A prominent exception is ESR (electron spin resonance) and EPR (electron paramagnetic resonance): these are equivalent terms that are both so well established in the literature that we have followed each author's preference for his particular chapter. We have also made the index as extensive as possible as an additional service to the reader; similarly, cross references between chapters have been inserted when they appeared to be helpful.

We should like to express our thanks to the many individuals who have assisted us in this undertaking and to the authors who have been most tolerant of our modifications of their chapters in the overall interest of the book. Helmut Beinert played a particularly prominent role from its inception: initially he helped to provide us with the incentive to take up the task, then aided in the recruitment of contributors, and finally provided many helpful comments on several of the chapters.

Harold M. Swartz
James R. Bolton
Donald C. Borg

Milwaukee, Wisconsin
London, Canada
Upton, New York
February 1972

Contents

Biological Applications of Electron Spin Resonance

Introduction

HAROLD M. SWARTZ

Departments of Radiology and Biochemistry
The Medical College of Wisconsin
Milwaukee, Wisconsin

JAMES R. BOLTON

Department of Chemistry
University of Western Ontario
London, Canada

DONALD C. BORG

Medical Research Center
Brookhaven National Laboratory
Upton, New York

Electron spin resonance is a technique that permits the investigator to detect and, in favorable cases, to characterize molecules with unpaired electrons without altering or destroying the molecules. More precise definitions of these types of molecules and how they are detected are covered in Chapter 1, but at this point we shall consider briefly why biologically oriented scientists might be interested in them and, in very general terms, introduce the underlying physical basis for the ESR technique.

Free radicals and biological compounds containing transition elements have turned out to be the types of molecules with unpaired electrons that have been most profitably investigated by ESR in biological research. Free radicals are characterized by high chemical reactivities—so high that they are rarely found, except as transitory chemical intermediates, unless special experimental procedures are employed. When such experiments have been performed, however, it has been possible with ESR to document that a large number of normal metabolic processes of cells do involve such intermediates. Naturally these intermediates occur principally in enzymatic reactions, and it is now recognized that a full understanding of many enzymes requires an investigation of their free radical intermediates. This is especially true of enzymes in electron transport and oxidation-reduction reactions. These are the enzyme systems that characteristically contain many of the transition-group "trace metals" that are essential microconstituents of tissue. In many cases trace metals participate in enzymatic reactions involving transfers of single electrons, and therefore unpaired electrons in the atomic orbitals of the metal constituents may also contribute to the ESR spectra of these enzymes. Thus the biochemistry of metalloenzymes has been an area of marked productivity for ESR spectroscopy and by means of this technique, combined with classical biochemical investigations, extremely detailed descriptions of the workings of some enzymes have been obtained.

Free radicals may also be important intermediates in other types of reaction. The actions of some drugs may include free radical intermediates as the reactive forms. Some authors feel that free radical reactions are important in many pathological processes such as aging and carcinogenesis. The latter has been an especially prominent field because several theories of carcinogenesis involve free radicals. In most of these areas, however, many of the investigations in which ESR is used have been impeded by a lack of full understanding of the biological problems, since so many of the investigators have had primary backgrounds in the physical sciences.

Another important field in which free radicals play a prominent role is radiation biology. Among the principal intermediates mediating the radiation damage of biological target molecules are free radicals, and ESR studies have made essential contributions to studies of the mechanisms of radiation damage to biomolecules and cells.

The understanding of the photosynthetic process has been greatly advanced by ESR studies. Photosynthesis proceeds by the photochemical conversion of light energy to electronic energy, and the chlorophyll molecule plays a critical role in this transduction. As chlorophyll absorbs light energy at the photoconvertor center, unpaired electrons result. ESR has provided a detailed account of a number of the steps in this energy-conversion process.

All of the preceding describes the use of ESR to detect and understand unpaired electrons that occur in cells as a result of normal or pathological processes. Most recently, a new type of biological ESR study has emerged in which the phenomenon of paramagnetism is used to probe normal structures and functions that ordinarily do not contain unpaired electrons. This experimental technique is termed spin labeling, and it utilizes the sensitivity of ESR spectroscopy to detect subtle changes in conformation of macromolecules and molecular aggregates such as membranes.

This, then, is a brief sampling of some of the areas of biology in which ESR investigations are currently playing a role. After an introduction to the principles of electron-spin resonance spectroscopy, we discuss each of the topics in more detail. Although some of the terminology and concepts are foreign to many biological scientists, it should be emphasized that they are not really difficult to master once the feeling of strangeness is overcome. Perhaps the most convincing argument that this is so is the fact that two of the three editors began their professional lives as physicians!

Before proceeding with the body of the text, the reader who is totally unfamiliar with the concepts and practices of ESR may appreciate a brief orientation, which is provided by the following simplified phenomenological description of the process. This reader may then find that he can scan Chapters 1 through 3 and then go on to the chapters that review ESR applications to different fields of biological research (Chapters 4 to 11). The need, however, for at least some conceptual grasp of the physical nature of the ESR phenomenon is stressed. To be sure, use of most of the conclusions based on ESR findings and comprehension of their import do *not* depend on complete familiarity with an ESR spectrometer. On the other hand, the biomedical investigator who is evaluating the potential of ESR applications in his field of research must appreciate the essence of the ESR experiment.

This point is emphasized because the interpretation and analysis of ESR data depend so much on an awareness of the basic principles. ESR differs significantly from most of the other spectroscopies used in the life sciences because the characteristics of its spectra are more strongly determined by the choices of instrumental settings and by subtleties of sample conditions than are those, for example, of optical absorption, infrared, or NMR spectra. ESR also lacks simple common rules of pattern analysis or group identification, such as are seen in infrared or NMR. On the contrary, in ESR studies, the selection of operating conditions (e.g., microwave power and modulation amplitude) and the properties of different samples (e.g., presence of water, type of paramagnetic species, and temperature) critically affect the spectra obtained and can even result in the lack of detection of some strong components, inappropriate emphasis of minor components, and serious distortion of signal shapes.

For ease of comprehension this simplified account describes ESR as applied only to free radicals. In fact, ESR has been as frequently used for the study of transition metals and other "paramagnetic" (see below for definition) components in biological and biochemical samples. This point is emphasized by the subject matter treated in the body of the book.

As the name of the technique implies, "electron spin" is important for our purposes. Crudely speaking, spin refers to rotation of the electron about its own axis like a top or tiny magnet. Quantum restrictions require that no two electrons in a molecule can have identical states; since there are only two possible spin states, two electrons in the same region of space (e.g., a bond) must spin in opposite ways. This is called an electron pair. Most organic and biological molecules contain an even number of electrons which are almost invariably "paired." If, however, a molecule contains an *odd* number of electrons, one electron is "unsatisfied" because it has no partner. Such a molecule is called a *free radical.*

Free radicals tend to undergo reactions in which one electron is gained or lost so that the final product will have all electrons paired—generally a more stable state. Thus free radicals are likely to be highly reactive, chemically aggressive, and—as a consequence—short-lived. Nonetheless, as the reader will realize from the material presented in this book, stable free radicals exist, and there are experimental techniques that can often make reactive free radicals "sit still" while their ESR "pictures" are taken (see, especially, Section 2.18).

For the purpose of constructing a naïve but useful mental picture the electron can be thought of as a spinning negative charge. Since a moving charge generates a magnetic field, the axis of each spinning electron has associated with it a magnetic moment; that is, the electron acts like a tiny

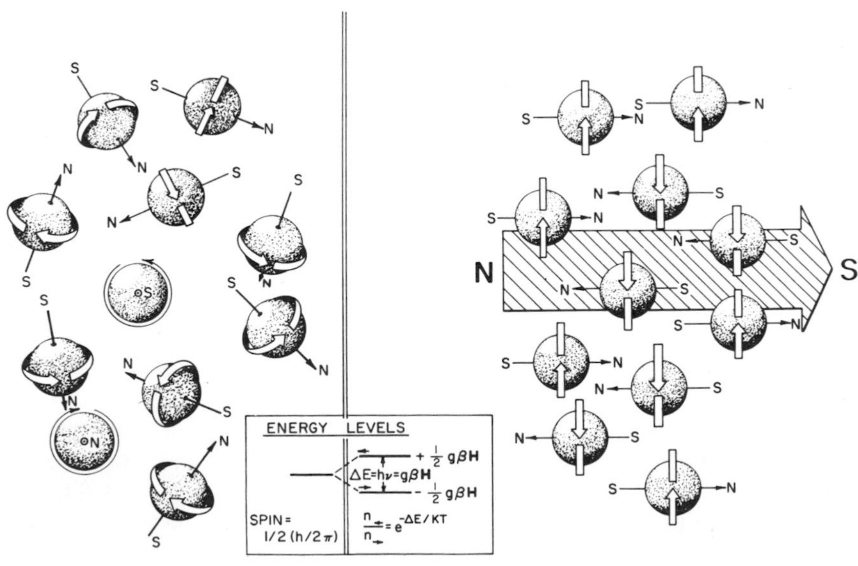

Fig. 1

bar magnet with a north and a south pole. Figure 1 diagrams electrons as spinning negative charges in various orientations, and each electron is drawn as though it had—as the earth has—a north and a south pole running through it. The restrictions of quantum mechanics, the world in which the electron lives, fix the magnitude of the spins of all electrons to be the same, and relative to any axis within a molecule only two orientations are allowed.

In this simple picture the magnetic dipoles produced by the electron spins are treated as though they were not coupled to any other magnetic influences within the molecule. When electrons are paired in chemical bonds or elsewhere, however, their spins are opposed. Hence the associated magnetic moments also are opposite and they effectively cancel each other out. For this reason most chemical and biochemical substances, which contain only paired electrons, have no net electron magnetic moments, but the "odd" electron of a free radical is not mutually compensated by an orbital partner, and the whole free radical molecule will carry an uncanceled electron-spin magnetic moment. Such a molecule is paramagnetic, meaning that it possesses a net electronic magnetic moment. Electron-spin resonance (ESR) spectroscopy (which is also known as electron paramagnetic resonance spectroscopy or EPR) takes advantage of the fact that *only* the paramagnetic molecules in a sample can be made to interact with a suitable external magnetic field. Hence a tiny population of free radicals (or other paramagnetic entities) can be detected and examined even in biological and chemical samples that are composed predominantly of other substances; this is an advantage that few other spectroscopies possess.

To portray rather crudely what is needed to obtain an ESR signal from a free radical sample a first approximation can be made that the electron-spin dipoles of free radicals interact with external magnetic fields as though they were *not* coupled to any internal fields. Thus the spin magnetic moment of an entire free radical molecular fragment can then be represented by that of the unpaired electron alone. The left side of Figure 1 represents the unpaired electrons belonging to a small population of free radicals (11 free radicals, to be exact), just as if these electrons were free in space. In the absence of an internal magnetic field the free radicals and their spin magnetic moments are randomly oriented and are in the same average energy state. If an external magnetic field is applied, the electronic magnets will become aligned—just as ordinary magnets would—and that is represented on the right side of the figure. In the case of the electronic magnets there are the laws of space quantization. So the electronic magnets can take only one of two orientations: either directed parallel to the external field (which is a slightly lower or more stable energy condition) or opposed to it (antiparallel). Thus the applied magnetic field segregates the system of equally energetic paramagnets into two subsets with a very small energy difference, ΔE.

Energy transitions are now possible in which the orientation of the electron spins will change. Such processes can occur if the spins, which are lined up by the applied (or external) magnetic field, are also coupled with electromagnetic waves of appropriate frequency. If the quantum energy of the second electromagnetic field—that is, the high-frequency field—just corresponds to the energy difference ΔE between the antiparallel and parallel electron magnetic moments, transitions will occur. In fact, the condition in which the electromagnetic field frequency brings about this energy exchange is a resonance condition. In other words, electrons can resonate with the radiation field: they can take energy from it and give energy to it. Some parallel magnetic dipoles will absorb a quantum of radiation energy to make them "jump" from the lower to the slightly higher energy states, and some of the antiparallel electrons will flip over to the parallel state, thus releasing the same amount of energy *to* the electromagnetic field.

Particles thermally distributed among quantized energy levels, however, always populate the more stable states to a slightly greater extent. Therefore at resonance there will be more parallel than antiparallel electrons; hence the resonance phenomenon will give rise to a *net* absorption of energy from the field. It is this net absorption of electromagnetic energy at resonance that is detected and amplified to provide the sample signal in ESR spectroscopy.

A simple equation that summarizes the resonance condition is given in the insert. In other words, for resonance to occur the energy difference ΔE between parallel and antiparallel alignments of the free electrons must equal the energy of just one quantum of the electromagnetic field, as given by $h\nu$, Planck's constant times the frequency of the field. This, in turn, is equal to the strength of the external magnetic field H times some physical constants, g and β, which need not be defined at this point.

In principle, the conditions for resonance to occur can be met at different combinations of magnetic-field strength and radiation frequency because a simple transposition of the resonance equation shows that the ratio of the frequency and the field equals a constant times a constant, which, of course, is a constant. Hence any value of frequency will have *some* value of field that corresponds to resonance. In practice, however, the net energy absorption, and thus the signal strength, increases with greater ΔE, and experimentally the highest practical frequencies are used; typically these are microwave frequencies in the radar range.

Figure 2 illustrates a commercial ESR spectrometer. On the left is a flat quartz container which is for liquid samples and in the center is the sample cavity between the poles of an electromagnetic. On the right is a partial view of the console. From what has just been said about the way in which energy absorption occurs in ESR it follows that detection requires several things. First, a stable magnetic field, and that is provided by the electromagnet.

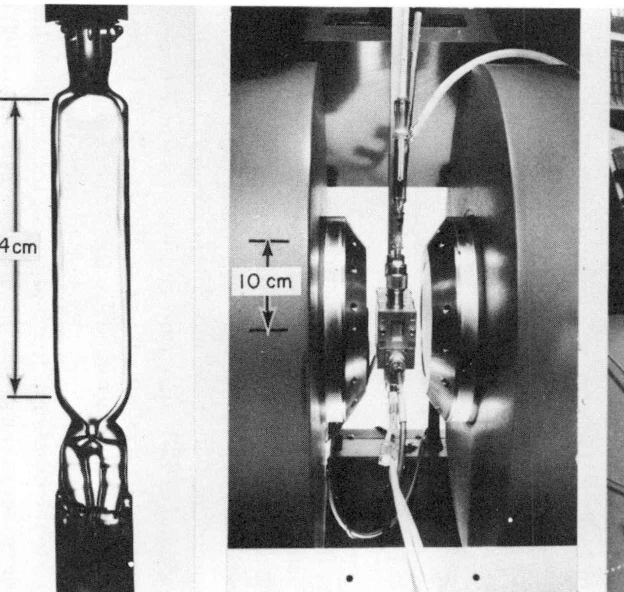

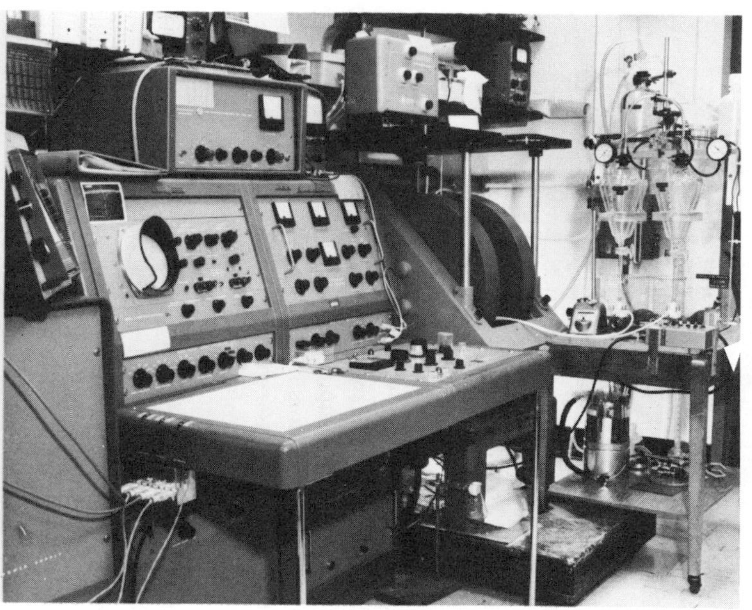

Fig. 2

Second, there must be a generator of electromagnetic waves at the required resonance frequency, and in the spectrometer the generator is a radarlike klystron electron tube which is in the box above the magnet. Third, there must be a device for exposing the sample to the proper orientation of both the magnetic field and the electromagnetic waves, and this is taken care of by the sample cavity, which holds the sample between the magnetic poles while irradiating it with microwaves that enter from a waveguide. That is to say, of the two main fields needed for resonance to occur the applied or external magnetic field is applied to the sample by the magnet, with the samples between its pole tips, whereas the microwave energy comes from its klystron generator through microwave plumbing (waveguide) into the sample cavity. Thus the sample is exposed to both fields. Additionally, of course, there must be detectors and recorders to measure the net absorption of energy at resonance and to record a signal, and these are provided by the rest of the machinery, which may also include a direct hookup to an on-line computer.

In the most favorable cases spectrometers like the one shown allow the detection of fewer than 10 billion free radicals (if the radicals are in solution, this corresponds to a concentration as dilute as 1-billionth molar). Despite this apparent sensitivity, with the limitations imposed on sample size, the confinement of the sample cavity (which is a small box), and the short lifetimes of most free radicals, a considerable fraction of free radicals of biochemical or biological interest still go undetected, regardless of the great advance represented by this type of spectroscopy over previous kinds of detection. This is discussed at greater length in Chapter 7.

In practice, samples are exposed to a constant frequency of the microwave field that is generated by the klystron tube, and the main magnetic field is varied with the electromagnet until the resonance condition is satisfied. In essence, then, an ESR spectrum consists of a measurement of absorbed microwave power plotted against the external magnetic field. Sensitive spectrometers, however, use phase-sensitive detection to enhance signal-to-noise ratios, with the result that most *real* ESR spectra represent essentially the first derivative of power absorbed plotted against magnetic field. This means that each line of resonance absorption is represented by a biphasic shape in the spectrum, as is seen in most of the spectra illustrated in this book.

The simplest kind of ESR spectrum consists of a single line. An ESR line can be characterized by its shape, by its width, and by its intensity, and also by the *g*-factor, which is determined by the ratio of field and frequency at the center of the resonance line. (Except to note that signal intensity *is* directly related to the number of free radicals in the sample, other conditions being equal, discussion of the properties of simple ESR lines is left to Chapters 1 to 3.) Unfortunately, however, these properties of single ESR lines do not vary much from one radical to another. Therefore, if all radicals gave only one-line spectra, ESR would be unable to identify or to describe them well. This can be a frustrating situation, and it applies to many of the biomedical examples treated in this book. In many other cases free radicals can be characterized by the detailed pattern of their ESR spectra and, in particular, by what is called the hyperfine structure.

Hyperfine structure is associated with the presence of nuclei that have net spins, hence *nuclear* magnetic moments of their own. In such cases the unpaired electrons are exposed to local magnetic fields produced by nearby magnetic nuclei. Because of this variable local field, the resonance condition is satisfied for electrons located on different free radical molecules at different values of the applied magnetic field, although the *total* field required for resonance remains the same, as expressed by the resonance equation. When resolved and analyzed, these hyperfine splittings may permit accurate determination of the orbital distribution of the unpaired electrons, hence the reactivities, spacial orientations, and structures of various positions in the free radical molecules. This, in turn, can often be rather directly related to molecular orbital calculations and thus to basic theory, but the main point is that the more detailed the line position and the spectral shape information in general, the greater the amount of analysis and the degree of identification obtained, which is hardly a surprising conclusion because it applies to *all* spectroscopies, not just ESR. It simply implies that spectral curvature and location data carry information, a point that is developed in some detail in Section 2.11.4.

At this point, the reader, previously unfamiliar with the concepts of ESR, should be able to approach the introductory chapters with a better conception of the general subject, although it should be stressed again that Chapters 1 to 3 do not require prior knowledge of ESR for their understanding. As an additional guide to the newcomer to ESR we have put some of the more advanced aspects in Chapter 1 into small type to indicate that they are not essential to an understanding of most of the text. We recommend that the reader go through the first three chapters once before proceeding to the applications chapters. He may later want to return to them for more detailed consideration in the context of particular applications of interest.

CHAPTER ONE

Electron Spin Resonance Theory

JAMES R. BOLTON

Department of Chemistry
University of Western Ontario
London, Canada

1.1 INTRODUCTION

Electron spin resonance (ESR) spectroscopy is a physical technique designed to detect species with unpaired electrons. Most molecules have all electrons paired; however, a respectable number of systems do contain unpaired electrons. These include the following:

1. Free radicals. A free radical is regarded as a molecule containing *one* unpaired electron.
2. Biradicals. These are molecules containing two unpaired electrons sufficiently remote from each other so that interactions between them are weak.
3. Triplet-state entities. These species contain two strongly coupled unpaired electrons. The triplet state may be the ground state or some optically or thermally excited state.
4. Entities with three or more unpaired electrons.
5. Point defects in solids or localized crystal imperfections. One or more electrons (or electron holes) may get trapped at or near these defects and thus give rise to an entity with unpaired electrons.
6. Most transition-metal ions and rare-earth ions.

Among the above systems the first and the last are found most commonly in biological systems.

This chapter is intended to provide a brief introduction to the principles of electron spin resonance spectroscopy. An attempt has been made to explain the phenomenon on a qualitative level and yet provide sufficient background for the chapters that follow. For the reader who has some background in quantum mechanics the sections in small type will provide further insight. For other readers, however, these sections may be omitted without breaking the continuity of the exposition.

No attempt has been made to be exhaustive and thus the reader is urged to consult some of the books (1–5) on electron spin resonance for further details.

1.2 THE RESONANCE PHENOMENON

ESR spectroscopy, like all other forms of spectroscopy, monitors the net absorption of energy from a radiation field when molecules change their energy state. Associated with the radiation field are oscillating electric and magnetic fields perpendicular to one another. In most forms of spectroscopy it is the electric-field component that interacts with molecules to cause the change in energy state; for instance, in visible spectroscopy absorption spectra result from transitions of electrons from their ground state to excited states. The energy required to achieve these transitions is absorbed in the form of light* quanta (a quantum of light has an energy $h\nu$, where h is Planck's

* We use the term "light" loosely to cover all types of electromagnetic radiation.

constant (6.625×10^{-27} erg-sec) and ν is the frequency of the light in hertz*). For absorption to occur two conditions must be met:

1. The packet of energy contained in the light quantum ($h\nu$) must correspond to the separation (ΔE) of energy levels between which a transition is to occur; that is,

$$h\nu = \Delta E. \tag{1-1}$$

This is known as the *resonance* condition; for example, in infrared spectroscopy the absorption lines observed correspond to separations between vibrational states of the molecules. It is not possible to excite these vibrational modes with visible light, even though the energy of visible-light photons is more *energetic* than that for infrared photons.

2. The oscillating electric (or magnetic) field component of the light must be able to stimulate an oscillating electric (or magnetic) dipole in the molecule. If this condition is fulfilled, then we say that the transition is "allowed"; for example, light in the microwave region will interact with molecules that have a permanent electric dipole moment (e.g., HCl); molecular rotation creates the required oscillating electric field; N_2, however, which has no dipole moment, does not absorb in the microwave region, even though rotational energy levels exist.

If a molecule contains a *magnetic* dipole (and therefore acts as a small magnet), we might expect an interaction with the *magnetic* component of a radiation field. Such absorptions are indeed observed but only in the presence of a static magnetic field. The reason for this will soon become apparent. The magnetic dipoles are provided by electrons and nuclei in the molecule. ESR spectroscopy deals primarily with the electron magnetic dipoles, whereas NMR (nuclear magnetic resonance) deals with the nuclear magnetic dipoles.

Although a rigorous description of the electron spin *resonance* phenomenon must come from quantum mechanics, useful analogies from classical physics may be drawn.

The magnetic dipole of an electron may be thought of as deriving from the fact that the electron is a charged particle and that a charge in motion creates a magnetic field. Two types of magnetic dipole are possible—one arising from the motion of the electron about the nucleus of an atom (called the orbital magnetic dipole), the other from spinning of the electron about an axis through its center (called the spin magnetic dipole). In the vast majority of cases 99 percent or more of the total electron magnetic dipole is due to the latter with only a small orbital contribution.

Magnetic dipoles are usually characterized by a quantity known as the

* 1 hertz = 1 cycle per second.

magnetic dipole *moment* $\boldsymbol{\mu}$* which is defined in terms of the interaction of a magnetic dipole with a magnetic field; $\boldsymbol{\mu}$, in effect, measures the "strength" of the magnetic dipole (or magnet) in a unit magnetic field. Like all dipoles the electron magnetic dipoles are vector quantities; that is, they have a direction as well as a magnitude.

Magnetic moments tend to be oriented by a magnetic field **H**. This is the familiar basis for the operation of a compass. From the fact that work must be done to disorient a magnet (or, alternatively, its magnetic moment) it can be inferred that there is a potential-energy difference between a condition of arbitrary orientation of $\boldsymbol{\mu}$ and **H** and one in which $\boldsymbol{\mu}$ and **H** are parallel (the state of minimum energy). The amount of work E required to disalign $\boldsymbol{\mu}$ from **H** is given quantitatively by

$$\begin{aligned} E &= -\boldsymbol{\mu}\cdot\mathbf{H} = -\mu H \cos(\boldsymbol{\mu}\cdot\mathbf{H}) \\ &= -\mu_z H, \end{aligned} \tag{1-2}$$

where μ = the magnitude of the magnetic moment $\boldsymbol{\mu}$,

μ_z = projection of $\boldsymbol{\mu}$ along the z direction (i.e., the direction of **H**),

H = the magnitude of the magnetic field **H**†,

$\cos(\boldsymbol{\mu}\cdot\mathbf{H})$ = the cosine of the angle between $\boldsymbol{\mu}$ and **H** [$\cos(\boldsymbol{\mu}\cdot\mathbf{H}) = 1$ at 0°].

As stated earlier, the electron-spin magnetic moment can be considered as arising from the spinning of an electron about its axis. All electrons have an intrinsic spin that is characterized by a spin angular momentum **P**. **P** and $\boldsymbol{\mu}$ are always proportional; that is,

$$\boldsymbol{\mu} = \gamma\mathbf{P}, \tag{1-3}$$

where γ is called the magnetogyric ratio. It is a unique result of quantum mechanics that the component of **P** (hence of $\boldsymbol{\mu}$) along a given direction

* Vector quantities are indicated by boldface type.

† The convention has grown in magnetic resonance to designate the magnetic field by **H** in units of gauss; despite the fact that the gauss is a unit of magnetic induction, **B**. **B** and the magnetic intensity **H** are related by $\mathbf{B} = \mu_0(1 + \chi)\mathbf{H}$. In mks units μ_0 (the permeability of free space) is $4\pi \times 10^7$ Webers/Amp-m or $4\pi \times 10^3$ G-m/A and χ is the magnetic susceptibility, the constant of proportionality between the magnetization $\mathscr{M}$ and the magnetic intensity **H** (i.e., $\mathscr{M} = \chi\mathbf{H}$). In cgs-gaussian units μ_0 = 1 gauss/oersted, so that, in the absence of magnetic material, $\mathbf{B} \approx \mathbf{H}$. Since this is true of most ESR samples, the habit has grown of designating the magnetic-field variable as **H** and using the units "gauss." Although this usage is not strictly correct, little confusion or error will result. We shall use the units of gauss for magnetic field intensity.

can have only two values. If P_z is this component, then

$$P_z = M_S \frac{h}{2\pi} = M_S \hbar, \tag{1-4}$$

where $M_S = \pm\frac{1}{2}$; M_S is called the spin quantum number. For classical motion

$$\gamma = -\frac{e}{2mc}, \tag{1-5}$$

where e = the charge on the electron,

m = the mass of the electron,

c = the speed of light.

Hence a combination of Eqs. 1-3 to 1-5 yields

$$\mu_z = -\frac{eh}{4\pi mc} M_S. \tag{1-6}$$

Equation 1-6 applies to the classical rotational motion of a charge about a fixed center; indeed, it applies to the orbital motion of an electron about the nucleus. Spin angular momentum, however, is a purely quantum mechanical effect and cannot be described accurately by classical analogs. Thus for the electron spin Eq. 1-6 must be rewritten as

$$\mu_z = -g \frac{eh}{4\pi mc} M_S = -g\beta M_S, \tag{1-7}$$

where $\beta = eh/4\pi mc$ is called the Bohr magneton and $g = 2.00232$* for a free electron. By substitution of Eq. 1-7 into Eq. 1-2 it is clear that the energies of electron-spin magnetic moments in a magnetic field are given by

$$E = g\beta H M_S = \pm\tfrac{1}{2} g\beta H. \tag{1-8}$$

These energies are displayed as a function of magnetic field in Fig. 1-1. Equation 1-8 is sometimes called the electron Zeeman energy.

Now if the sample is irradiated with light we shall find that at a certain magnetic field H_r absorption will occur. By applying the first condition for absorption it is apparent that at H_r the photon energy $h\nu$ must match that

* The g factor of the electron is actually 2.002319278 and is thus one of the most accurately known of the physical constants (6). It is remarkable that the theory of quantum electrodynamics is able to account for this factor within experimental error.

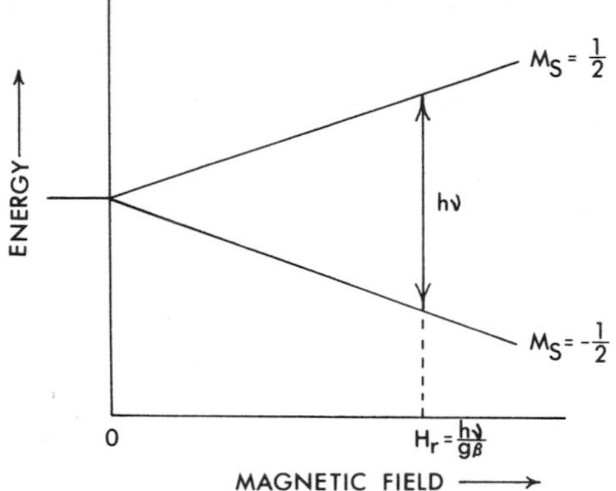

Fig. 1-1 Electronic energy levels as a function of the magnetic-field strength. H_r is the magnetic field at resonance; i.e., when $h\nu = g\beta H_r$; M_S is the quantum number for the z component of the electron spin.

separation of electron energy levels ($\Delta E = g\beta H_r$); thus the resonance condition is*

$$h\nu = g\beta H_r; \tag{1-9}$$

H_r is called the resonance magnetic field. The second condition is satisfied when the magnetic component of the microwaves is polarized perpendicular to the direction of the static magnetic field. This condition is easily met at microwave frequencies.

Equation 1-9 is satisfied over a wide range of frequencies and magnetic fields. For reasons of sensitivity, frequencies in the microwave region are used. Typically for $\nu = 9.5$ GHz†, $H_r = 3400$ G.

A quantum mechanical derivation of Eq. 1-8 begins with the Schrödinger equation

$$\hat{\mathscr{H}}\psi_i = E_i\psi_i, \tag{1-10}$$

where $\hat{\mathscr{H}}$ is the Hamiltonian operator for the energy of the system and E_i is the energy eigenvalue corresponding to the eigenfunction ψ_i.

The electron has an intrinsic angular momentum or spin. The operator for the z

* For a typical ESR experiment $h\nu$ corresponds to an energy of about 10^{-3} kcal/mole. Thus it is unlikely that radiation in the microwave region can cause any direct chemical effects. In NMR the analogous relation is $h\nu = g_N\beta_N H_r$, where g_N is the nuclear g factor, $\beta_N = eh/4\pi M_p c$ is the nuclear magneton, and M_p is the mass of a proton.

† 1 GHz = 10^9 Hz.

component of this spin is designated $\hat{S}_z$; the two possible spin eigenfunctions are $|\alpha\rangle$ and $|\beta\rangle$, that is

$$\hat{S}_z|\alpha\rangle = +\tfrac{1}{2}|\alpha\rangle, \tag{1-11a}$$

$$\hat{S}_z|\beta\rangle = -\tfrac{1}{2}|\beta\rangle. \tag{1-11b}$$

The eigenvalues of $\hat{S}_z$ are thus $M_S = \pm\frac{1}{2}$.

The electron spin and magnetic moments are also proportional in quantum mechanics, this is expressed as

$$\hat{\boldsymbol{\mu}} = \gamma\hat{\mathbf{S}}\hbar \tag{1-12}$$

For the electron $\gamma = -\dfrac{ge}{2mc}$ or

$$\hat{\boldsymbol{\mu}} = -\frac{geh}{4\pi mc}\,\hat{\mathbf{S}} = -g\beta\hat{\mathbf{S}}. \tag{1-13}$$

The Hamiltonian for this system is thus

$$\hat{\mathscr{H}} = -\hat{\boldsymbol{\mu}}\cdot\mathbf{H} = -\hat{\mu}_z H \tag{1-14a}$$

or

$$\hat{\mathscr{H}} = g\beta H\hat{S}_z. \tag{1-14b}$$

Now, since $g\beta H$ is a constant, $|\alpha\rangle$ and $|\beta\rangle$ are also eigenfunctions of $\hat{\mathscr{H}}$; thus

$$\hat{\mathscr{H}}|\alpha\rangle = g\beta H\hat{S}_z|\alpha\rangle = +\tfrac{1}{2}g\beta H|\alpha\rangle \tag{1-15a}$$

$$\hat{\mathscr{H}}|\beta\rangle = g\beta H\hat{S}_z|\beta\rangle = -\tfrac{1}{2}g\beta H|\beta\rangle \tag{1-15b}$$

or

$$E = \pm\tfrac{1}{2}g\beta H.$$

At this point it is worthwhile to elaborate on the statement that only species containing unpaired electrons will exhibit an ESR spectrum. Besides the quantization of the electron-spin angular momentum which leads to only two allowed values of μ_z, electrons also have the property that two and only two electrons may occupy a given atomic or molecular orbital; furthermore, these two electrons can be accommodated only if their spin magnetic moments are opposed; this is called the Pauli exclusion principle. Thus we use the term "electron pairs." Because of the complete cancellation of electron magnetic moments in such an electron pair, it is clear why only molecules with unpaired electrons will have an uncompensated electron magnetic moment and thus be detectable by ESR spectroscopy.

From Eq. 1-9 we may expect that there are two possible experimental approaches to the detection of resonant absorption by a paramagnetic sample. We may either fix H and vary ν or vice versa. The former case corresponds to fixing the energy-level spacing and adjusting the microwave photon energy to fit that spacing. In most forms of spectroscopy this is the procedure that must be followed, since energy levels are usually fixed by the molecular structure. The unique aspect of ESR and NMR spectroscopy is that the energy levels can be *tuned* (by varying H) to fit a fixed photon energy. For experimental reasons the latter method is preferred. Thus ESR spectra are plotted versus magnetic field rather than frequency.

1.3 RELAXATION AND LINEWIDTHS

1.3.1 Origins of Line Broadening

Any spectroscopic line has a finite width and ESR lines are no exception. The origins of this linewidth are complex, but an understanding of at least some of these mechanisms will allow valuable information to be gleaned from their study. In addition, lines that are too broad can interfere with the interpretation of ESR spectra, and therefore an understanding of the mechanisms of line broadening will also identify factors that can be altered to narrow the observed lines.

Two basic processes can lead to line broadening. The first is called *secular broadening*, which is caused by processes that generate varying local magnetic fields. By Eq. 1-8 this means that the separation in energy between the two electron spin states will vary. Hence for a given microwave frequency a range of fields will be found at which resonance will occur, and thus a broad line is generated. The variation in local magnetic fields can be dynamic or spatial: in the former case each paramagnetic center experiences a local magnetic field that *fluctuates in time*, whereas in the latter case the local magnetic field varies from one paramagnetic center to another but remains constant in time for a given paramagnetic center. The dynamic broadening is a *homogeneous* type of broadening, whereas the spatial type is termed *inhomogeneous broadening*. An example of a homogeneous type would be that introduced if an Mn^{2+} salt were added to an aqueous solution of a free radical. The paramagnetism of the Mn^{2+} would produce a strong but fluctuating local field. If, however, we were to freeze this solution, the broadening would become inhomogeneous because the local field would then be static for each radical. Generally, homogeneously broadened lines have a lorentzian shape, whereas inhomogeneously broadened lines have a gaussian shape (see Section 2.4 and Figs. 2-6 and 2-7).

The second source of line broadening is termed *lifetime broadening*. This concept is not so easy to visualize as that for secular broadening, since the mechanism has a purely quantum mechanical origin. By virtue of a finite lifetime (Δt) of a spin state the energy of that state will have a finite width (ΔE) determined by the Heisenberg uncertainty principle,* namely

* This principle is widely accepted and lies at the very foundations of quantum mechanics.

$$\Delta E \, \Delta t \sim \frac{h}{2\pi} \tag{1-16a}$$

or

$$\Delta \nu \, \Delta t \sim \frac{1}{2\pi}. \tag{1-16b}$$

From Eq. 1-9

$$\Delta \nu = \frac{g\beta}{h} \Delta H;$$

thus

$$\Delta H \sim \frac{\hbar}{g\beta \, \Delta t} = \frac{1}{\gamma_e \, \Delta t}, \tag{1-17}$$

where γ_e is the electron magnetogyric ratio.

Any process that increases the rate of transition between the two electron spin states will *decrease* Δt, hence *increase* the linewidth. Since this process applies equally to all members of the spin system, lifetime broadening is another type of homogeneous broadening.

1.3.2 Relaxation Times

In the absence of any external stimuli transitions are always occurring between the electron spin states. These are caused by interaction of the spin system with its surroundings through the random motion of molecules. The Δt that results from this transition rate will yield a linewidth termed "natural" or "inherent." This Δt is related to a time T_1 called the *spin-lattice relaxation time*. In fact, the inherent linewidth is given by*

$$\Delta H = \frac{\hbar}{g\beta}\left(\frac{1}{2T_1}\right). \tag{1-18}$$

The observed linewidth is defined in terms of a relaxation time T_2 such that

$$\Delta H = \frac{\hbar}{g\beta}\left(\frac{1}{T_2}\right), \tag{1-19}$$

where

$$\frac{1}{T_2} = \frac{1}{T_2'} + \frac{1}{2T_1}. \tag{1-20}$$

The relaxation time T_2', sometimes called the *spin-spin relaxation time*, encompasses all additional sources of broadening such as the secular sources

* An equal sign is permitted in Eq. 1–18 if ΔH is defined as the half-width between points of half-maximum amplitude on the absorption curve.

considered earlier. The relaxation time T_2 is simply a function of the observed linewidth.

T_1 varies strongly with temperature, almost always decreasing as the temperature increases. Many mechanisms contribute to T_1; one of the most important of these is the interaction between the spin and orbital motion of the electron. If the "spin-orbit coupling" is strong, T_1 may be so short that the line is many thousands of gauss wide and virtually undetectable. This is the case for many transition metal ions (see Section 1.10). The solution is to drop the temperature to lengthen T_1. Sometimes temperatures as low as 1 K are necessary.

1.3.3 Net Absorption as a Function of the Spin Populations

Clearly the detection of an ESR absorption requires that the paramagnetic system detectably interact with an electromagnetic field. When the sample is at "resonance," energy is exchanged back and forth between the electromagnetic field and the spin system such that transitions are induced upward and downward with equal probability. Thus a net absorption of energy requires a difference in population for the two levels between which transitions are being induced. Electrons are distributed between the two energy levels of Eq. 1-8 according to the Boltzmann distribution. If there are N^+ electrons in the upper level with energy E^+ and N^- electrons in the lower level with energy E^-, then

$$\frac{N^+}{N^-} = \exp\left[-\frac{(E^+ - E^-)}{kT}\right], \tag{1-21}$$

where k is Boltzmann's constant and T is the absolute temperature; *exp* means "exponential of." Substitution from Eq. 1-8 gives

$$\frac{N^+}{N^-} = \exp\left[-\frac{g\beta H}{kT}\right], \tag{1-22}$$

Since $g\beta H$ is about three orders of magnitude below kT, the exponential may be expanded*; that is,

$$\frac{N^+}{N^-} \simeq 1 - \frac{g\beta H}{kT} = 1 - \frac{h\nu}{kT}, \tag{1-23}$$

For $\nu \sim 10^{10}$ Hz and $T = 300$ K, $N^+/N^- = 0.9984$. Thus only a small fraction of the electrons actually contribute to the absorption. Sophisticated electronics are required to detect the signal.

* $e^{-x} \simeq 1 - x$, if $x \ll 1$.

1.3.4 Microwave Power and the Saturation Phenomenon

As noted above, the ESR signal amplitude depends on the existence of a *difference* in the populations of the two electron-spin energy levels. In the absence of an electromagnetic field this population difference in a static magnetic field **H** is achieved through the Boltzmann distribution Eq. 1-21. It is important to realize that for a two-level system (i.e., $S = \frac{1}{2}$) any change in the population difference n* can be achieved only by a net loss or gain in the total energy of the spin system. When $n = 0$, the spin system has its maximum achievable energy†; as n increases (i.e., more spins go to the lower state), the spin system loses energy. From a thermodynamic standpoint this implies that the spin system must be in thermal contact with its surroundings. This is illustrated in Fig. 1-2. The spin temperature T_S is

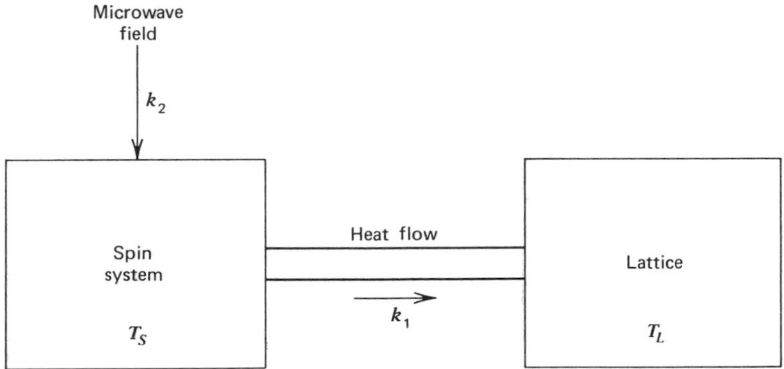

Fig. 1-2 Energy flow between the spin system and the lattice (surroundings). T_S is the temperature of the spin system and T_L is the lattice temperature. k_1 and k_2 are rate constants describing the rate of heat flow.

defined as that temperature at which a Boltzmann distribution would yield the observed population difference; the lattice temperature T_L is the normal temperature of the environment around the spin system. Suppose that we start with $T_S > T_L$. It is a simple matter to show that the rate of energy (heat) transfer from the spin system to the lattice will be given by

$$\frac{dE}{dt} = k_1 k(T_S - T_L); \tag{1-24}$$

* The population difference n is defined by $n = N^- - N^+$, where N^+ is the population of the $M_S = +\frac{1}{2}$ level and N^- is the population of the $M_S = -\frac{1}{2}$ level.

† A higher energy state is possible when more than two levels are present.

k_1 is a first-order rate constant and k is the Boltzmann constant. Since the units of k_1 are $\sec^{-1}$, we can represent it as an inverse time; that is, $k_1 = 1/T_1$. As above, T_1 is the spin-lattice relaxation time and characterizes the *efficiency* of thermal contact between the spin system and the lattice. Clearly, in the absence of other systems energy will flow from the spin system to the lattice until $T_S = T_L$. The total system will then be at thermodynamic equilibrium.

Now suppose we impose a microwave field such that the resonance relation Eq. 1-9 is satisfied. Energy will flow into the spin system at a rate due to the absorption of energy from the microwave field. The rate of energy input is characterized by k_2 (see Fig. 1-2), which in turn will be proportional to the microwave power P_0. As long as $k_2 \ll k_1$ the spin system can efficiently release this extra energy to the lattice; $T_S \approx T_L$ and little change in n from the unperturbed value will occur. When $k_2 \approx k_1$, however, the spin system can no longer release its extra energy to the lattice quickly enough; $T_S > T_L$ and n will decrease. This is the basis of the phenomenon known as saturation. Spin systems with short T_1's will not readily saturate and vice versa.

1.3.5 Relaxation Times from Transition Probabilities

The concept of a spin-lattice relaxation time can perhaps be seen more clearly in terms of transition rates. Let the probability of radiation induced upward transition be $P_\uparrow$ and a corresponding downward transition be $P_\downarrow$. Then the rate of change of the population of the lower state is given by

$$\frac{dN^-}{dt} = N^+P_\downarrow - N^-P_\uparrow. \tag{1-25}$$

If we define $n = N^+ - N^-$ and $N = N^- + N^+$, then

$$\frac{dn}{dt} = 2nP. \tag{1-26}$$

Note that $P_\uparrow = P_\downarrow = P$. The solution to this differential equation is

$$n = n(0)e^{-2Pt}, \tag{1-27}$$

where $n(0)$ is the value of n at the time when the radiation field is turned on. Clearly, in the absence of other processes n will decay exponentially to zero (i.e., the populations of the two states will equalize) and thus eventually no ESR signal will be detected. Note that P is related to the intensity of the microwave field.

We know that there must be another factor that causes transitions between the spin states, since in the absence of a radiation field the populations of the spin states will eventually reach that given by the Boltzmann distribution (Eq. 1-21). This can be done only if the surroundings (or lattice) cause transitions. Let the probability of these lattice-induced transitions be $W_\uparrow$ and $W_\downarrow$ for upward and downward transitions, respectively. Then in the absence of a radiation field

$$\frac{dN^-}{dt} = N^+W_\downarrow - N^-W_\uparrow. \tag{1-28a}$$

Equation 1-28a can be rearranged to give

$$\frac{dn}{dt} = (n - n_0)(W_\uparrow + W_\downarrow), \tag{1-28b}$$

where n_0 is the value of n for a Boltzmann distribution at the temperature of the surroundings. Note that in this case $W_\uparrow \neq W_\downarrow$; otherwise, n_0 would be zero. Since the W's are transition probabilities per unit time, we define a time T_1 such that

$$T_1 = (W_\uparrow + W_\downarrow)^{-1}; \tag{1-29}$$

hence

$$\frac{dn}{dt} = \frac{n - n_0}{T_1} \tag{1-30a}$$

or

$$n - n_0 = [n - n_0]_{t=0}e^{-t/T_1}. \tag{1-30b}$$

Thus, if any perturbation removes n from its equilibrium value n_0, $(n - n_0)$ will decay exponentially with a time constant T_1. The tighter the coupling of the spin system and the lattice, the shorter T_1 and the quicker the spin system will recover from a perturbation.

1.4 *g* FACTORS

The g factor in Eq. 1-9 is a universal constant and characteristic *of the electron* ($g_e = 2.00232$), provided that H_r is the magnetic field *at the electron.* The application of an external magnetic field, however, may generate an internal magnetic field in the sample which will add to or subtract from the external field. For matters of convenience H_r in Eq. 1-9 is defined as the *external* magnetic field at resonance. Any local magnetic fields are accounted for by allowing the g factor to vary; i.e.,

$$g_{\text{eff}} = \frac{h\nu}{\beta H_r}. \tag{1-31}$$

The g factor thus can be considered as a quantity characteristic of the molecule in which the unpaired electrons are located.* The measurement of the g factor for an unknown signal can be a valuable aid in the identification

* In NMR local fields are accounted for by the chemical shift σ. In this case the resonance condition is written $h\nu = g_N\beta_N H_r(1 - \sigma)$.

of the signal origin. Table 1-1 presents examples of g factors for some entities of biological interest.

Table 1-1 ***g* Factors for Some Representative Entities of Biological Interest**

Entity	Range of g
Magnesium and other porphyrin cations (e.g., the chlorophyll cation)	2.0024–2.0028
Flavosemiquinones (e.g., the lumiflavin semiquinone)	2.0030–2.0040
Benzosemiquinones (e.g., the plastosemiquinone)	2.0040–2.0050
Nitroxides (e.g., di-*t*-butyl nitroxide)	2.0050–2.0060
Peroxyl radicals	2.01–2.02
Sulfur-containing radicals	2.02–2.06
Cu^{2+} complexes	2.0–2.4
Fe^{3+} (low-spin) complexes	1.4–3.1
Fe^{3+} (high-spin) complexes	2.0–9.7

The principal source of the local magnetic fields, which cause g to deviate from the free-electron value g_e, is an orbital magnetic moment introduced by a mixing in of excited states into the ground state* (here the magnitude of the local field is proportional to the external field).

For most molecules the admixture of excited states is *not* isotropic (orientation-independent) but is anisotropic (orientation dependent); that is, the magnitude of the induced local field (hence the deviations of the g factor from g_e) depends on the orientation of the molecule with respect to the external magnetic field. If the molecules are oriented as in a single crystal, then H_r will vary as the crystal is rotated in the external magnetic field. Although this characteristic may increase the difficulty of analysis for ESR spectra, it can be used to advantage. This was elegantly demonstrated by Bennett, Gibson, and Ingram (7) when they determined the orientation of the four heme groups in a single crystal of hemoglobin. This type of study is

* This admixture is brought about by a coupling of the electron spin and orbital angular momenta as characterized by the atomic spin-orbit coupling constant λ. If the atomic shell is less than half full, $\lambda > 0$ and $g < g_e$. If the shell is more than half full, $\lambda < 0$ and $g > g_e$. See Ref. 5, Chapter 11.

nevertheless rather limited, for we are not often able to obtain biological paramagnetic entities in a single crystal state.

The anisotropy of the g factor is usually summarized in the form of a second-rank tensor. In a general Cartesian axis system, the g tensor is written as*

$$\mathbf{g} = \begin{pmatrix} g_{xx} g_{xy} g_{xz} \\ g_{yx} g_{yy} g_{yz} \\ g_{zx} g_{zy} g_{zz} \end{pmatrix} \tag{1-32}$$

The g tensor is almost always symmetric (i.e., $g_{xy} = g_{yx}$, etc.) and thus it contains only six independent elements.

There always exists a principal-axis system, X, Y, Z, in which the g tensor contains only diagonal elements; that is,

$$^{d}\mathbf{g} = \begin{pmatrix} g_{XX} & 0 & 0 \\ 0 & g_{YY} & 0 \\ 0 & 0 & g_{ZZ} \end{pmatrix} \tag{1-33}$$

There are still six independent quantities, since three direction cosines are required to specify orientation of the principal axes.†

If the molecule contains any elements of symmetry, some or all of the principal axes are fixed by the symmetry, for example, any twofold or greater axis of symmetry‡ is a principal axis; if the molecule contains only one twofold axis of symmetry, that axis is a principal one, and so on.

The elements of $^{d}\mathbf{g}$ are called the *principal values* of the g tensor. If X, Y, and Z are equivalent, as in an octahedron, tetrahedron, or cube, then $g_{XX} = g_{YY} = g_{ZZ}$. In such a case the g factor is isotropic and can be represented by a single value. This is also true if the paramagnetic entity is in a solution of low viscosity such as liquid water where molecular tumbling causes all the g-factor anisotropy to be averaged out.

If the molecule contains a single threefold or higher axis of symmetry (Z), then X and Y are equivalent. This is called axial symmetry and $g_{XX} = g_{YY} \neq g_{ZZ}$. It is common in such cases to designate the g factors as $g_{\parallel}$, the g factor parallel to the symmetry axis (i.e., $g_{\parallel} = g_{ZZ}$), and $g_{\perp}$ for the g factor perpendicular to this axis (i.e., $g_{\perp} = g_{XX} = g_{YY}$).

* A tensor of rank zero is a scalar; a tensor of rank one is a vector; a tensor of rank two is usually represented by a 3 × 3 matrix. Multiplication of a vector by a second-rank tensor results in a change both in magnitude and direction of the vector. Thus tensors are often employed to summarize anisotropic properties.

† See Ref. 5, Chapter 7, for a more thorough discussion of g anisotropy. A direction cosine is the cosine of the angle between one axis of the old set (e.g., X) and one axis of the new set (e.g., Z).

‡ An n-fold axis of symmetry is one in which a rotation by an angle $360/n°$ brings the molecule into itself again.

For molecules that contain no threefold or higher axis of symmetry, all three principal g factors are different (i.e., $g_{XX} \neq g_{YY} \neq g_{ZZ}$). Some authors refer to them as g_1, g_2, and g_3 or g_x, g_y, and g_z.

In most biological situations the paramagnetic entities are randomly oriented, hence the observed spectrum will represent a superposition of all possible values of H_r. In unfavorable cases (the anisotropy of the g factor causes a broadening comparable to the inherent linewidth) the result is a broad structureless line, and all information about the principal g factors [and about the hyperfine interactions (see Section 1.5)] is lost. However, when the principal g factors differ significantly, the individual values may be obtained even though the system is randomly disordered. This fact is illustrated for a system with $g_{\parallel} > g_{\perp}$ (see Fig. 1-3). Resonance can occur

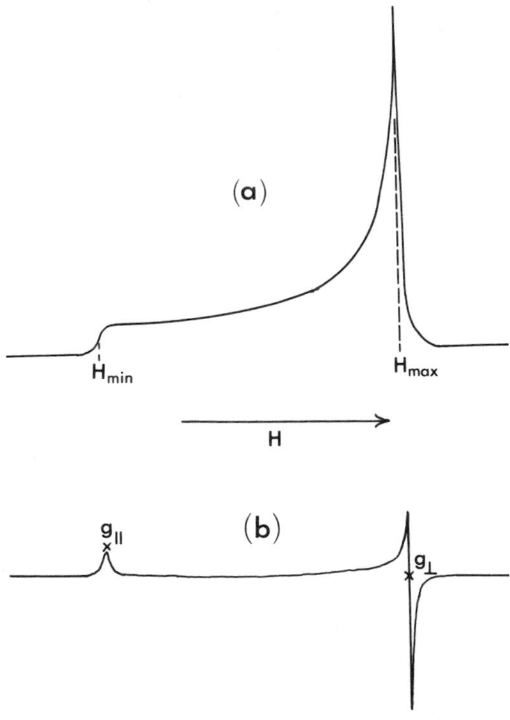

Fig. 1-3 Idealized ESR spectra for a system of randomly oriented entities exhibiting g anisotropy characteristic of a system with axial symmetry such that $g_{\parallel} > g_{\perp}$. Some broadening has been added to simulate a possible spectrum. (*a*) Absorption spectrum. Note that a significant resonance intensity is possible only between $H_{\min}$ and $H_{\max}$. (*b*) First-derivative spectrum. The x's mark the points at which $g_{\parallel}$ and $g_{\perp}$ occur.

only within a restricted range of field values, no matter what the orientation. The minimum field at which resonance will occur is given by

$$H_{\min} = \frac{h\nu}{g_{\parallel}\beta}. \tag{1-34a}$$

As H approaches $H_{\min}$ from below, no resonance occurs until $H = H_{\min}$. At that point the signal suddenly rises to a finite value. Only those molecules for which the symmetry axis (Z) is almost parallel to **H** will contribute to the signal, and therefore this part of the signal is relatively small.

The maximum field at which resonance will occur is given by

$$H_{\max} = \frac{h\nu}{g_{\perp}\beta}. \tag{1-34b}$$

As H approaches $H_{\max}$ from above, the signal will suddenly rise to a high value, much higher than at the $H_{\min}$ end. The reason is that many more molecules will have their symmetry axes almost in the *plane* perpendicular to **H** than those with their axes almost parallel to the axis of **H**. Hence we should observe an absorption signal as illustrated in Fig. 1-3*a*. The corresponding first-derivative signal is given in Fig. 1-3*b*. Note the points on the curve which characterize $g_{\parallel}$ and $g_{\perp}$.

The more complicated case of $g_{XX} \neq g_{YY} \neq g_{ZZ}$ is illustrated in Fig. 1-4. Again in favorable cases (i.e., in which the g anisotropy is sufficiently large) the principal g components can be obtained from the spectrum of the randomly oriented sample. Note our convention that X, Y, and Z be defined such that g_{ZZ} is the *most remote g* factor; g_{YY} is always the *intermediate g* factor.

For a system of axial symmetry g_{eff}, for an angle θ between the magnetic field and the symmetry axis, is given by

$$g_{\text{eff}} = (g_{\parallel}{}^2 \cos^2 \theta + g_{\perp}{}^2 \sin^2 \theta)^{1/2}. \tag{1-35}$$

Thus the resonant field is given by

$$H_r = \frac{h\nu}{g_{\text{eff}}\beta} = \frac{h\nu}{\beta} (g_{\parallel}{}^2 \cos^2 \theta + g_{\perp}{}^2 \sin^2 \theta)^{-1/2}. \tag{1-36}$$

All orientations are equally probable. Another way of stating this is to say that there will be equal numbers of molecules with their symmetry axes within any given element of solid angle.

For a circular element of area on a sphere for which the z axis is the field direction the area of this element is $2\pi r^2 \sin\theta\, d\theta$. Thus the solid angle $d\Omega$ subtended by this area is

$$d\Omega = \frac{2\pi r^2 \sin\theta\, d\theta}{4\pi r^2} = \frac{1}{2} \sin\theta\, d\theta. \tag{1-37}$$

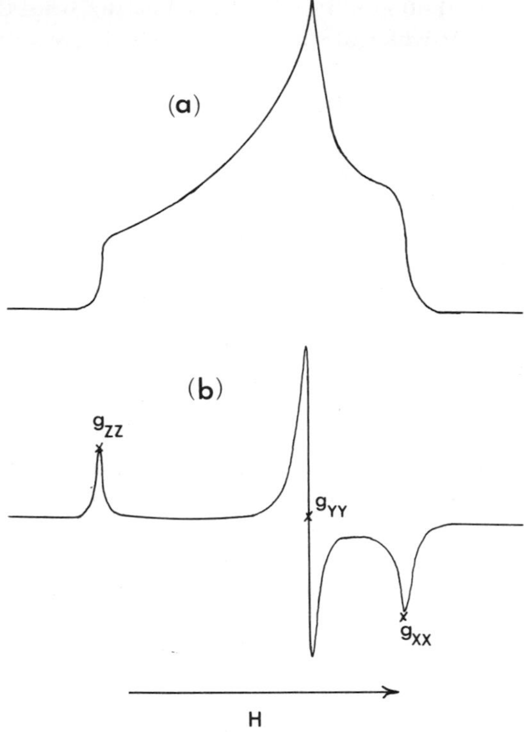

Fig. 1-4 Idealized ESR spectra for a system of randomly oriented entities exhibiting g anisotropy characteristic of a system with $g_{XX} \neq g_{YY} \neq g_{ZZ}$. Some broadening has been added to simulate a possible spectrum. (*a*) Absorption spectrum; (*b*) first-derivative spectrum; x's mark the points at which g_{XX}, g_{YY}, and g_{ZZ} occur. Note our convention that assigns g_{ZZ} to the most remote g factor; g_{YY} is always the intermediate g factor.

Since the probability that a molecule will have its symmetry axis within $d\Omega$ is proportional to $d\Omega$,

$$P(H)\, dH \propto \sin\theta\, d\theta \tag{1-38a}$$

or

$$P(H) \propto \frac{\sin\theta}{dH/d\theta}, \tag{1-38b}$$

where $P(H)\, dH$ is the probability that a molecule will have a resonant field between H_r and $H_r + dH_r$. By differentiating Eq. 1-36

$$P(H) \propto \frac{\beta}{h\nu} \frac{(g_{\parallel}^2 \cos^2\theta + g_{\perp}^2 \sin^2\theta)^{3/2}}{(g_{\parallel}^2 - g_{\perp}^2)\cos\theta} \tag{1-39}$$

or by substituting Eq. 1-36

$$P(H) \propto \left(\frac{h\nu}{\beta}\right)^2 \frac{1}{H_r^3(g_{\parallel}^2 - g_{\perp}^2)\cos\theta}. \tag{1-40}$$

The cos θ term in Eq. 1-40 means that $P(H)$ will increase to infinity as $\theta \rightarrow \pi/2$. Since $P(H)$ is also proportional to the intensity of absorption, we can see why Fig. 1-3*a* has the shape it has.

As noted earlier, paramagnetic entities in solution usually exhibit a single isotropic g factor. This results from an averaging process and

$$g_{\text{av}} = \tfrac{1}{3}(g_{XX} + g_{YY} + g_{ZZ}). \tag{1-41}$$

This averaging is effective only if the tumbling frequency is much greater than $\Delta g\beta H/h$, where Δg is the extreme variation of g. This condition is generally satisfied only for molecules with a moderate molecular weight ($M \sim 1000$) in solutions of low viscosity. Many systems of biological interest are much larger; hence even when in solution or liquid suspension they exhibit a "solid-state" type of spectrum with resultant line broadening due to g-factor anisotropy.

1.5 NUCLEAR HYPERFINE INTERACTION

In the preceding sections mention was made of the existence of local magnetic fields. Besides the local fields induced by the external field which lead to different g factors, there are local fields that are permanent and do not depend on the presence of an external field. These permanent local fields are generated by the presence of other magnetic moments, possibly those of other electrons but more commonly those of magnetic nuclei in the molecule. The interaction of an unpaired electron with a nuclear magnetic moment is termed nuclear hyperfine interaction.* It was first observed as a hyperfine splitting in the optical absorption spectra of atoms (8).

The appearance of nuclear hyperfine interactions greatly enhances the value of the ESR technique. ESR spectra can be split into many characteristic patterns of lines by the hyperfine phenomenon, and the resultant spectra have proved to be of great value not only in the identification of free radicals but also in providing an insight into the detailed electronic structure of free radicals.

It is not unreasonable that a proton should have a nuclear spin and concomitant nuclear magnetic moment, since, like the electron, it is a charged particle. It is rather surprising, however, that neutrons also possess a spin and magnetic moment. This is due to the fact that neutrons posssess a substructure, but that is a subject for nuclear physics and much beyond the scope of this book. It is enough to understand that many nuclei possess an

* *Fine* structure refers to the splitting of levels caused by other unpaired electrons (see Sections 1.9 and 1.10). The term *super*hyperfine structure is often applied to the hyperfine structure from ligands in a transition-metal complex.

inherent spin angular momentum (a result of all the angular momenta of the constituent nucleons).

The spin of a nucleus is characterized by the quantum number I which can take one of the values 0, $\frac{1}{2}$, 1, $\frac{3}{2}$, 2, ... As in the electron case, the z component of the nuclear spin is quantized and, characterized by the quantum number M_I. M_I can take on the values $-I, -I + 1, \ldots, I - 1, I$. Thus, if the nuclear spin is I, there are $(2I + 1)$ possible nuclear spin states. This is illustrated for $I = \frac{5}{2}$ in Fig. 1-5.

The spins and magnetic moments of some of the common nuclei encountered in biological systems are listed in Table A-1 in the appendix. Note that $I = 0$ for all nuclei for which the atomic mass *and* atomic number are *even*. This is a consequence of the fact that pairs of protons and pairs of neutrons cancel out their magnetic properties just like pairs of electrons. If the atomic number is *odd* and the atomic mass is *even*, I is an integer (i.e., 1, 2, 3, . . .); if the atomic mass is *odd*, I is a half-odd integer (i.e., $\frac{1}{2}, \frac{3}{2}, \frac{5}{2}, \ldots$).

The local magnetic field generated by a nuclear magnetic moment will add vectorially to the external magnetic field $\mathbf{H}_{\text{ext}}$ to give an effective field $\mathbf{H}_{\text{eff}}$; that is,

$$\mathbf{H}_{\text{eff}} = \mathbf{H}_{\text{ext}} + \mathbf{H}_{\text{local}} \tag{1-42a}$$

or

$$\mathbf{H}_{\text{ext}} = \mathbf{H}_{\text{eff}} - \mathbf{H}_{\text{local}}. \tag{1-42b}$$

Since there are $(2I + 1)$ possible values of M_I, there will also be $(2I + 1)$ possible values of $\mathbf{H}_{\text{local}}$. Thus resonance may be observed at $(2I + 1)$ values of the external magnetic field. The spectrum is thus split into a number of lines—termed *hyperfine splitting* (abbreviated as *hfs*).

The simplest system exhibiting hyperfine interaction is the hydrogen atom (one electron and one proton). An ESR spectrum of hydrogen atoms produced by irradiation in a crystalline solid is shown in Fig. 1-6. Instead of a single line characterized by $H_r = h\nu/g\beta$, with $g = 2.00232$, a pair of lines is observed at field values much removed from $h\nu/g\beta$. The average position of these lines (3353.5 G at 9.50 GHz) does correspond to $g \approx 2$. Since the proton has a spin $I = \frac{1}{2}$, M_I has the two allowed values $M_I = \pm\frac{1}{2}$. Hence there will be two possible local fields at the electron contributed by the proton. There will then be two possible values of the external magnetic field at which resonance may occur, that is, from Eq. 1-42*b*,

$$H_r = H' \mp \frac{a}{2} = H' - aM_I{}^* \tag{1-43}$$

where $a/2$ is the magnitude of the local field and H' is the resonant field when $a = 0$. Note that a represents the splitting (in gauss) between the two

* Equation 1-43 applies only when $H' \gg \frac{1}{2}a$. This condition is usually met and allows us to consider only the z components of the magnetic-field vectors.

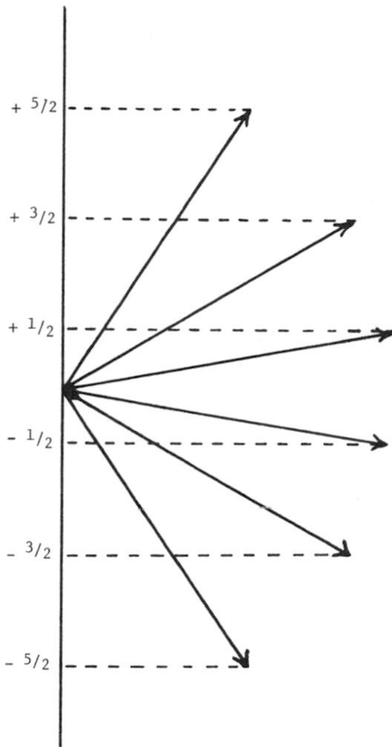

Fig. 1-5 Possible orientations of the nuclear-spin vector for $I = \frac{5}{2}$. The z component of the nuclear spin is quantized such that $M_I = \frac{5}{2}, \frac{3}{2}, \frac{1}{2}, -\frac{1}{2}, -\frac{3}{2}, -\frac{5}{2}$. The magnitude of the nuclear-spin vector is $\sqrt{\frac{5}{2}(\frac{5}{2} + 1)} = \sqrt{\frac{35}{4}}$ in units of $h/2\pi$.

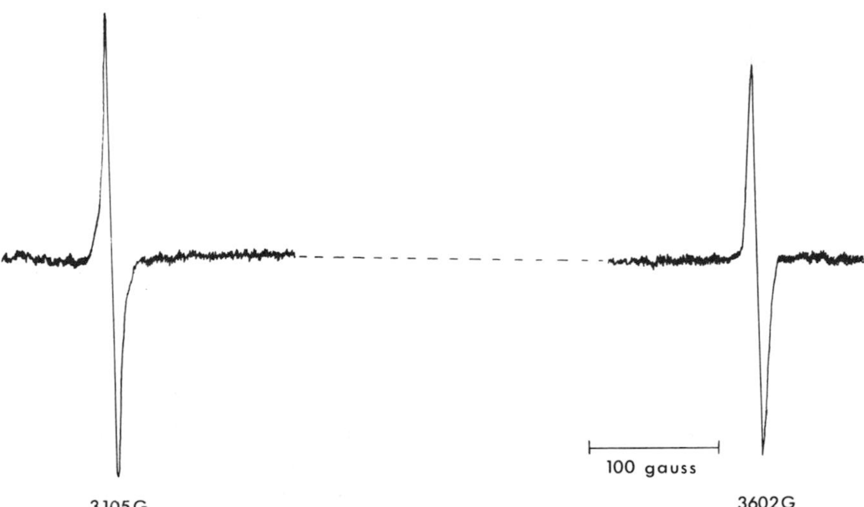

Fig. 1-6 ESR spectrum of hydrogen atoms in an X-rayed human tooth; $\nu = 9.495$ GHz. The numbers under each line are the resonant-field values. Resonances from other free-radical species occur in the dotted region. [Spectrum taken from T. Cole and A. H. Silver, Nature **200**, 700 (1963).]

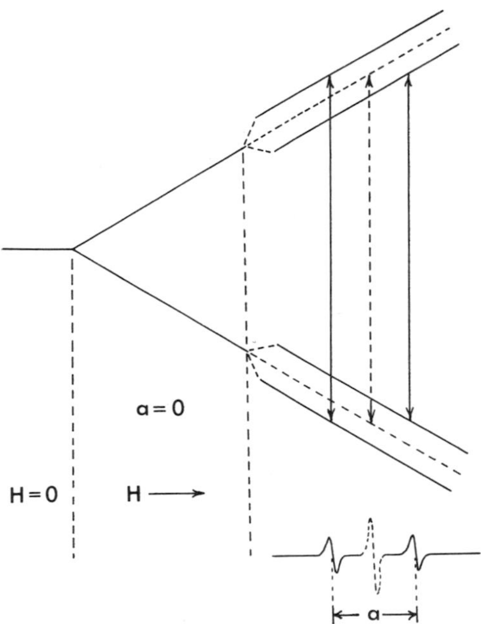

Fig. 1-7 Energy levels of the hydrogen atom as a function of magnetic field at constant microwave frequency. The dotted transition would be observed if a were zero; a is the proton hyperfine splitting. In the hydrogen atom it has the value 506.8 G. The hyperfine interaction is not shown as $H \rightarrow 0$, since the energy levels become nonlinear. (See Appendix C of Ref. 5.)

hyperfine lines. This interval therefore is called the hyperfine *splitting* constant.*

The nuclear hyperfine interaction splits each of the electron Zeeman levels of Fig. 1-1 into two levels, shown in Fig. 1-7. The allowed transitions correspond to $\Delta M_S = \pm 1$ and $\Delta M_I = 0$. These are called selection rules and may be interpreted as follows: the only effect of the proton is to create a local field at the electron; this should not change the selection rule for the electron spin resonance phenomenon, that is, $\Delta M_S = \pm 1$. It is possible to cause a change in the value of M_I by irradiation at the NMR frequency, but then $\Delta M_S = 0$. Thus, when *electron* spin resonance occurs, $\Delta M_I = 0$. Another interpretation is that during the time it takes for an electron to change its orientation the nuclear spin has no time to reorient.

Figure 1-8 exhibits an energy-level diagram for a free radical containing

* This term should not be confused with the hyperfine *coupling* constant A. See below.

a nucleus with $I = 1$. Three equally intense lines are predicted. The spectrum of the di-*t*-butylnitroxide radical in Fig. 1-9 is an example of this case. In general, if the nuclear spin is I, we expect $2I + 1$ equally intense hyperfine lines.

1.6 ORIGINS OF THE HYPERFINE INTERACTION

If the electron- and nuclear dipoles were to behave classically, an approximate expression for the hyperfine local field parallel to the external field would be

$$H_{\text{local}} = \mu_{N_z} \frac{(3 \cos^2 \theta - 1)}{r^3}, \tag{1-44}$$

where μ_{N_z} is the component of the nuclear magnetic moment along the

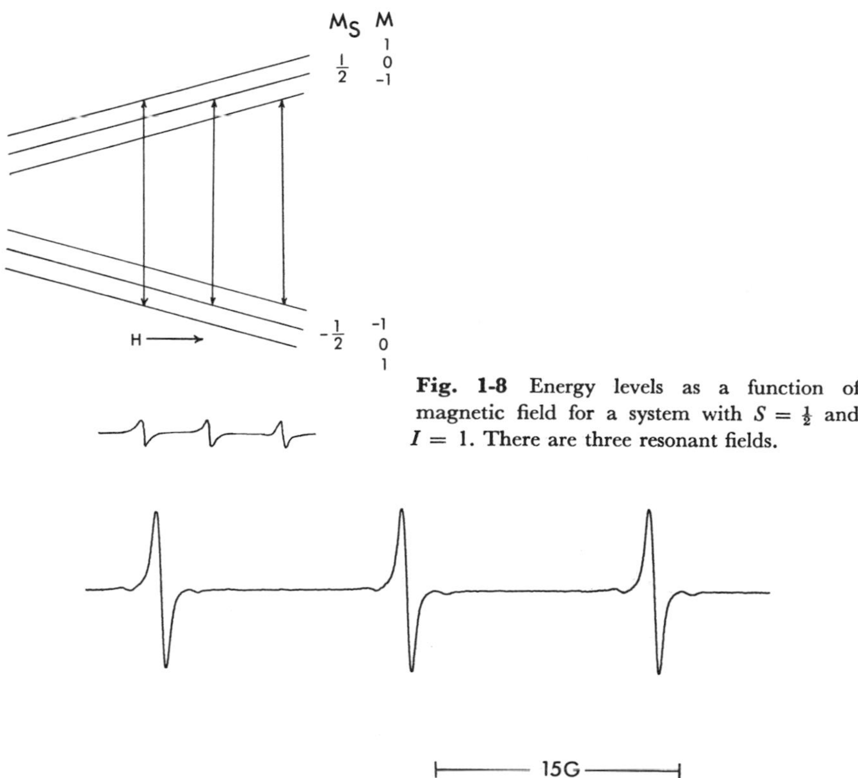

Fig. 1-8 Energy levels as a function of magnetic field for a system with $S = \frac{1}{2}$ and $I = 1$. There are three resonant fields.

Fig. 1-9 First-derivative ESR spectrum of the di-*t*-butyl nitroxide radical in a dilute ethanol solution at room temperature.

external-field direction, θ is the angle between the magnetic-field direction and a line joining the electron and nucleus, and r is the electron-nuclear distance. This classical system is illustrated in Fig. 1-10. It is apparent that $\mathbf{H}_{local}$ depends markedly on the value of θ and may aid or oppose the external field.

Electrons are not localized at one position in space; thus the effective value of $\mathbf{H}_{local}$ is obtained by averaging over all possible electron positions. If all orientations are equally probable (e.g., for an electron in an s orbital centered on nucleus N), the average value of $\cos^2\theta = \frac{1}{3}$ and the hyperfine interaction vanishes! It is strange then that a large hyperfine interaction is observed for the hydrogen atom for which the unpaired electron resides in a 1s orbital.

The answer to this paradox is that another type of hyperfine interaction,

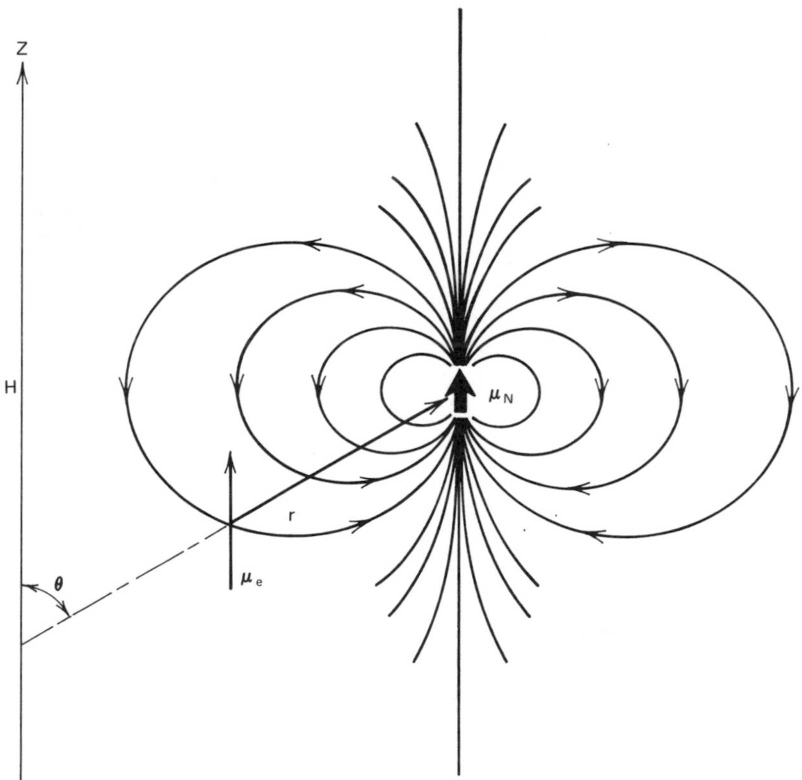

Fig. 1-10 Interaction of electron- and nuclear-spin dipoles. The curved lines represent the magnetic flux generated by the nuclear magnetic moment. This creates a local magnetic field $\mathbf{H}_{local}$ at the electron. $\mathbf{H}_{local}$ then adds vectorially to $\mathbf{H}$, the external magnetic field.

called the *isotropic* hyperfine interaction,* arises when the electron has a finite probability of being found *at the nucleus*. This property is found only for electrons in s orbitals. Electrons in $p, d, f, \ldots$ orbitals have a node at the nucleus. Thus there is a clear distinction: electrons in s orbitals will exhibit an isotropic hyperfine interaction, whereas electrons in $p, d, f, \ldots$ orbitals will exhibit only an *anisotropic* (i.e., orientation-dependent) hyperfine interaction.

In quantum mechanics the dipole-dipole interaction is represented by the operator

$$\hat{\mathscr{H}}_D = -g_e\beta g_N\beta_N\left[\frac{\hat{\mathbf{S}}\cdot\hat{\mathbf{I}}}{r^3} - \frac{3(\hat{\mathbf{S}}\cdot\mathbf{r})(\hat{\mathbf{I}}\cdot\mathbf{r})}{r^5}\right], \tag{1-45}$$

where g_N and β_N are the nuclear g factor and magneton, respectively, $\hat{\mathbf{S}}$ and $\hat{\mathbf{I}}$ are the electron and nuclear spin operators, respectively, and $\mathbf{r}$ is the vector joining electron and nucleus. By expanding the vectors into their components Eq. 1-45 may be transformed to

$$\hat{\mathscr{H}}_D = \hat{\mathbf{S}}\cdot g_e\beta g_N\beta_N\begin{bmatrix}\left\langle\dfrac{3x^2-r^2}{r^5}\right\rangle & \left\langle\dfrac{3xy}{r^5}\right\rangle & \left\langle\dfrac{3xz}{r^5}\right\rangle\\ \left\langle\dfrac{3xy}{r^5}\right\rangle & \left\langle\dfrac{3y^2-r^2}{r^5}\right\rangle & \left\langle\dfrac{3yz}{r^5}\right\rangle\\ \left\langle\dfrac{3xz}{r^5}\right\rangle & \left\langle\dfrac{3yz}{r^5}\right\rangle & \left\langle\dfrac{3z^2-r^2}{r^5}\right\rangle\end{bmatrix}\cdot\hat{\mathbf{I}} \tag{1-46a}$$

$$= h\hat{\mathbf{S}}\cdot\boldsymbol{T}\cdot\hat{\mathbf{I}}. \tag{1-46b}$$

The angular brackets represent an average over the wavefunction of the unpaired electron; $\boldsymbol{T}$ is a traceless (sum of the diagonal elements is zero) second-rank tensor. On rotation of the coordinate system a certain orientation may always be found in which $\boldsymbol{T}$ is diagonal (zero off-diagonal elements); that is

$$^d\boldsymbol{T} = \begin{pmatrix}T_{XX} & 0 & 0\\ 0 & T_{YY} & 0\\ 0 & 0 & T_{ZZ}\end{pmatrix}. \tag{1-47}$$

The X, Y, Z coordinate system is called the *principal-axis* system and need not be the same as the principal-axis system for the g tensor.

The isotropic hyperfine interaction is represented by the Fermi contact term in the Hamiltonian

$$\hat{\mathscr{H}}_{\text{iso}} = \frac{8\pi}{3}g_e\beta g_N\beta_N|\psi(0)|^2\hat{\mathbf{S}}\cdot\hat{\mathbf{I}} = hA_0\hat{\mathbf{S}}\cdot\hat{\mathbf{I}}; \tag{1-48}$$

$\psi(0)$ is the value of the wavefunction of the unpaired electron, evaluated at the nucleus, which is causing the hyperfine interaction. Thus only electrons in s orbitals

* This is also sometimes called the Fermi *contact* interaction, a purely quantum-mechanical effect which has no classical analog.

can contribute to A_0 as $p, d, f, \ldots$ wavefunctions all have nodes at the nucleus; A_0 (usually measured in megahertz) is called the *hyperfine coupling constant.*

The total hyperfine Hamiltonian is obtained by adding Eqs. 1-46*b* and 1-48 to obtain, in the principal axis system,

$$\mathscr{H}_{hf} = h\hat{\mathbf{S}} \cdot {}^{d}A \cdot \hat{\mathbf{I}} = h\hat{\mathbf{S}} \cdot \begin{pmatrix} T_{XX} + A_0 & 0 & 0 \\ 0 & T_{YY} + A_0 & 0 \\ 0 & 0 & T_{ZZ} + A_0 \end{pmatrix} \cdot \hat{\mathbf{I}}. \tag{1-49}$$

In solution the anisotropic (dipole-dipole) interaction averages to zero and thus only the Hamiltonian of Eq. 1-48 is operative.

The hydrogen atom will now be treated as an illustrative example. The proton has $I = \frac{1}{2}$; thus there are four possible spin functions:

$$|\alpha_e, \alpha_n\rangle, \qquad |\beta_e, \beta_n\rangle,$$

$$|\alpha_e, \beta_n\rangle, \qquad |\beta_e, \alpha_n\rangle.$$

Equation 1-48 is expanded as

$$\mathscr{H}_{\text{iso}} = hA_0[\hat{S}_z\hat{I}_z + \hat{S}_x\hat{I}_x + \hat{S}_y\hat{I}_y]. \tag{1-50}$$

At the high magnetic fields usually employed it can be shown* that the last two terms in Eq. 1-50 have a negligible effect. The first term must be added to Eq. 1-14*b* to obtain the complete Hamiltonian;

$$\mathscr{H} = g\beta H\hat{S}_z + hA_0\hat{S}_z\hat{I}_z. \tag{1-51}$$

Application of this Hamiltonian to the four spin functions yields the following energies:

$$E_{\alpha_e\alpha_n} = \tfrac{1}{2}g\beta H + \tfrac{1}{4}hA_0, \tag{1-52a}$$

$$E_{\alpha_e\beta_n} = \tfrac{1}{2}g\beta H - \tfrac{1}{4}hA_0, \tag{1-52b}$$

$$E_{\beta_e\beta_n} = -\tfrac{1}{2}g\beta H + \tfrac{1}{4}hA_0, \tag{1-52c}$$

$$E_{\beta_e\alpha_n} = -\tfrac{1}{2}g\beta H - \tfrac{1}{4}hA_0. \tag{1-52d}$$

The selection rules are $\Delta M_S = \pm 1, \Delta M_I = 0$; thus only two transitions are possible

$$\Delta E_1 = E_{\alpha_e\alpha_n} - E_{\beta_e\alpha_n} = g\beta H + \tfrac{1}{2}hA_0, \tag{1-53a}$$

$$\Delta E_2 = E_{\alpha_e\beta_n} - E_{\beta_e\beta_n} = g\beta H - \tfrac{1}{2}hA_0. \tag{1-53b}$$

It is usual to keep the microwave frequency constant (i.e., $h\nu_0$ is constant) and vary H. In this case resonance is observed at the two fields:

$$H_1 = \frac{h\nu_0}{g\beta} - \frac{1}{2}\frac{hA_0}{g\beta} = H' - \tfrac{1}{2}a, \tag{1-54a}$$

$$H_2 = \frac{h\nu_0}{g\beta} + \frac{1}{2}\frac{hA_0}{g\beta} = H' + \tfrac{1}{2}a. \tag{1-54b}$$

* See Appendix C of Ref. 5.

These equations are equivalent to Eq. 1-43; a (usually measured in gauss) is called the *hyperfine splitting constant.*

For the specific case of free radicals in a solution of low viscosity all orientations are made equally probable by virtue of the rapid molecular tumbling. Thus, although anisotropic hyperfine interactions may be present, only the isotropic interactions will be observed since the anisotropy is averaged out by the molecular tumbling. If the radicals are oriented as in a single crystal, then ESR spectra may be observed in which the spacing of the hyperfine components vary as a function of the orientation of the crystal in the magnetic field. Alternatively, if the solution of a free radical is frozen, then the spectrum observed may be a superposition of the spectra from all possible orientations. Unless the hyperfine splitting is large compared with the inherent linewidth (this is not often the case) much of the structure (and concomitant information) is lost in a broad, poorly resolved line. This is illustrated in Fig. 1-11 for the di-*t*-butyl nitroxide radical.

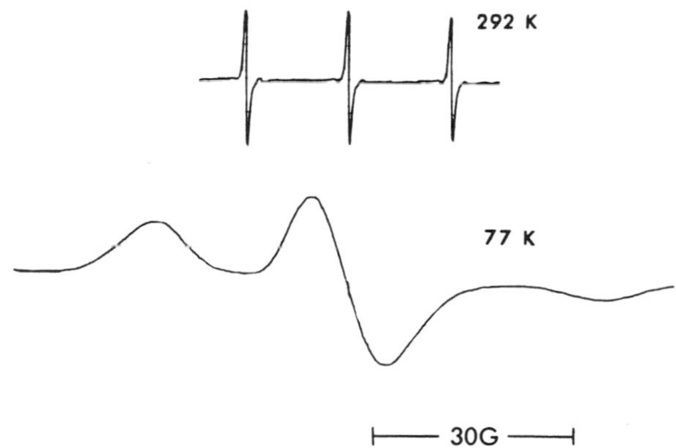

Fig. 1-11 First-derivative ESR spectra of the di-*t*-butyl nitroxide radical: (*a*) liquid ethanol solution at 292K; (*b*) solid glass at 77K.

In the cases in which the hyperfine interaction is large, some anisotropic and isotropic hyperfine parameters may be obtained from an analysis of the powder spectrum. Consider a radical which has axial symmetry (i.e., $x \equiv y$) and a single magnetic nucleus with $I = \frac{1}{2}$. Then from (1-44)

$$\text{for } \theta = 0°, H_{\text{local}} = \pm \frac{a_{\parallel}}{2}, \tag{1-55a}$$

$$\text{for } \theta = 90°, H_{\text{local}} = \mp \frac{a_{\perp}}{2}, \tag{1-55b}$$

where the top and bottom signs refer to $M_I = +\frac{1}{2}$ or $-\frac{1}{2}$, respectively. It is assumed that $a_{\parallel} > a_{\perp}$.

The local hyperfine magnetic field of the electron at the nucleus is usually much larger in magnitude than the external field. Thus we have the peculiar situation that the electron and nuclear magnetic moments *usually are not oriented along the same direction*. (For a discussion of this interesting phenomenon see Chapter 7 of Ref. 5.) The result is that resonance is possible only in the ranges $H' - a_{\parallel}/2$ to $H' - a_{\perp}/2$ and $H' + a_{\perp}/2$ and $H' + a_{\parallel}/2$. As in the case of g-factor anisotropy, the maximum absorption occurs for the perpendicular orientation. Figure 1-12 illustrates a possible absorption and first-derivative line shape. Unfortunately hyperfine interactions are usually not large enough to resolve these features. (However, see Section 2.11.4.)

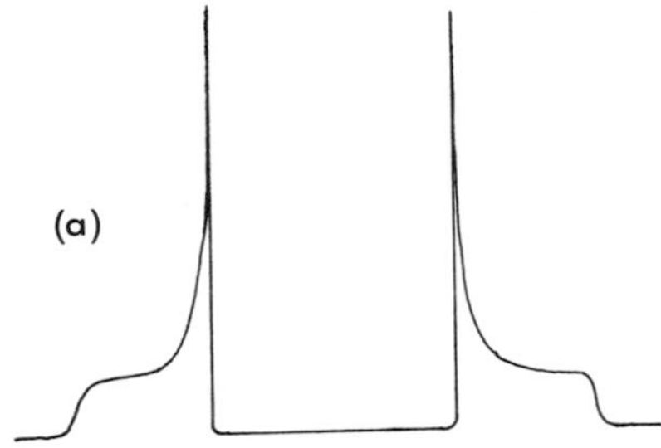

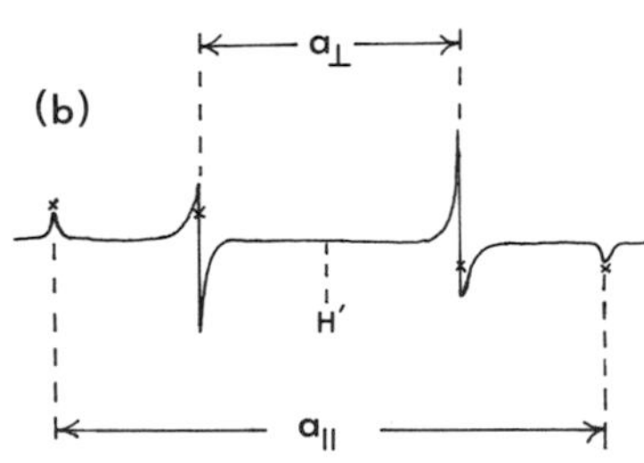

Fig. 1-12 Idealized ESR spectra for a system of randomly oriented radicals exhibiting hyperfine anisotropy characteristic of a system with axial symmetry such that $a_{\parallel} > a_{\perp}$. Some broadening has been added to simulate a possible spectrum. It is also assumed that the g factor is isotropic. (*a*) Absorption spectrum. Note that no resonance may be detected inside the field range from $H' - a_{\perp}/2$ to $H' + a_{\perp}/2$. (*b*) First-derivative spectrum. The x's mark the points from which $a_{\parallel}$ and $a_{\perp}$ should be measured.

When the symmetry is lower than axial, all three principal values of the hyperfine tensor may be different. These are designated as A_{XX}, A_{YY}, and A_{ZZ}. The corresponding hyperfine splittings are often referred to as a_1, a_2, a_3 or a_x, a_y, and a_z.

The arguments used in Section 1.4 concerning the rate of tumbling necessary to average out g anisotropy also apply to hyperfine anisotropy. Thus again for many systems of biological interest the size of the system may be too large; hence one must be content with a "solid-state" type of spectrum.

1.7 EFFECTS OF SLOW TUMBLING RATES

As pointed out in Sections 1.4 and 1.6, drastic changes in the ESR spectrum can occur when the paramagnetic entity is immobilized, compared with the spectrum obtained in which the paramagnetic entity is tumbling rapidly in solution. The reason for these changes lies, of course, in the fact that the anisotropic contributions to the g factors and hyperfine splittings are averaged out in the latter case. It is important to recognize why these contributions are not observed when the entity is tumbling rapidly. To do this we consider a model system consisting of a free radical R which can exist in two states, R_1 and R_2, such that the g factor is different in the two states. Consider, for the purposes of this example, that at $\nu = 9.5$ GHz the field separation between

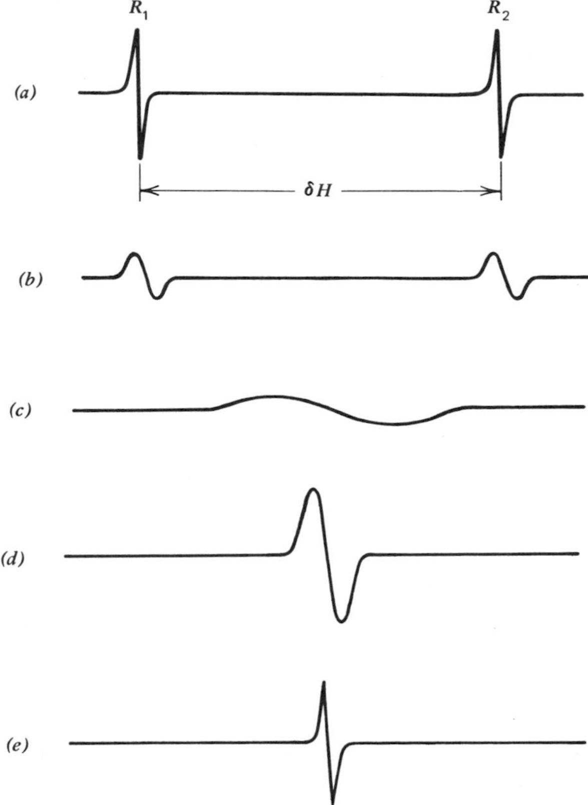

Fig. 1-13 Effects of the rate of exchange between R_1 and R_2 on the ESR spectra. (*a*) $\tau \to \infty$; $\Gamma = \Gamma_0$; (*b*) slow exchange rate region $\tau > 1/\gamma_e \delta H$; $\Gamma \sim \Gamma_0 + 1/\gamma_e \tau$; (*c*) intermediate exchange rate region $\tau \sim 1/\gamma_e \delta H$; (*d*) fast exchange rate region; $\tau < 1/\gamma_e \delta H$; $\Gamma = \Gamma_0 + \frac{1}{4}\gamma_e(\delta H)^2 \tau$ (*e*) $\tau \to 0$; $\Gamma = \Gamma_0$.

the two resonant fields for R_1 and R_2 is δH (see Fig. 1-13). We take the states R_1 and R_2 to represent (rather crudely) the *g*-factor anisotropy; i.e., we are allowing the system to exist in only two orientations. The spectrum that would be observed for this idealized system in a rigid matrix at low temperature is shown in Fig. 1-13*a*. The linewidth is Γ_0 (half-width at half-height of the absorption; see Figs. 2-6 and 2-7 and Table 2-1 for a definition of Γ).

Now as the temperature increases the matrix softens and R begins to exchange between the states R_1 and R_2; that is,

$$R_1 \rightleftharpoons R_2.$$

We assume that R_1 and R_2 have equal concentrations and that the rate of the forward or backward reaction is τ^{-1}, where τ is the average lifetime in state R_1 or R_2. From Eq. 1-17 additional lifetime broadening will be introduced because of the finite lifetime τ; that is, the effect of the exchange rate is to increase the linewidth to

$$\Gamma \sim \Gamma_0 + \frac{1}{\gamma_e \tau}. \tag{1-56}$$

Equation 1-56 will apply as long as $\tau > 1/\gamma_e \delta H$ (see Fig. 1-13*b*). This is called the slow exchange rate region. When $\tau \sim 1/\gamma_e \delta H$, however, we can no longer distinguish between individual states because of the "uncertainty principle" (see Section 1.3.1). This is the intermediate exchange rate region. The net result is that the ESR spectrum collapses toward the average *g* factor of the two states (see Fig. 1-13*c*). As τ becomes less than $1/\gamma_e \delta H$, a single line rises up in the center with a width

$$\Gamma \sim \Gamma_0 + \tfrac{1}{4}\gamma_e (\delta H)^2 \tau \tag{1-57}$$

(see Fig. 1-13*d*). This is called the fast exchange rate region and such a line is said to be exchange-narrowed. Finally in Fig. 1-13*e* the linewidth narrows to a limit Γ_0; that is, factors other than the exchange process determine the linewidth. This would be the case when the matrix becomes so fluid that essentially all of the anisotropy is averaged out by rapid motion of the radical.

The system we have considered is grossly oversimplified in terms of being able to explain real systems as they go from a rigid to a fluid state; the basic principles are the same, however. We have to consider both hyperfine and *g* anisotropy in terms of a continuous distribution of possible states in the rigid medium which then collapse into averaged states in the fluid medium; τ is called the *rotational correlation time* and, in fact, can be measured from equations such as Eqs. 1-56 and 1-57.

When both hyperfine and *g* anisotropy are of comparable magnitudes, the line shapes are complex and sensitive to small changes in τ. This is the case for the nitroxide radicals used as spin labels which are discussed in great detail in Chapter 11.

1.8 HYPERFINE INTERACTION WITH MORE THAN ONE MAGNETIC NUCLEUS

Since the orbital of an unpaired electron in a free radical is often delocalized over many atoms, the electron may be coupled to a number of magnetic nuclei. This leads to spectra more complicated than that seen when the coupling is made to a single magnetic nucleus as in the di-*t*-butyl nitroxide radical (see Fig. 1-8). Two cases lend themselves most easily to analysis:

1. The electron is coupled to a set of equivalent nuclei.
2. The electron is coupled more tightly to one nucleus (or several equivalent nuclei) and less tightly coupled to another. Both of these cases will be illustrated.

Consider first a molecule containing two equivalent magnetic nuclei with $I = \frac{1}{2}$ (e.g., two protons). The $\dot{C}H_2OH$ radical is an example of such a molecule in which the unpaired electron is equally coupled to the two hydrogen atoms, whereas no hyperfine interaction is observed for the OH proton (^{12}C and ^{16}O have no nuclear spin, hence no magnetic moment). Each CH_2 proton will contribute to H_{local} at the electron, as shown in Table 1-2. Figure 1-14 illustrates the corresponding splitting of energy levels as each hyperfine interaction is added. This is simply an extension of Fig. 1-7. Thus we illustrate only the high-field end of the diagram.

Table 1-2 Local-Field Contributions from Two Equivalent Protons

M_I		Total	H_{local}		Total	Resonant	Relative
1	2	M_I	1	2	H_{local}	field H_r	intensity
$\frac{1}{2}$	$\frac{1}{2}$	1	$\frac{1}{2}a$	$\frac{1}{2}a$	a	$H' - a$	1
$-\frac{1}{2}$	$\frac{1}{2}$	0	$-\frac{1}{2}a$	$\frac{1}{2}a$	0	H'	2
$\frac{1}{2}$	$-\frac{1}{2}$	0	$\frac{1}{2}a$	$-\frac{1}{2}a$	0	H'	
$-\frac{1}{2}$	$-\frac{1}{2}$	-1	$-\frac{1}{2}a$	$-\frac{1}{2}a$	$-a$	$H' + a$	1

Thus we expect a three-line spectrum with the center line twice as intense as the outer lines. The ESR spectrum of the $\dot{C}H_2OH$ radical is shown in Fig. 1-15.

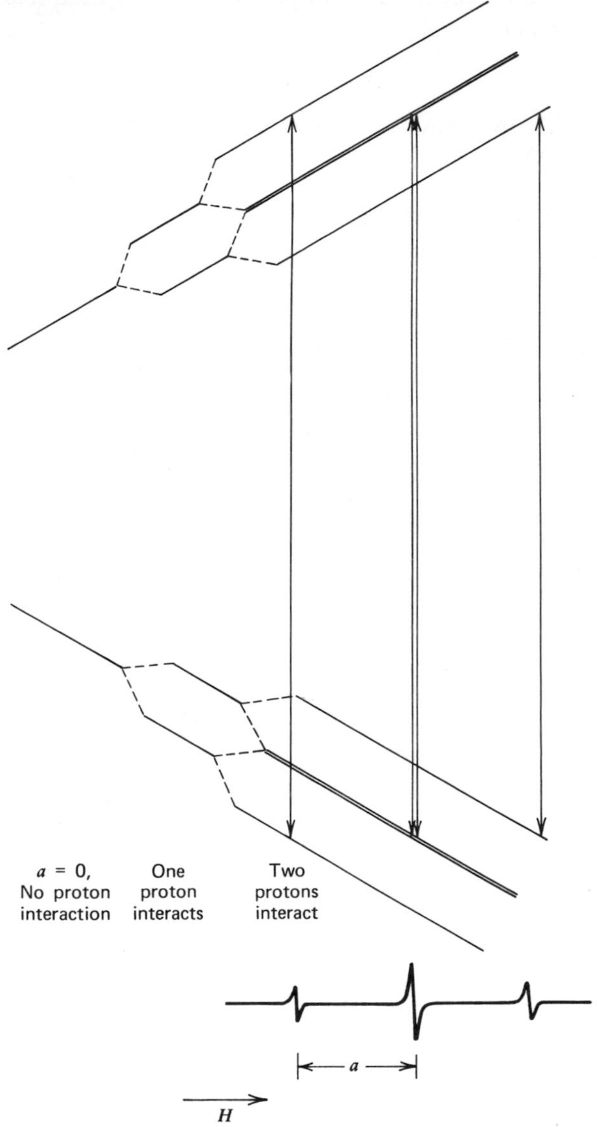

Fig. 1-14 Energy levels of a free radical with two equivalent protons. Each proton in turn splits each energy level in two.

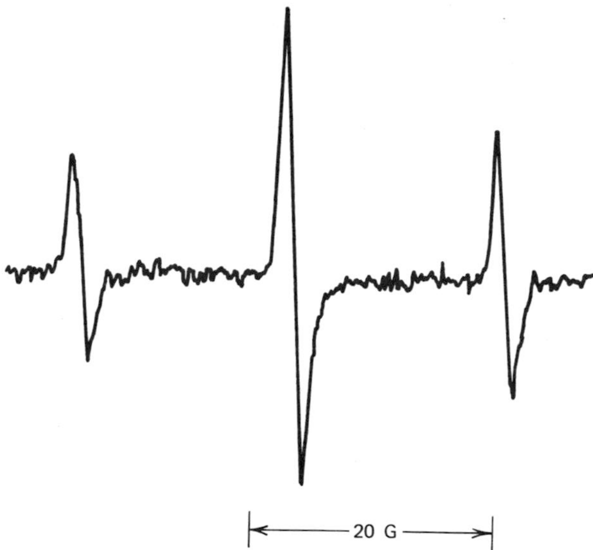

Fig. 1-15 First-derivative ESR spectrum of the $\dot{C}H_2OH$ radical at pH 1.03. Under these conditions no hyperfine splitting from the OH proton is resolved [taken from H. Fischer, *Mol. Phys.* **9**, 147 (1965)].

Table 1-3 illustrates the procedure for three equivalent nuclei with $I = \frac{1}{2}$. The extension to n equivalent nuclei is straightforward. The general result is that n equivalent nuclei with $I = \frac{1}{2}$ will result in $n + 1$ lines with intensities proportional to the coefficients of the binomial expansion of order n.*

Table 1-3 Local-Field Contributions from Three Equivalent Nuclei with $I = \frac{1}{2}$

M_I			Total	H_{local}			Total	Resonant	Relative
1	2	3	M_I	1	2	3	H_{local}	field H_r	intensity
$\frac{1}{2}$	$\frac{1}{2}$	$\frac{1}{2}$	$\frac{3}{2}$	$\frac{1}{2}a$	$\frac{1}{2}a$	$\frac{1}{2}a$	$\frac{3}{2}a$	$H' - \frac{3}{2}a$	1
$-\frac{1}{2}$	$\frac{1}{2}$	$\frac{1}{2}$	$\frac{1}{2}$	$-\frac{1}{2}a$	$\frac{1}{2}a$	$\frac{1}{2}a$	$\frac{1}{2}a$	$H' - \frac{1}{2}a$	
$\frac{1}{2}$	$-\frac{1}{2}$	$\frac{1}{2}$	$\frac{1}{2}$	$\frac{1}{2}a$	$-\frac{1}{2}a$	$\frac{1}{2}a$	$\frac{1}{2}a$	$H' - \frac{1}{2}a$	3
$\frac{1}{2}$	$\frac{1}{2}$	$-\frac{1}{2}$	$\frac{1}{2}$	$\frac{1}{2}a$	$\frac{1}{2}a$	$-\frac{1}{2}a$	$\frac{1}{2}a$	$H' - \frac{1}{2}a$	
$-\frac{1}{2}$	$-\frac{1}{2}$	$\frac{1}{2}$	$-\frac{1}{2}$	$-\frac{1}{2}a$	$-\frac{1}{2}a$	$\frac{1}{2}a$	$-\frac{1}{2}a$	$H' + \frac{1}{2}a$	
$-\frac{1}{2}$	$\frac{1}{2}$	$-\frac{1}{2}$	$-\frac{1}{2}$	$-\frac{1}{2}a$	$\frac{1}{2}a$	$-\frac{1}{2}a$	$-\frac{1}{2}a$	$H' + \frac{1}{2}a$	3
$\frac{1}{2}$	$-\frac{1}{2}$	$-\frac{1}{2}$	$-\frac{1}{2}$	$\frac{1}{2}a$	$-\frac{1}{2}a$	$-\frac{1}{2}a$	$-\frac{1}{2}a$	$H' + \frac{1}{2}a$	
$-\frac{1}{2}$	$-\frac{1}{2}$	$-\frac{1}{2}$	$-\frac{3}{2}$	$-\frac{1}{2}a$	$-\frac{1}{2}a$	$-\frac{1}{2}a$	$-\frac{3}{2}a$	$H' + \frac{3}{2}a$	1

* The binomial expansion is $(a + b)^n = \sum_{i=1}^{i=n} c_i a^{n-i} b^i$, where $c_i = n!/(n - i)!\,i!$.

Table 1-4 lists the binomial coefficients up to $n = 8$.

Table 1-4 Binomial Coefficients

n	Relative intensity of ESR lines	Number of lines
1	1 1	2
2	1 2 1	3
3	1 3 3 1	4
4	1 4 6 4 1	5
5	1 5 10 10 5 1	6
6	1 6 15 20 15 6 1	7
7	1 7 21 35 35 21 7 1	8
8	1 8 28 56 70 56 28 8 1	9

Sets of equivalent nuclei with $I = 1$ or greater can be handled in a manner similar to that illustrated in Tables 1-2 and 1-3. Table 1-5 presents the calculation for two equivalent nuclei with $I = 1$ (e.g., two equivalent ^{14}N nuclei).

Table 1-5 Local-Field Contributions from Two Equivalent Nuclei with $I = 1$

M_I		Total	H_{local}		Total	Resonant	Relative
1	2	M_I	1	2	H_{local}	field	intensity
1	1	2	a	a	$2a$	$H' - 2a$	1
1	0	1	a	0	a	$H' - a$	2
0	1	1	0	a	a	$H' - a$	
1	−1	0	a	$-a$	0	H'	
0	0	0	0	0	0	H'	3
−1	1	0	$-a$	a	0	H'	
0	−1	−1	0	$-a$	$-a$	$H' + a$	2
−1	0	−1	$-a$	0	$-a$	$H' + a$	
−1	−1	−2	$-a$	$-a$	$-2a$	$H' + 2a$	1

Figure 1-16 illustrates simulated ESR spectra for four equivalent protons and two equivalent ^{14}N nuclei, respectively.

We now consider the case of coupling to two inequivalent nuclei with $I = \frac{1}{2}$. If the first nucleus contributes a local field of $\pm\frac{1}{2}a_1$ and the second nucleus a field of $\pm\frac{1}{2}a_2$, the spectrum is easily constructed as in Table 1-6.

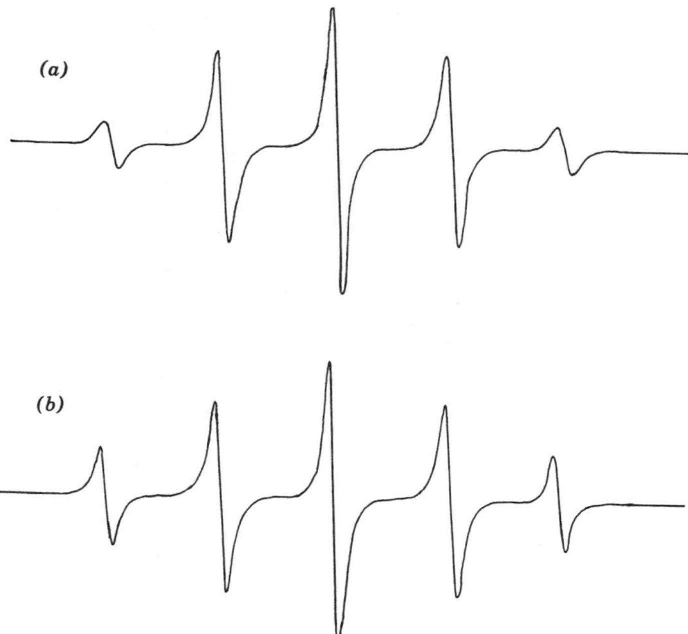

Fig. 1-16 Simulated first-derivative ESR spectra: (*a*) for the case of four equivalent protons ($I = \frac{1}{2}$); the relative intensities should be 1 : 4 : 6 : 4 : 1; (*b*) for the case of two equivalent ^{14}N nuclei ($I = 1$); the relative intensities should be 1 : 2 : 3 : 2 : 1.

Table 1-6 Local-Field Contributions for Two Inequivalent ($a_1 \neq a_2$) nuclei with $I = \frac{1}{2}$

M_I		H_{local}		Total H_{local}	Resonant field H_r	Relative intensity
1	2	1	2			
$\frac{1}{2}$	$\frac{1}{2}$	$\frac{1}{2}a_1$	$\frac{1}{2}a_2$	$\frac{1}{2}a_1 + \frac{1}{2}a_2$	$H' - \frac{1}{2}a_1 - \frac{1}{2}a_2$	1
$\frac{1}{2}$	$-\frac{1}{2}$	$\frac{1}{2}a_1$	$-\frac{1}{2}a_2$	$\frac{1}{2}a_1 - \frac{1}{2}a_2$	$H' - \frac{1}{2}a_1 + \frac{1}{2}a_2$	1
$-\frac{1}{2}$	$\frac{1}{2}$	$-\frac{1}{2}a_1$	$\frac{1}{2}a_2$	$-\frac{1}{2}a_1 + \frac{1}{2}a_2$	$H' + \frac{1}{2}a_1 - \frac{1}{2}a_2$	1
$-\frac{1}{2}$	$-\frac{1}{2}$	$-\frac{1}{2}a_1$	$-\frac{1}{2}a_2$	$-\frac{1}{2}a_1 - \frac{1}{2}a_2$	$H' + \frac{1}{2}a_1 + \frac{1}{2}a_2$	1

An ESR spectrum illustrating this case is shown in Fig. 1-17.

Obviously the more nuclei that interact with the unpaired electron, the more complex the ESR spectrum will become. However, because of the nature of biological systems (alluded to in Section 1.6), except for radicals of biological origin or interest, in solution, we rarely have the luxury of

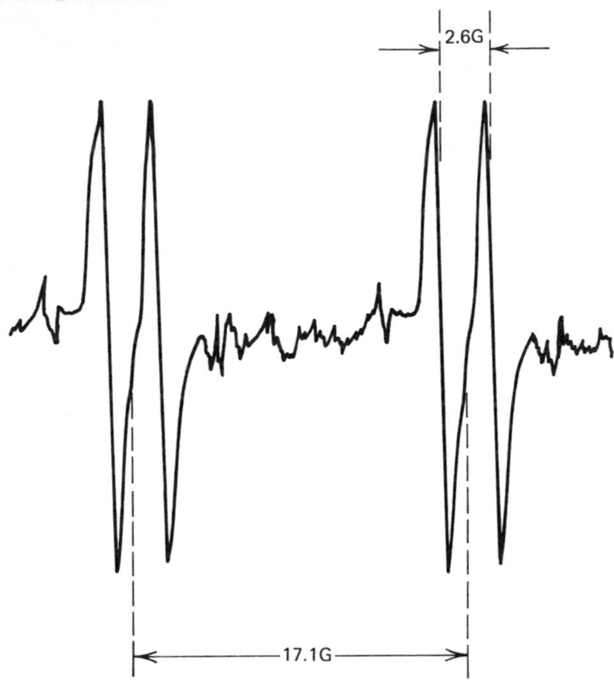

Fig. 1-17 First-derivative ESR spectrum of the HOĊHCOOH radical. The larger proton hyperfine splitting (17.1 G) is due to the CH proton; the smaller one (2.6 G) is due to the OH proton.

having to analyze such a spectrum! Nevertheless, if only for aesthetic purposes, we present the ESR spectrum of the naphthalene negative ion and its analysis in Fig. 1-18. This is a molecule with two sets of four equivalent protons. Historically, this was the first organic free radical studied by ESR in which proton hyperfine structure was observed (9). Analysis of such spectra can give information concerning the spatial distribution of the unpaired electron over the molecule (see Chapters 5 and 6 of Ref. 5).

When spectra such as that shown in Fig. 1-17 were first obtained, it was somewhat of a surprise that any hyperfine splitting was seen at all. The reason is that these are π radicals in which the unpaired electrons are located primarily in p orbitals. As noted in Section 1.5, an isotropic hyperfine interaction can be observed only if the unpaired electron has some s orbital character. Since the hydrogen atoms in π radicals are located in the nodal plane of the p orbitals, to a first degree of approximation no isotropic proton hyperfine splitting should be seen.

The reason that isotropic splittings are seen is that there is an interaction between the π and σ electrons by means of a mechanism called spin

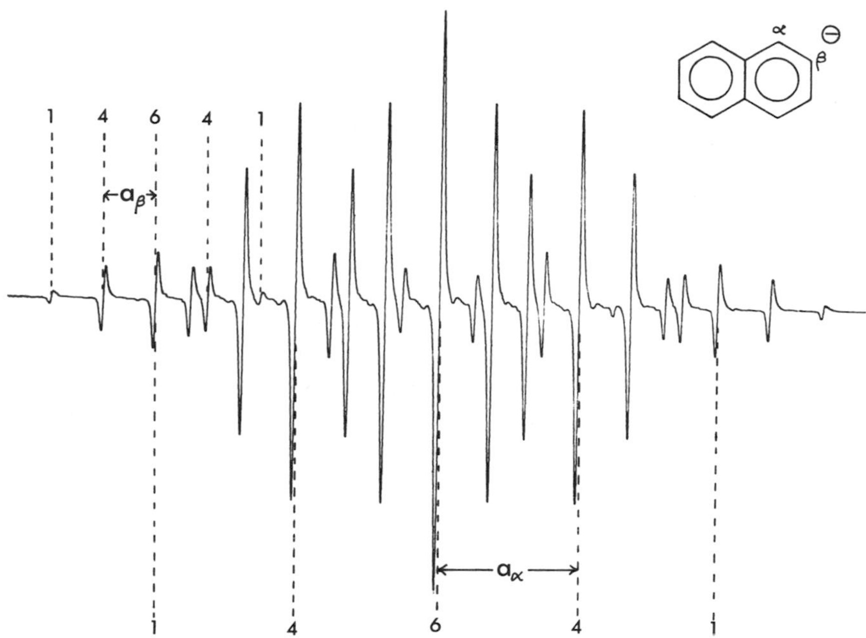

Fig. 1-18 First derivative ESR spectrum of the naphthalene anion. The numbers indicate the expected relative intensities within each group of lines a_α and a_β are the two basic proton hyperfine splittings for this molecule.

polarization. The magnitude of the proton hyperfine splitting proves to be a sensitive probe of the distribution of the unpaired electron as the relation

$$a_i^H = Q\rho_i^\pi \tag{1-58}$$

has been found to hold reasonable well. Here a_i^H is the proton hyperfine splitting for a proton adjacent to a carbon atom in a π system, ρ_i^π is the fraction of time the unpaired electron spends in the vicinity of carbon atom i and Q is a constant ($Q \sim 25$ G) (10).

1.9 TRIPLET-STATES

If a molecule contains more than one unpaired electron, there will be an additional contribution to the local field at the electron; this contribution is simply the dipolar magnetic field of one electron exerted at the position of the other. Qualitatively, the situation is the same as for the anisotropic hyperfine interaction considered in Section 1.5, but because the electron magnetic moment is about 10^3 times larger than nuclear magnetic moments the electronic local field is enormous and dominates the features of the spectrum.

Before considering the details of the ESR spectra of triplet-state systems let us determine how two electrons which are in different spatial orbitals* may interact. Since each electron has two states (corresponding to $M_S = \pm\frac{1}{2}$), there are four possible states for two electrons. It should not be surprising that the major interaction between two electrons is electrostatic in nature. This electrostatic (or exchange) interaction separates one of the four states from the other three. The unique state is called a singlet state (characterized by a total spin $S = 0$), whereas the other group of three is called collectively a triplet state (characterized by a total spin $S = 1$). The former is diamagnetic; the latter is paramagnetic. For two electrons in the same spatial orbital only the singlet state exists, since the triplet state is forbidden by the Pauli principle. Most molecules in their ground states have two electrons in each occupied orbital; thus only the singlet state is possible for these molecules. They may, however, have one or more *excited* triplet states which may be populated by absorption of light. Since triplet-singlet transitions are of very low probability, these excited triplet states are usually fairly long-lived (10^{-3} to 10 sec). A very few molecules have a triplet ground state (i.e., the triplet state is lower in energy than the singlet state); the oxygen molecule is the outstanding example.

The complete Hamiltonian describing the interaction of two electrons is

$$\mathscr{H} = hJ\hat{\mathbf{S}}_1 \cdot \hat{\mathbf{S}}_2 + \hat{\mathbf{S}} \cdot \boldsymbol{D} \cdot \hat{\mathbf{S}}. \tag{1-59}$$

Here $\hat{\mathbf{S}}_1$ and $\hat{\mathbf{S}}_2$ are the spin operators for electrons 1 and 2; $\hat{\mathbf{S}} = \hat{\mathbf{S}}_1 + \hat{\mathbf{S}}_2$; $\boldsymbol{D}$ is a traceless tensor analogous to the $\boldsymbol{T}$ tensor of Eq. 1-46*b* and

$$J = h^{-1} \int_{\tau_2} \int_{\tau_1} \psi(1)\ \phi(2)\ \frac{e^2}{r_{12}}\ \psi(2)\ \phi(1)\ d\tau_1,\ d\tau_2,$$

where ψ and ϕ are the respective wavefunctions for the two electrons and τ_1 and τ_2 refer to the coordinates of electrons 1 and 2, respectively.

The first term of Eq. 1-59 splits the four spin states into a singlet and a triplet with eigenfunctions

triplet state $S = 1$	singlet state $S = 0$
$\lvert\alpha(1)\alpha(2)\rangle$	
$\frac{1}{\sqrt{2}}[\lvert\alpha(1)\beta(2)\rangle + \lvert\beta(1)\alpha(2)\rangle]$	$\frac{1}{\sqrt{2}}[\lvert\alpha(1)\beta(2)\rangle - \lvert\beta(1)\alpha(2)\rangle]$
$\lvert\beta(1)\beta(2)\rangle$	

* Electrons in the same spatial orbital are subject to the Pauli principle. See above.

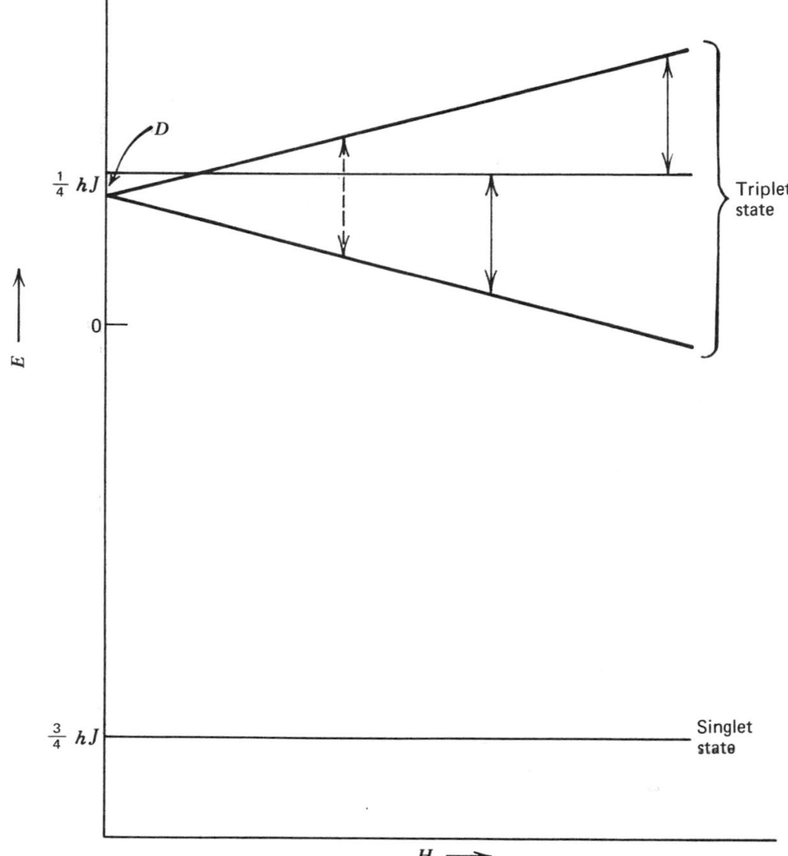

Fig. 1-19 The state energies of a system of two interacting electrons. The case illustrated is one in which the singlet state ($S = 0$) lies lower than the triplet state ($S = 1$). At zero magnetic field the singlet and triplets states are separated by the energy hJ. The separation D of the triplet levels at zero field is due to the dipole-dipole interaction between the two electron spins. The solid transitions are strongly orientation-dependent. The dotted transition is only weakly allowed, but because its position is relatively isotropic this "$\Delta M_S = 2$" transition may be the strongest in a randomly oriented sample.

The energies of the singlet and triplet states are illustrated in Fig. 1-19. The dipole-dipole interaction between the two electrons causes a splitting of the energies of the three states at zero magnetic field.* This splitting is highly orientation-dependent; hence the transitions shown in Fig. 1-19

* Spin-orbit coupling also contributes to the zero-field splitting.

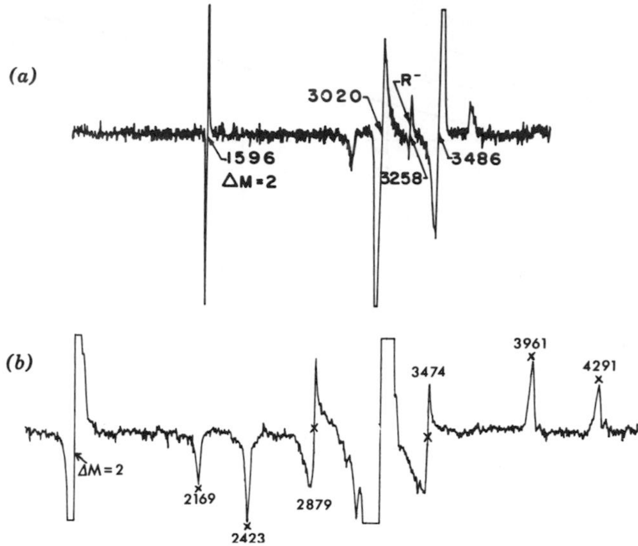

Fig. 1-20 First derivative ESR spectra of triplet-state systems. (*a*) A rigid solution of the dianion of triphenylbenzene. $\nu = 9.150$ GHz. The line marked R^- arises from the anion radical. This is an example of a system with axial symmetry [taken from R. E. Jesse, P. Biloen, R. Prins, J. D. W. van Voorst and G. J. Hoijtink, *Mol. Phys.* **6**, 433 (1963)]. (*b*) A rigid solution of naphthalene-d_8 excited to its lowest triplet state. The off-scale line in the center is presumably due to radicals produced by the UV irradiation [taken from W. A. Yager, E. Wasserman, and R. N. R. Cramer, *J. Chem. Phys.* **37**, 1148 (1962)].

usually occur over a very wide field range in a randomly oriented sample. As a result the lines due to the triplet state may be so broad that detection is difficult. The situation is analogous to but not exactly the same as that for nuclear hyperfine interaction. Fortunately the electronic dipole-dipole interaction is usually much larger than the inherent linewidth and thus the features expected at orientations near the principal axes are readily observed. Figure 1-20*a* illustrates the first-derivative ESR spectrum for the triplet state of the triphenyl benzene dianion (a ground-state triplet); Fig. 1-19*b* illustrates the analogous spectrum for the excited triplet state of naphthalene. The lines at low field (called the "half-field" transitions) correspond to transitions for which $\Delta M_S = 2$. They are only weakly allowed transitions but appear strong in the spectrum because they do not exhibit the large anisotropy that the $\Delta M_S = 1$ transitions do and thus are not spread out over so wide a field. *The observation of a half-field transition is a strong indication that the system is in a triplet state.*

At high field the three wavefunctions of the triplet state (see above) are eigenfunctions of $\hat{S}_z$ and may be represented as $|1\rangle$, $|0\rangle$, and $|-1\rangle$, where the numbers refer to the M_S quantum numbers.

The second term in (1-59), when combined with the electron Zeeman term, yields the spin Hamiltonian for a triplet state:

$$\hat{\mathscr{H}}_T = g\beta\mathbf{H}\cdot\hat{\mathbf{S}} + D_{XX}\hat{S}_x^{\,2} + D_{YY}\hat{S}_y^{\,2} + D_{ZZ}\hat{S}_z^{\,2} \tag{1-60a}$$

$$= g\beta H\hat{S}_z + D(\hat{S}_z^{\,2} - \tfrac{2}{3}) + E(\hat{S}_x^{\,2} - \hat{S}_y^{\,2}). \tag{1-60b}$$

Here

$$D = D_{ZZ} - \frac{(D_{XX} + D_{YY})}{2}, \tag{1-60c}$$

$$E = \frac{D_{XX} - D_{YY}}{2}. \tag{1-60d}$$

For $\mathbf{H}\|Z$, $\hat{\mathscr{H}}_T$ yields the energies*

$$E_1 = g\beta H_Z + \tfrac{1}{3}D, \tag{1-61a}$$

$$E_0 = -\tfrac{2}{3}D, \tag{1-61b}$$

$$E_{-1} = -g\beta H_Z + \tfrac{1}{3}D. \tag{1-61c}$$

For $\Delta M_S = \pm 1$ resonance will be observed at

$$H_Z = H' \pm D'. \tag{1-62}$$

Here $H' = h\nu_0/g\beta$ and $D' = D/g\beta$.

For $\mathbf{H}\|X$ resonance is observed at

$$H_X = H' \pm \frac{(D' - 3E')}{2} \tag{1-63}$$

and for $\mathbf{H}\|Y$

$$H_Y = H' \pm \frac{(D' + 3E')}{2}, \tag{1-64}$$

where $E' = E/g\beta$.

If the symmetry is axial (i.e., $X \equiv Y$), then $E = 0$ and the resonances for $\mathbf{H} \parallel X$ and $\mathbf{H} \parallel Y$ will coincide. This case is illustrated in Fig. 1-20*a* (i.e., $E' = 0$). The case of $E' \neq 0$ is illustrated in Fig. 1-20*b*.

A rigid matrix is required for the observation of the ESR spectra of triplet-state molecules; the reason is that the dipole-dipole interaction is so strong that molecular rotation provides a strong relaxation mechanism such that the lines are broadened beyond detection. An exception is the case in which the two unpaired electrons are sufficiently far apart (> 8 Å) so that

* These relations apply only when $g\beta H_Z \gg D$

molecular rotation averages out the dipolar fields as in anisotropic hyperfine splitting. Then the system behaves as if there were two weakly interacting doublet states. These molecules are called biradicals. They are considered briefly in Chapter 11.

1.10 TRANSITION-METAL IONS

The transition metals are those elements that have incomplete 3*d*, 4*d*, and 5*d* shells. Among them only V, Mn, Fe, Co, Cu, and Mo are found in significant amounts in biological systems and thus we restrict this section to those elements. They differ from the free radicals considered previously in that now there are unpaired electrons in *d* orbitals. This presents the following new features in the ESR spectra which are either not present or are not important for free radicals:

1. Spin-orbit coupling is usually strong and exhibits strong anisotropy so that *g* factors may vary over a wide range (an extreme range would be 0–9).
2. The features of the ESR spectrum depend strongly on the environment of the ion, especially the primary coordination sphere of ligands.*
3. We often require very low temperatures (77 K or lower) to observe resonance.
4. For ions with an even number of unpaired electrons it may be impossible to observe any ESR spectrum at all.

We shall not attempt to give a detailed and quantitative treatment of the theory of the ESR spectra of transition-metal ions, since it is a rather complex subject.† Instead we present a qualitative picture for each ion and simply quote results when needed.

We shall begin our discussion with the V^{4+} ion, since this ion has only one *d* electron. For the gaseous V^{4+} ion there are five *d* orbitals which, to a first approximation, have the same energy. In a solid or liquid, however, the ion is usually surrounded by a number of ligands which are either negatively charged or negatively polarized. Two basic arrangements of the ligands are found—the usual is six ligands arranged at the corners of an octahedron; a less common case has four ligands arranged at the corners of a tetrahedron. The effect of these ligands is to split the *d* orbitals into a set of two and a set of three separated by the energy Δ, as shown in Fig. 1-21; Δ is called "crystal-field" splitting. A distortion of either the octahedron or

* A ligand is any molecule or atom complexed to the transition-metal ion.

† Considerable further detail on iron is contained in Chapter 8 and on copper in Chapter 9 of this book. See Chapters 11 and 12 of Ref. 5 for a thorough treatment.

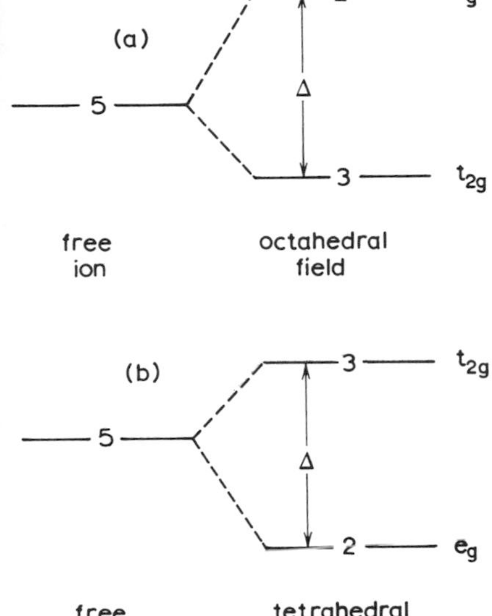

Fig. 1-21 Splitting of the energies of the five *d* orbitals. (*a*) In an octahedral crystal field; (*b*) in a tetrahedral crystal field. The numbers on the levels refer to the orbital degeneracy. The labels on the levels are group-theoretical designations.

the tetrahedron may cause a further splitting of levels; for instance, V^{4+} is usually found as the vanadyl ion VO^{2+} with five other more weakly bound ligands. The presence of the O^{2-} ion results in a strongly distorted octahedron such that all orbital degeneracy* is removed. (The ultimate distortion of an octahedron is a square-planar configuration.)

Although the electron orbital angular momentum is usually quenched in the ground state, excited states can mix with the ground states such that some orbital angular momentum is introduced. This creates a field-dependent local magnetic field and thus affects the observed g factor. It is found that for many transition ions a relation such as

$$g = g_e - k \frac{\lambda}{\Delta} \tag{1-65}$$

holds; g_e is the free electron g factor, λ is the spin-orbit coupling constant for the free ion, Δ is the crystal field splitting, and k is a factor that depends on orientation and the type of transition ion. For ions in which the d shell is less than half full $\lambda > 0$, hence usually $g < g_e$; for ions in which the d shell is greater than half full $g > g_e$. V^{4+} falls into the former class, and it is found that the g factors are slightly less than g_e.

* The degeneracy of a state is the number of independent wavefunctions which correspond to that state; for instance, if $L = 2$ (as for d electrons), the orbital degeneracy is five.

Spin-orbit coupling has another effect in that it strongly influences the value of T_1, the spin-lattice relaxation time, hence affecting linewidths. If Δ is large, spin-orbit coupling will be weak and T_1 long. This is the case for VO^{2+} and it is possible to see rather narrow lines even at room temperature.

An additional feature of V^{4+} is the prominent octet hyperfine splitting caused by the ^{51}V nucleus with $I = \frac{7}{2}$. A good example of V^{4+} is the vanadyl etioporphyrin shown in Fig. 1-22*a* in benzene solution at 20 C* and

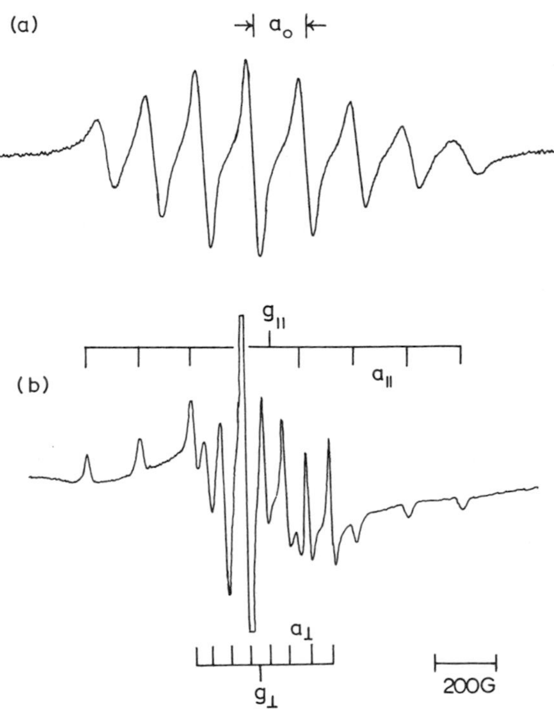

Fig. 1-22 First-derivative ESR spectra of vanadyl etioporphyrin II. (*a*) In benzene solution at 20°C the eight-line spectrum is due to hyperfine splitting from ^{51}V ($I = \frac{7}{2}$); the viscosity is low so that almost all anisotropy is averaged out; (*b*) In castor oil solution at 20°C; the viscosity is high so that a "solid-state" spectrum is observed. The anisotropic parameters are readily obtained from the spectrum [taken from E. M. Roberts, W. S. Koski, and W. S. Coughey, *J. Chem. Phys.* **34**, 591 (1961)].

* It may come as some surprise that an electron which is supposedly in a 3*d* orbital can give rise to an isotropic hyperfine splitting (see Section 1.6). However, a phenomenon known as spin polarization allows the electronic wavefunction to contain a small admixture of the 1*s*, 2*s*, and 3*s* orbitals. This is the origin of the isotropic hyperfine splittings in transition-metal ions.

in castor oil solution at 20 C in Fig. 1-22*b*. It is clear from Fig. 1-22*b* that the anisotropic hyperfine and *g* tensor components are readily obtained in this case from the "solid state" spectrum.

Mn^{2+} and Fe^{3+} are treated together, since they are isoelectronic ions, each with five *d* electrons. If the crystal-field splitting of the *d* orbitals is not too large, the ions will exist in the "high-spin" state with five unpaired electrons (see Fig. 1-23). For a large crystal-field splitting, however, spin pairing will lead to the "low-spin" state with one unpaired electron.

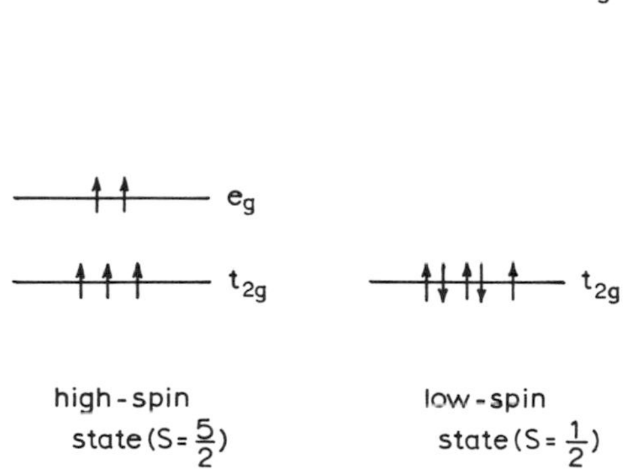

Fig. 1-23 Low- and high-spin states for a d^5 transition-metal ion. Note that the t_{2g} set of levels may hold six electrons whereas the e_g set may accept only four. The assignment of spins is governed by the Pauli principle and Hund's rules.

In the high-spin state all orbital angular momentum cancels out because there is one electron in each *d* orbital (a half-filled atomic shell usually has zero orbital angular momentum). Thus for purely octahedral symmetry the *g* factors are close to the free-electron value. There is, however, some additional fine splitting caused by dipolar interaction among the five unpaired electrons.

Mn^{2+} and Fe^{3+} in biological materials usually exist in a strongly distorted octahedral environment as in a porphyrin. The result is that the sixfold degeneracy resulting from five unpaired electrons ($S = \frac{5}{2}$) splits into three doubly degenerate states (see Fig. 1-24). If the splitting is much larger than the size of the microwave quantum (this is usually the case) and the symmetry is axial, only transitions between the bottom two states are possible. Thus the system behaves as if only two magnetic levels were present (it can be described by a spin Hamiltonian with an effective spin $S' = \frac{1}{2}$). However, the effective *g* factor is very anisotropic, varying between $g = 2$ and $g = 6$.

If the symmetry is less than axial, that is, rhombic, then mixing of states

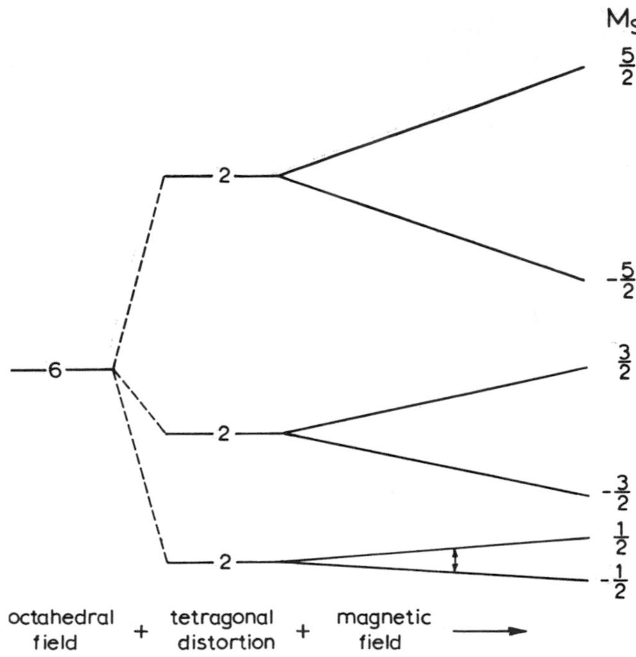

Fig. 1-24 Energy levels for the high-spin d^5 ion in an octahedral field with a strong tetragonal distortion. The numbers indicate the degeneracy of the levels. There is also a small splitting of levels in purely octahedral symmetry. This splitting has been neglected in this diagram. The double arrow indicates the only possible transition ($\Delta M_S = \pm 1$) for small microwave quanta.

occurs and transitions between each pair of states in Fig. 1-24 are allowed. Effective g factors (i.e., $g_{\text{eff}} = h\nu/\beta H$) between 2.0 and 9.7 are possible. In addition, one has the peculiar circumstance that the value of g_{eff} for a given orientation varies with the microwave frequency! For a randomly oriented sample a strong resonance is usually seen at $g \sim 4.3$. This system has been treated in detail by Aasa (11).

Mn^{2+} behaves in a similar manner to Fe^{3+} except that every line is split into six components from the hyperfine interaction with the ^{55}Mn nucleus ($I = \frac{5}{2}$). ESR spectra of Mn^{2+} can usually be detected at room temperature. If, however, the site symmetry around the Mn^{2+} is distorted, the resonances become anisotropic and thus a randomly oriented sample may exhibit such a broad resonance that detection becomes difficult.

Fe^{3+} is often found in the low-spin state in which the true spin is $S = \frac{1}{2}$. The g factors are usually found to be greater than 2, but the g anisotropy is not nearly so great as in the high-spin cases; for instance in *met*-myoglobin azide $g_z = 2.80$, $g_y = 2.25$, and $g_x = 1.75$.

Fe^{2+} has six d-electrons and can also exist in low-spin and high-spin states. For octahedral or distorted octahedral symmetry $S = 2$ for the high-spin state and $S = 0$ (diamagnetic) for the low-spin state (see Fig. 1-25a). For the paramagnetic states spin-orbit coupling is usually strong due to low-lying excited states so that temperatures of 20 K or less are required for observation of the ESR spectra.

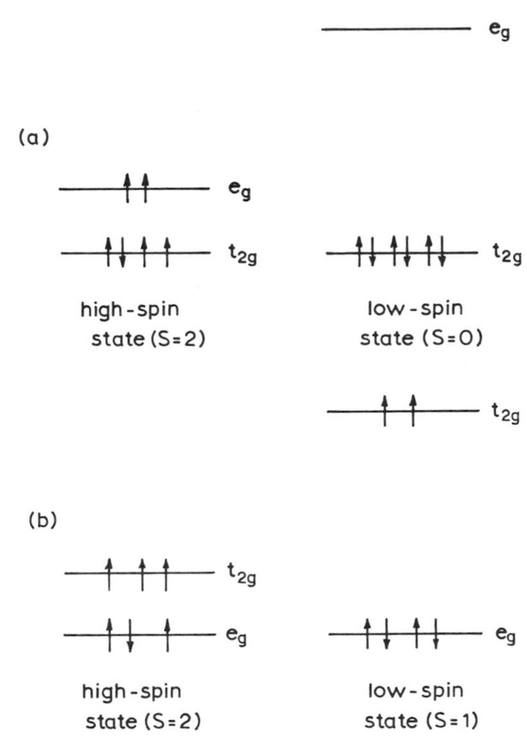

Fig. 1-25 Low- and high-spin states for a d^6 transition-metal ion: (*a*) octahedral symmetry; (*b*) tetrahedral symmetry.

Co^{2+} has seven d electrons. Again low spin ($S = \frac{1}{2}$) and high-spin ($S = \frac{3}{2}$) states are possible. In the low-spin case the g factors are slightly above 2 with $g_{\parallel} \sim 2.0$ and $g_{\perp} \sim 2.2$–2.3. In the high-spin case spin-orbit coupling and distortions from octahedral symmetry result in a system that behaves as if $S = \frac{1}{2}$; the g factors are usually near 4. ^{59}Co has $I = \frac{7}{2}$; thus an octet hyperfine splitting is expected.

Cu^{2+} has nine d electrons. Because the d shell holds only 10 electrons, all but one must be paired; thus this ion has $S = \frac{1}{2}$. ESR spectra are usually observable at room temperature; g factors are usually somewhat larger than the free-electron value ($g \sim 2.0$–2.4). ^{63}Cu and ^{65}Cu both have $I = \frac{3}{2}$ and similar magnetic moments. Thus hyperfine quartets are usually resolved in the ESR spectra.

Mo^{5+} has one $4d$ electron and its ESR behavior is similar to that of $3d^1$ ions such as V^{4+} or Ti^{3+}. In distorted octahedral environments g factors slightly less than 2 are found with $g_{\parallel} \sim 2.0$ and $g_{\perp} \sim 1.95$. Mo^{5+} ESR signals have been observed in xanthine oxidase (see Chapter 8).

1.11 DOUBLE RESONANCE

Double-resonance encompasses all techniques in which a sample is irradiated at more than one frequency. Two of these techniques have been used with ESR: electron-nuclear double resonance (ENDOR) in which the sample, in addition to being irradiated at the ESR frequency, is also irradiated at a frequency that will cause transitions between the nuclear spin levels and electron-electron double resonance (ELDOR) in which the sample is irradiated at two different microwave frequencies.

Of these two techniques only ENDOR has been applied successfully to important biological problems (see Section 8.2.1.4).

1.11.1 ENDOR

As noted in Section 1.6, much of the information about nuclear hyperfine splittings is not obtainable from the ESR spectra of biological systems because of the "solid state" nature of the spectra. The hyperfine splittings are there but are not resolved because of the anisotropy of the hyperfine splittings. The observed lines are a broad envelope of a multitude of individual line components. Even for radicals in the liquid state the number of hyperfine components may be so large that analysis is impeded by the extensive overlap of lines. In both cases the ENDOR technique may provide the missing information.

ENDOR was first proposed and demonstrated by Feher (12) in 1956. It is basically an ESR experiment in which one of the transitions in an ESR spectrum is subjected to partial power saturation. Then, by means of a coil around the sample, an intense radio-frequency (rf) field is applied. This field has a frequency such that transitions between the *nuclear* spin states may be induced. The frequency of the rf field is swept through a range appropriate to the nucleus being investigated. At points at which the photon energy ($h\nu$) matches the separation in energy of nuclear-spin states the partial saturation condition on the ESR line will be relaxed. This is indicated by an *increase* in the intensity of the ESR line.

For a given nucleus in a radical there will be *two* values of the rf frequency at which this increase in ESR intensity will occur. It occurs because there are *two* values of the hyperfine local field at the nucleus (one for $M_S = +\frac{1}{2}$ and one for $M_S = -\frac{1}{2}$). These two frequencies are given by

$$\nu_{N_1} = \left|\frac{A}{2} - \nu_0\right|, \qquad \text{(1-66}a\text{)}$$

$$\nu_{N_2} = \left|\frac{A}{2} + \nu_0\right|, \qquad \text{(1-66}b\text{)}$$

where A is the hyperfine coupling and ν_0 is the frequency at which the nucleus N would resonate in the absence of hyperfine coupling (i.e., $A = 0$).*

Thus the two rf frequencies ν_{N_1} and ν_{N_2} provide not only an accurate value of A but also a positive identification of the interacting nucleus (ν_0 is a function only of the magnetic moment of the nucleus).

To illustrate situations in which ENDOR may be applicable, the following points are given:

1. Resolution may be improved when a radical contains many nuclei that exhibit hyperfine interaction. In the ENDOR spectrum only two lines will be seen for each set of equivalent nuclei, whereas the ESR spectrum may have hundreds or thousands of lines; for instance, the ENDOR spectrum of the naphthalene anion (Fig. 1-18) would contain only four lines. This resolution improvement is usually possible only for free radicals in solution (13) and for paramagnetic entities oriented in single crystals. If, however, the g anisotropy is large, we may be able to obtain ENDOR spectra from a powder sample (14).
2. The sensitivity of ENDOR is rarely better than 10 percent that of ESR; the reason for this is that the intensity of the ESR signal changes by at best 10 percent when the rf field is applied. The ENDOR intensity is a *strong* function of the relaxation times of the system, both nuclear and electronic. Failure to detect an ENDOR signal (even though a strong ESR signal is seen) can usually be traced to an unfavorable set of relaxation times.
3. ENDOR spectra of powders or randomly oriented samples often exhibit a broad ENDOR signal at ν_0. This signal has been identified as arising from nuclei of the host and has been termed "matrix ENDOR." Such signals can be of value in establishing the environment of a paramagnetic entity.

* A more detailed description of ENDOR is given in Chapter 13 of Ref. 5.

1.11.2 ELDOR

This technique is similar to ENDOR in that a given ESR line is partially saturated. In this case, however, a *second* microwave frequency is employed. When the second frequency satisfies the resonance condition for a second transition, a reduction in the intensity of the first may be observed. This technique was introduced by Hyde et al. (15) who used a bimodal cavity. Its value in biological systems is yet to be established.

ACKNOWLEDGMENTS

I am indebted to Helmut Beinert, Donald Borg, Tore Vänngård, and Harold Swartz for their criticisms of this chapter. I am especially grateful to Dan Kohl for his guidance and suggestions on the approach to take.

REFERENCES

1. P. Ayscough, *Electron Spin Resonance in Chemistry*, Methuen, London, 1967.
2. M. Bersohn and J. Baird, *Electron Paramagnetic Resonance*, Benjamin, New York, 1966.
3. A. Carrington and A. McLachlan, *Introduction to Magnetic Resonance*, Harper and Row, New York, 1967.
4. G. Pake, *Paramagnetic Resonance*, Harper and Row, New York, 1967.
5. J. Wertz and J. Bolton, *Electron Spin Resonance—Elementary Theory and Applications*, McGraw-Hill, New York, 1972.
6. B. Taylor, W. Parker, and D. Langenberg, *Rev. Mod. Phys.*, **41,** 375 (1969).
7. J. Bennett, J. Gibson, and D. Ingram, *Proc. Roy. Soc. (London)*, **A240,** 67 (1957).
8. G. Herzberg, *Atomic Spectra and Atomic Structure*, Dover, 1944.
9. D. Lipkin, D. Paul, J. Townsend, and S. Weissman, *Science*, **117,** 534 (1953).
10. For further background in this field see J. Bolton in *Radical Ions*, E. Kaiser and L. Kevan, Eds., Wiley, New York, 1968, Chapter 1.
11. R. Aasa, *J. Chem. Phys.*, **52,** 3919 (1970); see also W. Blumberg in *Magnetic Resonance in Biological Systems*, A. Ehrenberg, B. Malmström, and T. Vanngård, Eds., Pergamon, New York, 1967, p. 119.
12. G. Feher, *Phys. Rev.*, **103,** 834 (1956).
13. J. Hyde and A. Maki, *J. Chem. Phys.*, **40,** 3117 (1964).
14. G. Rist and J. Hyde, *J. Chem. Phys.*, **52,** 4633 (1970).
15. J. Hyde, J. Chien, and J. Freed, *J. Chem. Phys.*, **48,** 4211 (1968).

APPENDIX

Table A-1 Spin and Magnetic Moments of Magnetic Nuclei Encountered in Biological Systems

Nucleus	Natural abundance(%)	Spin	Magnetogyric ratio (rad $sec^{-1}gauss^{-1} \times 10^{-4}$)
^{1}H	99.984	$\frac{1}{2}$	2.67510
^{2}H	0.016	1	0.41064
^{7}Li	92.57	$\frac{3}{2}$	1.03964
^{10}B	18.83	3	0.28748
^{11}B	81.17	$\frac{3}{2}$	0.85828
^{13}C	1.11	$\frac{1}{2}$	0.67263
^{14}N	99.64	1	0.19324
^{15}N	0.36	$\frac{1}{2}$	−0.27107
^{17}O	0.037	$\frac{5}{2}$	−0.36266
^{19}F	100	$\frac{1}{2}$	2.51665
^{23}Na	100	$\frac{3}{2}$	0.70760
^{31}P	100	$\frac{1}{2}$	1.08290
^{33}S	0.74	$\frac{3}{2}$	0.20517
^{35}Cl	75.4	$\frac{3}{2}$	0.26212
^{37}Cl	24.6	$\frac{3}{2}$	0.21818
^{39}K	93.1	$\frac{3}{2}$	0.12484
^{43}Ca	0.13	$\frac{7}{2}$	−0.17999
^{51}V	99.8	$\frac{7}{2}$	0.70323
^{53}Cr	9.5	$\frac{3}{2}$	−0.15120
^{55}Mn	100	$\frac{5}{2}$	0.65980
^{57}Fe	2.25	$\frac{1}{2}$	0.08644
^{59}Co	100	$\frac{7}{2}$	0.63171
^{63}Cu	69.1	$\frac{3}{2}$	0.70904
^{65}Cu	30.9	$\frac{3}{2}$	0.75958
^{77}Se	7.5	$\frac{1}{2}$	0.51008
^{79}Br	50.6	$\frac{3}{2}$	0.67021
^{81}Br	49.4	$\frac{3}{2}$	0.72245
^{85}Rb	72.8	$\frac{5}{2}$	0.25829
^{87}Rb	27.2	$\frac{3}{2}$	0.87533
^{95}Mo	15.8	$\frac{5}{2}$	0.17428
^{97}Mo	9.6	$\frac{5}{2}$	−0.17796
^{127}I	100	$\frac{5}{2}$	0.53522
^{133}Cs	100	$\frac{7}{2}$	0.35089

CHAPTER TWO

Experimental Aspects of Biological Electron Spin Resonance Studies

JAMES R. BOLTON

Department of Chemistry
University of Western Ontario
London, Canada

DONALD C. BORG

Medical Research Center
Brookhaven National Laboratory
Upton, New York

HAROLD M. SWARTZ

Departments of Radiology and Biochemistry
The Medical College of Wisconsin
Milwaukee, Winconsin

2.1 INTRODUCTION

In this chapter we consider experimental aspects of ESR spectroscopy, emphasizing in particular those areas of special interest to investigators of biological phenomena. (One aspect, quantitative measurements, is of sufficient importance and magnitude that it is covered separately in Chapter 3.) Several good general ESR texts (1, 2, 3) cover many experimental aspects in much greater depth than is possible here, and the reader is urged to consult them as well as the two periodicals (4, 5) that carry papers on specific ESR techniques and devices.

Since most life scientists will have access only to commercial ESR instruments, we limit our discussion to techniques and methods that can be employed with these instruments or that involve simple modifications. Only brief mention is made of techniques that require more extensive modifications.

We begin by outlining the minimum essential elements for a working ESR spectrometer and by pointing out an analogy with the more familiar optical spectrometer. We then add components one by one, showing how each improves the operation of the spectrometer, until we have completed a typical commercial ESR instrument. Some of these components are discussed in greater detail in subsequent sections.

2.2 THE SIMPLEST ESR SPECTROMETER

Any spectrometer involves three basic elements: a radiation source, a sample which absorbs some of the radiation and a detector which measures the intensity of transmitted radiation. In Fig. 2-1 we compare the operation of a simple optical spectrometer, using visible light, with the simplest type of ESR spectrometer. In the optical spectrometer the radiation source is usually a tungsten lamp followed by a monochromator (this may be a prism or a grating) which selects from the lamp's emission the light that has a given narrow band of wavelengths; in the ESR spectrometer the radiation source is a radio tube, called a klystron—no monochromator is necessary because the klystron output is monochromatic. The output of the klystron is in the microwave region (wavelength 0.1 to 10 cm).

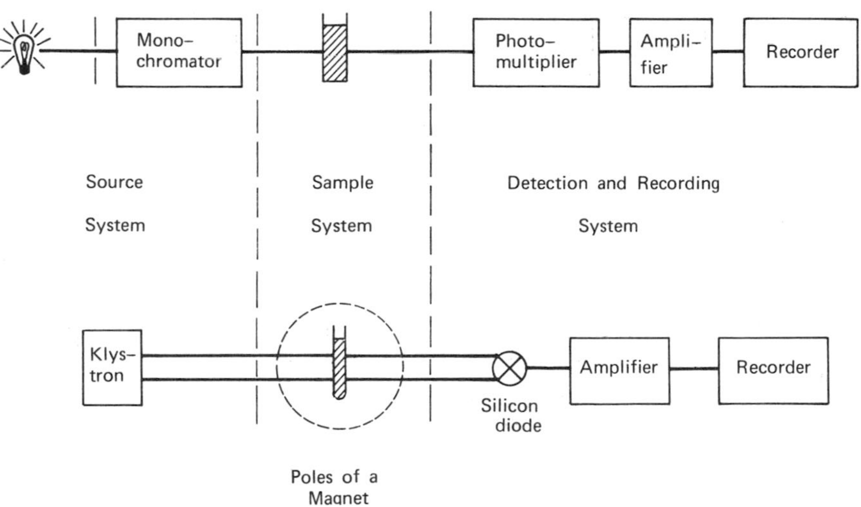

Fig. 2-1 Comparison of an optical spectrometer with the simplest type of ESR spectrometer. In the optical spectrometer a monochromatic beam of light passes through a sample and is detected by a photomultiplier; in the ESR spectrometer a monochromatic beam of microwaves passes through a sample in a magnetic field and is detected by a silicon diode.

In the optical spectrometer the collimated monochromatic light beam passes through the sample in a sample cell, where some of the light is absorbed; the remainder falls on a detector, usually a photomultiplier. The current generated by the photomultiplier is proportional to the transmitted light intensity. A comparison of this intensity with the sample in the cell versus a blank in the cell will allow a calculation of the percent absorption, or the optical density of the sample. A plot of either of these quantities versus wavelength will give the optical absorption spectrum of the sample.

In the ESR spectrometer shown in Fig. 2-1 a beam of microwaves from the klystron is transmitted to the sample through microwave plumbing (waveguide); the sample is held in the external magnetic field required for resonance to occur (see Eq. 1-9). The intensity of transmitted microwaves is determined by a microwave rectifier, usually a silicon crystal, which proportionately converts the microwave radiation to an electrical current that can be accurately measured. In principle an ESR spectrum could be obtained by plotting the percent absorption of microwave power versus the frequency (or wavelength) of the klystron output. In ESR spectroscopy, however, we have the advantage of being able to "tune" the separation of the energy levels to match the microwave photon energy. Thus an ESR spectrum can also be obtained by fixing the frequency of the microwaves and varying the magnetic field; in practice this is what is done for reasons noted shortly.

2.3 A TYPICAL ESR SPECTROMETER

Although the ESR spectrometer in Fig. 2-1 can be made to work, it is not a sensitive instrument. Through the years, since the first ESR experiment in 1945, various components have been added to improve both the sensitivity and operating convenience of the spectrometer. Figure 2-2 shows a block diagram of a typical modern ESR spectrometer to which we refer, as each element is described, in terms of how it works and why it is necessary or at least desirable.

2.3.1 The Source System

In principle the resonance equation, Eq. 1-9, can be satisfied for any frequency of electromagnetic radiation; as noted in Section 1.3.3, however, the population difference between the two energy levels allowed for the electron spin states increases linearly with the magnetic field. Thus for reasons of sensitivity we want to use a frequency as high as is practical. Limitations at the high-frequency end include sample size, geometry, magnetic field intensity, and homogeneity. For these and other reasons most commercial ESR spectrometers operate in the microwave region, primarily at X band ($\nu \sim 9.5$ GHz); although instruments are also available at K band ($\nu \sim 24$ GHz) and Q band ($\nu \sim 35$ GHz).

Microwaves have unique properties because they have wavelengths of the order of centimeters (e.g., X-band radiation has a wavelength of approximately 3 cm). One of these properties is that a polarized beam of microwaves can be transmitted most efficiently by means of a rectangular metal pipe called a waveguide. Waveguides can be bent or twisted at will, provided the bends are not too sharp. Most of the connections between components in the microwave system are thus made with sections of waveguide.

The output of the klystron can be tuned either by varying the "reflection" voltage applied to it or by a mechanical tuning stub. The reflector voltage can vary the frequency of the klystron by about ± 20 MHz about a center frequency determined by the tuning stub.

The klystron is one of the important sources of noise in the ESR spectrometer, and thus it is most important that a low-noise type of klystron be used. Solid-state microwave sources, that are much simpler to operate than a klystron and can operate on low voltages, have recently become available; the present devices, however, are still rather noisy. If the noise and a few other problems can be solved, these new sources will certainly replace the klystron.

To operate effectively a klystron must be protected from microwave energy reflected from the system it is feeding. This protection is provided by a nonreciprocal device called an *isolator*. It readily transmits microwaves in the forward direction but strongly attenuates any reflections in the reverse direction.

The wavelength or frequency of the microwaves is usually measured with a device called a *wavemeter*. Its operation is described in Section 2.10.

It is important to be able to vary the intensity of the microwave beam, commonly termed microwave power. This is accomplished by means of an absorbing element called an *attenuator*. The dial of the attenuator is calibrated either in *milliwatts* of microwave output or in *decibels* below the maximum output of the system. Decibels are defined by

$$\text{db} = 10 \log \frac{P_{\text{out}}}{P_{\text{in}}}, \tag{2-1}$$

where P_{in} is the input power to the attenuator and P_{out} is the output power; for example, if P_{in} is 200 mW, an attenuation of -20 db* would give P_{out} as 2 mW. Most commercial instruments have klystrons with outputs of 100 to 500 mW and attenuators ranging from 0 to 60 db. There are some situations in which greater attenuation is required (see discussion of power saturation in Section 2.7).

2.3.2 The Cavity and Sample System

One of the principal reasons that the ESR spectrometer shown in Fig. 2-1 is insensitive is that the percent absorption is small. In an optical system

* Most attenuator dials give only the absolute value of the decibels.

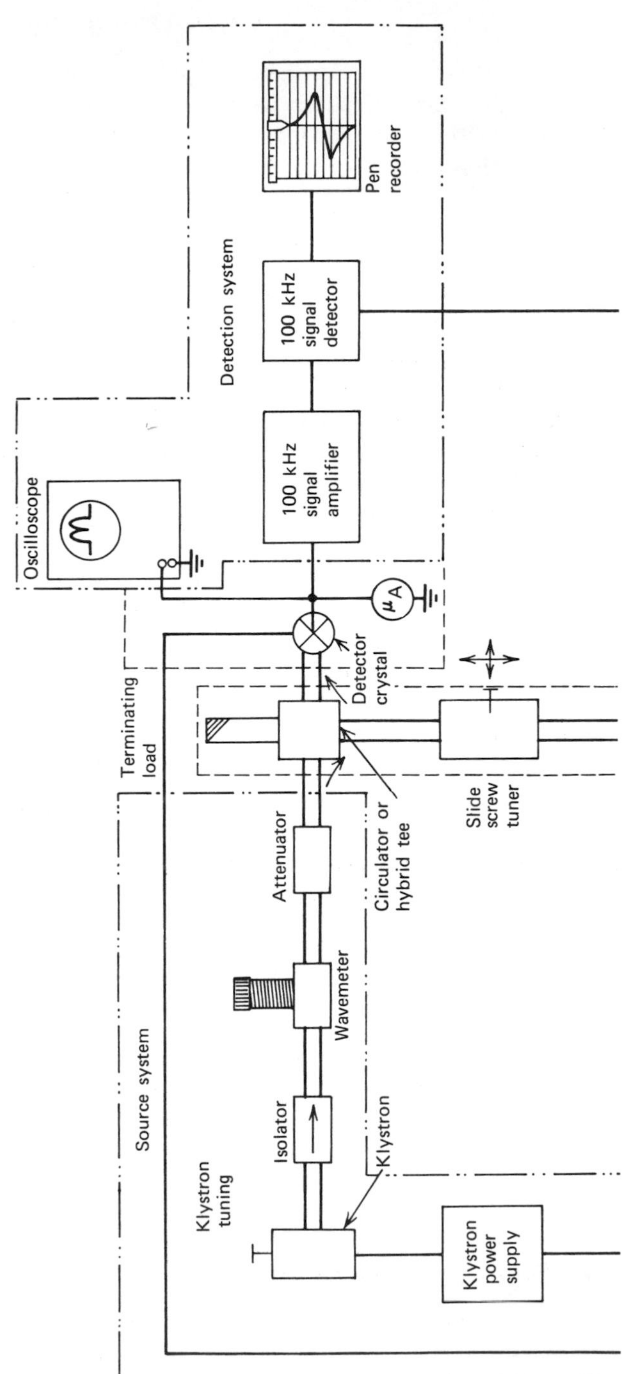

Detection system
Pen
recorder
100 kHz
signal
detector
100 kHz
signal
amplifier
Oscilloscope
μ_A
Detector
crystal
Terminating
load
Slide
screw
tuner
Circulator or
hybrid tee
Attenuator
Wavemeter
Source system
Isolator
Klystron
Klystron
tuning
Klystron
power
supply

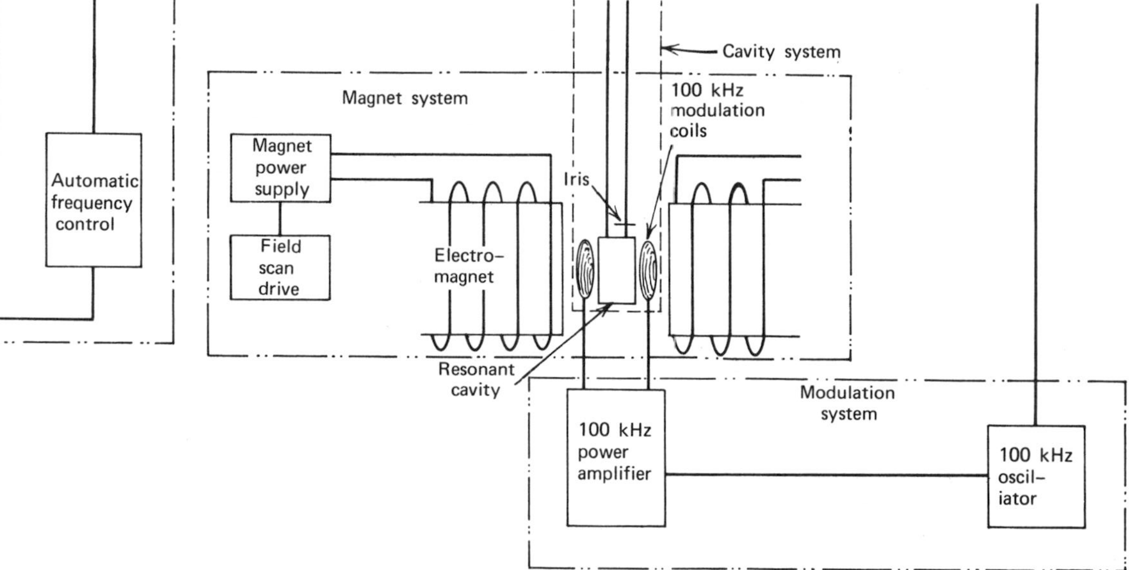

Fig. 2-2 Block diagram of a typical X-band ESR spectrometer employing 100 kHz phase-sensitive detection.

the percent of the source emission absorbed by the sample can be increased by concentrating the light beam with a lens. The analogous operation with microwaves is to place the sample in a power-collecting probe, usually a rectangular or cylindrical box called a *cavity*. There are two types of cavity: the *transmission* cavity has a coupling hole to a waveguide section at each end; a *reflection* cavity has a coupling hole in only one end. The cavity operates with microwaves in much the same way as an organ pipe does with sound waves. The cavity magnifies the intensity of the microwaves when the frequency is such that some of the dimensions of the cavity are multiples of half-wavelengths. The lowest frequency at which this occurs is called the *resonant frequency* of the cavity.

As noted in Chapter 1, electromagnetic radiation consists of two fields, the electric field $\mathbf{E}_1$ and the magnetic field $\mathbf{H}_1$, which are always perpendicular to each other. To provide the optimum absorption signal for ESR, a cavity should (a) provide a high energy density of microwaves, (b) allow placement of the sample at a maximum of $\mathbf{H}_1$ and a minimum of $\mathbf{E}_1$ [because resonance requires interaction with the magnetic field (see Section 1.2), whereas interaction with the electric field leads to non-resonant dielectric loss of power (see Section 2.9)] and (c) have $\mathbf{H}_1$ perpendicular to the static field $\mathbf{H}$, a condition required for the spin transitions to be "allowed" (see Section 1.2).

Most commercial ESR spectrometers employ a rectangular cavity, although cylindrical cavities are also available. Figure 2-3*a* illustrates a TE_{102} rectangular cavity; TE stands for transverse electric, that is, the $\mathbf{E}_1$ field is always oscillating perpendicular to the long axis of the cavity z. The subscripts refer to the number of half-wavelengths along the axes x, y, and z. The spatial distribution of the $\mathbf{E}_1$ and $\mathbf{H}_1$ fields is illustrated in Figs. 2-3*b* and *c*, respectively. It is seen that if the sample is placed along the x axis it will be at a maximum of $\mathbf{H}_1$ and a minimum of $\mathbf{E}_1$. The TE_{011} cylindrical cavity illustrated in Fig. 2-4*a* may also be employed. As seen in Figs. 2-4*b* and *c*, this cavity also satisfies the conditions of ESR if the sample is placed along the axis of the cylinder.*

The degree to which a cavity is able to amplify the intensity of the microwave field is described by a factor of merit called Q; Q is defined as

$$Q = \frac{2\pi\ (\text{maximum microwave energy stored in the cavity})}{(\text{energy lost per cycle})}. \qquad (2\text{-}2)$$

An alternative definition is

$$Q = \frac{\nu_r}{\Delta\nu}, \qquad (2\text{-}3)$$

* The discussion of cavities in this chapter must necessarily be limited. Reference 1, Chapter 8, contains an excellent discussion of cavities and their properties.

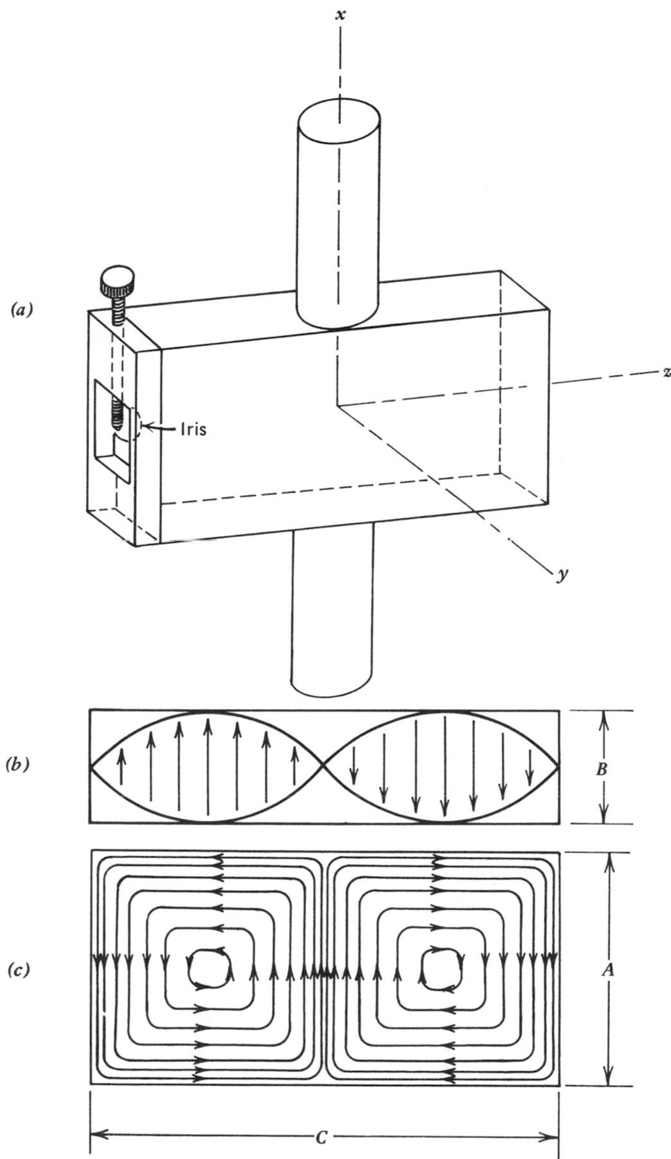

Fig. 2-3 A rectangular parallelepiped TE_{102} microwave cavity. (*a*) Cylindrical extensions ("stacks") above and below the cavity prevent excessive leakage of microwave radiation out of the cavity and act as positioning guides for the sample. The microwave energy is coupled into the cavity through the iris hole at the left. This coupling may be varied by means of the iris screw. (*b*) The electric field contours in the *yz* plane. One half-wavelength in the *z* direction corresponds to the shortest distance between points of equal field intensity but of opposite phase. (*c*) Magnetic field contours in the *xz* plane. *A* is approximately one half-wavelength and *C* is exactly two half-wavelengths. The *B* dimension is not critical but should be less than one half-wavelength.

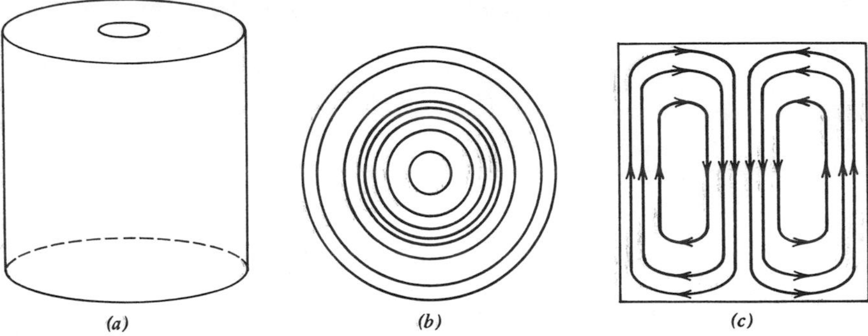

Fig. 2-4 Cylindrical cavity operating in the TE_{011} mode. (*a*) Cavity; the height and diameter of the cylinder govern the resonant frequency. (*b*) Electric field contours on a cylindrical cross section. (*c*) Magnetic field contours along a vertical cross section containing the axis of the cylinder.

where ν_r is the resonant frequency of the cavity and $\Delta\nu$ is the frequency difference between the points at which the microwave power in the cavity has dropped to one-half its maximum value at ν_r (Eq. 2-3 is generally used in measurements of Q); Q's of the order of 5000 to 10,000 are typical for rectangular cavities at X band, whereas Q's as high as 20,000 are obtained with cylindrical cavities. It is important to note that the intensity of microwaves at the sample is proportional to $P_0 Q$, where P_0 is the microwave power incident on the cavity. Factors that affect the Q of a cavity are discussed in Section 2.9.

The functioning of a high Q cavity is dependent on its construction, and experimenters are cautioned to avoid disassemblying a cavity unless they have the proper tools and training to reassemble it. Good cavities cost as much as $2000!

Since the Q of the cavity is a maximum when the microwave frequency is ν_r, it is important that the klystron output be accurately fixed at that frequency. This is accomplished by means of an automatic frequency control which locks the frequency of the klystron output to the resonant frequency of the cavity. This is one reason why ESR spectra are run at fixed frequency and variable magnetic field and not vice versa.

Microwave energy is coupled into and out of the cavity by means of a small hole called an *iris*. A brass-tipped Teflon screw in front of the iris permits the coupling to be varied to achieve an optimal impedance match of the cavity to the waveguide. In some spectrometers additional matching is provided by a small adjustable metallic probe, called a *slide-screw tuner*, inserted in the waveguide.

The cavities illustrated in Figs. 2-3 and 2-4 are both reflection cavities. Reflection cavities are used instead of transmission cavities because of their superior ability to discriminate against klystron noise. They do, however, require some means of coupling microwave energy into and out of the cavity. This is accomplished by the microwave bridge, which routes the klystron output to the cavity and routes the reflected power from the cavity to the detector. In most modern spectrometers this function is performed by a *circulator*, a nonreciprocal device similar to the isolator. Some older spectrometers use a hybrid T. The circulator is preferred because some signal is lost in the hybrid T, and the circulator also facilitates the design of microwave bridges that can operate with high attenuation of klystron power.

2.3.3 The Modulation and Detection Systems

Until recently most ESR spectrometers employed a small silicon crystal diode as a detector; newer models, however, are utilizing a semiconductor device called a "back diode."* Both types of detector act as a microwave rectifier by converting the microwaves into direct current. As the magnetic field approaches a resonant value, the sample will begin to absorb energy from the microwave field. This will cause a slight decrease in the cavity Q (see Eq. 2-2), hence a decrease in the reflected microwaves. Thus a resonant absorption will appear as a change in the detector current.

The straight dc detection of this change in current is accompanied by considerable noise. If, however, the signal information can be made to appear at only one frequency, all other frequencies can be filtered out, thus bringing about a considerable improvement in the signal-to-noise ratio. This trick is accomplished by a technique known as *phase sensitive detection*. To achieve this in ESR detection two Helmhotz coils driven by an oscillator are placed, one on each side of the cavity, so that a small-amplitude ac magnetic field at a frequency ν_m is superimposed on the dc field. When the sample is at or near resonance, a component of the detected signal will be modulated at the frequency ν_m. This signal is amplified in a narrow-band amplifier, the output of which serves as one input into the phase sensitive detector; the other input is a portion of the signal driving the modulation coils. The filtered output of the phase-sensitive detector is proportional both to the amplitude and phase difference of the two input signals.

The output of the phase-sensitive detector is rectified and sent to a chart recorder or the oscilloscope for display or to a computer input. If the amplitude of the field modulation is kept small compared with the linewidth of the ESR signal, the displayed signal will closely approximate the *first*

* The experimenter should be aware that both types of detector can vary considerably in noise characteristics from one component to another. Several detectors should be tried and selected for low noise.

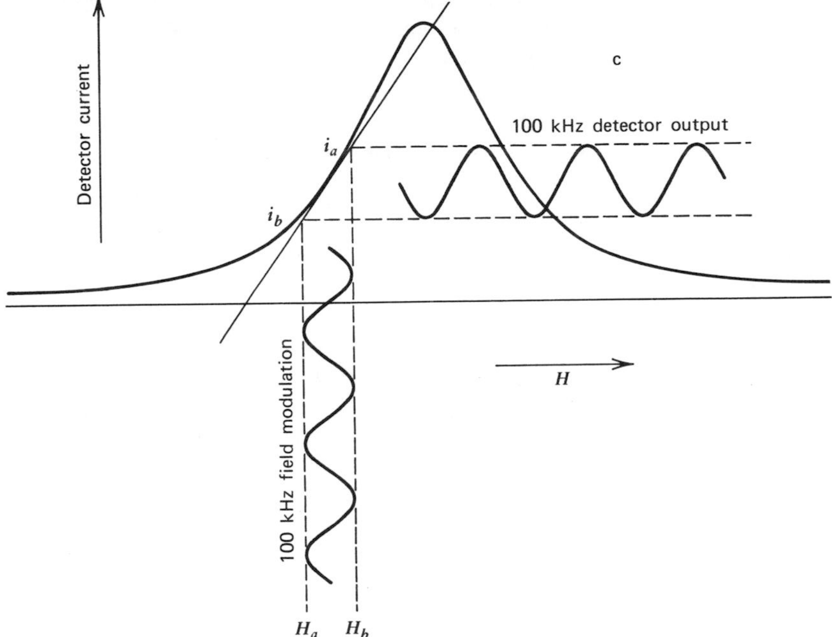

Fig. 2-5 Effect of small-amplitude 100 kHz field modulation on the detector output current. The static magnetic field is modulated between the limits H_a and H_b. The corresponding crystal current varies between the limits i_a and i_b.

derivative of the absorption signal* (see Figs. 2-6*b* and 2-7*b*). The reason for this is seen in Fig. 2-5. As the field varies between H_a and H_b, the detector current varies between i_a and i_b. If the excursion is small, $(i_a - i_b)$ will be proportional to the slope of the absorption curve.

The high noise rejection of the phase-sensitive detector arises from the fact that the noise "bandwidth" is reduced to a few hertz about the modulation frequency [the bandwidth is determined by the filter time constant used in the spectrometer output (see Section 2.11)].

Some spectrometers are equipped to display the *second derivative* of the absorption (Figs. 2-6*c* and 2-7*c*). This is accomplished either by detecting at $2\nu_m$ while modulating at ν_m or by using two modulation frequencies and two phase detectors; the output of one phase detector is then used as the input to the second.

* Although, strictly speaking, a first-derivative curve should have its first deflection in a positive direction, it is an accepted convention in ESR spectroscopy to present spectra with either a positive or a negative initial deflection. This convention is not carried over to absorption presentations that are always given as positive deflections.

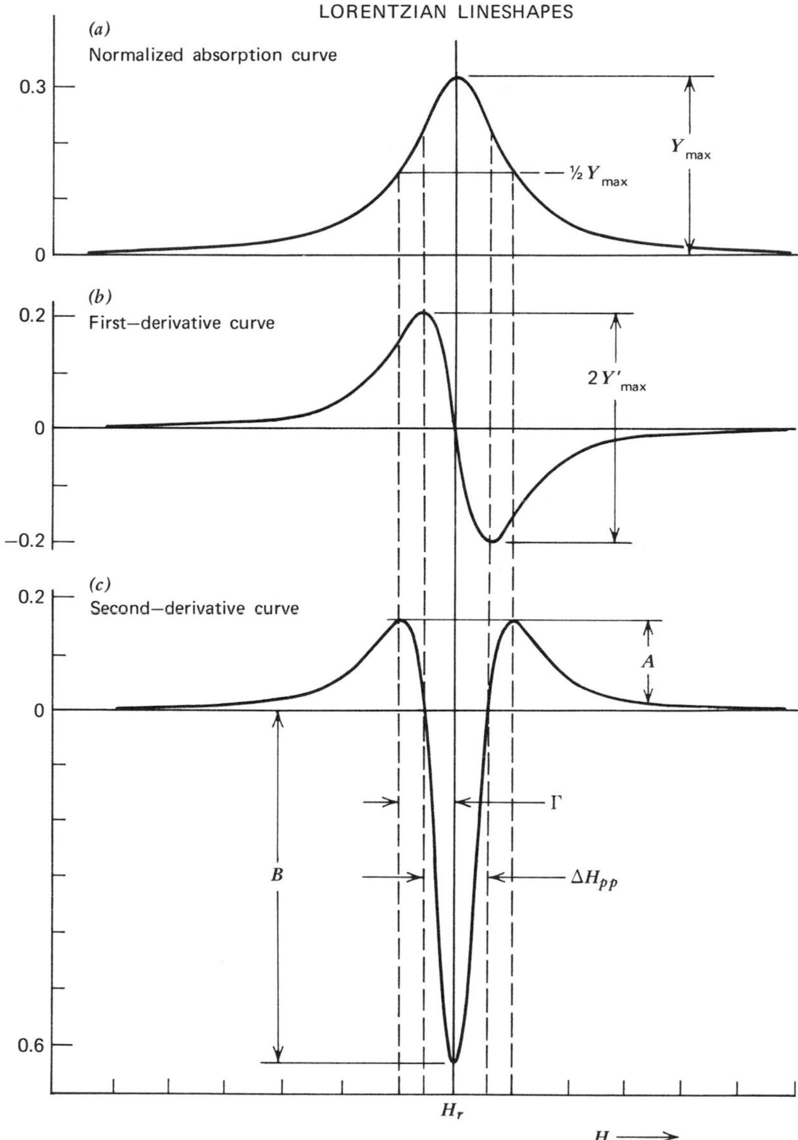

Fig. 2-6 Lorentzian lineshapes. (*a*) Absorption spectrum. (*b*) First-derivative spectrum. (*c*) Second-derivative spectrum. For an explanation of the symbols see Table 2-1.

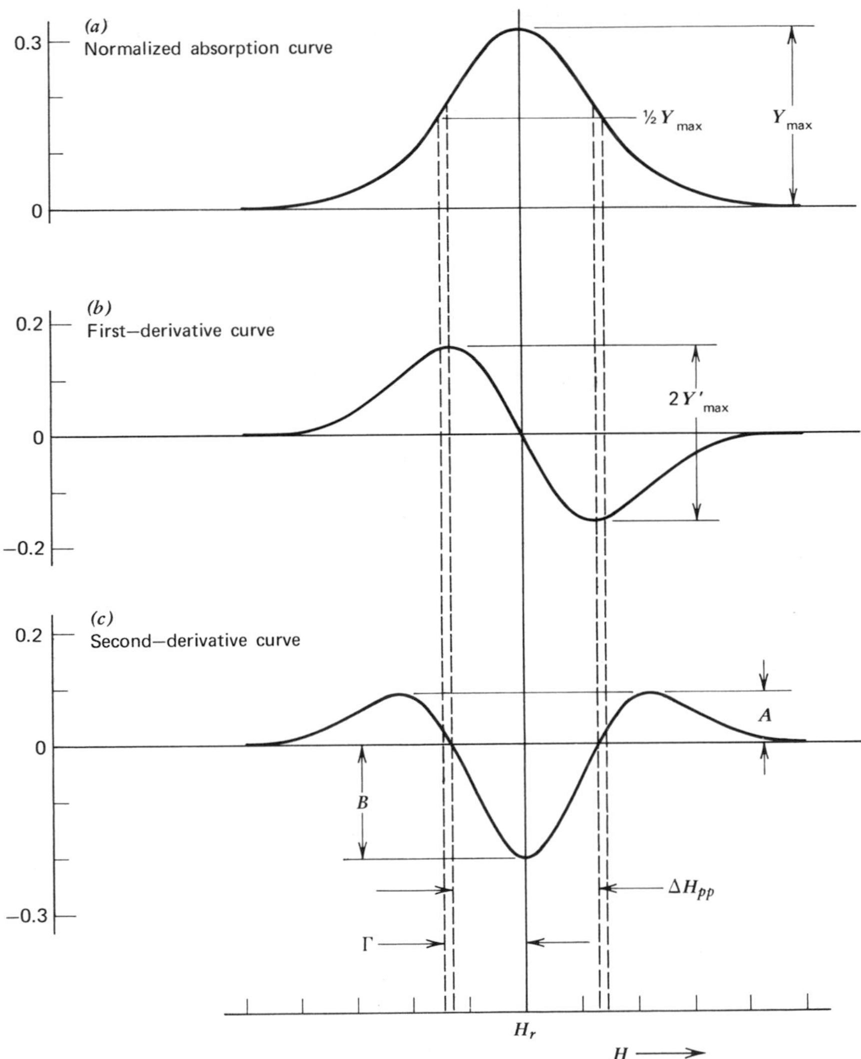

Fig. 2-7 Gaussian lineshapes. (*a*) Absorption spectrum. (*b*) First-derivative spectrum. (*c*) Second-derivative spectrum. For an explanation of the symbols see Table 2-1.

Although the phase-sensitive detector brings about a significant improvement in the signal-to-noise ratio, some noise still comes through from several sources. The crystal detector itself produces a noise that is approximately inversely proportional to v_m; also at low frequencies vibration can contribute noise. Thus the use of high modulation frequencies tends to minimize these noise sources; 100 kHz is a popular modulation frequency. This subject is treated in more detail in Section 2.6.

2.3.4 The Magnet System

The static magnetic field at the sample must be homogeneous and steady. Variations in the field (both in space and time) at the sample should be less than 10 mG for high resolution work. Variations as high as 100 mG, however, are generally acceptable for biological materials because of the inherently broad lines.

Stability of the field is achieved by a highly regulated power supply. Most systems now use a magnetic field-sensing device such as a Hall-effect crystal to stabilize the field. The voltage output of a Hall crystal is a linear function of the magnetic field and is used in a feedback to stabilize the field and allow for linear field sweeps.

The size of the magnet is a major economic factor in the choice of a spectrometer. Homogeneity is no longer a significant factor because modern shimming techniques provide adequate homogeneity for a magnet even as small as one with 4-in. diameter pole faces. The disadvantage of a small magnet is that the air gap employed must also be so small that only the cavity will fit between the pole faces. This limits the amount of apparatus that can be mounted around the cavity and prevents the utilization of dual cavities (see Section 2.15). Also the maximum field attainable may not be sufficient for signals with very low g factors. A larger magnet will certainly be required if operation at higher microwave frequencies is contemplated. Nevertheless, for many applications in biology the economic "desk-top" model ESR spectrometer with a 4-in. magnet has found wide acceptance and has obviously proved satisfactory for many investigations.

2.4 LINESHAPES AND LINEWIDTHS

Theoretically, ESR lines should be infinitely narrow; experimentally, they are broadened by various mechanisms, both intrinsic (determined by sample properties and the physics of the resonance experiment) and extrinsic (dependent on spectrometer operating conditions), as cited in Section 1.3. Lineshapes of ESR signals of biological materials are often asymmetric because of the "solid-state" or "powder spectrum" nature of the spectra.

When symmetrical lineshapes are obtained, however, they can usually be characterized by two main types: the lorentzian line or the gaussian line. Lineshapes were discussed in terms of line-broadening mechanisms in Section 1.3, but for the present purposes it suffices to recall that the lorentzian lineshape is often found for free radicals of low molecular weight in solution. A lorentzian lineshape usually implies that all radicals are resonating at the same field (homogeneous broadening). The gaussian lineshape is more common in biological systems. This shape may result from a system in which each paramagnetic entity resonates at a slightly different magnetic field, most commonly because the apparent line is really an envelope of unresolved hyperfine components of narrower intrinsic linewidths (see Section 1.3). Figures 2-6 and 2-7 illustrate these two lineshapes along with their first and second derivatives. It should be noted that the lorentzian line has a much longer tail than the gaussian line, and thus a longer segment must be considered for adequate quantification by integration (see Section 3.3.1). Table 2-1 contains the analytical forms of the two lines; definitions of the various quantities are given in Figs. 2-6 and 2-7.

2.5 SENSITIVITY

Since paramagnetic entities of biological interest usually occur in rather low concentrations, the sensitivity of an ESR spectrometer is of crucial concern. Sensitivity is usually expressed in terms of the minimum detectable number of paramagnetic centers N_{min}. For a signal-to-noise ratio of unity, N_{min} is given by*

$$N_{\text{min}} = \frac{3V_s k T_s \,\Delta H_{pp}}{2\pi Q_u \eta g^2 \beta^2 S(S+1) H_r} \left(\frac{3FkT_d b}{P_0}\right)^{1/2}, \tag{2-4}$$

where V_s = the sample volume,

k = Boltzmann's constant,

T_s = sample temperature,

ΔH_{pp} = peak-to-peak width of the first-derivative ESR signal,

F = a noise figure (>1) to take account of noise sources other than thermal detector noise (an ideal spectrometer would have $F = 1$),

T_d = detector temperature,

b = bandwidth (in sec^{-1}) of the entire detecting and amplifying system; b is usually determined by the time constant τ of the output filter; in this case $b = \tau^{-1}$,

* See Ref. 1, pp. 544 ff.

Q_u = effective unloaded Q factor of the cavity (see Section 2.9),

η = filling factor of the cavity; for a TE_{102} cavity $\eta \approx 2V_s/V_c$, where V_c is the cavity volume,

g = g factor of the signal,

S = spin quantum number for the paramagnetic center ($S = \frac{1}{2}$ for free radicals),

H_r = resonant magnetic field at the center of the signal,

P_0 = microwave power incident on the cavity.

Equation 2-4 applies only when microwave saturation (see Section 2.7) is negligible. All quantities are in cgs units.

We may obtain an estimate of N_{min} by inserting the following typical values of the quantities in Eq. 2-4:

$$
\begin{aligned}
V_s &= 0.1 \text{ cm}^3, & \eta &= 0.02, \\
T_s &= T_d = 300 \text{ K}, & g &= 2.00, \\
\Delta H_{pp} &= 1 \text{ G}, & S &= \tfrac{1}{2}, \\
F &= 50, & H_r &= 3400 \text{ G}, \\
b &= 1 \text{ sec}^{-1}, & P_0 &= 10 \text{ mW}. \\
Q_u &= 5000, & &
\end{aligned}
$$

With these values we obtain $N_{\text{min}} \approx 2 \times 10^{11}$ spins or the minimum detectable concentration is $\sim 3 \times 10^{-9} M$. Manufacturers of ESR spectrometers like to quote values of N_{min} for their instruments. Obviously these numbers are meaningless unless accompanied by a description of the conditions under which N_{min} was determined. It would be preferable if manufacturers would adopt a sensitivity standard (as in NMR); the sensitivity of an instrument would then be given as a signal-to-noise ratio under standard conditions of measurement. (When evaluating manufacturers' claims for sensitivities, it should be kept in mind that the type of sample, the type of cavity, and the sample holder are critical parameters.)

If the ESR spectrum contains many lines, as in the presence of hyperfine splitting, then N_{min} must be multiplied by the factor

$$R = \frac{\sum_j D_j}{D_k}, \tag{2-5}$$

where D_k is the relative intensity of the central line and $\sum_j D_j$ is the sum of the relative intensities of all the lines in the spectrum; for example, the di-*t*-butyl nitroxide radical (Fig. 1-10*a*) has $R = 3$, whereas the naphthalene anion (Fig. 1-17) has $R = 7.11$.

Table 2-1 Properties of Lorentzian and Gaussian Lines

	Lorentzian	Gaussian
Equation for normalized absorption line	$Y = Y_{\max} \frac{\Delta H_{pp}^2}{\Delta H_{pp}^2 + \frac{4}{3}(H - H_r)^2}$	$Y = Y_{\max} \exp\left[\frac{-2(H - H_r)^2}{\Delta H_{pp}^2}\right]$
Peak amplitude	$Y_{\max} = \frac{2}{\pi\sqrt{3}\, \Delta H_{pp}}$	$Y_{\max} = \left(\frac{2}{\pi}\right)^{1/2} \frac{1}{\Delta H_{pp}}$
Half-width at half-height	$\Gamma = \frac{\sqrt{3}}{2} \Delta H_{pp}$	$\Gamma = \left(\frac{ln2}{2}\right)^{1/2} \Delta H_{pp}$
Equation for the first-derivative line	$Y' = -Y_{\max} \frac{8\Delta H_{pp}^2 (H - H_r)}{3[\Delta H_{pp}^2 + \frac{4}{3}(H - H_r)^2]^2}$	$Y' = -Y_{\max} \frac{4(H - H_r)}{\Delta H_{pp}} \exp\left[\frac{-2(H - H_r)^2}{\Delta H_{pp}^2}\right]$
Peak-to-peak amplitude	$2Y'_{\max} = \frac{\sqrt{3}}{\pi} \frac{1}{\Delta H_{pp}^2}$	$2Y'_{\max} = 4\left(\frac{2}{\pi e}\right)^{1/2} \frac{1}{\Delta H_{pp}^2}$
Peak-to-peak width	ΔH_{pp}	ΔH_{pp}

Since the optimization of sensitivity is probably of most importance in biological ESR measurements, much of the rest of this chapter is devoted to a discussion of the various factors that affect sensitivity. Some are covered in more detail in Chapter 3 in connection with quantitative measurements.

2.6 EFFECTS OF THE MODULATION AMPLITUDE AND MODULATION FREQUENCY

Under the usual conditions of an ESR experiment, the magnetic field at the sample H is given by

$$H = H_0 + H_m \sin 2\pi \nu_m t, \tag{2-6}$$

where H_0 is the value of the dc magnetic field, H_m is the modulation amplitude, and ν_m is the modulation frequency. As noted earlier, H_m must be kept small compared with the linewidth ΔH_{pp} to avoid distortion of the derivative lineshape (see Fig. 3-3 for examples of this distortion). On the other hand, the derivative amplitude is a maximum when $H_m \approx 2\Delta H_{pp}$ for lorentzian lines and $H_m \approx \Delta H_{pp}$ for gaussian lines. At these settings the lines are considerably broadened and distorted (the linewidth is increased by a factor of $\sim$ 3 for lorentzian lines and $\sim$ 1.6 for gaussian lines).

If sensitivity is of prime concern, then H_m should be adjusted for maximum derivative amplitude; if, however, resolution is also important, some sensitivity will have to be sacrificed to achieve the desired resolution of line components. The optimum setting of H_m can be achieved only by a trial-and-error process.

The modulation frequency ν_m normally has no effect on the lineshape except when very narrow lines are encountered or modulation frequencies in excess of 1 MHz are used. Since these conditions are not normal to biological systems, we shall not pursue the effect on lineshape here.*

Since, in general, F in Eq. 2-4 increases as ν_m decreases, the value of ν_m has an effect on sensitivity. This is due to the noise characteristics of the detector and is the reason that most ESR spectrometers operate at a modulation frequency of 100 kHz. For higher values of ν_m it is difficult to get the modulation field into the cavity. Back-diode detectors do allow operation at ν_m as low as 1 kHz with little loss in sensitivity; however, there appears to be little reason for using lower modulation frequencies in most biological applications. One exception is when operation at 4 K or lower is necessary. Since the cavity is usually immersed in liquid helium, the modulation

* See Chapter 1, Ref. 1, Appendix D, for a discussion of this effect.

coils must be external to the dewars. The modulation field will then be highly attenuated if a frequency much higher than ~ 1 kHz is used.

2.7 MICROWAVE POWER AND SATURATION

For most detectors used in ESR the signal amplitude is proportional to $P_0^{1/2}$ below saturation. As saturation sets in, the population difference n decreases (Eq. 1–26) and eventually the signal amplitude will decrease with increasing power. This is illustrated in Fig. 2-8. Saturation has another effect which is related to the Heisenberg uncertainty principle. The increased microwave power results in an increased rate of transitions between the two energy levels—the spin lifetime is reduced, thus leading to line broadening through

$$\Delta H \sim \frac{1}{\gamma_e \tau}, \tag{2-7}$$

where ΔH is the linewidth, τ is the spin lifetime, and γ_e is the electron magnetogyric ratio.

Up to this point our discussion of saturation phenomena applies only to systems in which all the paramagnetic centers are identical; i.e., all centers resonate at the same magnetic field. As indicated before, such a line is said to be *homogeneously broadened.* This is usually the case for free

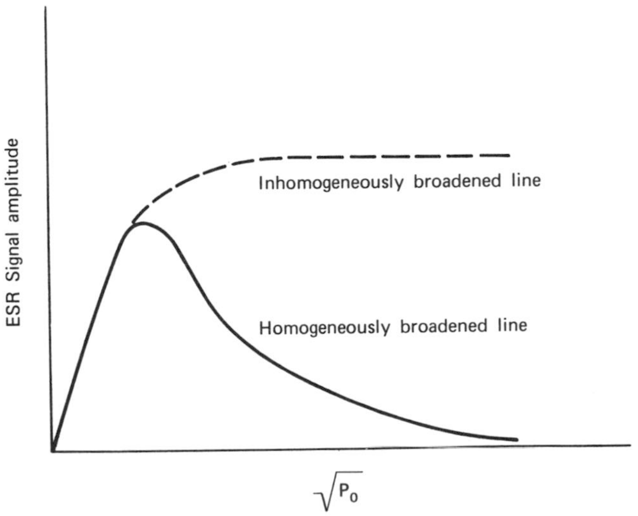

Fig. 2-8 Variation of ESR signal amplitude with microwave power (P_0) for a homogeneously broadened line (solid curve) and an inhomogeneously broadened line (dotted curve).

radicals in solutions of low viscosity. Most ESR signals of biological interest, however, are *inhomogeneously broadened*. Such a lineshape is an envelope of individual line components. Saturation phenomena for inhomogeneously broadened lines can be quite complex; nevertheless in most cases the derivative amplitude increases with increasing microwave power and then levels off when the saturation region is reached. This is illustrated as the dotted line in Fig. 2-8. Usually saturation has little effect on the linewidth of an inhomogeneously broadened line.

The two curves in Fig. 2-8 represent limits of the amplitude behavior. Real systems can exhibit saturation curves which lie anywhere between the two limits; for example, Castner (6) has shown that even if the linewidth of the individual components is only 1/100 as wide as the envelope of these components the saturation behavior is still close to that of a homogeneously broadened line.

It is often useful to compare the saturation behavior of two or more signals. This is best done by using a standard that does not saturate. Singer et al. (7) have described a method based on a ruby standard (Cr^{3+} in alumina). One may either tape the ruby crystal to the outside of the sample tube or use a dual cavity.

From a practical viewpoint microwave power saturation is extremely important. If the possibility of saturation is not considered, large errors in quantitation may result. Qualitative errors due to line broadening and/or suppression of a readily power-saturable signal by a minor nonsaturating component may also occur. When there is no saturation, the observed intensity (I) of a species varies with power as

$$I \propto P_0^{1/2}. \tag{2-8}$$

Obviously, then, we should like to operate at a power level as high as possible to get maximum intensity, but many of the ESR species of biological interest start to power saturate at power levels of less than 100 μW. If we consider operations at the upper power ranges of most commercial instruments (approximately 200 mW), the potential for error becomes apparent. (These aspects are discussed in more detail in Chapter 4.) The most practical solution is always to study a sample at different power levels to determine its particular power saturation properties and then select the best operational power level for that sample. If another paramagnetic species does not interfere and only qualitative spectra are desired, operation in a region of partial power saturation will give maximum sensitivity (homogeneous broadening in this situation will be less than 20 percent).

Saturation is a valuable technique when two signals overlap. If one signal saturates readily and the other does not, the use of high microwave powers will favor the signal that does not saturate. This technique is illustrated in Fig. 2-9.

It is important to note that the usual convention is to measure microwave power *incident* on the cavity (P_0) and not the energy density *in* the cavity (i.e., $H_1{}^2$, which is proportional to P_0Q). Thus the intensity of the microwave field that the sample encounters depends on the cavity Q, and that, in turn, will be affected by the sample and sample holder. For many samples of biological interest with high water contents the effect on Q is considerable and there is no simple way of calculating actual power. A good

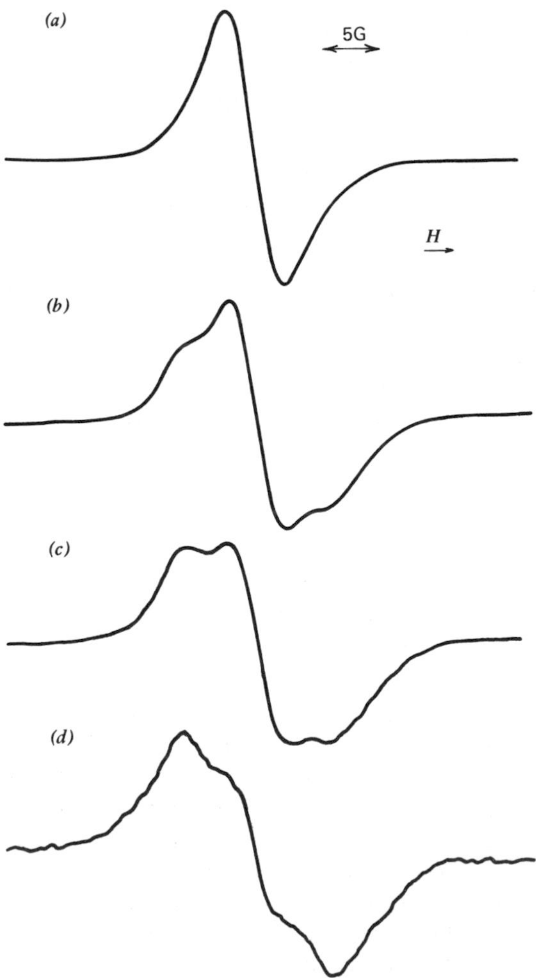

Fig. 2-9 ESR spectrum of two radicals at different microwave powers. Power increases from (*a*) to (*d*). The broad underlying spectrum appears only at higher power levels where the narrow signal is highly saturated.

alternative is to use a dual cavity with a standard sample that does not readily power saturate. "Effective" microwave power can then be determined by measuring the intensity of the spectrum of the standard. In this way accurate power saturation curves can be obtained on virtually all samples, as is developed in greater detail in Chapter 3.

Any ESR absorption line is accompanied by a shift of the cavity resonance frequency. This phenomenon is called *dispersion*. The dispersion signal can be detected by proper phasing of the microwave bridge. These signals can be advantageous when dealing with easily saturable ESR signals, since the dispersion signal does not saturate so readily as the absorption signal.

2.8 CONCENTRATION EFFECTS AND THE EFFECTS OF OTHER PARAMAGNETIC SPECIES

In some situations (at moderate concentrations) it is observed that ESR linewidths increase as the concentration of paramagnetic species increases.* There are two reasons for this. First, the proximity of another paramagnetic species creates a dipole local magnetic field which adds to the external field in a random fashion. Second, if the second paramagnetic species has a short value of T_1 it can cause a fluctuating local field at the first paramagnetic species and thus lead to line broadening and a resistance to saturation.

In biological systems we rarely have to worry about self-broadening due to concentrations of paramagnetic entities that are too high; however, we sometimes have a situation in which a free radical lies close to a transition metal ion in a protein. If the ESR spectrum of the free radical is seen at all, it will be broadened and will not readily saturate. This phenomenon has been observed in metal containing flavoproteins (see Chapter 8).

2.9 FACTORS AFFECTING THE Q OF THE CAVITY: THE PROBLEM OF AQUEOUS SOLUTIONS

It is clear from Eq. 2-4 that any factor that changes the Q of the cavity will affect sensitivity. It is thus important to understand how the Q factor can be adversely affected.

From Eq. 2-4 we see that any characteristic of the materials in the cavity that causes a dissipation of the microwave energy in the cavity will decrease Q. Given that the cavity has originally been designed and constructed for a high Q, the only variable factors are the sample and the sample holder. The major effect of the sample on the Q is the extent to

* At extremely high concentrations there may be line narrowing due to exchange effects (see Section 1.7).

which the sample interacts with the electric component of the microwave field. (It is precisely this interaction that cooks a roast in a microwave oven!) The interaction of the sample with the electric component of the microwaves increases with the dielectric constant of the sample and geometrically to the extent that the sample extends into the region of nonzero electric field (see the electric-field contours in Figs. 2-3 and 2-4). Since most samples of biological interest are in aqueous solution or suspension and since water has a high dielectric constant, this presents serious problems.

Several methods can be employed to minimize the reduction of the Q factor by aqueous samples.* Early workers used capillary tubes; this, however, has the disadvantage of small sample size and poor sample configuration if light irradiation is to be used or if solid tissues are to be studied. Other workers have used a long cavity (e.g., $TE_{1,0,10}$) in which the aqueous sample is placed at an electric field node at one end. This does allow larger samples but has the disadvantage of a small filling factor η. The technique most commonly used now places the aqueous solution in a sample cell consisting of two quartz plates separated by ~ 0.2 mm. This "aqueous solution sample cell" is then aligned by means of adjustment screws so that the aqueous sample lies along the nodal plane of the electric field of the microwaves in a TE_{102} or TE_{104} cavity. Optimum sensitivity is achieved when the volume of the aqueous sample is such that the Q factor is reduced to about one-half its value when no sample is in the cavity. It is difficult to calculate what this volume will be for any given sample and therefore it is advantageous to have a set of sample cells with thicknesses varying from 0.2 to 0.4 mm every 0.05 mm.† The sample tube exhibiting the best sensitivity (all other factors being equal) can then be selected.

A good solution to the water problem is to freeze the sample. This drastically reduces the dielectric constant; however, if the sample is sensitive to freezing damage, this method should not be used. One should be aware that freezing some samples can produce ESR signals.

The sample holder can also affect sensitivity, principally by distorting the distribution of the magnetic field of the microwaves. In general, the effect of quartz (the usual sample-holder material) is to concentrate the magnetic field so that the result is an increase in effective microwave power at the sample (see Fig. 3-8). If it is a nonsaturating sample, it can result in an appreciable increase in signal magnitude. It is therefore important that we compare samples in the same or equivalent sample holders (unscrupulous salesmen may attempt to show increased sensitivity by putting standard samples in large quartz containers).

* See Ref. 2, p. 504 ff, and Chapter 4 of this book for further discussions of the water problem.
† Thermal American Fused Quartz Co., Route 202 and Change Bridge Road, Montville, N.J., or James F. Scanlon Co., 11701 E. Washington Boulevard, Whittier, California 90606, will fabricate such cells from high-purity quartz such as "Spectrosil."

2.10 MICROWAVE FREQUENCY

Most commercial ESR spectrometers operate in the X band with the microwave frequency in the ~ 8.8 to 9.6 GHz range. A major change in the microwave frequency is not often contemplated, mainly because of the expense of a second microwave system that would be required. There are situations, however, in which a change in the microwave frequency ν_0 can be valuable.

When each component arises from a separate paramagnetic entity and two or more signals overlap, an increase in ν_0 can bring about a better resolution of these signals. This can be seen from the following relation

$$\Delta H = \frac{-\Delta g}{g_{av}} H_{av}. \tag{2-9}$$

Here ΔH is the field difference between two ESR signals, Δg is the difference in g factors, g_{av} is the average g factor, and H_{av} is the average resonant magnetic field. Since H_{av} increases in direct proportion to ν_0, resolution will improve at higher frequencies. It should be noted that if the field difference between two lines develops from hyperfine splitting *no change* will be observed on increasing ν_0. This is one way of distinguishing between a hyperfine splitting and a difference in g factors.

Generally sensitivity will increase with increasing ν_0; the exact dependence, however, is a strong function of the sample characteristics.* If the sample is of fixed size (as with a single crystal), higher frequencies are a decided advantage; for constant microwave power the sensitivity increases as $\nu_0^{4.5}$. If we have unlimited amounts of sample material, the improvement in sensitivity is only proportional to $\nu_0^{1.5}$. Also at the higher frequencies sample and sample-tube dimensions must be smaller, since the cavity dimensions are inversely proportional to ν_0. This can be a decided advantage when the amount of sample available is limited, as in enzyme kinetic studies (8).

For aqueous samples the advantages of a higher frequency are not great. In fact, if the signal saturates readily, there can actually be a decrease in sensitivity with increasing ν_0.†

In some applications it is important to have a direct measurement of ν_0. This can be accomplished most easily by means of a wavemeter (see Fig. 2-2). This is simply a cylindrical cavity with an adjustable end piece. The resonant frequency is directly proportional to the length of the cavity. Micrometer adjustment allows the measurement of ν_0 to a precision of ~ ±1 MHz with an accuracy of ~ ±3 MHz. Greater accuracy requires the use of frequency counters.

* See p. 551, Ref. 1.
† See Ref. 2, Table 3-7, p. 98.

2.11 FILTERING, SIGNAL AVERAGING, AND COMPUTERS

2.11.1 Filtering

Of all the factors in Eq. 2-4 we have direct control over only a few; the bandwidth b is one of these factors. All commercial spectrometers have a knob usually labeled "time constant." It is most often a simple RC filter which filters out high-frequency noise. The frequency at which the noise voltage is reduced by a factor of 2 by this filter is $(RC)^{-1}$; $\tau = RC$ (where R is in megohms and C in microfarads) is the filter time constant. In most situations the bandwidth b is determined by this filter, that is, $b = \tau^{-1}$.

The advantage of filtering the output signal is that the sensitivity, or, more commonly, "signal-to-noise" ratio, is increased by the factor $\tau^{1/2}$. This increased sensitivity is gained at the expense of the need for a slower scan rate. A good working rule is to adjust the scan rate so that the time required to go from peak to peak on a derivative is $\sim 10\,\tau$; otherwise the lines will be distorted (See Fig. 3-2 for an example of this distortion and Section 3.3.2 for further discussion.)

As long as the ESR signal and the spectrometer are stable, long time constants and scan times can certainly be used to improve sensitivity. In many situations, however, this is neither practical nor even possible. Over periods of very long scans (hours or overnight) the stability of most ESR spectrometers is not good enough to permit the recording of spectra without significant distortion caused by baseline drift and other slowly varying aspects of spectrometer performance.

Although it is true that some new spectrometers with solid-state electronics are remarkably stable and can produce accurate spectra with τ as long as 100 sec (authors' experience), most older machines manifest disturbing drift with τ greater than about 3 sec, when operated with weak signals at high gains. Furthermore, long scans are susceptible to adventitious disturbances, such as power shutdowns or operation in the laboratory of other apparatus that broadcasts noise; they also imply enough prior knowledge of the spectrum to be recorded so that the modulation amplitude, amplifier gain, scan range, scan time, and filter-time constant can be sufficiently optimized before the scan is begun. This is an important experimental consideration, for once a sizable fraction of a very slow scan with a long τ has been recorded we are usually committed to completing the scan without further changes in the operating conditions.

This limitation of preselecting spectrometer operating conditions may be partially relieved and the problem of slow background drift (effectively a very low frequency noise in the system) largely canceled out by routing the ESR signal output directly into a computer operated in the signal-averaging

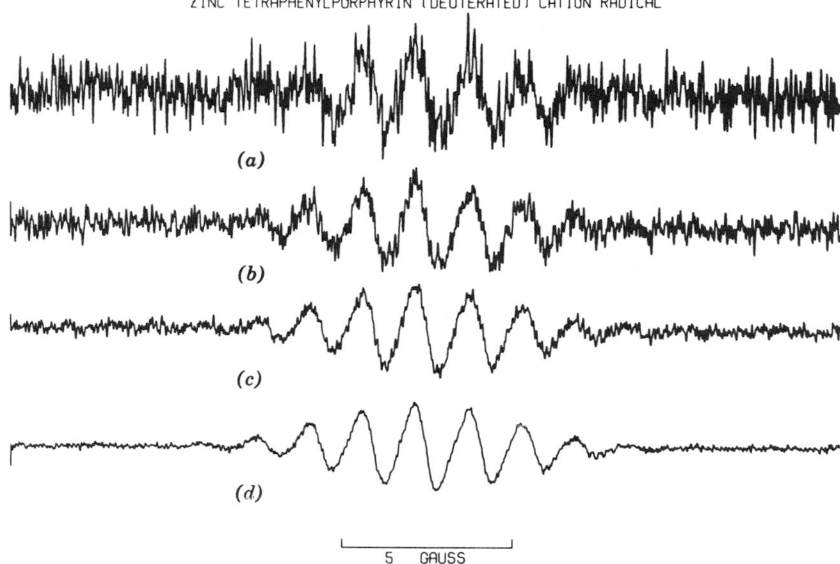

Fig. 2-10 Effect of a time averaging computer on the signal-to-noise ratio: (*a*) 1 scan, (*b*) 4 scans, (*c*) 16 scans, (*d*) 64 scans.

mode (see below) and recording spectra from the computer. In addition, in a number of instances weak ESR signals are obtainable from transient processes that are repeatable or may be recycled. Clearly long scan times and filter constants cannot be used to improve sensitivity in these cases, but signal averaging *is* applicable as a means of improving the signal-to-noise ratios (Fig. 2-10).

2.11.2 Signal Averaging

In recent years it has become increasingly common for ESR spectroscopists to employ small, special-purpose ("hard-wired") computers designed especially for signal averaging and/or pulse-height analysis. Computers of this kind with 256 to 4096 channels of memory, built-in analog-to-digital converters (ADC), monitoring oscilloscopes, chart-driving and digital outputs, and some limited capacity for data processing* are currently available for

* Usually segregation of the memory into two or more parts with data transfer, display comparison, and addition/subtraction between parts and sometimes extending to arithmetic scaling of spectra with addition/subtraction of constants, integration, differentiation, and some simple digital filtering.

about \$5000 to \$16,000. In a few laboratories somewhat larger and more flexible general-purpose computers are used for ESR applications, as noted below, and with these systems signal averaging is usually treated as a programmatic ("software") option.

As implied from the preceding paragraphs, the concept of signal averaging (also known as "time averaging") is applicable to phenomena that can be repeated over and over, either because they are intrinsically short-lived or because they can be optionally scheduled as the sums of multiple short runs rather than a single long one, such as the replacement of a long scan of an ESR spectrum by the repetition of a number of shorter ones. This is usually accomplished, in the ESR case, by converting the output signal from the spectrometer into digital form with an analog-to-digital converter (ADC) and storing the digital values sequentially in separate channels of computer memory as the spectrum is scanned. The process is then repeated, with the scan of computer memory channels synchronized with the scan of the ESR spectrum either by having the computer's scanning ramp amplified to drive the spectrometer's magnetic-field scan (or vice versa) or by using a triggering signal of some kind to lock the computer's independent time base ("ramp") to the identical phase of the spectrometer's scan with each cycle. The digital outputs of successive scans are added, and in this way the computer memory sums the total scan information. With proper synchronization the true signal components of the separate runs will add coherently in the same memory channels with each scan; the random noise components will add incoherently. The coherent signal will thus grow directly with n, the number of scans, whereas the incoherent or noise signal will increase only as $n^{1/2}$. Thus the overall improvement in signal-to-noise ratio or sensitivity is $n^{1/2}$. Hence the terms "time averaging" or "signal averaging."

When the computer's time base is locked to the field scan of the ESR spectrometer in the manner just described, the computer will signal-average the ESR spectrum. If, however, the spectrometer dwells at a constant magnetic field and the computer is triggered at the same phase in the cycle of some recurrent experimental variable (such as a shutter or radiation or heat pulse), the computer will time-average the time sequence of the ESR signal amplitude at that field value. This can be invaluable in kinetic studies in which very fast reactions occur. As pointed out earlier, small values of τ must be used in these cases because the changes in signal amplitude will be rapid; nevertheless time averaging will "buy back" a sensitivity equivalent to that obtainable with long filter time constants (see below), even though they cannot be used in the actual experiments.

As noted above, the overall improvement in sensitivity with signal averaging is $n^{1/2}$. Since the effect of a filter's time constant τ on sensitivity varies with $\tau^{1/2}$, there is no *theoretical* advantage in obtaining spectra by the use of signal averaging in place of a single scan with the optimum

τ, provided that the cumulative time for recording a given spectral scan range is the same in both cases. Several *practical* advantages, some of which were alluded to earlier, however, are noted in Sections 2.11.3 and 2.11.4.

2.11.3 Filter and Gain Considerations when Using Computers

The optimum filter and spectrometer gain need *not* be accurately known or estimated ahead of time when signal averaging. Provided only that the bandwidth b of the output filter be broad enough to pass all spectral features of interest on each single pass, the exact setting of τ will not otherwise be critical. The signal-to-noise ratio will improve as $n^{1/2}$, and data collection can be stopped at will when the ratio becomes acceptable, as determined by inspection. Thus the "effective" filter bandwidth may be adjusted to the experimental situation with a minimum foreknowledge of the actual signal-to-noise ratio or of the narrowest spectral features that can be resolved usefully (i.e., of the broadest b that is feasible).

The range of accessible "effective" bandwidths is broadened beyond the limit $n^{1/2}$ imposed by time averaging alone when digital filtering routines are available with the computer system employed. These routines permit optimal filtering to be achieved for any given accumulation of experimental data by trial-and-error filtering/observation cycles carried out by data processing alone, without destruction of the raw data, and with a resultant minimum restraint on the preselection of τ or even of "effective" b (which varies as $n^{-1/2}\ \tau^{-1}$).

In addition, digital filters have another advantage over RC or other analog filters in that they are usually symmetrical. An analog filter applied to a scanned spectrum or other time-dependent input could be truly symmetrical only by "predicting" the future, i.e., by making certain assumptions about the curvature of that part of the data envelope not yet recorded. The achievement of a narrow b by employing a long, asymmetrical τ results in a serious constraint on the maximum scan speed that can be used without significant distortion of lineshapes (or decay curves), intensities, and positions, as illustrated in some detail in Section 3.2.2.

From these advantages already listed for time averaging (especially in conjunction with computer filtering) it might be supposed that τ could be made arbitrarily short, with all adjustments necessary to narrow b made later by control of n, by determining the duration of the experiment, and by selection of an appropriate digital filter following completion of "real-time" data processing. Similarly, virtually any spectrometer gain setting might appear acceptable when the signal output is fed directly into a time-averaging computer because the scale of the spectrum displayed by a recorder can be so easily varied over an extremely broad range when data are stored in a computer. In practice, however, there are real limits on τ and spectrometer gain imposed by the nature of digital data-handling systems.

With regard to the independent (or x-axis) variable, e.g., the magnetic field scan, the limit of resolution is determined by the number of channels. Usually 1024 (2^{10}) or 2048 (2^{11}) channels are provided by commercial time-averaging computers, although 4096-channel averagers, most commonly used for high-resolution NMR with its intrinsically narrow lines, are available also. In any case, no frequency component of curvature can be recorded that is greater than b_c, the effective bandwidth cutoff, where $b_c = \tau_c^{-1}$ and τ_c is the time required to scan two successive channels. Hence for any selected scan rate and number of channels (that will determine τ_c) there is nothing to be gained from setting τ less than τ_c. In fact, a bandwidth greater than b_c at the computer input can serve only to admit high-frequency noise components without any compensating improvement in resolution. Therefore, when ESR spectrometers' output time constants are not conveniently adjustable over a sufficiently wide range, ESR-computer systems often employ continuously variable electronic low-pass or band-pass prefilters to process output signals before they are admitted to the computers' ADC's.

In light of the preceding remarks about the power of digital filtering, the use of a prefilter might appear redundant. This is not so because the dependent (or y-axis) variable, the ESR signal, is digitized by the ADC and thus integerized to a finite resolution. Commonly 2^8-bit to 2^{12}-bit signal resolution is used by the ADC components of time-averaging computers; for example, a 2^{10}-bit ADC will provide a *maximum* signal resolution of about 0.1 percent *of full-scale* per scan. Although in the presence of some random noise the effect of summing multiple scans (i.e., time averaging) may allow an overall resolution somewhat more defined than the minimum "granularity" achieved by a single passage, it is obvious that spectral shape information will be lost to the computer if the spectrometer signal is so weak that it is integerized into only a few steps by the ADC. To preserve maximum y-axis resolution with digitized data it is therefore desirable to set the spectrometer gain so that the maximum excursions of the signal are nearly full scale.* On the other hand, if noise components superimposed on the signal then exceed full scale, they will be truncated asymmetrically, and the averaging out of these incompletely recorded noise features will distort the spectrum. Thus it becomes clear why admitting "excess noise" (at frequencies above b_c) to a digital data system may produce signal distortion at one extreme

* In practice we usually back off from full-scale amplification to allow for some baseline drift during long runs without having signal components that then move off scale.

of gain setting or loss of signal resolution at the other; hence the value of prefiltering the experimental signal even before a digital filter is employed.

In fact, to use the full range of an ADC effectively a prefilter should be set to a time constant longer than τ_c when the highest frequency components of interest are less than b_c—in other words, when the curvature to be resolved does not require the full channel resolution provided by the computer scan. In the limit of the theoretical optimum, then, the prefilter time constant should be set with as much foreknowledge of the linewidths to be resolved as is demanded by the optimum setting of τ for a single slow scan. In practice, however, the range of adjustment of effective b provided by the experimental determination of n, the number of scans to be signal-averaged, and by the use of digital filtering following data recording allows considerable latitude in the preselection of τ for the spectrometer and/or prefilter.

When signal-to-noise ratios permit, it is often convenient to set $\tau = \tau_c$, depending entirely on n and digital filtering to achieve proper sensitivity. Similarly, the useful dynamic range provided by most ADC's is so much greater than that of the usual analog recorders that the preselection of spectrometer gain settings for time averaging is seldom critical. However, for very weak and noisy ESR spectra requiring long signal averaging, such as those from many tissues, or with highly complex spectra, such as those from some biochemicals in solution, successful application of signal-averaging ESR spectroscopy may call on an appreciation of those limitations of digital data recording discussed here.

2.11.4 Resolution Enhancement and Other Data Processing with Computers

From the preceding section (2.11.3) it is clear that the use of signal averaging and digital data filtering can in many instances relax the requirement for preselection of the filter time constant and spectrometer amplifier gain. Furthermore, in Section 2.11.1 it was stated that the effects of slow background drift and other low-frequency noise components are largely canceled out during signal averaging. This is so because background level changes, long in comparison with single scan times, will be evenly distributed over many scans to alter the baseline level of the summed spectra without significant spectral distortion, whereas distortions caused by baseline shifts that occur during single scans tend to be averaged out in the same way as high-frequency noise components (see Section 2.11.2).

On the other hand, there may be background features *un*associated with drifts or other transient phenomena that can distort even signal-averaged spectra: for example, broad signals from paramagnetic metals in the sample or cavity walls or intrinsic waveguide-coupling effects on signal baseline levels sometimes seen with high gains and wide scans (referred to occasionally as "potato"). General-purpose computers, which can process digitized spectral data in a more flexible manner than "dedicated" signal averagers, often can compensate for intrinsic background features such as these. Thus background spectra may be read in from magnetic tape, disk file, or other bulk storage, shifted to register the proper channel locations, scaled appropriately, and then subtracted from experimental spectra. It is also a trivial matter, with such computers, to correct for many of the recording errors that could otherwise interfere seriously with the quantitative evaluation of ESR spectra. Chapter 3 discusses at length the problems and difficulties that these errors lead to.

The loss of spectral detail either by necessary overmodulation or by inherent broadening can be partially rectified by computer processing in which resolution of spectra is enhanced by increasing signal curvature in general or by programs that enhance the curvature corresponding to desired signal frequencies at the expense of other frequencies.

According to the dictates of information theory, however, the total information content of a set of data cannot be increased by any manipulation, and resolution enhancement can increase curvature (or shape) information only at the cost of intensity or (signal-to-noise) information. Since, as will be shown, resolution enhancement can be a powerful technique of great utility in ESR spectroscopy, ESR/computer systems may generate requirements for obtaining data with much greater sensitivity than that needed to obtain "clean-looking" spectra. Consequently such systems will place a high premium on spectrometers and magnets that are sufficiently stable to permit prolonged runs with extensive signal averaging.

In principle, enhanced curvature can be obtained in a number of ways, including experimental methods that do not require digital data processing; for example, recording ESR spectra in the second derivative presentation (see Figs. 2-6*c* and 2-7*c* and Fig. 2-12) will increase curvature at the expense of sensitivity. Spectrometer components have also been designed to convert the output signal to approximate the third derivative of the ESR absorption signal (9) or to represent the effect of subtracting third and fifth derivative components (with adjustable weighting), thus effectively narrowing recorded linewidths in a first derivative-type presentation (10). These procedures, however, require intense signals, and the same effective treatment of data can be achieved more easily (and as an option *not* requiring prior commitment) by computer processing of conventional first-derivative spectrometer outputs.

Furthermore all resolution enhancement methods are not equally effective. Since apparent line narrowing by sharpening curvature reduces sensitivity, it is important with all but the strongest signals to utilize a procedure that does not also enhance noise components of the spectrum excessively. In other words, the effective bandwidth of the "enhancement filter" should be narrow enough to include only the frequencies corresponding to the signal components of greatest interest. This subject has been reviewed extensively by Ernst (11), but it is pertinent to note that the use of higher derivative presentations (second or third) is broad-banded and thus inefficient in this regard. Subtracting higher order derivatives from a first-derivative output is better but still noisy in comparison with filter shape functions that can be adjusted flexibly and set to enhance selected linewidths (or their corresponding frequencies).

Different methods of specifying complex filter functions and processing data with them are discussed by Ernst (11). One successful approach involves computer conversion of spectra into the frequency domain by using Fourier transformations. The transformed ESR data are then treated with the selected filter function, back-transformed by Fourier methods, and displayed as resolution-enhanced spectra. Although this method has been applied in a spectacular way by Hedberg and Ehrenberg (12) and efficient fast Fourier transform packages are now available for small computers, it requires twice as many data locations in the computer memory as there are spectral channels. The executive program is also extensive. In any case, Hedberg and Ehrenberg (12) (using a large off-line computer) enhanced the resolution of a spectrum with very high signal-to-noise (from extensive signal averaging) so that hyperfine structure from gaussian lines previously inapparent to the eye could be readily visualized, the hyperfine splitting determined, and a successful analysis completed (Fig. 2-11).

In theory, however, a convolutional integral exists for any shape function that can be defined in the frequency domain, although occasionally an exact analytical expression cannot be found (11). Since convolutional methods (11) are simpler to code and operate with small computers, resolution enhancement by convolutional methods may appear more attractive to many ESR spectroscopists.

In the laboratory of one of the authors an ESR/computer system has access to a program that employs a convolutional function to sharpen spectral lines. The shaping function (11) may be used successfully on spectra with undetermined lineshapes, but it is optimized to transform lorentzian lines into gaussian lines of a desired width, usually narrower. Two parameters are controlled independently to scale the function: the width of the spectral lines to be enhanced the most (determined by the convolutional window) and the degree to which the program sharpens the lines. Excessive sharpening or choice of too narrow a window results in undue amplification of noise, but trial-and-error adjustments are readily made while monitoring the computer display. Figure 2-12 illustrates this method. Use of this convolutional method on the raw data of Hedberg and Ehrenberg (12) (kindly provided by them) provided resolution enhancement comparable to that discussed in the preceding paragraph (Fig. 2-11).

2.11.5 Interfacing of Computers to ESR Spectrometers and Other Apparatus

Commercial systems are available to interface ESR spectrometers with small laboratory computers. Usually, however, these are expensive devices, dedicated to interfacing with only one line of ESR spectrometers. To avoid these costs and restrictions many spectroscopists have elected to employ only small signal-averaging computers (see Section 2.11.2). When the data processing facilities described in Section 2.11.4 are needed, the output of the signal averager is transcribed onto magnetic tape, punched paper tape, or cards and the data processing is performed off-line at a central computing facility. Of course, there is then a loss of the ready access to data processing provided by an on-line connection to a small computer, so there is good reason to seek relatively inexpensive and generalized spectrometer/computer interfacing.

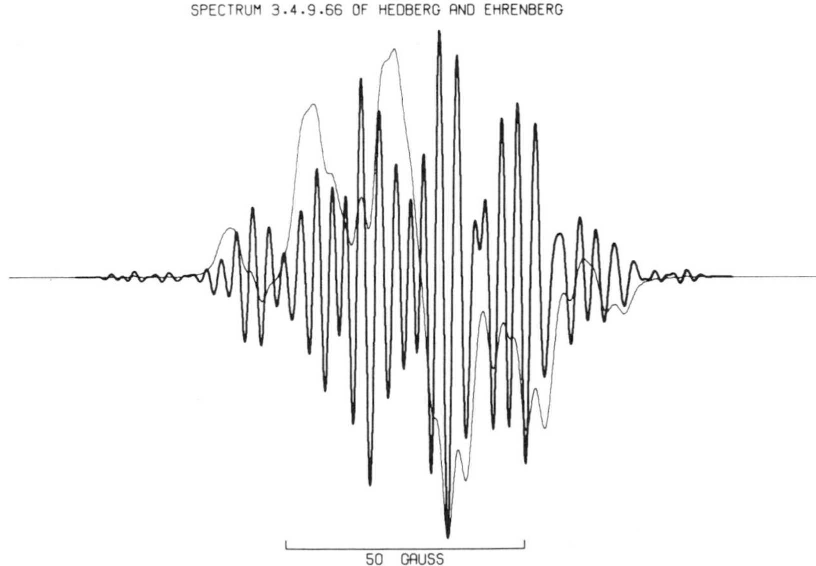

Fig. 2-11 An example of resolution enhancement by Fourier transform analysis. The light trace is the original spectrum; the heavy trace represents the result of the resolution enhancement [taken from A. Hedberg and A. Ehrenberg, *J. Chem. Phys.* **48**, 4822 (1968)].

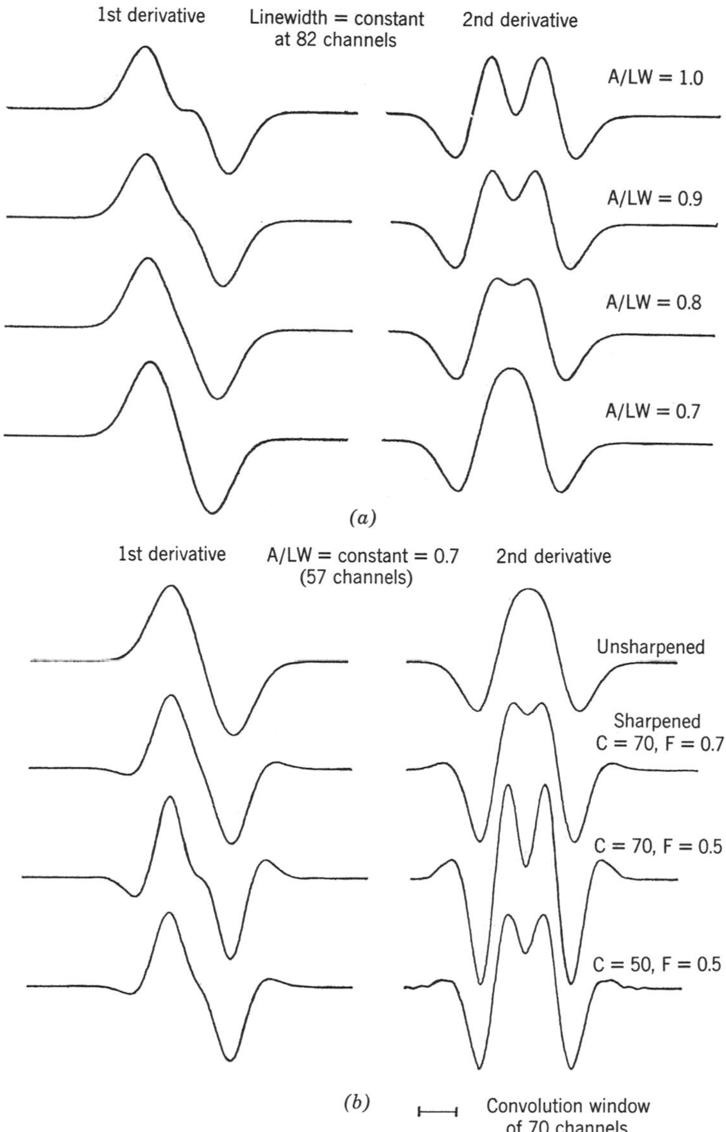

Fig. 2-12 (*a*) First- and second-derivative presentations of two overlapping gaussian lines at different values of the ratio A/LW, where A is line separation (splitting) and LW is linewidth (peak-to-peak for first derivative). The presence of two lines is largely obscured in the first-derivative spectrum at $A/LW = 0.8$, although two peaks remain clearly discernible in the second-derivative display. (*b*) At $A/LW = 0.7$ even the second derivative fails to disclose the two components, but resolution enhancement then partially separates them. The convolutional shape function used is optimized to convert lorentzian lines of C-channels into gaussian lines which are further sharpened to a LW only a fraction, F, as great as C (see Ref. 11); however, it can be seen that resolution is enhanced even when the assumed linewidth and line shape do not correspond exactly to those of the experimental lines.

A general-purpose interface can also be of inestimable value in making the best use of an on-line computer in a laboratory with other spectrometers and apparatus. This is so because the data-processing routines described in Sections 2.11.2–4, although described in terms of ESR spectroscopy, are basically general in format and can be applied to spectra and data arrays of many kinds, including NMR,* optical, beta or gamma spectra, and chromatographic data. Since most recording laboratory instruments put out a voltage signal, even though the voltage ranges are far from uniform and may or may not be referenced to ground, it is convenient to include in a general-purpose computer interface an operational amplifier component that can then be set to match the fixed input requirements of the ADC.

In addition to the data-processing capabilities already described (signal averaging, scaling and shifting of data arrays, adjustments of base-line levels and slopes, curve smoothing and digital filtering, addition and subtraction of spectra, obtaining (multiple) integrals or derivatives, and curve shaping and resolution enhancement), small computers can also be used to perform spectrum simulation, especially of solution spectra. Direct intercomparison of experimental and simulated spectra can greatly facilitate spectral analysis. For all these reasons and because digital recording and storage of experimental data allow previous spectra to be accessed for reworking or comparison with subsequent data, as desired, it seems likely that computerized methods of handling ESR data will become more and more prevalent.

2.12 MAGNETIC-FIELD CALIBRATION

Absolute magnetic-field measurements are usually carried out by measuring the frequency at which a water sample exhibits proton magnetic resonance. Such an "NMR fluxmeter" can measure magnetic fields to at least 1 ppm or better. However, with the availability of good g factor standards and samples with well-established hyperfine separations, one rarely has to measure an absolute magnetic field. For field scan widths less than 100 G Wurster's blue (N,N,N',N'-tetramethyl-p-phenylenediamine cation) perchlorate is a good standard (13). Table 2-2 lists the field positions for the

* In passing, the question arises as to why NMR spectroscopists have not made greater use of resolution enhancement. Resolution of partially overlapping lines is of signal importance in NMR, especially in the proton resonance spectra of biological macromolecules. Furthermore, many NMR spectrometers are already operating with signal averagers or with general-purpose computers that provide the fast Fourier transforms so vital to the powerful and increasingly popular Fourier-transform NMR spectroscopy. Resolution enhancement requires only minor additional programming of such systems.

Table 2-2 Field Positions of the Strong Lines in Half the ESR Spectrum of Wurster's Blue Perchlorate in (Degassed) Absolute Ethanol at 23°C[a]

$$a^{H}_{CH} = 1.989 \pm 0.009 \text{ G}$$
$$a^{H}_{CH_3} = 6.773 \pm 0.005 \text{ G}$$
$$a^{N} = 7.051 \pm 0.007 \text{ G}$$

$g = 2.003015 \pm 0.000012$ (corrected for second-order shifts)
$= 2.003051 \pm 0.000012$ (uncorrected)

Line position (G) relative to the center[b]	Relative Intensity	$\tilde{M}^{H}_{CH}$	$\tilde{M}^{H}_{CH_3}$	$\tilde{M}^{N}$
0.000	16,632	0	0	0
0.278	9.504	0	−1	1
1.711	6,336	1	1	−1
1.989	11,088	1	0	0
2.267	6,336	1	−1	1
2.796	2,376	−2	1	0
3.978	2,772	2	0	0
4.785	9,504	−1	1	0
5.062	7,392	−1	0	1
6.496	5,940	0	2	−1
6.773	14,256	0	1	0
7.051	11,088	0	0	1
7.329	4,752	0	−1	2
8.762	9,504	1	1	0
9.040	7,392	1	0	1
11.558	5,940	−1	2	0
11.836	6,336	−1	1	1
13.547	8,910	0	2	0
13.824	9,504	0	1	1
14.102	5,544	0	0	2
15.536	5,940	1	2	0
15.813	6,336	1	1	1
18.609	3,960	−1	2	1
18.887	3,168	−1	1	2
20.598	5,940	0	2	1
20.875	4,752	0	1	2
22.587	3,960	1	2	1
22.864	3,168	1	1	2
25.382	1,760	−1	3	1
25.660	1,980	−1	2	2
27.371	2,640	0	3	1
27.649	2,790	0	2	2
29.360	1,760	1	3	1
29.638	1,980	1	2	2
32.433	880	−1	3	2
34.422	1,320	0	3	2
36.411	880	1	3	2
41.195	396	0	4	2
43.184	264	1	4	2

[a] W. R. Knolle, Ph. D. Thesis, University of Minnesota, 1970.
[b] Any line position is given by $\Sigma_i\ a_i\tilde{M}_i$.

major lines in this spectrum. Fremy's salt [potassium peroxylamine disulfonate, $K_2NO(SO_3)_2$] may also be used. Table 2-3 gives the pertinent data

Table 2-3 Fremy's Salt Standard
[potassium peroxylamine disulfonate, $K_2NO(SO_3)_2$]

Method of sample preparation

Samples should be freshly prepared from solid $K_2NO(SO_3)_2$ kept in a refrigerator. Dissolve sufficient $K_2NO(SO_3)_2$ in a saturated solution of K_2CO_3 to give $[NO(SO_3)_2^{2-}] \sim 10^{-4}$ *M*.

Hyperfine Splitting

The three lines in this spectrum are not equally spaced because of a second-order effect. If the center line is taken as zero field, the field positions (at X band) are

$$-13.118 \text{ G} \qquad 0.000 \text{ G} \qquad +13.064 \text{ G}$$

The position of the center line relative to the other two depends on the microwave frequency; the separation of the two outer lines, however, is always 26.182 G.

Data taken from R. J. Faber and G. K. Fraenkel, *J. Chem. Phys.*, **47,** 2462 (1967).

for this standard. For field scan widths less than 500 G, Mn^{2+} in SrO powder is convenient, and its line positions are listed in Table 2-4. For larger scan widths it is best to use direct field measurements.

Table 2-4 Mn^{2+} Standard[a]

SrO powder invariably contains sufficient Mn^{2+} to give a strong ESR signal. Fortunately this signal has very narrow ($\sim$ 1.5 G) lines and is spread over a wide field range. When the spectrum is taken at X band (ν = 9.5 GHz), the six ^{55}Mn hyperfine lines appear at the fields

$$-212.1 \text{ G} \qquad -132.3 \text{ G} \qquad -50.8 \text{ G} \qquad +33.2 \text{ G} \qquad +119.4 \text{ G} \qquad +207.0 \text{ G}.$$

The reference field (0.000 G) is the field at which the g factor should be measured. The pertinent data for this spectrum are $g = 2.0012 \pm 0.0002$ and $|A| = 78.21 \times 10^{-4}\ \text{cm}^{-1}$.

[a] Taken from J. Rosenthal and L. Yarmus, *Rev. Sci. Inst.*, **37,** 381 (1966).

Field-scan calibrations are most conveniently made if a dual cavity is available (see Section 2.15). The standard and unknown can then be run at the same time. If a dual cavity is not available, a run of the standard before and after the unknown should suffice.

For most biological ESR studies the usual Hall sensor-regulated magnetic-field controls will provide adequate measurement and control of magnetic fields, provided that they are checked occasionally with a standard sample.

2.13 MEASUREMENT OF *g* FACTORS

The absolute measurement of a *g* factor requires knowledge of the microwave frequency and the resonant magnetic field. A number of systematic errors can enter (14); hence absolute measurements are rarely attempted. Instead we employ standards for which the *g* factors are well known. Table 2-5 lists the *g* factors for some of these standards. The unknown *g*

Table 2-5 *g*-factor Standards

Substance	*g* Factor
DPPH (α,α-diphenyl-β-picrylhydrazyl) powdcr	2.0037 ± 0.0002[a]
Wurster's blue perchlorate in degassed ethanol	2.00305 ± 0.00002[b]
Perylene cation in 98 percent H_2SO_4	2.00258 ± 0.00002[c]
Tetracene cation in 98 percent H_2SO_4	2.00260 ± 0.00002[c]

[a] J. A. Weil and J. K. Anderson, *J. Chem. Soc.*, **1965**, 5567; D. E. Williams, *ibid.*, **1965**, 7535.
[b] W. R. Knolle, Ph.D. Thesis, University of Minnesota, 1970.
[c] B. G. Segal, M. Kaplan, and G. K. Fraenkel, *J. Chem. Phys.*, **43**, 4191 (1965).

factor g_X is then calculated from

$$g_X = \frac{g_S H_S}{H_X} = \frac{g_S H_S}{H_S - \Delta H} \approx g_S\left(1 + \frac{\Delta H}{H_S}\right). \qquad (2\text{-}10)$$

Here g_S is the *g* factor of the standard and H_S and H_X are the resonant magnetic fields for standard and unknown, respectively, and $\Delta H = H_S - H_X$. If the *g* factors of the standard and the unknown do not differ greatly, then ΔH will be small compared with H_S and accurate results will depend only on an accurate measurement of ΔH. Equation 2-10 should not be used when *g* factors deviate markedly from that of the standard. Then either a standard with a *g* factor close to that of the unknown should be used or both the microwave frequency and the magnetic field should be measured.

2.14 ISOTOPIC SUBSTITUTIONS

The ESR spectra found in most systems of biological interest often contain multitudes of hyperfine components, most of which are not resolved. In this situation specific or even general isotopic substitution can be a great aid in the assignment of hyperfine splittings and in the very identification of the radical species. Several examples are to be found in this book; for instance, much of the width of Signal I seen in photosynthetic systems was shown to be due to proton hyperfine structure by growing the algae or bacteria on a fully deuterated medium (see Chapter 6). Also, one of the ESR signals seen in reduced iron-sulfur proteins was shown to come from two iron atoms by substituting ^{57}Fe for ^{56}Fe (see Chapter 8).

For radicals in solution which are of biochemical interest, the hyperfine structure may be well resolved, but ambiguities may exist in assignment. Specific isotopic substitution (D [or ^{2}H] for ^{1}H, ^{15}N for ^{14}N, ^{33}S for ^{32}S, etc.) can provide the additional information necessary for assignment. Even when the resolution is not complete, changes in the total width of the ESR spectrum may allow not only an assignment to a given position but also a measurement of a specific hyperfine splitting. The classic example of this type of analysis is for the flavin semiquinones (see Chapter 8). Obviously this technique requires the services of a good synthetic chemist.

In the above vein a nucleus with a spin may also be substituted for one without a spin and new hyperfine splitting information obtained; for instance, ^{13}C$(I = \frac{1}{2})$ can be substituted for ^{12}C$(I = 0)$.

Isotopic replacement can also be used to advantage in improving sensitivity and resolution. Replacement of all hydrogens by deuterium will narrow the ESR signal by a factor of 2 to 4 if proton hyperfine structure contributes significantly to the width. This will increase the signal (derivative) amplitude (thus improving sensitivity) and help to separate that signal from other signals (thus improving resolution).

2.15 DUAL CAVITY OPERATIONS

The use of a dual cavity offers many experimental advantages for biological ESR studies. The price paid for these advantages is monetary (about \$1000) and some loss of sensitivity due to a lower filling factor; however, some sensitivity due to a higher Q is regained. The usual dual cavity consists of two TE_{102} cavities coupled to form a TE_{104} cavity. Each part of the cavity can be modulated separately so that a standard and an experimental sample can be studied simultaneously. The experimental virtue of this arrangement is that both samples have identical microwave environments except for the different modulations applied and local distortions of the microwave field by the samples and their holders.

With a suitable standard and a dual cavity, effective microwave power, magnetic field position, and overall operation of the various components of the spectrometer can then be continuously monitored. Some of these parameters can also be measured with single cavities by measuring standard samples before and after experimental samples and assuming that (a) the spectrometer operated in exactly the same way during this interval and (b) the standard and the sample perturbed the operations identically. These assumptions are of doubtful validity for some typical "lossy" biological samples and for most spectrometers, which usually "drift" somewhat during a day's operation. The need for extra operations to run the standards also increases the time needed to analyze each sample. More detailed considerations of dual cavity operations will be found throughout this book and especially in Section 3.4.

2.16 EFFECT OF OXYGEN

Oxygen is one of the most important experimental factors in free radical chemistry and ESR spectroscopy. The reason for this is that the oxygen molecule normally contains two unpaired electrons and so reacts quite readily with other molecules that have unpaired electrons.* Because

* A complete explanation of why the oxygen molecule has two unpaired electrons requires quantum mechanical calculations that we have not considered here. Briefly, there are two orbitals (each able to accommodate two electrons) available for the last two electrons of molecular oxygen. It turns out that the total energy of the molecule is less if each electron goes into a different orbital rather than into the same orbital with different spins. This, however, leaves oxygen with two unpaired electrons, and so when it comes in contact with another molecule it tends to attract electrons from that molecule to complete the pairing of its electrons. When a molecule loses electrons it is said to be oxidized, a term obviously arising from this tendency of the oxygen molecule to take on electrons. A molecule with two unpaired electrons is often called a biradical, although when the two unpaired electrons interact sufficiently the molecule is better described as being in the triplet state (see Section 1.9). (Thus oxygen's stable or "ground" state is triplet in contradistinction to the triplet states of most other molecules, which are excited states, as noted in Section 1.9.) When a biradical reacts with another radical (1) and only one of its electrons becomes paired the resultant product is a free radical in contrast to the usual radical-radical reactions (2).

(1) $$O_2^{:} + R\cdot \rightarrow R\text{—}O_2^{\cdot}$$

(2) $$R\cdot + R\cdot \rightarrow R\text{—}R$$

of these properties oxygen can affect ESR spectra in at least six ways, several of which are of special importance in biological studies.

1. The oxygen molecule itself has an ESR spectrum. This is a broad spectrum extending over several thousand gauss. Occasionally gaseous oxygen may affect room temperature operations, and most workers circulate dry nitrogen gas through the waveguide to keep it out (also to prevent condensation of water vapor). Liquid oxygen may cause more significant disturbances in studies carried out in liquid nitrogen. Because the boiling point of liquid nitrogen is 77 K and oxygen boils at 96 K, liquid nitrogen will rapidly condense oxygen from air, so that liquid nitrogen that is initially oxygen free can rapidly accumulate it in significant amounts. The liquid oxygen will have an intense ESR absorption that will appear as a large baseline drift over much of the region usually studied with biological samples. Simple precautions to avoid large liquid nitrogen-air contact surfaces will eliminate this problem.

2. Many radicals will react rapidly with oxygen to form peroxy radicals. Unless we are studying peroxy radicals, this will, of course, prevent the study of the desired radicals. The occurrence of peroxidation can usually be detected experimentally by the asymmetry of the organoperoxy radical (see Section 10.3.2).

3. Another effect, perhaps related to No. 2, is the reactivity of oxygen with lyophilized preparations. In this case, however, the complication is not a radical-radical reaction but a generation of a new radical which lacks the typical shape of a peroxy radical. Extremely small traces of oxygen are sufficient for this reaction. This phenomenon is discussed in detail in Chapter 5.

4. The presence of oxygen can also result in a reduction of relaxation times, especially in frozen solutions. If this effect occurs in a sample in which some radicals are power saturating, the result is an apparent increase in the intensity of the spectrum. This is an example of the effects discussed in detail in Section 2.7.

5. The presence of oxygen may also alter hyperfine structure, again by affecting relaxation times. The result is a loss of hyperfine structure in certain circumstances, although the overall intensity is not affected. One example is the loss of secondary hyperfine structure in DPPH solutions in the presence of oxygen; this line-broadening effect of dissolved oxygen is actually quite common with free radicals in solution and must be kept constantly in mind.

6. Another effect of oxygen of potential importance in biology is the increase in damage observed in bacteria frozen in the presence of oxygen. This appears to involve free radical reactions but the mechanism has not been worked out. This effect is discussed in more detail in Chapter 4.

Oxygen undoubtedly can affect experimental ESR results in other ways not enumerated above. The solution to this problem is to consider explicitly the possible role of oxygen in all such experiments and attempt to control its concentration or at least equalize it in all samples. It should be noted that many of the effects of oxygen described here can occur at very low oxygen concentrations (even as low as $\sim 10^{-10}$ M) and that simple precautions such as the use of ordinary nitrogen gas sources often will not properly exclude oxygen.

2.17 OVERLAPPING SPECTRA

The problem of overlapping spectra is especially important in biological studies, compared with physical and chemical studies. This is because biological samples are generally more complex and contain many paramagnetic species in multiple environments. In addition, many of these species are located on large molecules, which usually prevents complete averaging out of anisotropic hyperfine components by rapid tumbling, and so the lines are broad. As a consequence, the usual simple methods of resolving overlapping spectra (chemical separation and/or analysis of hyperfine structure) are generally not applicable to biological samples. There are, however, many other techniques that can be utilized to resolve, at least in part, some of the overlapping spectra in biological samples. These techniques are discussed in depth throughout the book and therefore are not covered in detail here. The purpose of this section is to draw the reader's attention to this problem and to outline briefly some possible approaches to it.

One of the most useful approaches is the use of power saturation (see Section 2.7): many otherwise indistinguishable spectra can be resolved almost completely by this approach. Another useful technique is observation at different temperatures to take advantage of the fact that many inorganic paramagnetic species have such broad lines at room temperature that they are undetectable. The use of higher operating frequencies for ESR spectroscopy (e.g., K band or Q band) can also help to separate overlapping spectra whose g factors are different (see Section 2.10). Computer techniques offer another set of approaches to the problem, especially if there are paramagnetic species with any components that can be separately resolved (e.g., the low-field component of the organosulfur radical) (see Section 2.11). Another approach utilizes biological and/or biochemical conditions that may differentiate species on a functional rather than a spectroscopic basis. Physical separation of subcellular structures and/or molecular components may also be useful, but care must be taken to be certain that on fractionation signals are neither lost nor generated. Other techniques include the use of double resonances (ENDOR and ELDOR) (see Section 1.11) and isotopic substitutions (see Section 2.14) to resolve the participation of given inorganic elements or to narrow certain components selectively.

2.18 FAST REACTIONS AND TRANSIENT PARAMAGNETIC INTERMEDIATES

Free radicals are odd-electron species that are intrinsically stable, but because of the strong tendency of unpaired electrons to pair up they are characteristically highly reactive entities with short lifetimes in most chemical milieux. Other labile paramagnetic intermediates of biological interest also exist: reactive valence states of certain metalloenzyme complexes (see Chapters 8 and 9) and triplet excited states produced by some photochemical and radiation-induced reactions of biochemicals (possibly involved in photobiology as well) (see Sections 1.9 and 8.2.3). However, on the time scale of fast chemical and biochemical reactions ESR spectroscopy is very slow; the fastest response times of most commercial spectrometers is 0.1 to 1.0 msec and time intervals of several seconds to many minutes are required to scan most ESR spectra [even many hours with weak signals (see Section 2.11.1–2)].

Despite the fact that some free radicals and most metal complexes and metalloproteins are chemically stable, special preparative procedures are required before ESR spectroscopy can be carried out with many materials of biological interest (see Chapters 4, 5, 8, and 10). Therefore the experimental techniques discussed in this section are those that allow time-consuming ESR measurements to be made on sufficient quantities of short-lived paramagnetic particles; the problem of dealing with labile free radicals receives greatest emphasis.

Two general approaches have been successfully exploited to achieve this end: (a) trapping normally reactive products and sequestering them in an unreactive matrix and (b) using regenerative procedures to produce a dynamic steady-state whose stationary concentration is maintained long enough for ESR spectra to be scanned. Of course, for kinetic analyses alone ESR measurements of transient, repeatable phenomena may be effected with the signal-averaging techniques noted in Section 2.11.2, thus requiring neither trapping nor steady-state methods.

2.18.1 Trapping Techniques

Normally reactive species may be trapped when they are formed by physical means in the solid state, in a dehydrated environment, in an aprotic or relatively apolar solvent, at low temperature, or under any other conditions that inhibit their characteristic reactivity. The physical means by which free radicals are formed under such circumstances include photochemical reactions, ionization by irradiation, or by atomic bombardment from a low-pressure gas subjected to microwave discharge (see Chapter 10). Reactive species in mixtures containing equilibrium or pseudoequilibrium concentrations of transient paramagnetic intermediates may be trapped by rapid freezing.

Alternatively, high velocity streams containing paramagnetic products of chemical (or biochemical) reactions initiated within liquid mixing reactors may be cooled rapidly to very low temperatures, thereby quenching the decay of free radical or other reactive species. As first put forward by Bray (15), the aqueous reaction jet is impinged at high velocity (up to 30 m/sec) on cold isopentane (ca. −140 C). As a result, very fine droplets are formed with a high surface-to-volume ratio conducive to efficient heat transfer; heat transfer is also facilitated by the use of the isopentane, which remains fluid at sufficiently low temperature, yet is not so volatile that it will form an insulating gas blanket, as liquid nitrogen would. The freezing time with this technique is in the range of 5 to 10 msec (16), which is fast enough to "stop" many reactions of biochemical interest.

As Beinert points out (Section 8.4), changes may occur on freezing so that the species observed are not exactly the same as those present in solution before quenching. Nonetheless, the quick-freeze approach has the advantage of providing samples that are stable as long as they remain deeply frozen, and therefore ESR measurements can be made at leisure. Furthermore, with the most advanced apparatus of this type, which employs a high-powered ram to drive a push-block that expresses the contents of syringes into a reaction mixer at virtually constant velocity (to ensure homogeneity of the dead time from reaction to quenching) (17), submilliliter volumes are required for each sample. This small volume consumption is an important consideration when studying enzyme reactions or otherwise using scarce biochemical reactants.

At the cost of wasting some materials, flow mixers designed for continuous flow (see Section 2.18.2) may be readily adapted for quick-freeze applications. In an improvisation used by one of the authors (DCB) (see Fig. 7-15) a small micromixer fabricated for ESR flow work at Q band (Fig. 2-13) is fitted with a polyethylene outlet tube drawn out to form a fine nozzle. Although the velocity profile of the product stream (propelled by gas pressure or by a syringe drive) does not approach the step function approximated by the syringe ram of Hansen and Beinert (17), a uniform quench time for the ice droplets collected is obtained by moving the tube containing the cold isopentane to intercept the high-velocity outlet stream only during an interval of steady-state operation.

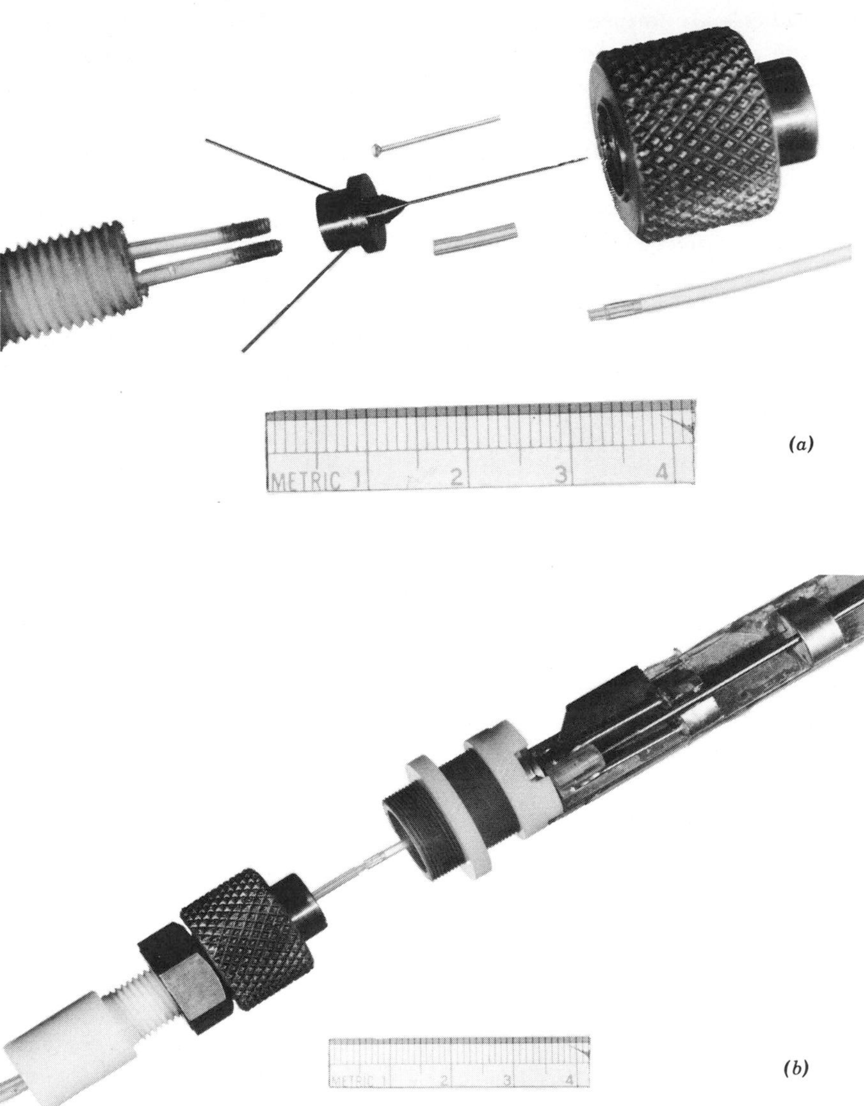

Fig. 2-13 (*a*) Disassembled continuous-flow micromixer for Q-band ESR. Stylets placed in the stainless steel mixer indicate the simple Y-junction flow path. The knurled bottom of the cylindrical TE_{011} microwave cavity is at the upper right. The 0.24-mm I.D. plastic outflow tube (with flared end and located just above the mixer) can be replaced with a jet nozzle for quick-freeze applications. (*b*) Mixer assembled and in place within the bottom of the cavity, which remains open to show the outflow tube surrounded by its stiff collar.

The quick-freeze method allows labile products of chemical or biochemical reactions to be examined, whereas more conventional trapping procedures require that the paramagnetic species be generated *in situ*, usually by one of the physical techniques noted earlier in this section. A straightforward example is the freezing of a solution, with the resulting glassy or polycrystalline ice then exposed to a light source capable of producing a photochemical product from the solute. Frozen in the solid state, normally reactive paramagnetic photoproducts may be accumulated and studied by ESR, as typified by the trapping of free radicals from the chromophores of visual pigments irradiated with visible light (18).

A variant of this photolysis *in situ* replaces the ice with mixtures of condensed gases (propane/propene) which remain liquid even down to 77 K. For those solutes that can be taken up this system allows charge-transfer and other reactions to be monitored by ESR as solutions are mixed or annealed. The cold liquids, however, are sufficiently viscous that the remaining thermal solvent motion is insufficient to provide typical room-temperature solution ESR spectra with well-resolved isotropic hyperfine structure (see Section 1.8).

Even without cryogenic liquid solvents, it has been common to use annealing in conjunction with low-temperature trapping techniques. In this way secondary paramagnetic products may be observed as reactions of successively higher activation energy are brought into play. Although the competitive reactions that may occur in solution at room or body temperatures are not well reproduced in this way, nor are other properties of the liquid state properly represented, the procedure of sequential warming and recooling for ESR observation of newly trapped species is easy to carry out and has proven to be useful in many cases. It has been especially popular in studies of free radicals produced by ionizing radiations (see Chapter 10).

Recently a specialized kind of trapping has been developed for use with room-temperature solutions wherein some degree of ESR isotropic hyperfine structure may be retained to provide partial identification of reactive free-radical intermediates. In what is basically a variation of the spin-label concept treated in detail in Chapter 11, nitroso compounds are added to reaction solutions in which transient free radicals are formed by chemical or physical means. The radicals may then be scavenged by the nitroso moiety to form a paramagnetic nitroxide free-radical complex, but unlike stable spin labels, whose nitroxide sites are strongly shielded sterically (see Chapter 11), the unpaired electron distribution of the complex may delocalize over adjacent regions of the compound so that the ESR spectral detail is influenced by magnetic nuclei that make up proximal portions of the scavenged radical component. Analysis of the smaller splittings of the nitroxide complex's hyperfine structure may then help to identify or characterize the "spin-trapped" free radical (19).

2.18.2 Regenerative or Steady-State Techniques

Trapping procedures are usually simple and do not require large samples. Although more complicated, the quick-freeze method is still conservative of materials, as noted, and has been used with great success in studies on enzyme reactions involving transient paramagnetic valence states of some metalloenzymes (see Section 8.4). Because ESR spectra are often much better resolved from liquid samples, in which anisotropic line-broadening interactions may average out (see Section 1.6), steady-state methods can provide significant advantages over trapping in solids. This is especially true for free radicals, but with transition-metal compounds for which the ESR spectra are so broad (typically hundreds of gauss: Chapters 8 and 9) that anisotropic interactions smear out few, if any, spectral features, trapping may be easier and more economical.

2.18.2.1 Electrolysis

Electrochemical generation of free radicals is possible with many of the redox reactions that give indications of one-electron intermediate steps on potentiometric or amperometric (polarographic) analysis. If the effective half-life of the paramagnetic reaction intermediate is about 100 msec or longer,* a steady-state population of free radicals sufficient for ESR measurements may be established near the electrode surface. This is the result of competition between electrolytic radical formation, due to diffusion of solute molecules from the bulk solvent into the electroactive region, versus free-radical decay reactions.

Maki and Geske (20) were the first to show that electrolysis could be carried out within the walls (*intra muros*) of flat ESR aqueous solution cells. Subsequently, electroreductions were made by using mercury pool cathodes and oxidations at gold foil or platinum gauze anodes. Aprotic polar solvents may stabilize some free radicals, and this permits the use of flat chambers somewhat thicker than those of typical aqueous solution cells because these solvents are less "lossy" than water (see Section 2.9). With metal electrodes it is also possible to flow solutions slowly through the cells; this can maintain a higher steady-state population of electrolysis products in cases in which rapid reactions deplete the bulk solvent of available reactant or can prevent a change in the free-radical concentration due to slow depletion during prolonged measurements. When the paramagnetic products are relatively long-lived (seconds or more), the use of closed-loop flow systems may even be superior to electrolysis *intra muros* because electro-

* In the case of reactions of order greater than one the "effective" half-life refers to the concentration range necessary for ESR spectroscopy (see Section 2.5).

lysis cells with efficient mixing and with larger and more effective electrode geometries can be used.

Although electrolysis is a relatively efficient regenerative procedure in that it can be performed with small volumes of solution, it may be complicated by electrode surface reactions and diffusion effects. Furthermore, since reaction products are not removed, secondary reactions can occur, and in some cases the steady-state concentrations of their products may vastly exceed those of the primary free radicals, which may not even be observed by ESR. However, even if these complexities do not intervene, many free-radical reactions of interest cannot be initiated by electrolysis, and others give rise to free radicals that are too ephemeral to satisfy the empirical criterion cited before, namely, a decay time on the order of 100 msec or longer.

In addition to these intrinsic constraints on the employment of electrolysis as a regenerative method, the prospective user should be apprised of some idiosyncrasies imposed by the characteristics of the electrolysis cells designed to obtain ESR from lossy solutions. Of course, an ionic medium is required to carry out electrolysis; yet with some of the aprotic solvents often used with electrolysis *intra muros*, the supporting electrolyte (most often a tetra-alkyl ammonium salt) is only weakly ionized. In these cases there is a significant internal resistance to the flow of current. The impact of this feature is exaggerated by the use of flat chambers to optimize cavity Q with such solutions (see Section 2.9); for example, a representative aqueous solution cell has a cross-sectional area of about 2.5 mm^2 throughout a chamber 4 to 5 cm long, and with a weak electrolyte, as just described, electrical resistance of 1 to 10 $\times$ 10^4 Ω is not uncommon. With a platinum gauze electrode in the flat cell, a typical electrolyzing current might be a few to 40 or 50 μA. Hence the voltage drop due to IR loss across the cell may often be a significant fraction of a volt.

For these reasons the applied electrode potentials required for an electrochemical reaction may be much greater than the potentials indicated by polarography. Even when a reference electrode is inserted as close as possible to the flat cell, the indicated potential may still exceed the effective solution potential at the working electrode. Although these strictures do not apply to aqueous solutions with strong electrolytes, it is a common practice when performing ESR electrolysis *intra muros* to raise the applied potential empirically until an increased current flow or the appearance of an ESR signal indicates that an electrochemical reaction has occurred.

2.18.2.2 Continuous Flow

A dozen years ago Hartridge and Roughton's continuous flow method, initially developed for optical studies of hemoglobin oxygenation (21), was adapted to obtain ESR of free radicals in aqueous solutions by Yamazaki, Mason, and Piette (22) (see Section 7.2.2.1). The principle is simplicity itself: solutions of reactants are forced by pneumatic pressure or by a syringe ram (which must press forward evenly to avoid oscillation of the effluent stream) into a reactor/mixer and the output flow is observed downstream. As long as the flow is continuous and constant, the composition of the product mixture at a given distance downstream corresponds to a fixed time interval following reaction.

This method of regenerating the population of short-lived products to maintain a steady state can provide concentrations of free-radical products that are acceptable for ESR spectroscopy even when the radical decay times are much too short to permit detection by electrolysis *intra muros* (see Section 2.18.2.1). Furthermore, with high-velocity flow, observational dead times are so short that they obviate complications from secondary reactions. On the other hand, the continuous-flow method tends to be prodigal of reactants, and this has limited its application to biochemicals or to enzymic reactions.

The pioneering application of continuous flow to ESR of lossy solutions [by Yamazaki et al. (22)] was for X-band ESR. A flat aqueous solution cell was affixed to a 12-jet lucite mixer. The dead space for flow from the mixer to the center of the microwave cavity was 0.14 ml, which provided a dead time of about 12 msec at a maximum flow rate of 12 ml/sec. Subsequently others modified the ESR flow apparatus to provide higher stationary concentrations of short-lived radicals within that portion of the flat chamber in which ESR detection sensitivity is greatest. This was achieved by minimizing flow dead time largely by reducing dead space and secondarily by allowing maximum volume flow rates compatible with the flat ESR cells required to optimize detection sensitivity of aqueous solutions (see Section 2.9).

In the most successful modifications (23, 24) small dead space results from the use of a simple two-jet mixer fashioned as an integral part of a quartz flow cell to adjoin the flat portion of the cell (Fig. 2-14). The jets are offset to impart a rapid swirl to the reacting solutions while they are in the short chamber that flares smoothly into the flat cell (Fig. 2-14). The dimensions of the reaction chamber and inlet jets permit the maximum flow rate to be determined by the intrinsic flow resistance of the flat portion of the cell. Interior contours are carefully shaped, with the jet orifices ground and polished, to supply approximately equal volumes of the two reaction mixtures at different rates of pneumatically actuated flow and to prevent cavitation with fast flow.

Volume flow rates above 20 ml/sec can be produced in flat chambers of 0.25×9 mm cross section by gas overpressure or by a syringe drive. This

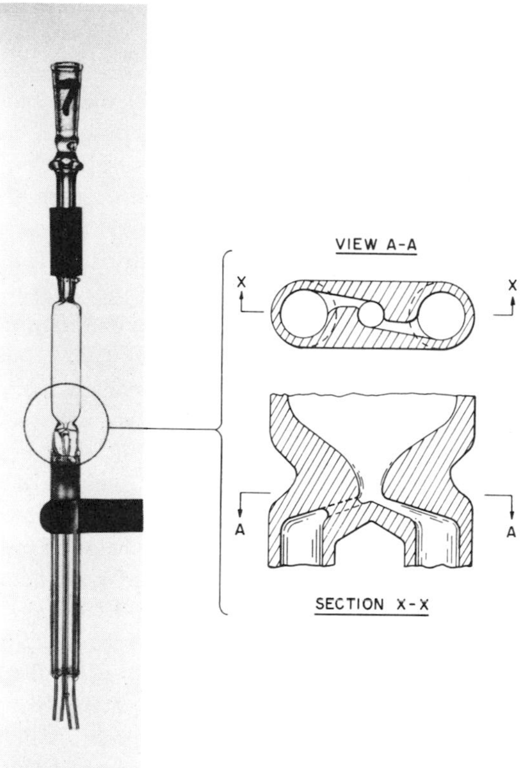

Fig. 2-14 Two-jet, quartz, aqueous-solution flow cell for X-band ESR. The flat portion of the cell is about 4-cm in length and 1-cm wide, and the slit between the flat sides is 0.25-cm deep.

corresponds to an average linear flow of about 900 cm/sec. The resulting dead time is roughly 0.25 msec through the 0.005 ml dead space from the mixer to the bottom of the flat compartment and less than 1.4 msec through the overall 0.027 ml dead space to the level at which ESR detection sensitivity is greatest.

With a fast recording system (see Section 2.11) these cells have provided ESR spectra with signal-to-noise ratios sufficient to resolve moderately complex hyperfine structure (ca. 20 lines) from very short-lived free radicals; for example, with free radicals whose second-order decay constants are roughly 10^9 $M^{-1}\text{sec}^{-1}$ spectral scans lasting less than 3 sec have sufficed when approximately 25 ml of each of the two reactant solutions of 0.02 M

concentration were consumed (25). Although it represents significant conservation of materials in comparison with the 1 liter-per-scan consumption of continuous flow ESR experiments in physical organic chemistry, even this reduced utilization rate is prohibitively high for many biochemicals.

Further savings of substantial magnitude in material consumption have been secured by fabricating high-velocity continuous-flow apparatuses for use with ESR at Q band. Because of the small dimensions of Q-band cavities, micromixers with dead spaces of less than 0.001 ml suffice. Commercial Q-band microwave cavities are of the cylindrical TE_{011} type, and the observation cells are simple capillary tubes of about 0.27 mm ID. Although several Q-band mixer designs have been tested, including multijet models (8), the small bores of the fluid paths ensure turbulent flow, and therefore there will be efficient reaction even when mixing through a simple Y junction; Q-band mixers of this kind (Fig. 2-13) with two or three inlet ports have been made and used with success.

With apparatus of this sort, driven by a gas pressure head of 3 to 4 atm or by a special syringe pump, linear-flow velocities of more than 10 m/sec are easily obtained with bulk flow rates well below 1 ml/sec. The corresponding dead times from mixing to the locus of ESR detection are 1 msec or less. In addition to being able to study the ESR of unstable free radicals at more than one microwave frequency (see Section 2.10), these Q-band micromixers permit ESR spectra from short-lived free radicals to be recorded with sensitivities comparable to those of the best X-band systems (see above) but with only 3 to 7 percent as much material (8), despite greater restrictions concerning microwave power saturation at Q band. They have also made feasible ESR continuous-flow studies with scarce biochemical reactants.

2.18.2.3 Stopped Flow

Analyses of the stopped flow kinetics of chemical and biochemical reactions measured by optical absorption spectrometers have been in common use for many years. Monitoring appropriate peaks of ESR spectra can also lead to kinetic analysis (see Section 2.11.2), and, in principle, ESR continuous flow apparatus should be readily adaptable to stopped flow applications. In fact, slow kinetics (decay half-lives on the order of 100 msec or more) *can* be readily determined by ESR stopped flow when pneumatically driven systems are equipped with fast solenoid valves or when syringe pumps have magnetic clutches.

Despite the short dead times of high-velocity continuous flow cells for ESR at X band (see Section 2.18.2.2), decay kinetics of very short-lived free radicals cannot be obtained reliably from operation in the stopped flow mode. This is so not only because of the finite closing times of valves and clutches and the difficulties of stopping a rapid flow abruptly without oscillations and eddy currents but because the region of ESR detection within the microwave cavity is relatively extensive, being effectively 1 cm long at X band. As a result the time coherence of the free radical population giving rise to the ESR signal is smeared out, an effect made even greater by the fact that the velocity profile of the flow path through the sensitive region of the aqueous solution flat cell is certainly *not* flat, but probably resembles a two-dimensional laminar flow.

The small Q-band flow cells (see Section 2.18.2.2 and Fig. 2-13) have rather sharply defined regions of ESR detection, and their thin capillary observation tubes give rise to turbulent flow. Hence stopped flow with Q-band apparatus might appear less encumbered by uncertainties regarding the time-histories of the free radicals that are detected than is the case at X band. In practice, however, it is not possible to stop a high velocity liquid column suddenly without reverberations which are large in comparison with the tiny detection volume (ca. 0.0001 ml) of the Q-band system. So with present apparatus high-resolution stopped flow analysis is not feasible with Q-band ESR either.

2.18.3 Flash Photolysis and Pulse Radiolysis

There are many reactions of biological interest that can be initiated by light or high-energy radiation. In these cases the use of flash-photolysis techniques for light and pulse radiolysis for high-energy radiation has proved to be of immense value in the study of the primary processes. In most studies to date the kinetic course of the transients so produced has been followed by optical absorption spectroscopy. There is no reason why ESR should not be applied as well, and indeed recent work has demonstrated the feasibility of such studies. Hales and Bolton (26) and Atkins et al. (27) have developed the flash-photolysis ESR interface. The experiment consists of fixing the magnetic field at a value at which ESR signals might be expected and then repetitively flashing with a flash tube which puts out a short-duration but very intense pulse of light (usually 5 to 100 μsec). Alternatively, we may use a laser flash (pulse duration < 1 μsec). The use of a time-averaging computer (see Section 2.11.2) is absolutely essential, since very short time constants must be used to record the rapid changes in signal that occur. At the current state of this field we may resolve radical kinetics with half-times as short as ~ 5 μsec. Similar techniques have been developed for pulse radiolysis (28), the only difference being that the reaction is initiated by a pulse of electrons. There is no doubt that these techniques will become increasingly popular in biological investigations, especially in photosynthesis.

2.19 LOW TEMPERATURE STUDIES

Many biological investigations are carried out at low temperatures (usually ~ 77 K) to trap reactive intermediates (usually free radicals) and to enhance sensitivity. Reactions are stopped primarily by a "cage" effect as the radicals become immobilized in the frozen matrix. The usual reaction-rate-retarding effect of low temperatures also plays a role. It should be kept in mind, however, that some reactions can proceed at 77 K and even at lower temperatures. (In fact, a few reactions, such as hydrogen atom diffusion in some crystals, will go faster in the frozen state, presumably due to geometrical factors). The factors that can enhance detection sensitivity at low temperature include a more favorable Boltzmann distribution of electron spins between the two allowed energy levels (see Section 1.3.3 and Fig. 1-1) and sometimes the elimination of nonresonant absorption of microwaves by liquid water (i.e., ice is less "lossy" than liquid water, as discussed in Section 2.9). Low temperatures may also be necessary to obtain sufficiently narrow linewidths to make them observable when spin-lattice relaxation times are extremely short e.g., some Fe(II) compounds (see Chapter 8).

Several experimental problems may occur in low-temperature studies. If the sample is kept in liquid nitrogen during the ESR observation, the bubbling that results as the liquid nitrogen boils may cause significant noise, especially at high power operations. A variety of techniques can be used to minimize this noise, including placing the equivalent of boiling chips in the sample-holding dewar, bubbling a small stream of helium (to form nuclei for very fine bubbles which do not make much noise) in the dewar, or supercooling the liquid nitrogen by pumping on it and thus lowering its temperature for a time below its boiling point. Another alternative is to cool the sample in a stream of cold, dry, gaseous nitrogen. This will give a somewhat higher observation temperature and cost more in terms of expenditure of nitrogen but it will eliminate the bubbling problem. Some types of samples (e.g., cylinders of frozen tissues) cannot be readily accommodated with this kind of cooling, which is usually done in an apparatus similar or identical to the Varian variable temperature accessory. Freezing may introduce artifacts by breaking bonds and generating radicals. It will also change the relaxation times of many paramagnetic species, making some more observable and causing others to power saturate. The solid matrix will prevent molecular tumbling and therefore many lines will be broadened. The most important point is that the use of low temperatures may affect the results obtained, so we must carefully determine what these effects are for the samples being studied.

We shall not consider in detail the use of very low temperatures (i.e., in the region of 4 K and lower). These experiments may often provide much additional information but they do require special cryogenic apparatus. One of the major problems at these low temperatures is that T_1 as a rule is very long (1 msec to several seconds). This means that ESR signals will strongly saturate at the power levels usually employed at higher temperatures. We must have power levels of 1 μW or less to avoid these saturation problems. On the other hand, one of the major advantages of the use of low temperatures is greatly improved sensitivity (see Eq. 2-4) and the narrowing of lines, especially for transition metal ions.

The reader is urged to consult the experimental textbooks (1, 2) for a thorough discussion of the problems, advantages, and techniques of very low temperature experiments. Some examples of the results of such studies are cited in Chapter 8.

2.20 RECENT SPECTROMETER DEVELOPMENTS

The balance of this book deals with the operation of and the results obtained with existing commercial instruments. In this section we consider briefly some of the recent and proposed developments in ESR spectrometers.

From a strictly biological viewpoint perhaps the most exciting concept is the proposed development of a highly sensitive *in vivo* ESR spectrometer by Commoner's group at Washington University in St. Louis. They are attempting to build an instrument capable of producing spectra via a small probe (a slow-wave structure instead of a microwave reflection cavity) that could be inserted inside a living animal or even a human being. Such a development would overcome many of the experimental difficulties described in detail in Chapter 4.

Another instrumental development, from the same laboratory, is an ESR spectrometer capable of giving good spectra at X band in the presence of significant amounts of water. This has been developed to the point that they have published one paper on results with this instrument in which they irradiated "living" tissues in the cavity and simultaneously obtained ESR spectra. This may eventually lead to significant new information, but its potential has not yet been fully tested.

Also related to radiation studies is the development of X-band spectrometers capable of resolving very short-lived species produced by electron irradiation of aqueous solutions within the microwave cavity. The problems associated with the electronics of resolution at times of 1 msec or less have been solved by at least one group, Smaller et al., at Argonne National Laboratory (28), and this type of apparatus is now being actively utilized in radiation chemistry studies. Presumably it could also be useful in radiobiological investigations.

REFERENCES

1. C. Poole, Jr., *Electron Spin Resonance—A Comprehensive Treatise on Experimental Techniques,* Wiley-Interscience, New York, 1967.
2. R. Alger, *Electron Paramagnetic Resonance Techniques and Applications*, Wiley-Interscience, 1968.
3. T. Wilmshurst, *Electron Spin Resonance Spectrometers*, Hilger, London, 1967.
4. *Review of Scientific Instruments.*
5. *Journal of Physics E: Scientific Instruments* (before 1968 *Journal of Scientific Instruments*).
6. T. Castner, *Phys. Rev.*, **115,** 1506 (1959).
7. L. Singer, *J. Appl. Phys.*, **30,** 1463 (1959); L. Singer and J. Kommandeur, *J. Chem. Phys.*, **34,** 133 (1961); L. Singer, W. Smith, and G. Wagoner, *Rev. Sci. Instr.*, **32,** 213 (1961).
8. D. Borg and J. Elmore, Jr., in *Magnetic Resonance in Biological Systems*, A. Ehrenberg, B. Malmström, and T. Vänngård, Eds., Pergamon, New York, 1967, p. 383.
9. T. Halpern and W. Phillips, *Rev. Sci. Instr.*, **41,** 1038 (1970).
10. L. Allen, H. Gladney, and S. Glarum, *Rev. Sci. Instr.*, **40,** 3135 (1964); S. Glarum, *Rev. Sci. Instr.*, **36,** 771 (1965).
11. R. Ernst, *Adv. Mag. Res.*, **2,** 1–135 (1966).
12. A. Hedberg and A. Ehrenberg, *J. Chem. Phys.*, **48,** 4822 (1968).
13. W. Knolle, Ph.D. Thesis, University of Minnesota, 1970.
14. B. Segal, M. Kaplan, and G. Fraenkel, *J. Chem. Phys.*, **43,** 4191 (1965).
15. R. Bray, *Biochem. J.*, **81,** 189 (1961).
16. R. Bray, *Rapid Mixing and Sampling Techniques in Biochemistry*, B. Chance Ed., Academic, New York, 1964, p. 195; G. Palmer and H. Beinert, *ibid.*, p. 205.
17. R. Hansen and H. Beinert, *Anal. Chem.*, **38,** 484 (1966).
18. F. Grady and D. Borg, *Biochem.*, **7,** 675 (1968).
19. S. Forschult, C. Lagercrantz, and K. Torssell, *Acta Chem. Scand.*, **23,** 522 (1969); E. Janzen and B. Blackburn, *J. Am. Chem. Soc.*, **91,** 4481 (1969).
20. A. Maki and D. Geske, *J. Chem. Phys.*, **30,** 1356 (1959).
21. Hartridge and Roughton, *Proc. Royal Soc.* (*London*), **A-104,** 376 (1923).
22. L. Yamazaki, H. Mason, and L. Piette, *J. Biol. Chem.*, **235,** 2444 (1960).
23. D. Borg, *Nature*, **201,** 1087 (1964).
24. D. Borg, *Rapid Mixing and Sampling Techniques in Biochemistry*, B. Chance Ed., Academic, New York, 1964, p. 135.
25. D. Borg and J. Elmore, Jr., *Magnetic Resonance in Biological Systems,* A. Ehrenberg, B. Malmström and T. Vänngård, Eds., Pergamon, Oxford, 1967, p. 341.
26. B. Hales and J. Bolton, *Photochem. Photobiol.*, **12,** 239 (1970).
27. P. Atkins, K. McLauchlan, and A. Simpson, *Nature* **219,** 927 (1968); *Chem. Commun.* **179,** (1968); *J. Phys. E: Sci. Instr.*, **3,** 547 (1970).
28. B. Smaller, J. Remko, and E. Avery, *J. Chem. Phys.*, **48,** 5174 (1968).

CHAPTER THREE

Quantitative Considerations in Electron Spin Resonance Studies of Biological Materials

MALCOLM L. RANDOLPH

Biology Division
Oak Ridge National Laboratory
Oak Ridge, Tennessee

Research sponsored by the U.S. Atomic Energy Commission under contract with Union Carbide Corporation.

3.1 INTRODUCTION

Next in importance to the observation that an electron spin resonance (ESR) signal exists in a sample and to an identification of the responsible molecular species is a quantitative measurement of how many ESR centers are present. Absolute spin concentration values are especially needed in photochemical and photobiological studies for the determination of quantum yields and in radiochemistry and radiobiology for G values.* In heterogeneous spin systems spin concentration values may be the only possible quantitative measurement and may be useful when the molecular species are unidentified. Concentrations are also needed for higher than first-order kinetic studies. In this chapter emphasis is on the aspects and problems of estimating spin concentrations by ESR. The treatment is oriented toward free radical work with conventional X-band spectrometers, although similar considerations often apply for other circumstances. The discussions emphasize simple basic considerations.

An ESR signal may be quantitated in various ways, with the method and degree of rigor employed depending on the purpose of the measurement. At least five useful degrees of sophistication can be distinguished.

1. For some relative intralaboratory work, measurement of the derivative signal amplitude under standard conditions of sample bulk, modulation, microwave power, scan rate, etc., may be sufficient.
2. For relative studies of extended duration measurement of the derivative signal may be normalized against a standard sample containing stable free radicals, thus compensating for variations caused by instrumental drifts in sensitivity.
3. For order of magnitude estimates of spin concentrations comparison of the product of [derivative signal height] times [the square of signal width] versus the same product for a standard sample may suffice.
4. For quantitative estimates absolute numbers of spins may be calculated by applying first principles to measurements of the signal and all pertinent instrumental parameters (see Eq. 2-4).
5. For quantitative estimates of spin concentrations usually the computed first moment or second integral of the derivative curve is compared with that for a standard sample.

Each approach has characteristic advantages and disadvantages, some of which are common to several approaches.

Of these five approaches for estimation of spin concentrations the first two

* A G value is the number of specified events produced per 100 electron volts absorbed from ionizing radiation.

are obviously oversimplifications because they give no consideration to the width or shape of the spectra. Thus only relative values can be obtained and these are valid only if the spectrum remains unchanged in width and shape. Although estimation by the third approach includes a measurement of width, the failure to consider spectral shape reduces the method's absolute significance for single-line spectra perhaps to order of magnitude estimates; this method is of doubtful applicability for multiline spectra. The fourth approach has an obvious attraction for purists because it affords absolute values from "first principles." As Yariv and Gordon (34) described this method, one must determine 11 parameters (albeit several may come from a priori knowledge of the radical species) and several assumptions, including alignment of the crystal symmetry axis along the dc magnetic field and a known (e.g., lorentzian) curve shape. Although high precision may be obtained in this way, this approach has been employed only by workers with strong interests in instrumentation (see Section 2.5).

The fifth approach, comparisons of first moment or second integral for a test sample versus that for a standard sample is the method most commonly used in quantitative ESR studies, and analysis of it constitutes a major portion of our discussion. We describe the elementary evaluation of ideal derivative data and then consider the effects of phenomenological deviations from ideality and of random errors in obtaining data. Considerations pertinent to this aspect of ESR spectroscopy may also apply to other aspects.

In the ideal case the number of spins in an unknown sample, N_x, is related to the number of spins in a standard sample, N_s, by

$$N_x = \frac{H_{m_s}\sqrt{P_s}\, G_s \Sigma_x}{H_{m_x}\sqrt{P_x}\, G_x \Sigma_s} N_s \,, \tag{3-1}$$

where sub s and x designate the standard and unknown samples, respectively, H_m, the modulation amplitude, P, the microwave power, G, the overall spectrometer gain, and Σ, the integral of the ESR absorption (or its equivalent) over the entire signal. Only for distortion-free lines is Σ simply inversely proportional to $H_m\sqrt{P}$. In practice Σ depends on H_m and P in more complex ways and on other variables (26) such as scan width, sample geometry, and signal errors, all of which we discuss. Determination of Σ is the crucial experimental problem.

An ESR measurement is basically a measure of number of spins rather than their concentration. If the effective sample size is known, we may estimate the concentration of spins. With this mental reservation we often speak of numbers of spins and their concentration interchangeably. (Direct comparisons in terms of concentrations may be made when solutions contain both sample and standard.) In this chapter and elsewhere in this book we consider only the bulk or average concentration of spins in samples rather than the much greater local concentrations which, for example, occur in microscopic volumes in the "spurs" and around the tracks of ionizing particles. The local concentration may be crucial in radiation damage studies. Furthermore the local rather than bulk concentration is, of course, the concentration that determines spin-spin interactions and power saturation characteristics. Wyard (33) has reviewed methods for estimating local concentrations.

3.2 EVALUATION OF RECORDED SIGNALS

The usual output of an ESR spectrometer is an approximation of the derivative of the resonance absorption with respect to magnetic field (see Section 2.3.3). Signal distortions, aside from random noise and drifts, are produced by application of microwave power on the test sample and by magnetic-field modulation, both of which are inherent in contemporary instrumentation. On the other hand, the signal amplitude, at low power and modulation, is directly proportional to the field modulation and increases with microwave power. Hence the setting of these parameters is a compromise between faithful reproduction of the lineshape and discrimination against noise and drifts (see Section 2.3.3). In the context of this chapter, which is devoted to concentration measurements, experimental demonstration of lineshapes is trivial; hence we can advantageously use power levels and modulation amplitudes that distort the signal. How far we can go in these approaches is discussed at length in later sections. Meanwhile we consider the idealized distortion-free cases in which integrations are assumed to extend to infinity.

Since the recorded ESR signal usually is approximately the first derivative of the absorption signal, an estimate of the spin concentration must involve evaluation of the *second* integral of the spectrometer output. Burgess (5) has shown that the second integral is equivalent to the first moment. His derivation is equivalent to

$$\text{second integral, } I = \int_{-\infty}^{+\infty} A(h)\, dh\,, \tag{3-2}$$

where $A(h)$ is the amount of microwave power absorbed at h, and h is the field at resonance minus the variable field. By integrating by parts we obtain

$$I = h\,A(h)\Big|_{-\infty}^{+\infty} - \int_{-\infty}^{+\infty} h\,D(h)\, dh\,, \tag{3-3}$$

where $D(h)$ is the derivative of $A(h)$. [The usual signal presentation is an approximation to $D(h)$.] For lineshapes such as gaussian or lorentzian

$$h\,A(h) = 0 \text{ at } h = \pm\infty;$$

hence

$$I = -\int_{-\infty}^{+\infty} h\,D(h)\,dh = \text{first moment}, \tag{3-4}$$

where the moment is taken as positive for a counterclockwise rotation.

In cases of overlapping or split lines we usually integrate over all the lines, thus leading toward a measurement of the total number of spins present. In this chapter we assume that all resonant species have but one unpaired electron per molecule and that with a spin angular momentum of $S = \frac{1}{2}$. The ratio of the number of molecules with spin S required to produce a given signal to the number with spin $\frac{1}{2}$ required to produce the same signal is $3/[4S(S + 1)]$ (see Eq. 2-4). Our analytical treatments are confined to singlet lines for simplicity, but the principles are largely the same for multiple lines.

Once we have reliable data the integral or moment calculation can be made in any of a variety of ways—for example, by schemes based on analog computers (12, 24), desk calculators (32), moment balances (5, 16, 17), and combinations of hand and automated devices. With currently available commercial spectrometers the most sophisticated solution seems to be to convert the analog spectrometer output to digital form and do computations on a dedicated or perhaps a time-shared computer (see Section 2.11).* The computational choice is one of convenience and speed. The crucial problem in obtaining accuracy remains in the input data and not in the computation. Practical concerns in the choice of first-moment or double-integral calculations are discussed in Section 3.5.

3.3 OPTIMIZING THE SPECTROMETER SETTINGS

In this section we discuss qualitatively and quantitatively how spectrometer settings, hence deviations from the simple idealized circumstances, influence attempts to measure spin concentrations. Parameters involved include magnetic-field scan width, scan rate, modulation amplitude, and microwave power. We assume that the linewidth (in MHz) (see Section 1.2) is large

* We can conceive of a computer-controlled spectrometer that repetitively scans a spectrum and from past scans selects and sets the best instrumental parameters to obtain a desired accuracy in the least time, perhaps displaying results while approaching this goal. Such an instrument would probably convert to digital form as soon as possible rather than develop an analog curve before computation.

compared with the modulation frequency, so that we may ignore modulation side bands, and negligible compared with the microwave frequency. For reasons of simplicity we treat scan rate independently and scan width, modulation, and power both separately and jointly. Our theoretical calculations are for lorentzian and gaussian lineshapes, although observed lines may lie between these idealizations. The lorentzian lineshape results from spin-lattice relaxation (30) and the gaussian lineshape from spin-spin interactions (4) (see Section 1.3.1 and Figs. 2-5 and 2-6). Essentially these lineshapes have the form

$$A(h) = \frac{A(0)}{1 + Bh^2} \quad \text{(lorentzian)}, \tag{3-5}$$

$$A(h) = A(0)e^{-Kh^2} \quad \text{(gaussian)}, \tag{3-6}$$

where $A(h)$ is the microwave power absorbed and $h = H - H_r$ where H is the external magnetic field strength and H_r, the value of H at resonance (see Table 2-1). We shall consider the shapes given by Dyson (7) and Posener (22) as not applicable to our problems.

3.3.1 Scan Width, $2S$

Inspection of the equations for lorentzian and gaussian lineshapes reveals that the shapes are symmetric about $h = 0$ and that the absorption approaches zero asymptotically as h approaches infinity. Since experimental data cover only a finite scan, we must consider the effect of this scan width. Usually the results are based on a calculation of the first moment or second integral of the derivative signal $D(h)$, assuming that the derivative and moment or the derivative, absorption, and integral are zero at the start of the scan. The significance of these assumptions is shown in Fig. 3-1, from which

Fig. 3–1. ESR curves (for a lorentzian line), as used for quantitative studies. (*a*) The derivative signal $D(h)$ versus external magnetic field h. (*b*) The true absorption curve $A(h)$ versus h, obtained by integrating $D(h)$ from $h = -\infty$ to h. The experimental absorption curve is obtained by assuming $A(h) = D(h) = 0$ at the initial value of $h = -S$ and integrating $D(h)$ from $-S$ to h. The experimental baseline (BL) differs from the true baseline initially by $A(-S)$ and has a slope $D(-S)$ and a finite width from $-S$ to S. (*c*) The true second integral curve I versus h, obtained by integrating $A(h)$ from $h = -\infty$ to h. The desired result is the value when the integration extends from $-\infty$ to ∞. The experimental value is smaller by $2SA(-S) + 2S^2D(-S)$ than $\int_{-S}^{S} A(h)\,dh$. (*d*) The moment elements versus h. The initial assumption that $D(-S) = 0$ makes the effective experimental baseline BL. (*e*) The moment curves M versus h, obtained by integration from panel (*d*). The effective experimental baseline is BL. $V(S)$ is defined as $\int_{-\infty}^{S} hD(h)\,dh$. The final moment equals $\int_{-S}^{S} hD(h)\,dh$. (*f*) The experimental values versus h. A corrected integral, *CI*, curve is also shown. It is obtained by assuming a horizontal baseline in panel (*b*).

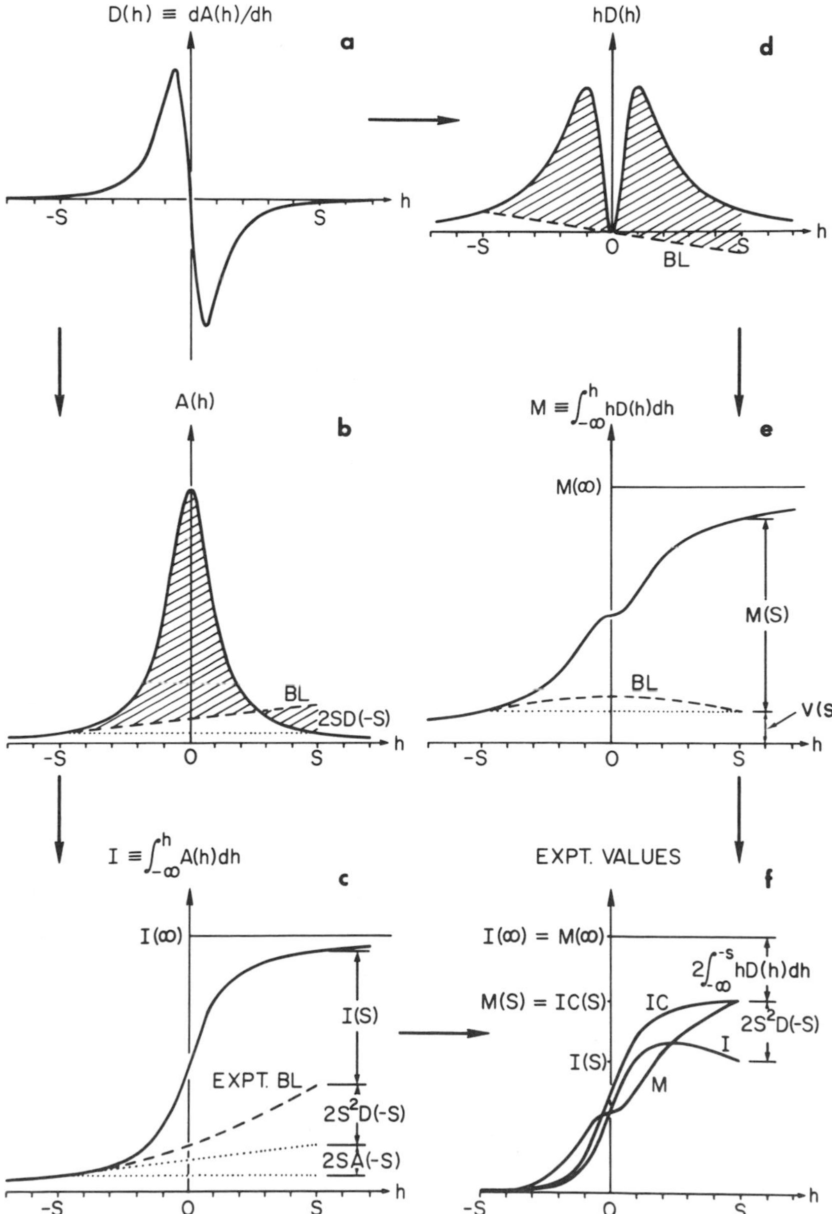

D(h) ≡ dA(h)/dh
a
-S
S
h
hD(h)
d
-S
O
BL
S
h
A(h)
b
BL
2SD(-S)
-S
O
S
h
M ≡ ∫_{-∞}^{h} hD(h)dh
e
M(∞)
M(S)
BL
V(S)
-S
O
S
h
I ≡ ∫_{-∞}^{h} A(h)dh
c
I(∞)
I(S)
EXPT. BL
2S²D(-S)
2SA(-S)
-S
O
S
h
EXPT. VALUES
f
I(∞) = M(∞)
2∫_{-∞}^{-S} hD(h)dh
M(S) = IC(S)
IC
2S²D(-S)
I
I(S)
M
-S
O
S
h

the experimentally determined values of the second integral, $I(S)$, and first moment, $M(S)$, for a scan from $-S$ to S are

$$I(S) = \int_{-S}^{S}\int_{-S}^{h'} D(h)\,dh\,dh' = \int_{-S}^{S} A(h)\,dh - 2SA(-S) - 2S^2D(-S)$$

$$= I(\infty) - 2\int_{-\infty}^{-S} A(h)\,dh - 2SA(-S) - 2S^2D(-S), \qquad (3\text{-}7)$$

$$M(S) = -\int_{-S}^{S} h\,D(h)\,dh$$

$$= M(\infty) + 2\int_{-\infty}^{-S} h\,D(h)\,dh. \qquad (3\text{-}8)$$

We have already (Eqs. 3-3 and 3-4) shown that $I(\infty)$ and $M(\infty)$ are equal. By very similar analysis we can show that the correction terms $-2\int_{-\infty}^{-S} A(h)\,dh - 2SA(-S)$ and $2\int_{-\infty}^{-S} h\,D(h)\,dh$ in Eqs. 3-7 and 3-8 are identical; hence $M(S) = I(S) + 2S^2D(-S)$.

For first-moment calculation of the lorentzian and gaussian lineshapes given by Eqs. 3-5 and 3-6 the fractional errors for the first moments E_L and E_G caused by finite scan $-S$ to S become

$$E_L = 1 - \frac{M(S)}{M(\infty)} = 1 - \frac{2}{\pi}\left(\tan^{-1} S - \frac{S}{1 + S^2}\right) \qquad (3\text{-}9)$$

and

$$E_G = 1 - \operatorname{erf}(S) + \frac{2}{\sqrt{\pi}} Se^{-S^2}, \qquad (3\text{-}10)$$

where for the lorentzian line S is half the scan width in units of half the absorption width at half maximum; for the gaussian line S is half the scan width in units of half the absorption width at $1/e$ times the maximum and erf (S) is the error function $= (2/\sqrt{\pi}) \int_0^S e^{-x^2}\,dx$. Some numerical results are given in Table 3-1. Köhnlein and Müller (18) and Judeikis (15) have given similar values for moment calculations. Obviously for comparable accuracy the scan must be much wider for a lorentzian with its long "tails" (see Section 2.3) than for a gaussian curve of the same linewidth. Hence baseline stability and noise are much more important for lorentzian than for gaussian curves. The errors become greater if the resonance is broadened by power saturation or field modulation. We shall consider these combined effects later. Table 3-1 also shows that, as expected from Eqs. 3-7 and 3-8, the first moment calculation gives smaller errors for finite scan than the second integral calculation. However, the corrected integral calculation, which we describe and discuss in Section 3.5.2, yields at all scan widths the same values that the first moment yields.

Table 3-1 Combined Effect of Finite Scan and Initial Zero Assumptions on Second Integral *I*, Moment *M*, and Corrected Integral *CI*[a]

$$\text{Percent error} = \left(1 - \frac{\text{value for scan}}{\text{value for } \infty \text{ scan}}\right) 100$$

	Lorentzian		Gaussian	
Scan, $2S$[b]	I	M or CI	I	M or CI
3				21.1
4		55	37.6	4.6
5			7.4	0.6
6	74	39.6	0.8	<0.1
10	48	24.8		
20	25.1	12.7		
40	12.7	6.4		
80	6.4	3.2		
120	4.2	2.1		
200	2.5	1.3		

[a] These results do not allow for power saturation or line broadening.
[b] Units of scan are half-width of true absorption at half-maximum for lorentzian or half-width of true absorption at $1/e$ times maximum for gaussian. Scans go from $H_0 - S$ to $H_0 + S$, where H_0 is the field at resonance.

3.3.2 Scan Rate and Integration Time

The derivative output of most spectrometers incorporates an adjustable filtering circuit with a time constant τ for suppression of noise. As discussed by Strandberg, Johnson, and Eshback (28) and Poole (20, p. 854), the product of this time constant and the scan rate (expressed in terms of linewidth per unit time) must be much less than one to avoid distortions of the recorded signal. The reduction of signal amplitude, the shift in crossover from positive to negative derivative value, the broadening of the recorded line, and asymmetry are shown in Fig. 3-2. Ernst (9) has discussed these problems, using figures similar to our Fig. 3-2. Distortion is obviously most important where the derivative is changing value most rapidly. For infinite width of scan the second integral or first moment is, in theory, independent of these distortions. For the obvious gross distortion of a lorentzian line and finite scan width, shown in Fig. 3-2, the moment or corrected integral is calculated as 31.4 percent smaller than expected for an infinite scan with no distortion, whereas with this scan width and no distortion the difference is 24.8 percent (Table 3-1). If signals are broadened by

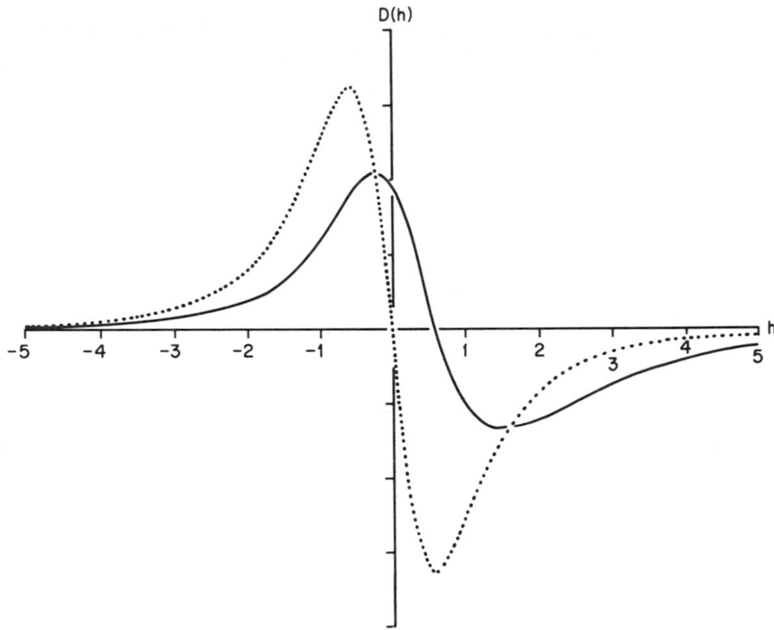

Fig. 3-2. Distortion of lorentzian derivative curve by scan rate. Dotted curve with negligible scan rate; solid curve with scan rate equals (half-width of absorption at half maximum)/(filter time constant). Abscissa units are half-width of absorption at half maximum; ordinate units are arbitrary.

power saturation or overmodulation, the effect of scan rate should be reduced. Henceforth we assume that corrections for scan rate with curves which superficially appear undistorted by the rate of scan are negligible compared with other corrections. Except when using computer techniques (see Section 2.11), the time required for a scan is obviously independent of linewidth, since the optimum scan rate is proportional to linewidth.

3.3.3 Dispersion

The magnetic resonance susceptibility, expressed analytically, is the difference between a real and an imaginary term. The imaginary term corresponds to changes in cavity Q, hence results in power absorption on which spin numbers are usually based. The real term corresponds to a change in frequency or dispersion. If, as is common when we operate a spectrometer at high power, the microwave frequency is stabilized on the sample cavity resonant frequency, the dispersion signal is automatically suppressed. If, as is likely at low power, the microwave frequency is stabilized otherwise, such as on a reference cavity, we may observe the absorption signal, the dispersion signal, or a mixture of the two, depending on phase adjustments of the spectrometer. The derivative of the dispersion signal is symmetrical and resembles the shape of the second derivative of the absorption curve. Hence a mixed dispersion-absorption output is asymmetric (20, p. 530). If the scan is symmetric about the center of the resonance, the contribution of dispersion to the first moment or corrected second integral is zero. For simplicity we assume that dispersion can be ignored for our purposes. This assumption may be questionable for asymmetric derivative curves obtained at low power and analyzed over an asymmetric scan.

3.3.4 Modulation Amplitude, H_m

The recorded output is an approximation of the derivative of the ESR absorption curve with respect to externally applied magnetic field or time (see Section 2.3.3). Field modulation of finite amplitude limits the precision of this approximation. For small modulation amplitude* (i.e., much less than the linewidth) the recorded derivative curve shape is constant and its amplitude is directly proportional to the modulation. This proportionality disappears at larger modulation. When sinusoidal modulation is about equal to the linewidth, a maximum value of the recorded derivative amplitude is obtained; when the modulation amplitude is still greater, the recorded derivative amplitude decreases and the width of the recorded derivative curve increases. Typical results are shown in Fig. 3-3. For measurements of the area under absorption curves the effects of overmodulation on signal amplitude and width are compensatory. Hence, both theoretically (3) and experimentally, the area is directly proportional to the modulation amplitude, regardless of the lineshape, if the scan is infinitely wide. Figure 3-4 demonstrates this experimentally (24) for a single- and a double-line spectrum. Obviously, for concentration measurements, overmodulation is a means of increasing "signal-to-noise." However, since overmodulation puts more significance on values in the wings of spectra, more care is needed in evaluating information in the wings, baseline corrections, and finite cutoff.

With finite scan widths the signal distortion produced by modulation reduces the values obtained by second-integral or first-moment calculations.

* The dials of some instruments give modulation in terms of peak-to-peak modulation of the modulated magnetic field. Mathematically, the modulation amplitude is the maximum excursion from the mean value or half the peak-to-peak value. In this chapter we use *modulation, modulation amplitude,* and H_m interchangeably to mean the mathematically defined term.

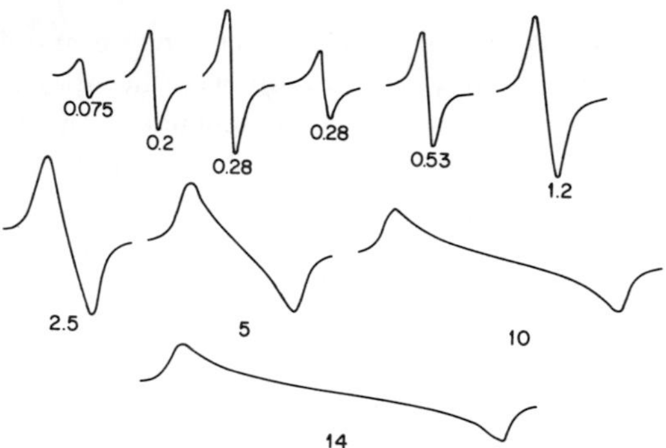

Fig. 3-3. Distortion of lorentzian derivative curves by overmodulation. Modulation indicated in units of undistorted peak-peak width of derivative curve (27).

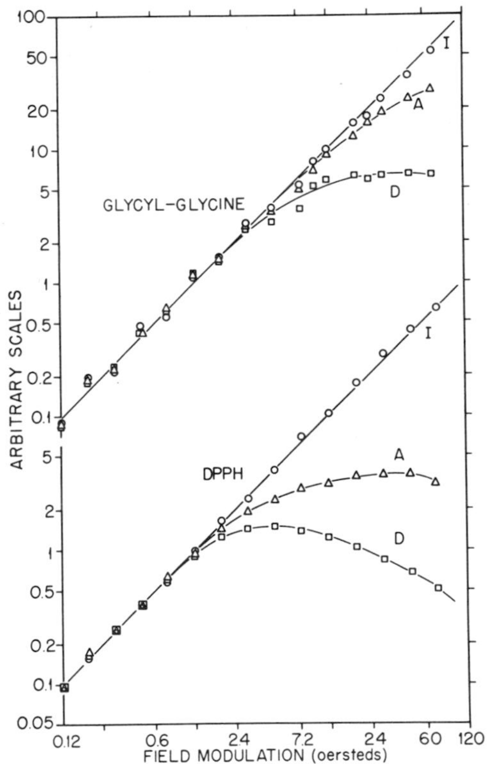

Fig. 3-4. Experimental demonstration of dependence of derivative *D*, absorption, *A*, and second integral, *I*, on modulation. Glycyl-glycine, irradiated with X-rays, gives a doublet with peaks about 17 oe apart and crystalline DPPH gives a singlet with linewidth about 2.5 oe (24).

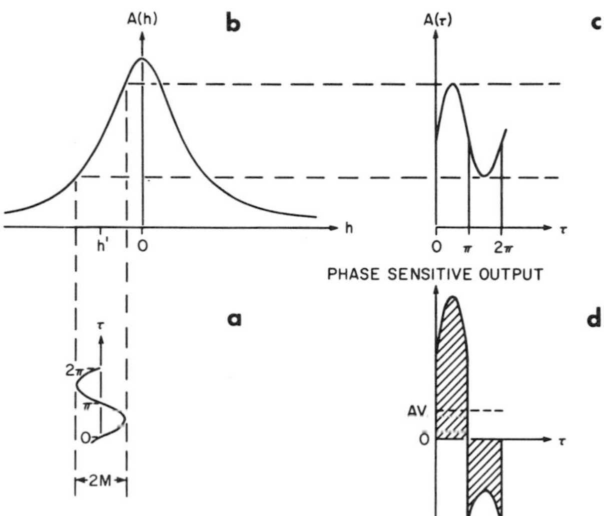

Fig. 3-5. Demonstration of how signal amplitude depends on modulation amplitude. (*a*) One cycle of the sinusoidal variation of field caused by modulation, H_m, shown as a function of time, τ. Typical modulation frequency is 100 kHz. (*b*) Absorption, $A(h)$, plotted versus magnetic field. Going from part (*a*) to (*b*) to (*c*), we see that modulation about an average field value h' causes the variation of absorption with time shown in part (*c*). The phase-sensitive circuitry reverses the polarity of the signal at times $\gamma = \pi, 2\pi, 3\pi$, so that for 1 cycle of modulation the output of the phase-sensitive circuit is as shown in part (*d*). Finally this variation is averaged over many cycles to give a final value such as "AV." in part (*d*).

The operation of modulation and phase-sensitive detection is shown graphically in Fig. 3-5. Mathematically, the signal at field H is given by

$$\text{sig}\,(H) = \int_0^{\pi} A(H + H_m \sin \tau)\, d\tau - \int_{\pi}^{2\pi} A(H + H_m \sin \tau)\, d\tau, \tag{3-11}$$

where $A(h)$ is the true absorption at field h. For infinite scan widths the second-integral or first-moment values for this signal expression are directly proportional to the modulation. We have seen that the values of integrals and moments are reduced at finite scan widths. Application of modulation reduces these values still more. Results of computer calculations for this effect are given in Tables 3-2 and 3-3. The effects of modulation broadening have been treated in more elegant mathematical ways (20, p. 695, 23, 31), but brute-force integrations have seemed more convenient here, especially when we wish to extend the calculations to allow for power saturation.

Table 3-2 Effect of Modulation H_m and Finite Scan $2S$ on Spin Concentration Estimates for Lorentzian Curves[a]

	Percent error $= 100 - M(S, H_m)/H_m M(\infty, 0.01)$						
Modulation[b]	$S^b = 3$	5	10	14	20	28	40
→0	39.3	24.7	12.6	9.0	6.3	4.6	3.2
2	46.7	26.4	12.8		6.3		
3.5		31.7					
5	85.6	46.7	14.2	9.5	6.5	4.6	3.2
7			16.7	10.2			
10			33.7	12.2	7.2		
14			72.5	27.6	8.5	5.1	
20					23.0	6.1	3.6
25					61.3		
28						18.3	4.2
40							15.2

[a] Identical results are obtained by first-moment $M(S, H_m)$ and corrected second-integral calculations.

[b] Units of modulation amplitude and S are half-width of true absorption curve at half maximum. To express either in units of full-width between peaks of true derivative curve multiply values by $\sqrt{3}/2 = 0.866$. Note that full scan width equals $2S$.

Table 3-3 Effect of Modulation H_m and Finite Scan $2S$ on Spin Concentration Estimates for Gaussian Curves[a]

	Percent error $= 100 - M(S, H_m)/H_m M(\infty, 0.01)$				
Modulation[b]	$S^b = 1$	2	3	4	5
→0	56	4.2	0.04	0.00	0.00
0.5	61				
1	71	12.5	0.4	0.00	
1.5			1.8		
2		44	6.3	0.2	
2.5					0.01
3			32	4.5	0.11
4			64	27	3.5
5					23.4

[a] Identical results are obtained by first-moment $M(S, H_m)$ and corrected second-integral calculations.

[b] Units of modulation amplitude and S are half-width of true absorption curve at $1/e$ times the maximum. To express either in units of full width between peaks of true derivative curve multiply values by $1/\sqrt{2} = 0.7071$. Note that full scan width equals $2S$.

Inspection of the results for lorentzian curves given in Table 3-2 reveals that if the modulation is half the scan width the error $E_L(S, H_m = S/2)$ for all scan widths tested is very nearly

$$E_L\left(S, H_m = \frac{S}{2}\right) = \left(\tfrac{9}{8}\right)E_L(S, H_m \to 0)$$

$$= \frac{9}{4\pi}\left(\tan^{-1} S - \frac{S}{1 + S^2}\right), \qquad (3\text{-}12)$$

where $E_L(S, H_m \to 0)$, obtained from Eq. 3-9, is the fractional error for finite scan with negligible error caused by modulation.

For gaussian curves inspection of Table 3-3 reveals that combined scan width and modulation errors are negligible if the half-scan width S is greater than 3.5 and the modulation is half the scan. These wide modulations may grossly distort the lineshapes, especially the derivative, and markedly reduce the peak observed value of the absorption from that expected. Figure 3-6 shows the error in concentration estimates if the modulation is

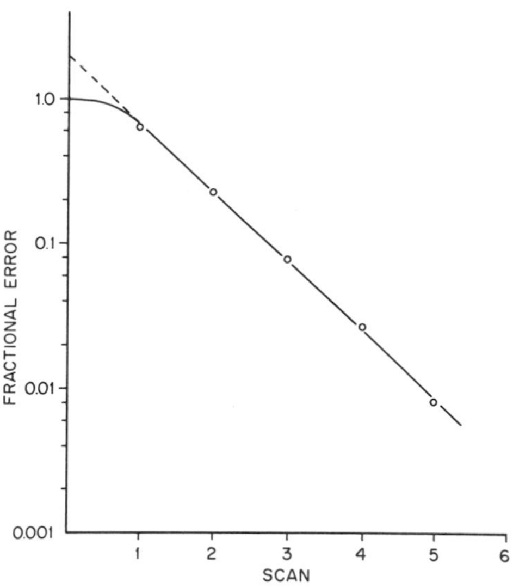

Fig. 3-6. Plot of [fractional error $= 1 - \int_{-S}^{S} A(h)\, dh / \int_{-\infty}^{\infty} A(h)\, dh$] for gaussian curves with modulation $= 0.7S$ versus scan (S). Line is an empirical fit. Scan units are full width of absorption at $1/e$ times maximum.

made 0.7 of the scan width (where modulation and scan are measured in units of half the field width of the true absorption curve at $1/e$ times its maximum). The empirical result over the range of interest ($1 \leq S \leq 5$) is that the percent error E is well approximated by

$$E = 2e^{-1.09S}. \tag{3-13}$$

3.3.5 Power, *P*

Lineshape, relaxation time, and power saturation are bound together in the theory of ESR (see Section 1.3). Here the theory of these subjects is treated only briefly; a more complete treatment is given in Chapters 1 and 2 of this book and in various other places [(20), p. 695].

An ESR experiment consists basically of measuring that portion of the energy of a microwave beam that is absorbed by the sample at resonance. At and near resonance conditions there is a net absorption proportional to the difference in populations of electrons in upper and lower energy states. Normally the relation between upper state n_1 and lower state n_2 electron populations is

$$n_1 = n_2 e^{-\Delta E/kT}, \tag{3-14}$$

where ΔE is the difference in energy between the two states, k is the Boltzmann constant, and T, the absolute temperature (see Section 1.3.3). If the microwave power is great enough, it will increase the upper state population, thus decreasing the difference in populations, the power absorbed, and the observed signal. These phenomena are known as saturation.

There are two physically different mechanisms of line broadening, each with different experimental manifestations (21) (see Section 1.3.1). For *homogeneously* broadened lines the observed lineshape is distorted on power saturation and its amplitude is less than otherwise expected, whereas for *inhomogeneously* broadened lines the lineshape is constant, although its amplitude on power saturation is less than otherwise expected. Since for homogeneously broadened lines the saturation effect is greatest at resonance conditions the experimentally observed linewidth increases with microwave power. We would normally expect a lorentzian line to be homogeneously broadened and a gaussian line to be inhomogeneously broadened. In general, free radicals are much more susceptible to saturation than are paramagnetic transition-metal ions. Although this may cause difficulties in interpretation when both types of ESR signal are present in a sample, it may also allow the two types of signal to be measured separately by varying the power (see Section 2.7).

For homogeneous broadening (10, 14, p. 128, 20, p. 705, 21) the detector signal with linear detection* and constant average power incident on the detector is

$$\text{sig}(h) = \frac{C_1 A(h)\sqrt{P}}{1 + C_2 P A(h)}, \tag{3-15}$$

where C_1 and C_2 are (for a particular resonant species) constants involving terms of no concern to our present discussion, $A(h)$ is the absorption-curve lineshape, as given typically by Eqs. 3-5 and 3-6, and P is the microwave power. The usual spectrometer output is the derivative of Eq. 3-15 with respect to h, or more precisely an approximation of that derivative because of finite modulation and scan rate, as already discussed. The signal distortion produced by power saturation, unlike the distortions produced by modulation or scan rate, always diminishes the estimate of spin concentrations, regardless of scan width. Table 3-4 shows the dependence of various

Table 3-4 Form of Dependence of ESR Outputs on Microwave Power (P) with Infinite Scan and Negligible Modulation

	Homogeneous broadening	
Signal type	Lorentzian	Gaussian
Derivative maximum	$\frac{\sqrt{P}}{(1+P)^{3/2}}$	—
Absorption maximum	$\frac{\sqrt{P}}{1+P}$	$\frac{\sqrt{P}}{1+P}$
First moment or second integral	$\frac{\sqrt{P}}{\sqrt{1+P}}$	$\sqrt{P}\left(\frac{1.4}{\sqrt{1+P}} - 0.4\right)$[a]

[a] Empirical relation applicable in most practical cases—see Table 3-6 and text.

resonance characteristics on microwave power. Obviously at low power the signal corresponding to spin concentration increases as $\sqrt{P}$. An experimental verification of the dependence of second integral on power is shown in Fig. 3-7.

* By "linear detection" we mean use of a detector (e.g., a crystal diode) with the characteristic that, in normal use, the rectified current is proportional to the square root of the incident power.

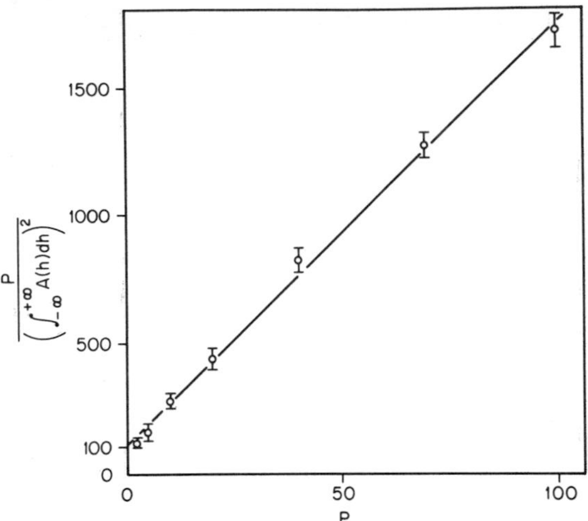

Fig. 3-7. Experimental verification for lorentzian curve of dependence of second integral, $\int_{-\infty}^{\infty} A(h)\, dh$, on power P, both in relative units. $P/(\int_{-\infty}^{\infty} A(h)\, dh)^2 = A + \mathrm{B}P$ (29).

3.3.6 Combined Effect of Scan Width, Modulation, and Power

The most practical cases of the effects of spectrometer settings are those in which scan width, modulation, and power are all finite. If homogeneous broadening applies, the lorentzian and gaussian derivative curves $D_{\mathrm{L}}(H)$ and $D_{\mathrm{G}}(H)$, can be calculated from

$$D_{\mathrm{L}}(H) = H_m \sqrt{P} \times \int_0^{\pi/2} \frac{H \sin \tau \, d\tau}{[1 + P + (H - H_m \sin \tau)^2]\,[1 + P + (H + H_m \sin \tau)^2]}, \tag{3-16}$$

$$D_{\mathrm{G}}(H) = H_m \sqrt{P} \int_0^{\pi/2} \left[\frac{e^{-(S - H_m \sin \tau)^2}}{1 + Pe^{-(S - H_m \sin \tau)^2}} - \frac{e^{-(S + H_m \sin \tau)^2}}{1 + Pe^{-(S + H_m \sin \tau)^2}} \right] d\tau, \tag{3-17}$$

where modulation H_m and scan S are in units used before (see Tables 3-1 and 3-2) and the units of power P are such that the absorption is reduced to half the expected value when $P = 1$. (Expressed this way, the magnitude of P depends on both the physical microwave power and the relaxation times T_1 and T_2 for the resonance. Furthermore, in these expressions we assume constant cavity Q and coupling and suppress a proportionality constant.) Equations 3-16 and 3-17 are, of course, derived from Eqs. 3-5, 3-6, 3-11, and 3-15. Results of calculations of the second integrals, corrected integrals, and first moments from these expressions are given in Tables 3-5 and 3-6.

Inspection of Table 3-5 reveals that for lorentzian lines, homogeneously broadened, the "percent error," or deviation from predicted value in

Table 3-5 Combined Effect of Modulation H_m, Scan Width ($2S$), and Power (P) on Concentration Estimates for Lorentzian Curves Homogeneously Broadened[a]

		Percent error $= 100 - 0.1\, M(P, S, H_m)/H_m \sqrt{P} M(0.01, \infty, 0.01)$			
Power[b]	Scan, $2S$[c]	H_m[c] $\to 0$	$H_m = 0.5S$	$H_m = 5$	$H_m = S$
$\to 0$	10	25	28	47	47
	20	12.6	14.2	14.2	34
	40	6.3	7.2	6.5	23
	80	3.2	3.6	3.2	15.2
0.1	10	29	32	52	52
	20	17.2	18.9	18.9	38
	40	11.0	11.8	11.2	27
	80	7.8	8.2	7.9	20
0.3	10	37	40	57	57
	20	26	27	27	44
	40	18.6	19.4	18.8	34
	80	15.5	15.9	15.5	27
1	10	53	56	69	69
	20	42	43	43	58
	40	36	36	36	49
	80	32	33	33	43

[a] Identical results are obtained by evaluating first moments $M(P, S, H_m)$ and corrected second integrals.

[b] Units of microwave power are the power required (for a particular radical species) to reduce the peak value of the absorption to half that expected from the $\sqrt{P}$ dependence which obtains at low power.

[c] Units of S and modulation are half-width of true absorption curve at $\frac{1}{2}$ times its maximum value.

Table 3-6 Combined Effect of Modulation (H_m), Scan Width ($2S$), and Power (P) on Concentration Estimates for Gaussian Curves Homogeneously Broadened[a]

		Percent error $= 100 - 0.1\, M(P, S, H_m)/H_m \sqrt{P} M(0.01, \infty, 0.01)$			
Power[b]	Scan, $2S$[c]	H_m[c] $\to 0$	$H_m = 0.5S$	$H_m = 2$	$H_m = S$
$\to 0$	4	4.2	12.5	44	44
	6	0.04	1.8	6.3	32
	8	0.00	0.2	0.2	27
	10	0.00	0.01	0.00	23
0.1	4	11.0	19.4	48	48
	6	6.5	8.3	12.7	37
	8	6.5	6.7	6.7	32
	10	6.5	6.5	6.5	29
0.3	4	22.5	30	55	55
	6	17.1	18.8	23	45
	8	17.1	17.3	17.3	40
	10	17.1	17.1	17.1	37
1	4	40	51	69	69
	6	40	41	51	61
	8	40	40	40	57
	10	40	40	40	55
	16				39

[a] Identical results are obtained by evaluating corrected second integrals and first moments $M(P, S, H_m)$.

[b] Units of microwave power are the power required (for a particular radical species) to reduce the peak value of the absorption to half that expected from the $\sqrt{P}$ dependence which obtains at low power.

[c] Units of S and modulation are half-width of true absorption curve at $1/e$ times its maximum value.

concentration measurements, is uniformly increased by $100(1 - 1/\sqrt{1 + P})$ as the microwave power is increased with constant scan and modulation. This is, of course, a reflection that homogeneous broadening is important only near the center of resonance lines; hence its full effect obtains for all practical scan widths. Thus for lorentzian lines, homogeneously broadened with $H_m = 0.5\,S$ (see empirical equation 3-12), the general relation for the percent error is

$$E_{\mathrm{L},H} = 100\left[\frac{9}{4\pi}\left(\tan^{-1} S - \frac{S}{1 + S^2}\right) + 1 - \frac{1}{\sqrt{1 + P}}\right]. \quad (3\text{-}18)$$

Similarly, for gaussian curves inspection of Table 3-6 indicates that the percent error is increased by about $140(1 - 1/\sqrt{1 + P})$, as the microwave power P is increased with constant scan and modulation. Hence, using Equation 3-13, a general empirical equation for the percent error for gaussian lines, homogeneously broadened with $H_m = 0.7\ S$, is

$$E_{\mathrm{G},H} = 200e^{-1.09\ S} + 140(1 - 1/\sqrt{1 + P}). \quad (3\text{-}19)$$

3.4 DUAL CAVITIES

In order to compare quantitatively the numbers of spins in standard and test samples, the experimental conditions, especially the microwave power, must be quantitatively known or known to be equal. Sample insertion into the ESR cavity tends to alter the microwave system. As pointed out long ago by Ehrenberg and Ehrenberg (8), the problems of errors caused by introduction of the sample can, in principle, be solved experimentally by using samples of various sizes and extrapolating to zero sample size. This is obviously a tedious method that becomes impractical for samples which at optimal conditions are near the limit of instrumental sensitivity. Another solution is the use of a dual cavity, as introduced by Köhnlein and Müller in 1960. In such cavities we measure the standard and test samples simultaneously with the intent of measuring both samples with the same coupling Q and microwave field.

Use of a dual cavity, however, is not quite a cure-all. Casteleijn, ten Bosch, and Smidt (6) show by theoretical and experimental methods that if the two samples in a dual cavity (operated in the TE_{104} mode) are distinctly different, especially in bulk and dielectric constant, the microwave magnetic fields they experience are different for two reasons: (a) fields within an ideal cavity are nonhomogeneous and average values will depend on sample geometry and placement; (b) insertion of samples and sample tubes (especially quartz dewars) distorts the field distribution.

3.4.1 Sample Size

Classical electromagnetic theory for an ideal empty cavity predicts that the average microwave field integrated over the volume of a large sample is less than at the optimal (central) position. For a plane sample of radius 3 mm at the optimum height the average of the quasi-stationary and microwave magnetic fields in their (typical) case was 5 percent less than at the axis. At the ends of a long sample the effect may be greater. The variation of fields along the length of the sample is such that signal amplitude per unit length, sig, for a point sample follows the simple relation

$$\text{sig} = \cos^2\left(\frac{\pi l}{2l_0}\right)\text{const.,} \tag{3-20}$$

where $2l$ is the sample length and $2l_0$, the cavity height (about 2.3 cm in typical X-band spectrometers) (19). Averaged over the length of a centrally positioned sample, this becomes

$$\text{sig} = \left(\frac{1}{2} + \frac{l_0}{2\pi l}\sin\frac{\pi l}{l_0}\right)\text{const.,} \tag{3-21}$$

which has limiting values of 1 for zero length and 0.5 for $l = l_0$. For the idealized case the effective correction is taken as the product of the radial and length corrections, which may be an underestimate. Note that these considerations tend to reduce the measured signal of the large unknown sample. Empirical corrections to compensate for this effect may be obtained by measuring signal amplitudes of a point source (e.g., a DPPH crystal) placed at various points in the volume used for experimental samples.

3.4.2 Field Distortion

The second kind of error caused by sample insertion is the more difficult problem of microwave magnetic-field distortion. The effect, as explained by Casteleijn, ten Bosch, and Smidt (6), is shown exaggerated in Fig. 3-8. The results: the optimum position for the negligibly small, standard sample shifts; the resonant frequency of the cavity is decreased; and there is a compression of magnetic field lines in the physically large unknown sample. This compression of field lines in the sample increases the signal amplitude and gives an illusion of greater spectrometer sensitivity, which is merely a reflection of greater microwave inductive field intensity at the sample site, thus causing saturation at a lower apparent power.* The last effect seems the most serious and tends to increase the ratio of signal from the large unknown sample to that from the small standard sample. The shifts in optimum position and resonant frequency are comparable; that is, Casteleijn

* Furthermore, if the inductive field intensity is not constant over the sample, saturation will be reached at different measured power levels for different parts of the sample.

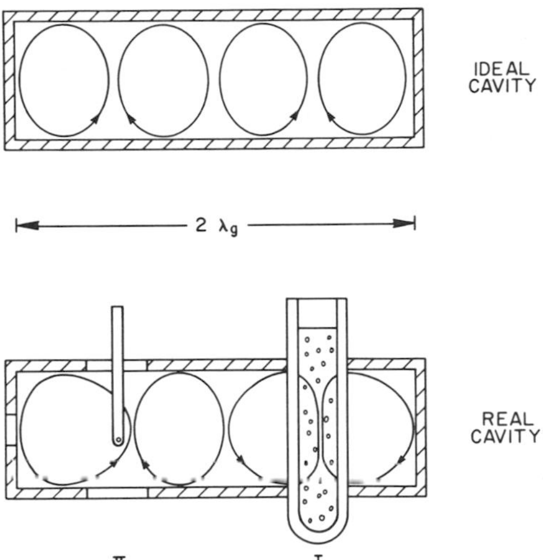

Fig. 3-8. Magnetic field lines in ideal ESR cavity and in real cavity showing exaggerated distortion caused by insertion of large sample with high dielectric constant in sample position *I*. λ_g is the wavelength in the metal waveguide.

and co-workers found that insertion of a standard dewar in one side of the dual cavity produced a shift of about 1.5 mm in optimum position or 4 percent of λ_g, the wavelength in the guide, and a 4 percent change in resonant frequency. For the more common shift of resonant frequency by less than 10 MHz the corresponding shift in optimal positioning is of the order of usual positioning uncertainties.

To evaluate the magnitude of the field compression effect Casteleijn, ten Bosch, and Smidt (6) resorted to an experimental technique. They note that the effective value of the quasi-stationary and microwave magnetic fields can be measured by the ESR technique, and they use a negligibly small DPPH sample in "free space," in empty tubes, at the center of test samples, etc., in both halves of the cavity. They then define a field compression factor f which amounts to

$$f = \left(\frac{Y_{\mathrm{II}}}{Y_{\mathrm{I}}}\right)_0 \left(\frac{Y_{\mathrm{I}}}{Y_{\mathrm{II}}}\right)_s \simeq \left(\frac{Y_{\mathrm{I}}}{Y_{\mathrm{II}}}\right)_s \geq 1, \tag{3-22}$$

where the Y's are signal amplitudes measured at the optimum position in sample holes I and II, with (s) and without (0) a sample in hole 1. The magnitudes of f they found in typical cases are plotted against changes in resonant frequency for an X-band spectrometer in Fig. 3-9. The size of the "points" represents experimental uncertainties and the line is only a crude

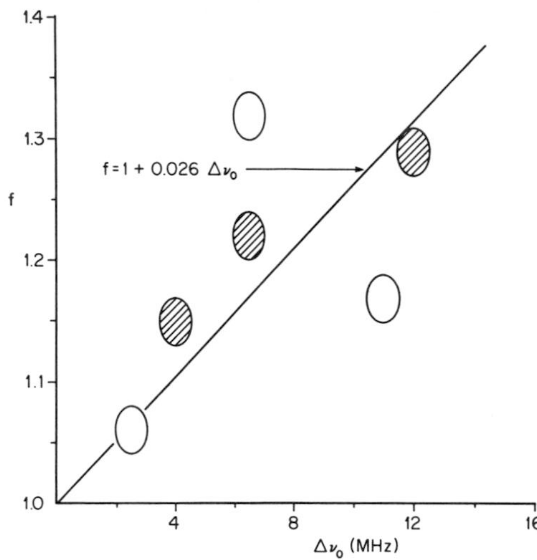

Fig. 3-9. Change in field compression factor f versus change (i.e., reduction) in resonant cavity frequency $\Delta\nu_0$, for X-band cavity (6).

empirical fit, but the conclusion seems to be that if the resonant frequency shifts by 10 MHz we may expect a 25 percent error because of the field compression effect. Note that frequency shifts of 1 MHz can be measured with relatively simple frequency meters such as an HP X532B.

Casteleijn and co-workers (6) then recommend that the overall effect of sample insertion be taken as the product of the radial effect, the length effect, and the field compression factor. This may be sufficiently refined for most uses but remains an incomplete analysis because the radial effect has been evaluated only at $l = 0$ rather than integrated over l; the length effect has been evaluated only at $r = 0$, rather than at all r; and f has been evaluated only at l and r both zero. The assumptions are indicated by the mathematical approximation

$$\frac{\int R(r, l)\, L(r, l)\, f(r, l)\, dv}{\int_v dv} \approx \bar{R}(r, 0)\, \bar{L}(0, l)\, f(0, 0), \qquad \text{(3-23)}$$

where dv is a volume element and v the sample volume. We do not really know how good this approximation is, but the first two factors tend to decrease and the last factor to increase estimates of spins in unknown samples.

3.4.3 Inequality of Sample Positions

Hyde (13) has indicated that errors caused by instrumental differences between the two sample positions (a and b) in a cavity may be minimized experimentally by interchanging the positions of standard (subzero) and unknown samples. If the amplifier gains (G and G_0) for the samples are constant, the unknown spin concentration is

$$N = \frac{N_0 G}{G_0}\left(\frac{M_{0a}M_{0b}}{M_a M_b}\right)^{1/2}, \tag{3-24}$$

where the M's are first moments or second integrals. This procedure removes instrumental differences between sample positions but obviously does not reduce the problems caused by finite versus infinitesimal sample size or by microwave field distortion.

3.5 SIGNAL ERRORS

3.5.1 Kinds of Error

To determine the number of spins in a sample we usually compute results from the approximate derivative output of the ESR spectrometer versus magnetic field. We have discussed how instrumental settings such as power level, scan width, and modulation influence derived results, but our analysis so far has ignored all the possibilities for experimental errors in the signals from the spectrometer. These errors, unlike the considerations already discussed, can lead to differences in the values obtained by first-moment and corrected second-integral calculations. These effects all depend on finite scan width S and, contrary to all previous considerations, generally increase as some power of S. Since both positive and negative effects may occur, cancellation of errors is possible. This section discusses these errors, their effects, and some methods of compensating for them. Implicit in all calculations of this section are the assumptions that true derivative curves are ideal and that the observed curves are free from distortions caused by power saturation, modulation, or scan rate. Here we do not consider signal-to-noise problems, which are discussed by Ernst (9) and elsewhere in this volume (see Section 2-5).

Possibilities for errors in the output of the spectrometer are suggested in Fig. 3-10, in which the real axes are $D(h) = dA/dh$ and h and the false experimental axes are da/dx and x. The errors are α, the initial error in the baseline, β, the tangent of the angle of baseline drift, here assumed to be a constant, γ, the difference between the true and experimentally accepted field for cross-over (i.e., field at which derivative changes sign), and δ, the error in centering the scan on the assumed field cross-over. The error α usually includes $[D(h)]_{\min h}$, the initial value of the real derivative. With the exception of $[D(h)]_{\min h}$, all these errors may be positive or negative. In these terms the experimental approximation da/dx to the true derivative

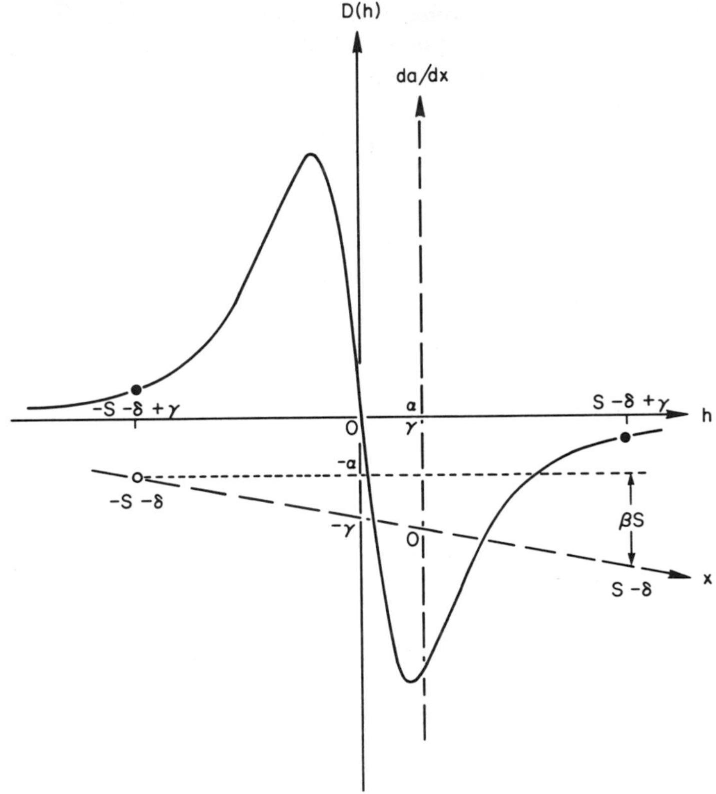

Fig. 3-10. Possible errors in ESR derivative signal versus magnetic field. See text for explanation.

$D(h)$ becomes

$$\frac{da}{dx} = [D(h)]_{h=x+\gamma} + \alpha + \beta(x + S + \delta), \tag{3-25}$$

the limits of integration become

$$- S - \delta \leq x \leq S - \delta \tag{3-26}$$

or

$$- S - \delta + \gamma \leq h \leq S - \delta + \gamma, \tag{3-27}$$

and the moment arm

$$x = h - \gamma. \tag{3-28}$$

We shall consider the effects of these errors, which can be expressed as transformations of axes, separately and in concert.

3.5.2 Corrected Second Integral

The effect of the α error on the calculated absorption curve is shown in Figs. 3-1 and 3-11. Since this tends to be a large error numerically (see Section 3.5.4) and since, when doing double integrations, we usually have the final absorption value available, many workers have compensated for the α error by adding or subtracting an amount proportional to the appropriate triangular area [equal to $SA'(S)$ or $SA''(S)$] in Fig. 3-11.

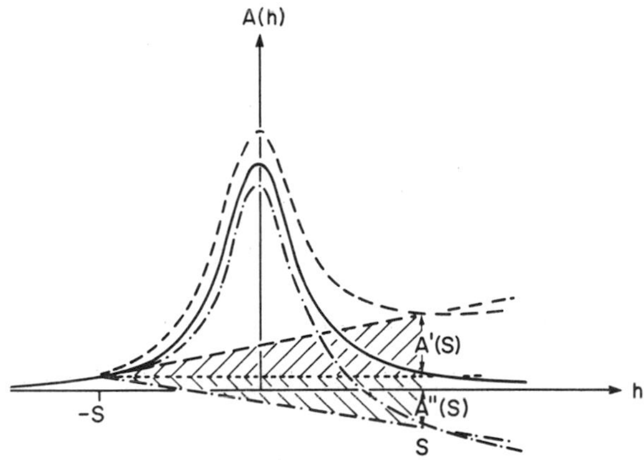

Fig. 3-11. Effect of α error on absorption curve. In calculating area of absorption curve, this may be compensated for by the addition (or subtraction) of shaded triangle.

Since this is a common and very helpful procedure, we consider it as a third computational method, which we call "corrected second integral" or simply "corrected integral."

3.5.3 General Solutions

The effects of the signal errors—α, β, γ, and δ—on the computed first-moment, second-integral, and corrected-integral values are the sum of individual effects plus interaction terms. Here we present the general solutions. A prime purpose of this subsection is to compare the three computational methods.

From Eq. 3-25, basic principles, and some algebra given in the appendix, we can obtain the following expressions for the second integral I, the first moment M and the corrected integral CI.

$$I(S, \alpha, \beta, \gamma, \delta) = \int_{H_i}^{H_f} A(h)\,dh - 2SA(H_i) + 2\alpha S^2 + \frac{4\beta S^3}{3}, \quad (3\text{-}29)$$

$$M(S, \alpha, \beta, \gamma, \delta) = -\int_{H_i}^{H_f} hD(h)\,dh + \gamma[A(H_f) - A(H_i)] + 2\alpha\delta S + 2\beta\delta S^2 - \frac{2\beta S^3}{3}, \quad (3\text{-}30)$$

$$CI(S, \alpha, \beta, \gamma, \delta) = \int_{H_i}^{H_f} A(h)\,dh - S[A(H_i) + A(H_f)] - \frac{2\beta S^3}{3}. \quad (3\text{-}31)$$

3.5.4 Magnitude of Effects of Individual Errors

In subsection 3.5.3 we have developed the general expressions for the results of signal errors. Here we present the magnitude of effects for those errors treated separately. We shall rely on Eqs. 3-29, 3-30, and 3-31.

The effect of the α error is most prominent for the integral method, the moment calculation is independent of α unless δ is also nonzero, and the corrected integral is always independent of α; for example, if α is 1 percent of the maximum peak-to-peak derivative for a lorentzian curve scanned over a range $S = -5$ to $+5$ (of our units), the error in the second integral is more than 20 percent of the expected value in addition to the error due to finite scan. Likewise, for a gaussian curve scanned from $S = -2$ to 2, the error is almost 14 percent. (See Table 3-1 to compare these effects with the effects of finite scan.) The magnitude of this effect dictates good signal-to-noise ratios. Bigger effects would, of course, obtain if the line were broadened by power saturation or field modulation.

A β error alone influences the result for all three methods, as shown in Eqs. 3-29, 3-30, and 3-31. These errors depend on the cube of scan width and may be positive or negative, depending on the sign of β. For a given error ($\pm 2\beta S$) in the final derivative the effect for an integral calculation is the same as for an α value of $2\beta S/3$. This dictates that the spectrometer yield stable baselines.

As a countermeasure to the possibility of β errors it may be desirable to follow the suggestion of Schmidt and Solomon (25) that the development of a high-sensitivity spectrometer with bolometer detection is feasible with good baseline stability or to follow the ESR cavity designs of Franconi (11) with their promise of exceptional baseline stability. Linear corrections for baseline drifts may be obtained by adding to the spectrometer output a properly phased voltage proportional to the voltage controlling the field scan. The constant of proportionality is made such that initial and final values of the derivative signal are equal. Such circuitry is easily devised, but rigorous justification of the use of such a correction is difficult because the baseline drift may be nonlinear or inconsistent. The problem of random, but not systematic, baseline drift is largely mitigated when data are recorded by summing multiple scans ("time-averaging") on a computer, as discussed in Section 2.11.

The γ and δ errors enter into the results through the scan limits H_i and H_f. The magnitude of these effects for various typical cases is given in Tables 3-7 and 3-8. The moment and corrected integral computational methods are much less sensitive to these experimental errors than is the integral computation. For cross-over errors the corrected integral and moment

Table 3-7 Percentage of Errors Caused by Crossover Errors γ at Various Scan Widths[a]

			Percent error = 100[value (S, γ) − value $(S, 0)$]/value $(\infty, 0)$	
Curve shape	Scan, $2S$	Cross-over error	I	M or CI
Lorentzian	10	0.5	7.6	−0.5
		1.0	13	−1.9
		−0.5	−11	−0.5
		−1.0	−27	−1.9
	20	1	4.1	−0.3
		2	6.9	−1.1
		−1	−6.1	−0.3
		−2	−15	−1.1
Gaussian	4	0.2	20	−1.4
		0.5	31	−9.2
		−0.2	−35	−1.4
		−0.5	—	−9.2
	6	0.5	0.7	−0.3
		1.0	0.6	−3.3
		−0.5	−10	−0.3
		−1.0	−80	−3.3

[a] The units of S and cross-over error for lorentzian are half-width of absorption at half maximum and for gaussian, half-width at $1/e$ times maximum.

[b] Positive value indicates that the cross-over occurs before the assumed cross-over.

Table 3-8 Percentage of Errors Caused by Centering Errors δ at Various Scan Widths[a]

Shape	Scan, $2S$	δ (percent of S)[b]	Percent error = 100[value (S, δ) − value $(S, 0)$]/value $(\infty, 0)$		
			I	M	CI
Lorentzian	10	10	7.6	−2.0	−0.5
		20	13	−3.7	−1.9
		30	16	−5.4	−4.6
		−10	−11	3.0	−0.5
		−20	−27	8	−1.9
		−30	−53	17	−4.6
	20	10	4	−1.0	−0.3
		20	7	−2.0	−1.1
		30	9	−2.9	−2.6
		−10	−6	1.6	−0.3
		−20	−15	4.3	−1.1
		−30	−30	9.5	−2.6
	40	20	3.5	−1.0	−0.5
		30	4.4	−1.5	−1.3
		50	5.2	−3.0	−4.9
		−20	−8	2.2	−0.5
		−30	−16	4.9	−1.3
		−50	−54	23	−4.9
Gaussian	4	10	20	−2.6	−1.3
		20	29	−5.4	−5.7
		30	32	−10	−14
		−10	−35	5.4	−1.4
		−20	−92	18	−5.7
		−30	—	44	−14
	6	20	0.8	−0.4	−0.5
		30	0.7	−1.6	−2,2
		50	−0.9	−10.6	−19.5
		−20	−16	2.7	−0.5
		−30	−55	14	−2.2
		−50	—	—	−20

[a] The unit of S for lorentzian is half-width of absorption at half maximum and for gaussian, half-width of absorption at $1/e$ times the maximum.

[b] Positive value indicates that the center of resonance curve occurs before center of scan.

methods yield identical results. For centering errors the corrected integral seems generally, but not always, preferable.

Overall, the corrected integral seems to be the method of choice because it is less or equally dependent on the experimental errors α, β, γ, and δ than are the other methods. The second integral method is clearly most dependent on these same errors.

Extraneous paramagnetic species in impurities or "dirt" in the spectrometer cavity or in dewars or sample tubes may be significant. Even if these species do not yield peaks in the range of observation, they may cause apparent nonlinear baseline drifts that cannot be precisely compensated for by the corrections previously discussed. If apparent baseline drifts are highly reproducible, subtraction of a blank signal from the experimental signal may be an effective correction. Each case, however, must be considered separately and with caution.

It should also be noted that computer processing of ESR spectral data, discussed briefly in Section 2.11, allows ready compensation to be made for experimental errors of the kind described here, before (or even after) spectra are integrated. Random baseline drift, as noted above, tends to average out in the time-averaging mode of data accumulation and background signals may be dealt with in a flexible manner that can involve scaling, shifting, etc.

3.6 STANDARDS

Comparison of a first moment, second integral, or corrected integral value for a test sample versus that for a known standard is the usual method for precise quantitative ESR measurements, as pointed out in the introduction. Most of the complexities in evaluation of results, which we have discussed in this chapter, would disappear if the test and standard samples were measured under identical conditions (e.g., measured simultaneously, using a dual cavity) and if the samples had the same crucial characteristics—bulk dielectric constant, linewidth and -shape, relaxation time (power saturation), similar number of spins, etc. No single standard, obviously, can satisfy all these conditions for all test samples. Presumably crucial characteristics of the standard will be at least as well known as those of the test sample so that the uncertainty in the result will be primarily that in the test sample. To ensure this condition the standard should have an easily detectable number of spins and, if a dual cavity is to be used, should impose no more severe limitations on scan width, modulation, scan rate, or power than the test sample. Stability with respect to time and temperature are also desirable properties of a standard.

DPPH (α,α-diphenyl-β-picryl hydrazyl) has been the most popular standard despite the fact that it does "decay" with time. Paramagnetic salts (e.g., $CuSO_4.5H_2O$) and spin labels also make good standards. If the purity and molecular weight are known, the number of spins present in a fresh sample may be calculated from the sample weight. An indication of the sensitivity of ESR measurements is that practical standards weigh but a few micrograms at most, which may force us to resort to indirect calibrations, such as by optical absorption measurements or titrations with standardized reagents, when absolute values are needed. To obtain volume and dielectric losses comparable to test samples the actual sample may be distributed in an inert material. Hyde (13), Anderson (2), Poole (20, p. 589), and Alger (1, p. 202) have discussed standard samples rather thoroughly.

3.7 CONCLUSIONS

There are numerous applications in biology and other fields for which quantitative ESR values are needed. In doing such work we must first decide what accuracy is required. When samples with identical lineshape, saturation characteristics, and geometry are to be compared in a dual cavity, accurate relative values may be obtained from measurements of derivative peak heights. If, however, the samples to be compared have dissimilar geometry, saturation characteristics, or lineshape or if absolute values are needed, more sophisticated calculations must be made and more attention must be given to such factors as scan width, microwave power, modulation, instrument drifts, and seemingly small measurement errors. How these factors affect absolute quantitative measurements have been discussed in this chapter.

The spin concentration in a sample may be estimated by second-integral, first-moment, or corrected second-integral calculation from the usually presented derivative output of an ESR spectrometer. The uncertainty of the results depends in different ways on possible systematic and random signal errors, with the corrected second integral being the most reliable method; computer data processing may markedly facilitate the correction procedure.

The best compromises in instrument settings differ for quantitative work and maximum sensitivity or determination of lineshape. For quantitative work scan width must generally be greater than for other work, but restrictions of low power and modulation can be relaxed. Scan rate and dispersion are relatively unimportant. Although dual cavities reduce many instrumental problems, they do not eliminate all that might be expected.

The ideal quantitative ESR standard is a stable material with a well-known number of spins having lineshape, -width, and power saturation characteristics similar to those of the test sample. Although a variety of standards have been proposed, a single universal standard seems impractical.

General understanding of the problems discussed in this chapter should enable workers to appraise realistically the importance of various parameters of quantitative measurements, hence to obtain more accurate concentration values.

ACKNOWLEDGMENTS

J. J. ten Bosch and the editors of this book have contributed valuable discussions to this presentation.

APPENDIX

Here we derive Eqs. 3-29, 3-30, and 3-31 from Eqs. 3-25 through 3-28. Integrations with respect to x extend from $x_i = -S - \delta$ to $x_f = S - \delta$ and with respect to h from $H_i = -S + \gamma - \delta$ to $H_f = S + \gamma - \delta$. The second integral, by definition, is

$$I(S, \alpha, \beta, \gamma, \delta) = \int_{x_i}^{x_f} \left(\int_{x_i}^{x} \frac{da}{dx}\, dx \right) dx.$$

From Eq. 3-25 and using Eqs. 3-26, 3-27, and 3-28 we obtain

$$\begin{aligned}
I(S, \alpha, \beta, \gamma, \delta) &= \int_{x_i}^{x_f} \left[\int_{H_i}^{h} D(h)\, dh \right] dx + (\alpha + \beta S + \beta\delta) \int_{x_i}^{x_f} \left(\int_{x_i}^{x} dx \right) dx \\
&\quad + \beta \int_{x_i}^{x_f} \int_{x_i}^{x} x\, dx\, dx \\
&= \int_{H_i}^{H_f} A(h)\, dh - \int_{x_i}^{x_f} A(x_i)\, dx + (\alpha + \beta S + \beta\delta) \\
&\quad \left(\int_{x_i}^{x_f} x\, dx - \int_{x_i}^{x_f} x_i\, dx \right) + \beta \int_{x_i}^{x_f} \frac{x^2}{2}\, dx - \beta \int_{x_i}^{x_f} \frac{x_i^{\,2}}{2}\, dx \\
&= \int_{H_i}^{H_f} A(h)\, dh - 2S\left[A(x_i) + \alpha x_i + \beta S x_i + \beta\delta x_i + \frac{\beta x_i^{\,2}}{2} \right] \\
&\quad - 2S\delta(\alpha + \beta S + \beta\delta) + \frac{\beta}{3}(S^3 + 3S\delta^2) \\
&= \int_{H_i}^{H_f} A(h)\, dh - 2SA(H_i) + 2\alpha S^2 + \frac{4\beta S^3}{3}. \qquad (3\text{-}29)
\end{aligned}$$

The equation for the first moment is developed similarly. By definition

$$M(S, \alpha, \beta, \gamma, \delta) = -\int_{x_i}^{x_f} x \frac{da}{dx}\, dx$$

$$= -\int_{H_i}^{H_f} (h - \gamma)\, D(h)\, dh - (\alpha + \beta S + \beta\delta) \int_{x_i}^{x_f} x\, dx - \beta \int_{x_i}^{x_f} x^2\, dx$$

$$= -\int_{H_i}^{H_f} h\, D(h)\, dh + \gamma[A(H_f) - A(H_i)] + 2\alpha\delta S + 2\beta\delta S^2 - \frac{2\beta S^3}{3}. \tag{3-30}$$

The corrected integral involves, by definition, the following correction term

$$C(S, \alpha, \beta, \gamma, \delta) = S\int_{x_i}^{x_f} \frac{da}{dx}\, dx.$$

On substitution of Eq. 3-25 and integration, we get

$$C(S, \alpha, \beta, \gamma, \delta) = S[A(H_f) - A(H_i)] + 2\alpha S^2 + 2\beta S^3.$$

The corrected second integral is

$$CI(S, \alpha, \beta, \gamma, \delta) = I - C = \int_{H_i}^{H_f} A(h)\, dh - S[A(H_i) + A(H_f)] - \frac{2\beta S^3}{3}. \tag{3-31}$$

REFERENCES

1. R. Alger, *Electron Paramagnetic Resonance: Techniques and Applications*, Wiley-Interscience, New York, 1968.
2. R. Anderson, Electron Spin Resonance, in *Methods in Experimental Physics*, Vol. 3, D. Williams, Ed., Academic, New York, 1962, pp. 440–500.
3. E. Andrew, *Phys. Rev.*, **91,** 425 (1953).
4. N. Bloembergen, *Phys. Rev.*, **109,** 2209–2210 (1958).
5. W. Burgess, *J. Sci. Instr.*, **38,** 98–99 (1961).
6. G. Casteleijn, J. ten Bosch, and J. Smidt, *J. Appl. Phys.*, **39,** 4375–4380 (1968).
7. F. Dyson, *Phys. Rev.*, **98,** 349–358 (1955).
8. A. Ehrenberg and L. Ehrenberg, *Arkiv. Fysik*, **14,** 133–141 (1958).
9. R. Ernst, Sensitivity Enhancement in Magnetic Resonance, in *Advances in Magnetic Resonance*, J. Waugh, Ed., Academic, New York, 1966, pp. 1–135.
10. G. Feher, *Bell System Tech. J.*, **36,** 449–484 (1957).
11. C. Franconi, *Rev. Sci. Instr.*, **41,** 148–149 (1970).
12. A. Gibson and R. Raab, *Rev. Sci. Instr.*, **40,** 410–413 (1969).

13. J. Hyde, Experimental Techniques in EPR, in *Proc. 6th Ann. NMR-EPR Workshop*, Varian Associates, Palo Alto, California, November 5–9, 1962.
14. D. Ingram, *Free Radicals as Studied by Electron Spin Resonance*, Butterworths, London, 1958.
15. H. Judeikis, *J. Appl. Phys.*, **35,** 2615–2617 (1964).
16. W. Köhnlein and A. Müller, *Z. Naturforsch.*, **15b,** 138–139 (1960).
17. W. Köhnlein and A. Müller, A Double Cavity for Precision Measurements of Radical Concentrations, in *Free Radicals in Biological Systems*, M. Blois, Jr., et al., Eds., Academic, New York, 1961, pp. 113–116.
18. W. Köhnlein and A. Müller, *Phys. Med. Biol.*, **6,** 599–604 (1961).
19. C. Montgomery, *Technique of Microwave Measurements*, McGraw-Hill, New York, 1947, p. 295.
20. C. Poole, Jr., *Electron Spin Resonance*, Wiley-Interscience, New York, 1967.
21. A. Portis, *Phys. Rev.*, **91,** 1071–1078 (1953).
22. D. Posener, *Australian J. Phys.*, **12,** 184–196 (1959).
23. E. Putzer and O. Myers, *J. Appl. Phys.*, **37,** 458–459 (1966).
24. M. Randolph, *Rev. Sci. Instr.*, **31,** 949–952 (1960).
25. J. Schmidt and I. Solomon, *J. Appl. Phys.*, **37,** 3719–3724 (1966).
26. H. Slangen, *J. Sci. Instr.*, **3,** 775–778 (1970).
27. G. Smith, *J. Appl. Phys.*, **35,** 1217–1221 (1964).
28. M. Strandberg, H. Johnson, and J. Eshbach, *Rev. Sci. Instr.*, **25,** 776–792 (1954).
29. J. ten Bosch, "Radiation Effects in Collagen, A Quantitative Electron Spin Resonance Study," Ph.D. thesis, University of Utrecht, 1967.
30. J. Van Vleck, *Phys. Rev.*, **57,** 426–447 (1940).
31. H. Wahlquist, *J. Chem. Phys.*, **35,** 1708–1710 (1961).
32. S. Wyard, *J. Sci. Instr.*, **42,** 769–770 (1965).
33. S. Wyard, The Measurement by Electron Spin Resonance Spectroscopy of Local Concentrations of Radiation Produced Radicals, in *Charged Particle Tracks in Solids and Liquids* (Second L. H. Gray Conference) S. Wyard, Ed., the Institute of Physics and the Physical Society, London, 1969, pp. 86–92.
34. A. Yariv and J. Gordon, *Rev. Sci. Instr.*, **32,** 462–463 (1961).

CHAPTER FOUR

Cells and Tissues

HAROLD M. SWARTZ

Departments of Radiology and Biochemistry
The Medical College of Wisconsin
Milwaukee, Wisconsin

4.1 INTRODUCTION

The study of ESR spectra of whole cells and tissues is the most direct approach to determining the existence, role, and importance of free radicals and paramagnetic metal ions in cellular processes. The existence of free radicals in cells was postulated before the introduction of ESR spectroscopy so it was natural that cellular ESR studies began quite early in its development. By 1954 ESR spectra were demonstrated in several normal tissues (18). Since then ESR signals of a bewildering variety have been found in virtually all types of animal and plant preparations, in both normal and pathological states. Unfortunately, because of the complexity of cells and the relatively nonspecific spectroscopic information contained in ESR spectra, interpretation of these spectra in molecular terms is very difficult, and some investigators feel that studies of whole cells and tissues at this time are scientifically unproductive. On the other hand, many other investigators feel that some important biological phenomena can be investigated only by ESR studies of whole cells and tissues (e.g., Ref. 2); that is, once we go below this level of organization, information is lost because some ESR phenomena depend on interactions that occur only in intact cells. This dependence may be in terms of the type of paramagnetic species present or in terms of the stability and reactions of these species (see also Section 7.1).

The question of the wisdom of performing cellular ESR studies is somewhat muted by the fact that many such studies have been performed, more are being performed, and many apparently useful observations have emerged—especially when the experimenters were sophisticated in both ESR and biological techniques. It should also be noted that many published ESR studies have been performed without adequate understanding of the experimental artifacts that can occur in such studies and their results therefore are uninterpretable. This is especially true in regard to studies that utilized lyophilized preparations (see Chapter 5) and in general they are not covered in this chapter. We shall consider in some detail the principal experimental problems encountered in attempting ESR studies of cells and tissues and then critically review some of the results that have been obtained as examples of what has been and can be accomplished.

4.2 EXPERIMENTAL CONSIDERATIONS

The operational goal of tissue ESR studies is to examine paramagnetic species as they occur and change in the unperturbed organism. We have not yet established a means of studying cells *in situ* in the animal with adequate sensitivity and so must make experimental compromises. The experimental methods chosen should be carefully analyzed to determine how much they affect the observations we make. These turn out to be formidable problems because of the interplay of several experimental difficulties. Several useful approaches, however, have evolved over the last few years. Important experimental factors include nonresonant absorption of microwaves by water, spectrometer restrictions on sample size and shape, the nature and low level of paramagnetic species in cells, and the sensitivity of cellular functions to perturbations in the cellular environment. We shall consider each of these factors in turn with the understanding that they are in reality all closely interrelated.

4.2.1 Nonresonant Absorption of Microwaves by Water

Most existing spectrometers utilize 9 GHz electromagnetic radiation to observe spin transitions. This radiation (X-band microwaves) is readily absorbed by polar substances such as liquid water. The interaction is between the electrical component of the electromagnetic field and free polar groups such as the OH portion of the water molecule. The nonresonant absorption process is very efficient and significant amounts of water (0.1 ml or less) will effectively absorb all of the incident microwave from the usual ESR spectrometer microwave sources, thus reducing ESR sensitivity to nil (see Chapter 2). There are several ways in which this difficulty can be overcome but each solution brings with it several complications. Before discussing them in detail, however, we should briefly consider the state of water in biological systems.

Most functional cells are 50 to 90 percent water, although highly specialized cells or structures (such as hair, insect skeletons, and seeds) may contain much less water. Within a cell the water is not randomly distributed and there may be relatively dry regions. Also, much of the water in the cell is not really free but oriented or bound to various extents. The dielectric properties, hence the microwave absorbing properties of the cell, depend on freedom of motion of the water molecule and are also affected by the presence of ionic species such as Na^+, K^+ and Cl^-. As a consequence it is not possible to calculate accurately the nonresonant microwave absorption by cells. Average dielectric properties of cells can be measured and calculations made, but the usual and most practical procedure for ESR spectroscopy is to determine empirically the effect of cellular water on the particular experimental preparation being utilized (see Section 2.9). The general experimental observation has been that nonresonant absorption has been less than expected on the basis of the water and salt content alone, probably because a significant fraction of the intracellular water is bound tightly enough so that its dipolar motion in the oscillating electric field of the microwave radiation is restricted, much as in ice which is less "lossy" than liquid water.

Some electromagnetic frequencies above and below X band are not so readily absorbed by water (95) and spectrometers have been built to utilize these frequencies of exciting radiation. The size of the sample cavity and the strength of the magnetic field required for resonance are both affected by the choice of frequency. Lower frequencies allow larger samples and require lower strength (but larger size) magnetic fields. The overall sensitivity (in terms of minimum total spins that are detectable) is a direct function of frequency (see Section 2.10) and so low frequency spectrometers are less sensitive. For studies in which the concentration of spins cannot be changed, such as tissue, the effect of the larger sensitive volume may be a gain in effective sensitivity; for example, if an X-band spectrometer could detect 10^{12} spins/ml and a lower frequency spectrometer could detect only 10^{14} spins/ml and they took samples of 1 and 1000 ml, respectively, a sample with 10^{11} spins/ml could not be detected in X band but could be detected by the lower frequency instrument). Several low-frequency spectrometers have been built and used for tissue studies, but the results to date have been disappointing and have not approached theoretical sensitivity limits. They do offer advantages in ease of sample handling, however, and have even been used to study whole animals. The results to date and the lack of commercially available low-frequency instruments suggest that such instrumentation will not be a practical alternative in the near future.

There are commercially available higher frequency instruments (35 GHz: *Q* band) that operate in a region in which nonresonant absorption is not quite so severe a problem. The principal difficulty here is the very small sample size that must be utilized with this frequency. This feature, however, also offers a potential advantage: Q-band cylindrical tissue samples for TE_{011} cavities are small enough to be readily filled by needle biopsies of organs and this could prove valuable *if* clinical applications of ESR should eventuate. Nevertheless, there have been few reports of tissue studies with this frequency. It does offer an additional advantage in that some signals which overlap at X band may be separated at 35 GHz (see Section 2.10). The higher frequency spectrometer may be more expensive because of the higher strength magnet required, but the availability of these instruments is rapidly increasing and their utility for tissue ESR will probably be rapidly explored in the near future.

Another, more useful, set of alternatives is to continue to utilize X-band spectrometers but to eliminate the nonresonant absorption of water by (a) removing it (lyophilization or drying), (b) positioning it to minimize its interaction with the electrical field (oriented tissue slices), or (c) changing the water to a low-microwave-absorbing state (ice).

Lyophilization and/or drying are discussed in detail in Chapter 5, with the conclusion that this technique is of limited utility for tissue ESR studies.

If we use thin slices of tissue and carefully orient them in a rectangular microwave cavity, a position can be found in which the water in the tissues will not drastically affect the *Q* of the cavity. Many data have been obtained with such preparations. This is possible because it is the electrical component of the electromagnetic radiation that interacts with water and results in nonresonant absorption, whereas it is the magnetic component that interacts with unpaired spins and results in resonant absorption. Within rectangular microwave cavities (see Fig. 2-2) there is a plane at the center of the cavity at which the magnetic field is a maximum and the electrical field a minimum. The sample, in the form of a thin flat slice, is placed so that it occupies this region. Careful alignment is required because the actual region of minimum electrical field is quite small and large differences in nonresonant absorption can result from small changes in positioning. The use of the flat cell causes several other experimental difficulties as well. The preparation of thin tissue slices may cause functional changes in cells due to the slicing process. In addition, the small volume available precludes regulation of metabolic exchange. Oxygen and nutrients cannot be supplied to the tissue and its metabolic products cannot be removed. With single-cell or subcellular organelle preparations some of these difficulties might be overcome with a flow system, but there have been few published reports of such experiments. Putting too much tissue in the cell may result in pressure effects, whereas failure to fill the tissue cell completely will affect sensitivity. Some authors (22, 54) have suggested that the use of long multimode cavities may offer some practical advantage if flat cells are used. These advantages include less dependence on tissue placement position and perhaps some ease in sample preparation. Long cavities and long flat cells are not commercially available, however, and they do result in a decrease in sensitivity due to poor filling factors (see Section 2.9).

An analogous microwave situation exists in cylindrical cavities in which there is an electrical minimum and a magnetic maximum down the longitudinal axis. In this situation a capillary tube is used, which is adequate for single-cell preparations but not for tissues that have not first been homogenized. Cylindrical capillary tubes can also be used in rectangular cavities but they are less efficient than flat cells for lossy samples such as tissue.

The requirement of small sample sizes and the low levels of paramagnetic entities in tissues require prolonged observation times for adequate sensitivity (see Section 2.11). As indicated in later sections, the tissue ESR spectra change with time and temperature so that the prolonged observation times required lead to considerable experimental difficulties.

Many of these problems can be resolved by the use of frozen samples (without subsequent removal of water). When water is frozen, its dielectric constant drops from 80 to $\sim$ 2; hence there is a much reduced problem of nonresonant absorption by the water. This means that the sample size is restricted only by the usual sample limitations of the cavity employed and allows a sample more than 10 times larger than the sample used for the aqueous state methods. The use of a lower temperature also increases the sensitivity as a result of a more favorable ratio between the two possible spin states (see Section 2.19). Because of the increased sensitivity with frozen samples, averaging techniques are often not required and samples can be run much more quickly. The fact that fast freezing to 77 K stops virtually all cellular processes also allows us to take many more samples in a short time and then examine them by ESR when it is convenient. Samples can also be re-examined as desired.

Several potential problems may emerge when frozen samples are used. In aqueous-state samples at 273 K or higher, transition metal ions are often not observable because of their low concentration and the width of their lines. At 77 K most transition metal ions are readily detected and may overlie the free radical areas and complicate the interpretation of the data. At 77 K, however, the relaxation times of the transition-metal ions are much shorter than those of the usual tissue free radicals, and so the two types of ESR signal can be differentiated by means of power-saturation studies (see Section 2.7). (In fact, if one is interested in the transition-metal ions contained in cells, the use of frozen preparations is virtually a necessity.) Another drawback in the use of frozen materials is the elimination of the possibility of performing dynamic studies on the same sample. An available alternative is to take a number of different samples sequentially from similarly treated populations. Finally, there is the possibility that the process of freezing causes artifacts in the free radical spectra. This last point has been investigated, and except for the factor discussed above (paramagnetic ions and relaxation time effects) freezing was found to have little effect on preexisting free radicals (53, 99); that is, quick freezing appears to stabilize indefinitely the radicals existing in the cell just before freezing (see Section 2.18.1). One possible exception is free radical generation if oxygen is present at the time of freezing (97, 98).

4.2.2 Sample Size and Configuration Requirements

As indicated in the preceding section, each alternative sample-preparation method carries with it limitations on sample size and configuration. In X-band studies, the most extreme limitations are associated with attempts to observe tissue in the wet functional state. In rectangular cavities this means very thin oriented samples must be utilized with resulting small sample size, large surface area subjected to trauma, and limitations on metabolic exchanges. Cylindrical cavities require homogenization of tissues, thus vitiating one of the principal reasons for attempting whole-tissue studies. The least stringent sample size and configuration limitations are associated with frozen samples, but, even in this situation, considerable tissue trauma occurs in sample preparation and standard techniques limit the samples to 5 to 6 mm diameter cylinders 1 to 2 cm long. (Significantly larger volumes may be utilized with special cavities which allow the use of larger dewar inserts*; samples of several grams may be studied with these techniques.)

4.2.3 Sensitivity of Biological Processes to Environmental Changes

The sensitivity of biological processes to environmental changes seems so obvious that it should not need to be mentioned, except that this factor seems to have been ignored in many studies. There is currently no sample preparation technique that does not subject cells to an unphysiological environment. With X-band spectrometers the least disturbance may be obtained by the use of quickly frozen samples which give a sort of snapshot of the state of the cell before freezing. Particular caution must be used in interpreting the results of tissue-slice preparations because of the physical trauma involved in their preparation and the long observation times required. The last is especially important because of the inability to regulate the environment of tissue slices. [Mallard and Kent (65) have suggested that instead of the term "surviving tissues," often applied to such preparations, "dying tissues" might be more appropriate.]

The effects of various environmental factors on these and other preparations are considered in detail in the experimental result sections. A particularly important point is the temperature dependence of the free-radical signals seen in aqueous samples. The number and type of free radicals seen in these samples varies with temperature and the time a preparation is held at a particular temperature. The usual experimental compromise has been to study tissues at about 15 C, at which temperature there are still a detectable number of radicals that do not disappear too quickly.

4.2.4 Nature of the Paramagnetic Species in Cells

The properties of different types and amounts of paramagnetic species in cells give rise to certain experimental considerations. First, unlike pure chemical solutions, cells contain several paramagnetic species, many of which have overlapping spectra. Second, the concentrations of many of these species are quite low, requiring large amplifications and thus raising the possibility that paramagnetic species extrinsic to the sample will interfere. Third, the power saturation characteristics of different species vary widely and may easily lead to large quantitative and qualitative errors

* The usual X-band cavity has a stack diameter of 11 mm. A TE_{011} special cavity is available with a 25-mm stack diameter and a TE_{102} cavity with a 20-mm stack.

As noted before, organic free radicals in cells, especially in frozen preparations, power saturate readily, whereas transition element ions, which are usually also present in cells, power saturate much less readily, and so at higher power levels they may dominate the experimental spectra, although their concentrations are less than those of the free radicals. There is no simple solution to these problems but several approaches may be tried.

Careful power saturation studies must be done to find the level at which power saturation is negligible for the most readily saturable species (which is usually a free radical); this is especially important in studies with frozen samples. Such studies may also indicate whether there are paramagnetic species present which have overlapping spectra but which can be differentiated on the basis of their power saturation properties. Power may have to be reduced to 10 μW or less to eliminate power saturation completely in frozen samples (Fig. 4-1). Most commercial ESR spectrometers do not readily reach power levels this low and therefore many reported quantitative results with tissue are suspect. Measurement of effective power levels at the locus of tissue samples is quite difficult because of the nonresonant absorption of power by water. Measurements of incident power will be misleading because of variations in the Q factor of the cavity. One solution is to use a dual cavity with a nonpower-saturating standard in the second cavity and to base power measurements on the intensity of the standard signal (e.g., Ref. 98; see also Sections 2.7 and 3.4).

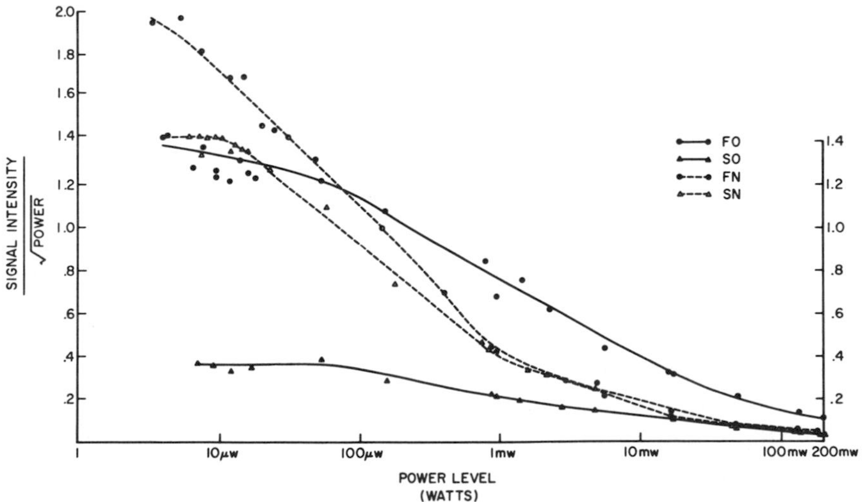

Fig. 4-1 Power saturation behavior of frozen *E. coli*. FO = fast frozen from oxygen-saturated solution, SN = slow frozen from nitrogen-saturated solution, etc. A negative slope indicates power saturation. (Data from Ref. 98, with permission of the publishers.)

Quantitative calculations of signal intensities and/or qualitative evaluation of spectra can be made in the presence of contaminants by subtracting that portion of the spectra due to the contaminants. The shape of the spectra due to the contaminants must be known and computers are essential if more than a few spectra are to be so analyzed (see Section 2.11). The most elementary of these procedures—subtraction of background signals in the cavity and/or sample holder—has been used by several groups but great caution must still be exercised to ensure that the presence of the sample does not significantly alter effective power levels. One approach is to use a dual cavity with identically contaminated sample cells and balance out the signal due to the sample cell by changing the phase of the standard cavity by 180° (93).

The contribution due to transition elements within the sample cannot be corrected for by any simple procedure. The best approach is probably to vary microwave power to determine the shape of the contributions due to the transition elements (which should predominate at high power levels) and then use a computer to subtract this signal shape at low power levels. This procedure assumes either that there is a spectral component of the transition element species sufficiently separated from the free-radical area to permit evaluation of the quantity present at a given power level or that extrapolation down from high power will give quantitatively and qualitatively accurate results at low power. To date few studies have used such techniques to evaluate data, and therefore many data must be considered semiquantitative at best. Such data may be useful if their nature is understood, but they can lead to considerable error if the approximations involved are not recognized.

The problem of resolving overlapping spectra, implicit in the preceding paragraph, is a profound one for biological investigations, but several approaches are possible. In addition to power saturation studies, thermal annealing, observations at different temperatures, phase shifting, observation at different frequencies, isotopic substitution and computer processing for resolution enhancement have all been used with varying degrees of success in studies of biological material. These techniques are discussed in more detail in Sections 2.11 and 2.17. Other, more sophisticated instrumental methods, such as double resonance techniques, may also be useful, but they have not yet been applied in tissue studies.

4.2.5 Artifactual Signals

While attempting to observe ESR spectra of cells and tissues we may detect signals, extrinsic to biological processes, which must be clearly differentiated. The most obvious source of these signals is paramagnetic contamination of the cavity and/or sample holders. Because of the high amplification frequently employed in biological ESR studies, such contamination is a constant problem and background spectra must be run frequently. Occasionally it may not be possible to remove the contaminant or to obtain a contaminant free sample holder and we must resort to subtraction techniques. These procedures are not only time consuming but also potentially inaccurate if instrumental conditions are not precisely duplicated while obtaining the background. The presence of the sample may influence cavity Q, dielectric loss, etc., and make reproduction of instrumental conditions quite difficult, although computer techniques may allow some of these changes to be compensated before background spectra are subtracted (see Section 2.11.4).

A second set of possible artifactual signals can develop in sample preparation. The problems associated with lyophilization are discussed in detail in Chapter 5. A considerable part of the signal seen in lyophilized samples does not reflect pre-existing unpaired spins and is due to interaction of cell contents with oxygen; whether the capacity of cell contents to interact with oxygen to form detectable ESR signals reflects some basic biological parameter is not clearly established. Several other preparation artifacts can occur. Rubbing, mixing, and grinding can mechanically induce resonances in many biopolymers, including DNA (1, 114) and probably in tissues as well. Pressures generated by freezing may also rupture molecular bonds producing unpaired electrons, although this does not appear to be a problem under the usual conditions used for tissue studies (53, 99). The presence of oxygen in the freezing media does, however, affect radical formation in bacteria (97, 98), and this effect could occur in tissues that were reoxygenated before freezing (*re*oxygenation is stressed because tissue preparation techniques ordinarily result in anoxia due to continued cellular metabolism without adequate perfusion). Oxygen can also lead to apparent artifacts by changing relaxation times in frozen solutions but this effect can be avoided by careful determination of the power saturation characteristics of each type of sample and by operating well below the saturation level (44).

Finally, care must be taken that external paramagnetic impurities are not brought into the sample during preparation. Several such instances are described in the literature with contamination from such sources as a compression apparatus and washing solutions.

4.2.6 Summary

In summary, considerable difficulties have been encountered in attempting to perform reliable tissue ESR studies but often these can be overcome by using existing techniques with reasonable caution. As indicated in the following sections, many interesting and potentially valuable facts have been elucidated by tissue ESR. The findings to date suggest that even more useful results may be obtained in the future by careful workers.

4.3 EXPERIMENTAL FINDINGS IN TISSUE ESR STUDIES

The current, generally accepted experimental findings are summarized here without any attempt to be exhaustively complete. [A list of studies of individual tissues has recently been published by Wyard (129).] In general, we consider only the results of unfrozen and quick-frozen samples, omitting reference to work based on lyophilized preparations for the reasons given in Chapter 5. Although the discussion centers on signals seen near $g = 2.0$, some comments are made also on pertinent findings in other parts of the spectrum. When pertinent, unpublished findings from our laboratory are indicated if the literature has not covered a particular topic.

4.3.1 ESR Spectra of Normal Tissues

Most normal tissues have qualitatively similar spectra, with prominent broad peaks at $g = 2.00$*, $g = 1.97$, and $g = 1.94$. Some tissues also have peaks at $g = 2.01$, $g = 2.03$, and $g = 4$. The positions of these peaks are relatively consistent, but their nomenclature is not, and the result is some confusion. Some, such as the $g = 2.00$ peak, are designated by their "apparent" g factors, the points of zero slope corresponding to the cross-over points near the middle of the first derivative curves. Some of the other peaks have their g factors assigned to the points of first-derivative maxima or minima. The situation is further confused by presentations of data as absorption or second-derivative curves as well as the usual first-derivative curves. The actual g factors cannot be determined readily in complex spectra with broad lines, but since in theory, absorption, and first- and second-derivative curves all contain the same information, there is no reason to prefer one system over another so long as it is clear what system is being used. Unfortunately this is not always the case, and care must be exercised in referring to the literature.

Different tissues vary markedly in the relative prominence and shape of these peaks. Within a single tissue the relative intensities of the different peaks may vary with environmental changes (118) and power level (100). The latter can result in quite dramatic differences, as indicated in Fig. 4-2. As already stated, this variation with power is due to the fact that the spectra observed in tissues usually derive from several components with different relaxation times and some may power-saturate at the usual microwave power levels used with commercial instruments.

The origin and meaning of the different peaks are incompletely under-

* More precisely, $g = 2.0035 \pm 0.0008$, but we use the less precise designation $g = 2.00$ in in the following to avoid confusion with reports in the literature of values that vary in the last two decimal places for a variety of reasons, some experimental, some instrumental.

stood. In general, organic free radicals occur at $g = 2.00$ (organosulfur radicals may have a component at $g = 2.06$ and organoperoxy radicals may have a component at $g = 2.03$, but these rarely occur in nonirradiated tissues), whereas signals from paramagnetic transition element ions (including those in organic matrices) occur at various g factors and account for virtually all lines away from the $g = 2.00$ area, as well as part of the $g = 2.00$ signal. Studies of pure enzyme systems and subcellular particles have provided detailed information about many of the lines due to paramagnetic ions, but some are still incompletely understood. This is especially true in malignant tissues which may have ESR spectral components that differ qualitatively and quantitatively from normal tissue.

Our primary interest is in the $g = 2.00$ area where organic free-radical signals occur, yet our understanding of this region is incomplete because of the complex composition of tissues and the unresolved spectral character of the composite "free-radical peak." At low microwave power levels, especially in wet preparations, the $g = 2.00$ peak predominates (20, 67, 109),

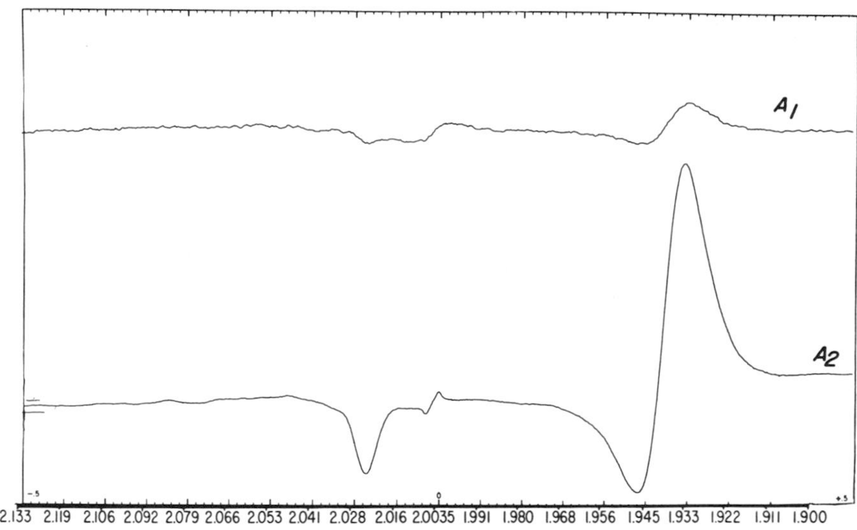

Fig. 4-2 ESR spectra of quickly frozen normal canine tissues. Instrumental settings selected to produce maximum signal/noise at 77 K without distortion. The g-factor scale is indicated on the abscissa. $\nu \sim 9.25$ GHz, using a Varian E-9 dual cavity spectrometer. Incident microwave power in milliwatts, relative amplification, modulation amplitude (100 kHz) in gauss, time constant, and scan time (for the 400-G-wide area shown in these figures) are listed under each figure.

A_1 = adrenal, 0.01 mW, ×40, 10 G, 1 sec, 4 min.
A_2 = adrenal, 200 mW, ×2.5, 8 G, 1 sec, 16 min.

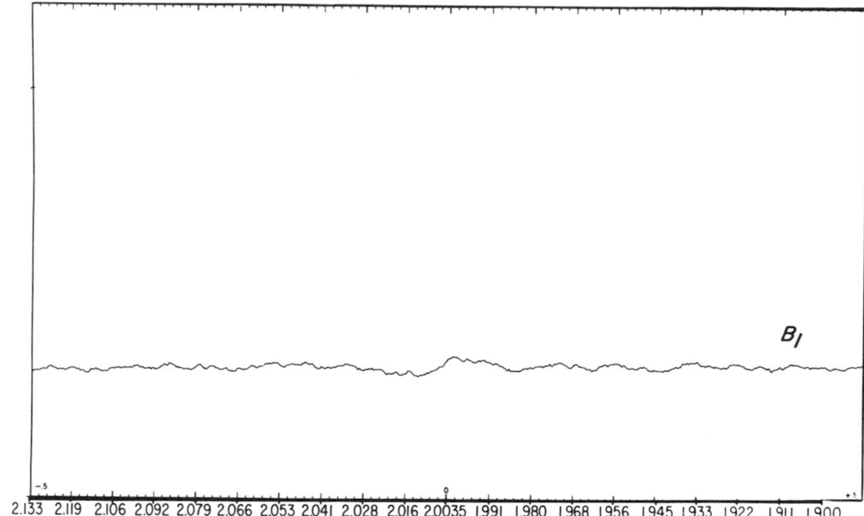

B_1 = bone, 0.01 mW, ×250, 8 G, 10 sec, 16 min.

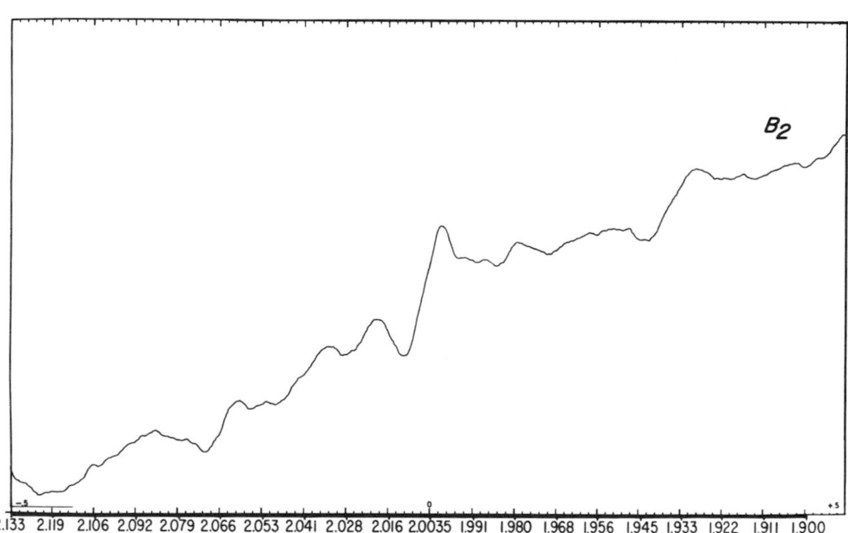

B_2 = bone, 200 mW, ×10, 10 G, 10 sec, 30 min.

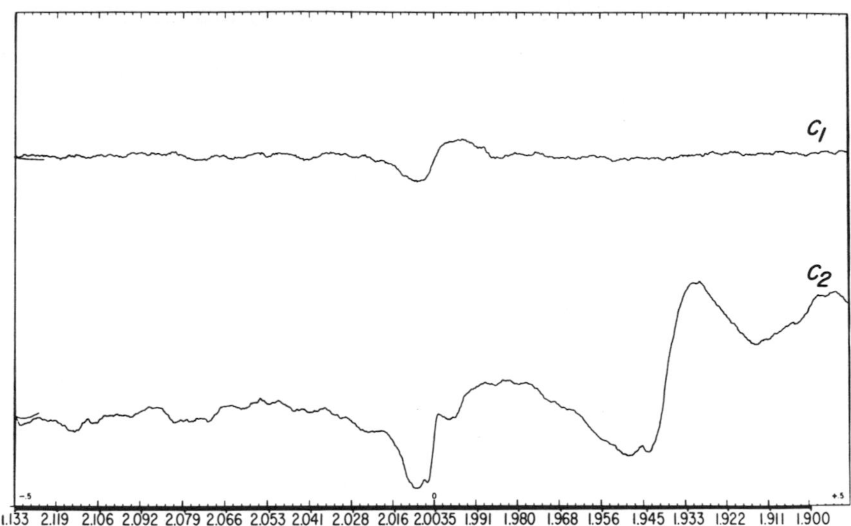

C_1 = brain, 0.01 mW, ×250, 8 G, 10 sec, 16 min.
C_2 = brain, 200 mW, ×32, 8 G, 3 sec, 16 min.

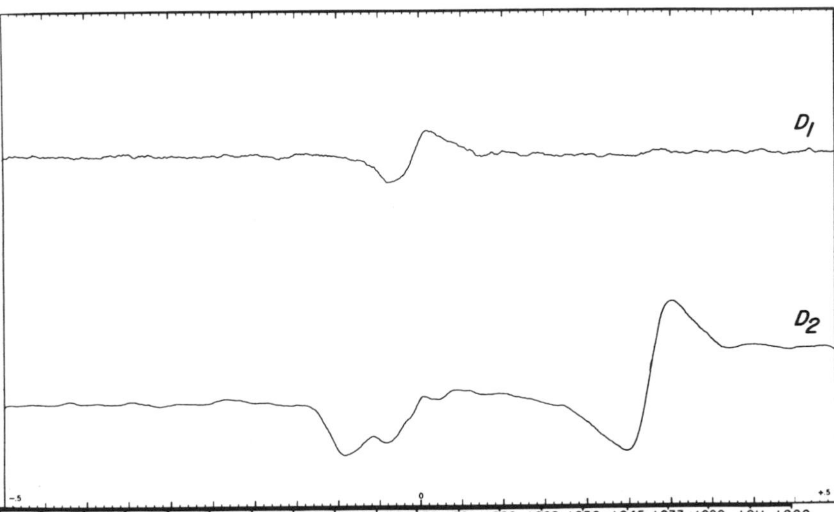

D_1 = heart, 0.01 mW, ×80, 8 G, 3 sec, 8 min.
D_2 = heart, 200 mW, ×10, 8 G, 3 sec, 16 min.

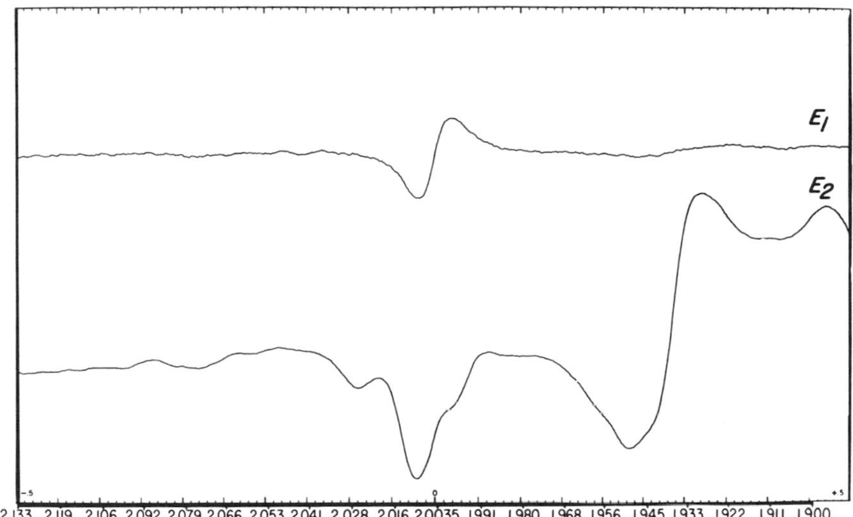

E_1 = kidney, 0.01 mW, ×63, 8 G, 3 sec, 8 min.
E_2 = kidney, 200 mW, × 10, 8 G, 10 sec, 30 min.

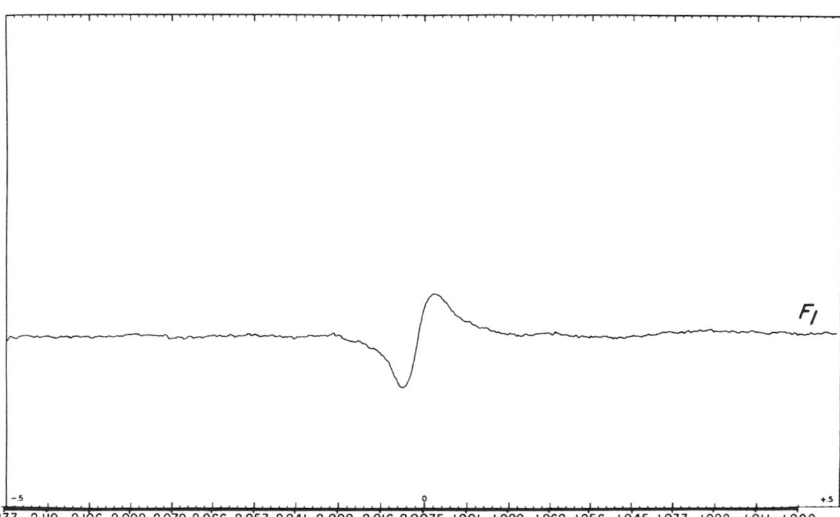

F_1 = liver, 0.01 mW, ×63, 8 G, 3 sec, 16 min.

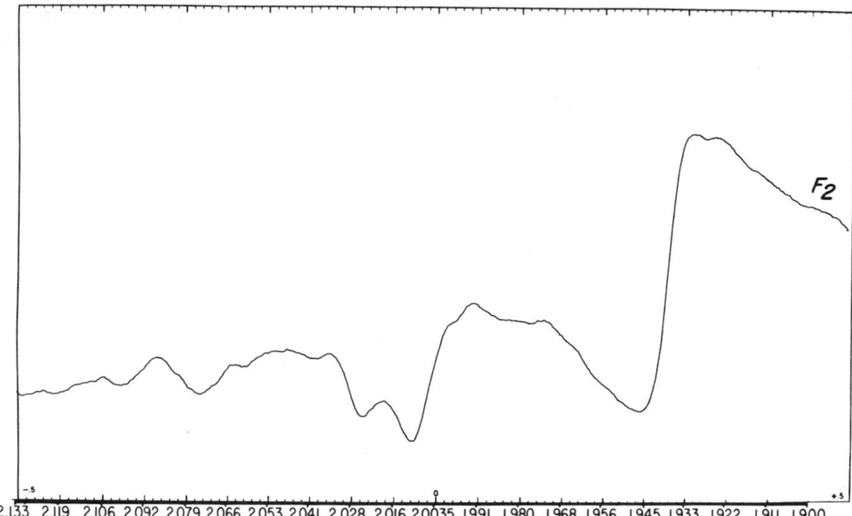

F_2 = liver, 200 mW, ×20, 8 G, 3 sec, 16 min.

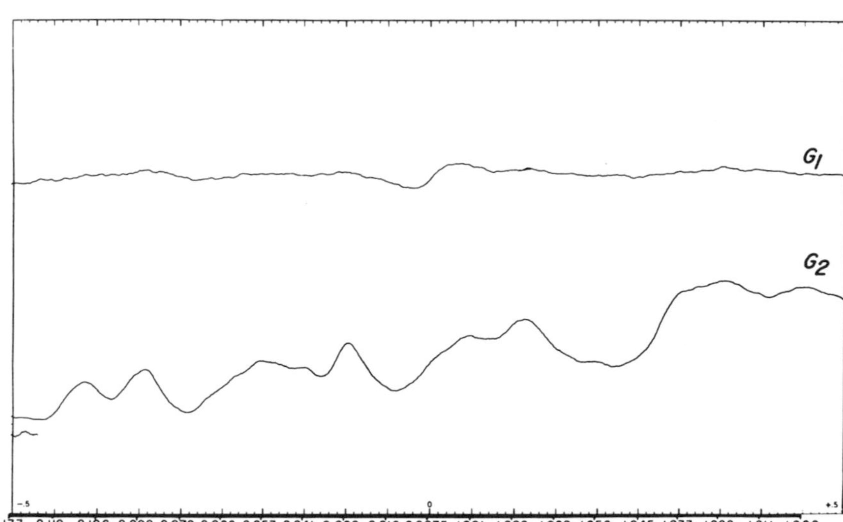

G_1 = pancreas, 0.01 mW, ×10, 12.5 G, 3 sec, 2 min.
G_2 = pancreas, 200 mW, ×10, 12.5 G, 3 sec, 16 min.

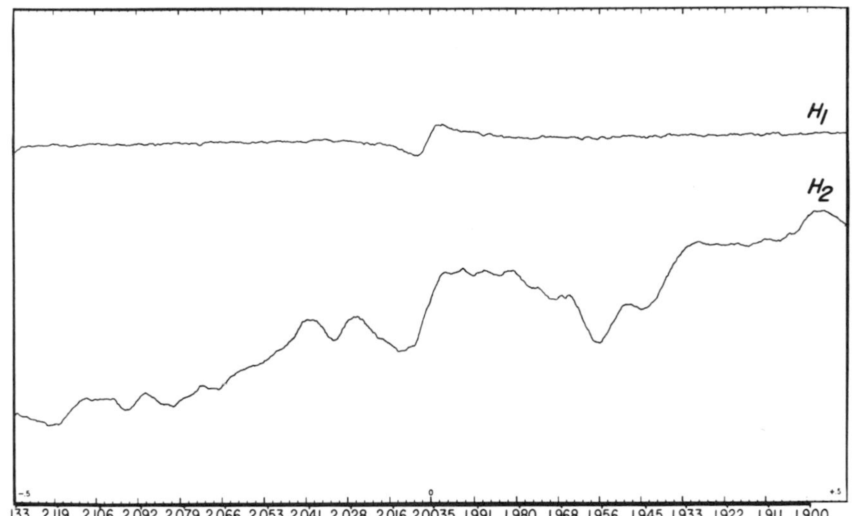

H_1 = spleen, 0.01 mW, ×125, 10 G, 10 sec, 30 min.
H_2 = spleen, 200 mW, ×50, 12.5 G, 10 sec, 30 min.

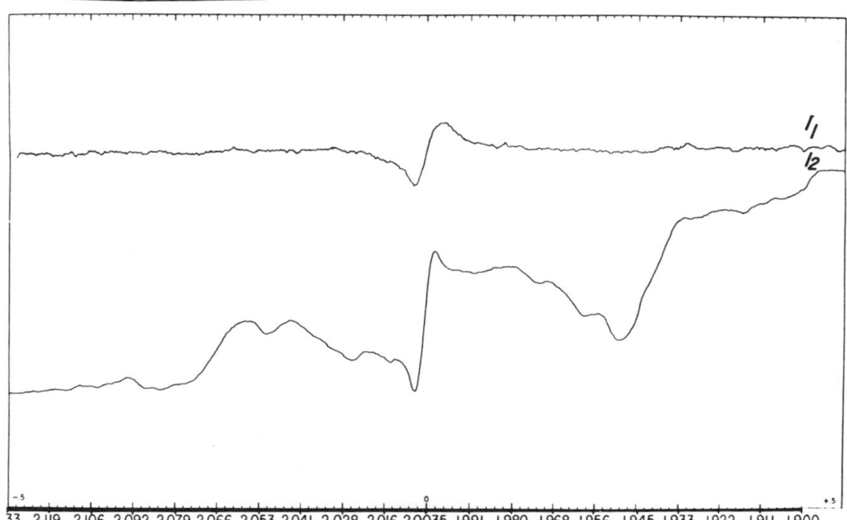

I_1 = stomach, 0.01 mW, ×200, 10 G, 10 sec, 30 min.
I_2 = stomach, 200 mW, ×40, 10 G, 10 sec, 30 min.

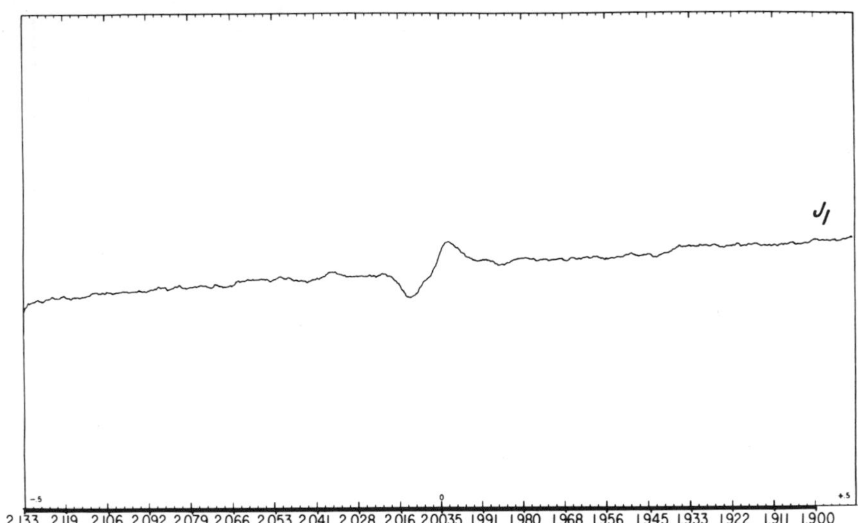

J_1 = testicle, 0.01 mW, × 160, 10 G, 10 sec, 30 min.

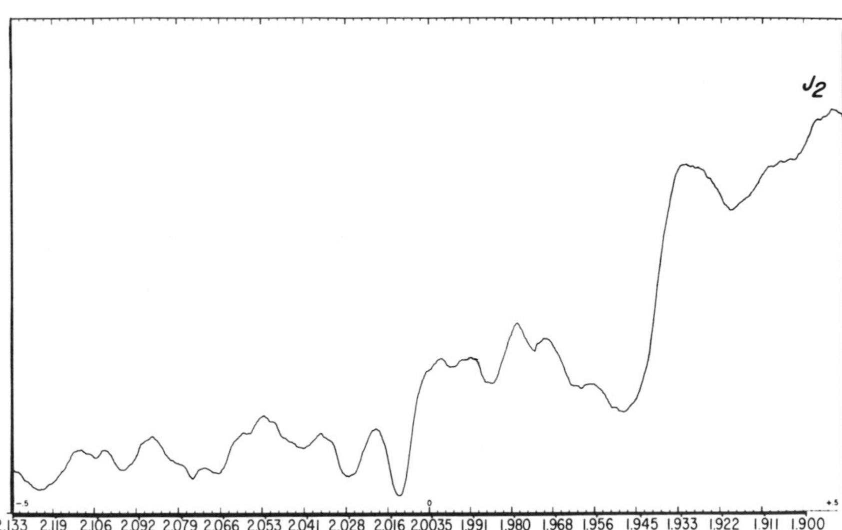

J_2 = testicle, 200 mW, × 50, 10 G, 10 sec, 60 min.

and it appears that many different organic free radicals may contribute to form the observed peak. At higher microwave power levels ($\sim$ 1 mW) the apparent contribution from free radicals may decrease due to power saturation and there may be a significant contribution from transition metals with components in the $g = 2$ area.

The type of signals dominating the $g = 2.00$ area of tissue also appear to change with time, as indicated in Fig. 4-3. The dramatic changes seen in this figure are probably due to changes in the ligand fields and/or to changed valence states of paramagnetic elements with components in the $g = 2.00$ area. When free radicals are the principal components of the $g = 2.00$ peak, the type of free radical predominating in the tissue may change without any such change in lineshape. This occurs because the observed peak is really an envelope of the spectra of different radicals that occur at almost the same g factor; hence they overlap one another. Changes in power saturation are easier to determine, however. They are also a reliable

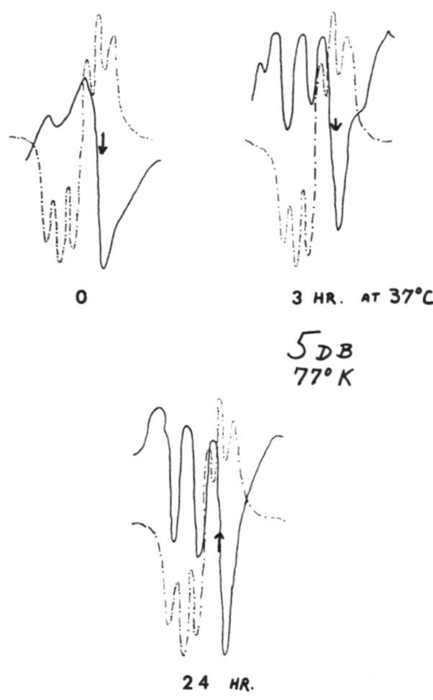

Fig. 4-3 ESR spectra of dog liver, held at 37 C for 0, 3, and 24 hr. Direct tracing of dual channel output of modified Varian V-4500 (6 in.) spectrometer. A DPPH in benzene standard (400-Hz modulation) is shown as a dotted line. The corresponding position of the center of the DPPH spectrum (to correct for pen displacement) is indicated by the arrow. The solid line is the 100-kHz modulated signal from the liver at 77 K; incident microwave power $\sim$150 mW (5 dB attenuation of full output power).

indicator of a change in radical species (if the environment has not changed greatly).

As shown in Fig. 4-4, the power saturation characteristics of ESR from fresh liver change with temperature and time, thus indicating a change in species even though the spectral shape has not changed. If we were to follow just the amplitude of the $g = 2.00$ signal, it is apparent that erroneous conclusions regarding changes in radical concentrations could result if the complex nature of the signal were not considered. Additionally, extension of such experiments for one to two days indicates that some of the $g = 2.00$ signal that appears to be due to free radicals is quite persistent, perhaps because it really originates from inorganic transition elements. Truby and Goldzieher (113), in a brief study that utilized three samples, also found

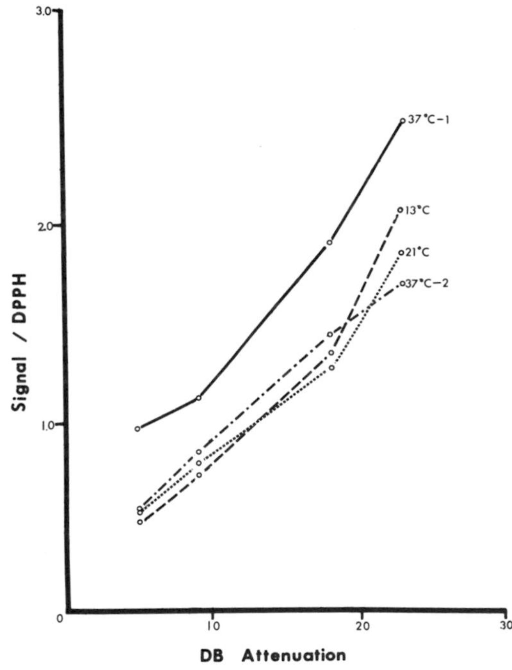

Fig. 4-4 Power saturation studies of a rat liver slice at various temperatures. The same sample was used for the entire study. It was placed in a tissue cell in the 100-kHz modulated cavity of a modified Varian V-4500 Dual Cavity X-Band Spectrometer, with a DPPH in benzene standard in the 400-Hz modulated cavity. Incident microwave power was progressively attenuated during each series of studies at an indicated temperature. The signal shape did not change; therefore first derivative peak-peak heights were utilized for quantification. These values were adjusted for changes in cavity Q by means of the observed signal intensity of the DPPH standard. The sample was observed first at 37 C, then at 21 C, then at 13 C, and finally at 37 C again; the latter is labeled 37 C-2.

that about 60 percent of the $g = 2.00$ signal in rat liver persisted for at least two weeks. Such findings indicate that we cannot interpret the $g = 2.00$ signal purely in terms of equilibrium concentrations of unstable organic radicals. Other experimental data on the nature of the components giving rise to the observed $g = 2.00$ signal are considered in detail in some of the following sections.

4.3.2 Multicellular Whole Organisms

A few intact multicellular organisms have been studied by ESR. The obvious limitations of these studies are size of the organism and its water content. The use of low-frequency ESR spectrometers to study tissues is discussed in Sections 4.2.1 and 2.17. Insects and other invertebrates have been studied (58, 94, 101) with conventional X-band instruments (9 GHz). The resulting spectra are usually simple single peaks in the $g = 2.00$ area. In some cases there are additional lines due to transition-metal ions, especially Mn^{2+}. The $g = 2.00$ signal appears to be due to both metabolic free radicals and, in pigmented tissues, melanin.

Nonresonant absorption due to water has not limited studies so much as might have been anticipated, probably because much of the water content of cells is "bound" in such a way that it interacts less efficiently with microwave quanta. This may account for the successful observation of resonances from the tail of a living rat in an X-band spectrometer in our laboratory.

An advantage of such whole organism studies is that they allow the observation of ESR parameters under physiological conditions with the possibility of further experimental manipulation also remaining. Development of instrumentation that would permit high-sensitivity ESR studies of intact mammals is proceeding in several laboratories. Commoner's group has reported preliminary specifications for such an instrument that utilizes a slow-wave detector instead of a microwave reflection cavity.

4.3.3 Microorganisms

ESR signals have been noted from a variety of microorganisms (31, 48, 86, 103, 127). These signals closely resemble those seen from mammalian tissues and include free radicals and trace elements. Manganese (II), copper (II), and iron are especially prominent in some species (108, 110, 111). The Mn^{2+} hyperfine structure may disappear when the ion is part of an aggregate or macromolecular complex. Failure to realize this fact can lead to highly erroneous results, such as those of Fischer et al. (31), who ascribed the unpaired electron content of the Mn complex to free radicals and who therefore claimed an apparent 100-fold increase in free radicals in an Arthrobacter species in the presence of Mn. In general, the shape of trace-element spectra from microorganisms suggests that the metals are bound to macromolecules. Data on the nature of this binding and on the function of the trace elements may prove to be some of the most valuable information obtainable by ESR studies of cells.

Isenberg and Baird (48) demonstrated ESR signals in anoxic thick suspensions of *E. coli* and found that they were related to viability, killed cells having no detectable signal. The signal was a 24-G wide singlet centered at $g = 2.00$. It should be noted, however, that in frozen bacteria the type of gas in the freezing medium can affect the number and type of radicals observed (97, 98, and Fig. 4-1). Similar gas effects may occur in frozen tissue but they have not been studied.

Microorganisms have also been used to study free-radical intermediates produced by biogenic oxidation or reduction (49, 126). Such studies provide information on metabolic capacities and pathways of cells, including the availability of electrons for reduction. Variations in the hyperfine structure of the free radicals produced by microorganisms may lead to information on the binding of the radicals to macromolecules. This kind of information may be especially important to an understanding of the mechanism of action of certain inhibitors (see Section 7.5.4).

The action of certain fungicides has been studied by ESR with observation of the production of a free-radical form of one fungicide and an apparent effect on trace-element oxidation states by another (Ref. 86 and Section 7.5.8).

4.3.4 Plants and Seeds

ESR signals (in addition to those associated with photosynthesis, see Chapter 6) have been reported in a variety of plants and seeds (21, 27, 36, 60, 77, 107), usually small in magnitude and quite long-lived. The usual seed spectrum is 5 to 25 G wide and without distinctive shape. In lettuce seeds the approximate number of spins per seed was 2×10^{13} (36). Wetting reversibly decreased the intensities of the observable resonances (83). At room temperature power saturation began at about 25 mW. Small signals have also been reported in several types of fruit (84). Changes of free-radical concentrations in seeds with storage time were investigated as a possible explanation of the increase in mutations noted in aged seeds, but no such increases were found (21, 107).

Trace metals may also contribute to the observed spectra seen in plant materials (21, 83, 90). A definite Mn^{2+} signal was detected in a variety of plant materials, including pine needles and cones, oak leaves, and ivy stems, and a probable Cu^{2+} signal was found in oak leaves and cotton. A broad signal reported at $g = 4$ (21, 82) may be due to iron or Co^{2+}.

Although most studies of plants have been done on dried materials, a few reports have been made on moistened or wet seeds on which a 0.3 GHz spectrometer was used (23, 92), but the low sensitivity of this instrument prevented the study of resonances except those induced by ionizing radiation. Malinovski and Kafalieva (64), using S-band (2.4 GHz) found readily detectable signals in living leaves and roots of several plants and directly demonstrated that they disappeared during lyophilization. A new signal was generated during or after the lypholization or drying process (see Chapter 5). All parts of the living plants had single peaks 10 to 13 G wide.

Borg (unpublished), using a flat cell in a standard X-band spectrometer, observed the six line Mn hfs plus photosynthetic free radical signals in intact leaves of the pond plant *Elodea canadensis*. Both components varied with light exposure, and the Mn^{2+} signal decreased with circulation of oxygenated medium in the dark.

4.3.5 Cell Components

To help us understand the findings from intact tissue samples, some of the studies done on cell components, including subcellular organelles, are reviewed. Additional discussions of particular paramagnetic species (such as enzymes) are given in other parts of the book, but the coverage here is limited to cell components that may play a significant role in the observed tissue ESR spectra.

4.3.5.1 Subcellular Organelles

A large portion, or (in the view of some authors) *all* the signals obtained from normal whole cells comes from the microsomes and mitochondria. This is especially true of the signals occurring away from the free-radical area. Microsomal fractions give prominent signals at $g = 2.41$, 2.25, and 1.91, whereas mitochondrial preparations have prominent lines at $g = 2.004$ and 1.94 (41). Each type of organelle may also show a number of other lines, including easily saturable $g = 2.0$ signals in some microsomal preparations (57). Most of the microsomal and mitochondrial preparation signals show little power saturation at 77 K, but they do broaden considerably at higher temperatures.

Mason et al. (71) separated liver cells into mitochondrial, microsomal, and "supernatant" fractions and demonstrated that all the qualitative features of whole-cell preparations at high microwave power could be accounted for by the fractions (Fig. 4-5). Their findings included a prominent signal in the $g = 2.0$ area in the supernatant. The contributions of the various subcellular elements to whole-cell ESR was also studied by Brzhevskaya et al. (15). Using fairly crude separations, they reported that at least

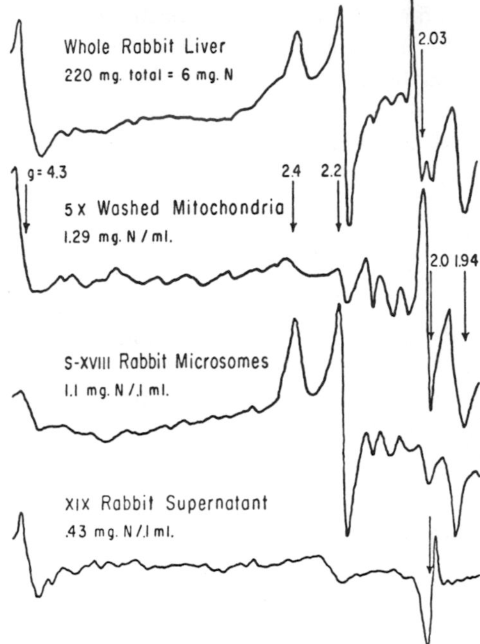

Fig. 4-5 ESR spectra of whole rabbit liver and homogenates at 113K, modulation amplitude 32 G at 100 kHz, scan speed 132 G/min. Samples suspended in 0.2 ml of 0.01 *M* tris-phosphate buffer, pH 8.2. (From Ref. 71, with permission of the publishers.)

50 percent of the intact-cell ESR signal was in the mitochondria. They found little signal in the nuclei or cytoplasm, but there was essentially the same signal in homogenized and whole cells.

In vitro manipulation of whole mitochondrial preparations indicates that the ESR spectra are relatively stable to environmental manipulations (14, 124). The signals remain stable at ice-bath temperatures for at least 24 hr but decay slowly at higher temperatures. Heating to 60 C irreversibly destroys the $g = 2.00$ signal. The use of inhibitors was reported by one author to result in about a 20 percent decrease in the intensity of the $g = 2.00$ signal (124); another found no change (14). Some changes appeared to occur with the use of uncoupling agents, but these were quite complex and had no definite pattern (see Sections 7.5.4 and 7.5.5).

Mason et al. concluded that the $g = 2.25$, 2.41, and 1.91 peaks belonged to the same species in rabbit liver because they showed similar temperature dependencies. This species appears to be a low-spin ferric hemoprotein (Fe_x). Much of the mitochondrial signal also appears to be due to iron-containing proteins (see Chapter 8). Microsomes of pig thyroid and rat brain (57) do not show the Fe_x signal but have a $g = 2.004$ signal. A similar signal has been reported in other microsomal preparations.

In general, the ESR properties of cell organelles indicate that they contribute importantly to the ESR signal seen in intact cells, especially at high microwave power, but the spectra of these organelles vary with physiological conditions and organ type. Therefore simple generalizations on the contributions of organelles to cell ESR spectra are likely to be misleading and each type of preparation must be individually investigated.

4.3.5.2 Melanin

The term *melanin* describes a number of related pigmented materials with definite chemical characteristics, including considerable chemical and physical stability. Commoner's (18) original observations included the fact that melanin contains stable free radicals. In pigmented tissues this signal may overwhelm other free radicals and it must always be considered when evaluating the ESR spectrum of a tissue. A detailed consideration of ESR studies of melanin is beyond the scope of this chapter, but several reviews are available (e.g., Ref. 9) and some additional aspects are covered in Section 7.3.7. The origin and role of the unpaired electron has been the subject of considerable speculation and several hypotheses have been put forward to suggest that the free radical nature of melanin accounts for some of its biological properties such as radiation protection. These speculations have been supported by the fact that melanin reacts readily with most free radicals. Recent studies in our laboratories, however, indicate that the reactivity of melanin with free radicals is unrelated to its unpaired electrons. Melanin has been reacted with a model free radical, DPPH, to completion and the number and type of unpaired spins in the melanin was found to be the same before and after, although all of the DPPH was consumed. The reactions of the added free radicals apparently occur with the quinoid part of the melanin polymer subunits. The unpaired electrons of melanin do not appear to be readily available to react, which is consistent with the fact that the number of unpaired electrons in melanin is unchanged after very drastic chemical treatments such as boiling for 24 hr in concentrated acid or base. The spins will apparently react more readily with paramagnetic elements, the apparent concentration changing in the presence of copper (9). In any case, some reduction of the melanin signal by NADH has been observed by Van Woert and a reduced melanin was hypothesized (115).

In addition to the spins normally found in melanin, it is also possible to induce additional unpaired electrons by visible or UV light (70). These spins appear to be much more reactive, possibly because they are located nearer surfaces, although they are spectroscopically indistinguishable from those seen in the ground state. A physiological role of these light-induced spins has been postulated, especially in visual processes (25).

4.3.5.3 Nucleic Acids

Although a number of early reports indicated unique ESR properties of nucleic acids and nucleoproteins (7, 8, 73, 74), it now appears that these spectra were due to contaminating paramagnetic metals (6, 47, 63, 91, 125). Very pure preparations generally do not show reproducible ESR signals. It is still possible that some of the "contaminants" represent functional additions to nucleic acids, but the bulk of the evidence is to the contrary. Part of the confusion regarding the origin of the observed ESR signals in nucleic acids was due to the assumption that the signals originated from paramagnetic species, whereas they actually appear to have originated from ferromagnetic constituents which give an apparent 1000-fold larger signal intensity per atom (91). The ferromagnetism may arise from chemical conversion during processing of constituents that normally do contain iron, but the iron *in vivo* is not in a ferromagnetic state and is too low in concentration for its possible paramagnetism to be determined (125).

4.3.5.4 $g = 2.03$ and $g = 1.94$ Signals

A considerable volume of literature, especially Russian, has built up concerning a peak seen at $g = 2.03$ (30, 117, 120–122). This signal is convenient to observe and follow because it is located away from the free radical area ($g = 2.00$) and therefore is not obscured by it. Early studies suggested that this signal might be due to an organic free radical with a high unpaired electron density on a sulfur atom (analogous to the organo-sulfur free radical seen in some sulfur containing compounds after irradiation) (see Chapter 10). The bulk of the evidence now indicates that this signal is associated with a paramagnetic ion complex rather than a true free radical. The signal appears to be related to the $g = 1.94$ signal seen in many tissues and ascribed to the iron in sulfur proteins.

A role of sulfur in the $g = 2.03$ signal is suggested by its location, temperature dependence, and the effects of thiol inhibitors on it (121, 122). Hollocher et al. (41), using ^{33}S proved that the $g = 2.026$ peak seen in *A. vinelandii* iron-sulfur proteins involved a sulfur atom. This and other work also suggested a close relationship to the $g = 1.94$ signal. On the other hand, a 1:1 relationship appears unlikely because the $g = 2.03$ signal and the $g = 1.94$ signals do not always change together and only the $g = 2.03$ signal can be observed at room temperature (122). Vanin et al. (117) feel that they may have now resolved this question, suggesting that the $g = 2.03$ and $g = 1.94$ signals arise from the same type of iron-sulfur proteins and represent different configurations of the same molecules. They do not indicate the nature of these conformational changes (see Section 7.3.12).

A prominent signal in the $g = 1.94$ area is usually found in many biological samples. In mammals it arises in mitochondria, and it has been shown to be due to iron in an unusual ligand field that includes a sulfur atom. The identification of this signal by isotope substitution studies (26, 43, 89) is a prime example of how sophisticated techniques can be successfully applied to complex samples. This signal is considered in greater detail in Chapter 8.

4.3.6 Whole Tissues and Cells

4.3.6.1 Physiological Variations

Variation of both *in vivo* and *in vitro* environmental factors can affect the observed ESR spectra of "healthy" cells and tissues. Neither type of variation has been fully studied, yet knowledge of these environmental effects appears essential if we are to interpret ESR studies of pathological parameters. Our current knowledge is summarized below.

A. IN VITRO VARIATIONS

Oxygen. The initial studies of "surviving" tissue by Commoner and Ternberg (20) established some of the important *in vitro* parameters. They found that the tissue signal was independent of oxygenation. This important finding would appear to have profound implications in the interpretation of the origin and significance of tissue ESR studies, but there has been little further work reported on this subject. The use of thin tissue slices makes adequate oxygenation quite difficult and most workers have not attempted to attack this problem, settling for hypoxic or anoxic samples.

Temperature. Commoner et al.'s original wet-tissue report (20) included the observation that the $g = 2.00$ tissue signal persisted for at least hours or days if held near 0 C; later they found (109) that they could retain the signal by freezing tissue and thawing just before observation. Other authors have reported similar findings (67). Raising the temperature of the tissue sample above 20 C leads to an irreversible loss of intensity, although the literature varies in regard to the precise rate of disappearance (55, 67).

Boiling was reported to have caused loss of all signals in either mitochondria or whole tissue (19, 20), although in our laboratory we have found that some signals due to transition metal ions do persist after boiling for 5 min. Prolonged boiling for 60 min may lead to generation of new signals due to changes in paramagnetic ions (17). Moderate temperature elevations (to about 15 C) may reversibly increase signal intensity and a transient increase will probably occur at higher temperatures. The effect of the suspending media on these temperature-intensity effects is not clear. It seems inevitable, in view of the limited metabolic interchange possible in flat tissue cells, that the tissues are quickly subjected to unusual environments, with a build-up of metabolic products at temperatures permitting even moderate cellular activity. Therefore the composition of the suspending medium is not really known for experiments with long observation times.

Time Between Sample Removal and ESR Observation or Freezing. Recent studies indicate that the early findings that tissue could be held for long periods of time without changing the ESR spectra may not apply in all cases, and it now appears that ESR spectra can change significantly as a function of time and temperature after biopsy. Because there is currently no sufficiently sensitive method to observe animal tissues *in vivo*, all studies must involve biopsy procedures for tissue sampling. These procedures introduce time delays before observation. The effect of the biopsy techniques and sample processing per se have already been considered, but, in addition to these factors, the passage of time is also important.

Figure 4-3 shows the qualitative changes seen over a period of hours in tissue from organs removed from healthy animals and held at 37 C for various times before biopsy and freezing. These changes have been studied in livers of several species (rats, mice, dogs, rabbits, sheep, and swine) and are quite reproducible. Similar changes have been observed in kidneys and may occur in other tissues. The changes appear as a function of the time and temperature of holding. By combining qualitative and quantitative parameters the interval between tissue removal (or death of the animal) and freezing can be estimated, a technique that may have potential medical-legal applications.

The long persistence of signals in the $g = 2.00$ area beyond the time of tissue viability has important implications in interpretation of experimental data. The assumption, often made, that all the $g = 2.00$ signals represent metabolic intermediates seems less tenable in view of its persistence for a matter of days. The results of power saturation studies suggest that this persistent signal is due, at least in part, to paramagnetic transition-metal ions rather than solely to organic free radicals. The results also imply that even in fresh tissue part of the $g = 2.00$ signal is due to such ions.

Perhaps changes in the environment of these ions explain the data shown in Fig. 4-4. In this experiment power saturation studies were made on tissue while it was fresh and after holding at various temperatures. Of special interest is the change in power saturation characteristics seen at the same observation temperature in the same tissue slice when it is observed at different times. Apparently unpaired species with different power saturation characteristics are contributing to the observed spectrum, although the spectra do not differ qualitatively. As noted earlier, such results imply that considerable caution must be employed in the interpretation of quantitative changes of tissue signals because changes in radical species can occur without changes in qualitative spectra.

B. IN VIVO VARIATIONS

This is an area that is especially in need of further work to ensure that changes observed in pathological processes are due to these processes and not to an unrecognized physiological effect.

Various Tissues. Most of the different organ systems have now been studied to at least some degree with regard to the $g = 2.00$ signal. Many of the available studies simply compare apparent intensities. It is generally recognized, however, that the $g = 2.00$ signal is due to several different species and probably does vary in composition between tissues (66). A list of relative intensities of ESR signals from some tissues is shown in Fig. 4-6 (66). These data give a good estimate of apparent relative differences for wet tissue slices, but we must remember the many applicable reservations discussed in this chapter in regard to absolute quantitation of such spectra. In addition, possible power saturation effects have not been ruled out.

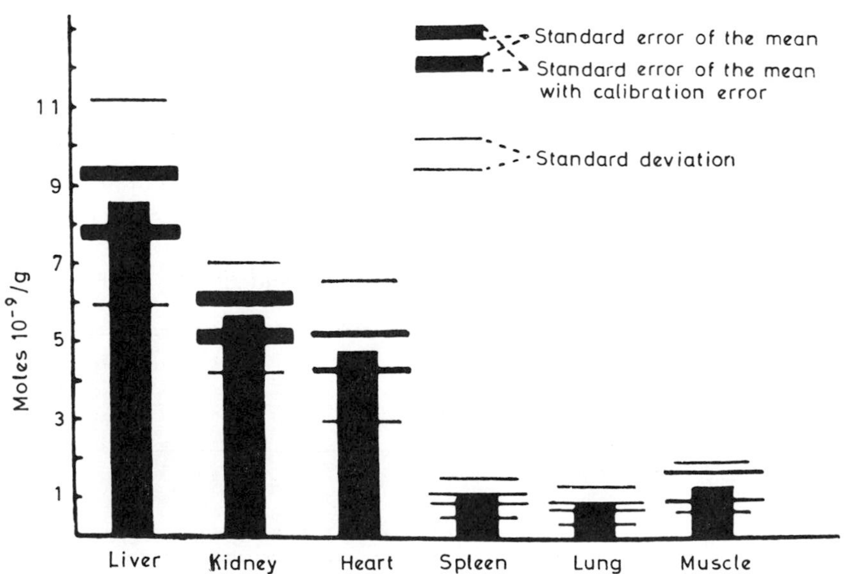

Fig. 4-6 Relative signal intensities at 37 C of normal rat tissues. (From Ref. 66, with permission of the publishers.)

It is of interest to note the very low concentration of free radicals in blood and spleen in contrast to the high values reported for these tissues when lyophilized samples are studied (e.g., Ref. 72 and Chapter 5).

The ESR spectra of bony materials appear to be somewhat different from those of other tissues, and several theories concerning the type of spectrum expected in bone have been proposed. A small but definite signal in the $g = 2.00$ area can be found in bone (96) as well as a variable number of other peaks with different g factors. The latter are probably due to transition-metal ions and may reflect the tendency of many trace elements to be deposited in bone.

The $g = 2.00$ signal increases with time after removal, especially if the bone is kept dry and exposed to air. Power saturation studies of the ESR signal in rat bones (11, 96) reveal that the signal power saturates less readily than long-lived radiation-induced ESR signals, perhaps indicating that some of the $g = 2.00$ signal is also due to sources other than organic free radicals. Becker (5) has suggested that the observed resonances may be due to a free charge-carrier population. Long-lived radiation-induced resonances in bone have been localized mainly within the inorganic matrix of bone (96). Similar attempts to identify the origin of the ESR signal in unirradiated bone have not been successful, perhaps because of the low level of resonances. Artifactual signals arising from trace elements (copper) in processing solutions (67) or mechanically induced by processing (68) have resulted in some confusion. At the present time no firm conclusions concerning the number, type, or significance of ESR signals in native bone seem possible.

Diet. Food intake appears to affect free radical levels significantly in liver but not in kidney. As shown in Table 4-1, prolonged starvation of rats led to a 20 to 30 percent increase in free-radical levels. Inasmuch as rats

Table 4-1 The Effects of Short-Term 80% N_2O and 20% O_2 on Free Radicals[a] in Fasting Rats

	Four-hour fast		Nine-hour fast	
	Liver	Kidney	Liver	Kidney
Control	102.3 ± 3.8	74.5 ± 4.2	106.0 ± 4.1	79.0 ± 4.7
Experimental	94.1[b] ± 2.8	79.1 ± 6.4	84.0[b] ± 1.3	72.8 ± 2.4

[a] Recorded as peak-peak heights of first-derivative curves ± SD of quick-frozen tissue samples observed at 77 K.

[b] Significant difference from control values (0.05 level). (From Ref. 50 with permission of the publishers.)

eat primarily at night, it is quite possible in some experiments to subject them inadvertently to starvation of this magnitude; this effect must then be considered. It is not known whether the increase in radicals simply reflects a quantitative change or whether qualitative changes are also involved. The effect of starvation in mice is opposite to that seen in rats: the levels of liver free radicals decrease in mice within 2 to 4 hr after withdrawal of food. There have been no published studies on the effect of different types of diet (except for carcinogenesis experiments) on tissue free radicals.

Metabolic Activity. The effect of metabolic activity on free-radical content has been discussed frequently, but rarely has it been directly investigated. In one study in which guinea pig adrenals were used (112) ACTH-stimulated adrenals had a small decrease in free-radical concentration compared with normal adrenals, whereas cortisone-suppressed animals had no change in their free-radical content. The observed differences were quite small. This is an area that requires considerably more data before any general conclusions can be made.

Oxygen. Holding animals in 100 percent or 5 to 10 percent oxygen atmospheres for 1 to 3 days did not lead to detectable changes in ESR spectra of quick-frozen biopsies in studies performed in our laboratory. With the experimental procedure employed, each sample was subjected to a 5 to 10 min period of anoxia while being processed and this could have obscured some changes. Studies of hyperoxia are of special interest in regard to some theories of oxygen toxicity that propose a free-radical mechanism as a cause. A critical test of these theories, however, would require experimental conditions that can detect very short-lived radicals and that do not change the oxygen tension from the *in vivo* situation.

4.3.6.2 Changes in Pathological States

A. CARCINOGENESIS

This has been and continues to be the problem that attracts the most interest in tissue ESR studies. The impetus came from theoretical considerations of the possible role of free radicals in carcinogenesis (13, 32, 62, 123). Interest has been sustained by experimental findings of differences in ESR spectra of tumors compared with normal tissues, although few of the experimental findings bear on the original hypotheses that led to the prediction of a role of free radicals in carcinogenesis.

The theoretical aspects are based on the high reactivity of free radicals, hence on the possibility of their drastically altering cellular processes. Free-radical processes have been invoked to explain carcinogenesis by ionizing radiation, which produces large amounts of free radicals. These considerations also predict that carcinogens may form free-radical intermediates and have been supported, at least to some extent, by the chemical nature of carcinogens. Studies of several carcinogens indicate that many of them do readily form complexes with acceptors, giving up a single electron and thereby forming free radicals (60, 104). These considerations do not necessarily imply any effect on the level or type of free radicals in malignant tissues but apparently led to their ESR study (see Section 7.5.1).

Starting with these considerations, many tumor tissues have been studied by ESR. Unfortunately a great number of these studies have been performed on lyophilized tissues and their significance is unknown. By using unfrozen and quick-frozen tissues and cells, however, a number of pertinent findings have been made. One of the earliest findings (20, 56), generally confirmed by later studies, was that tumor tissues usually have fewer free radicals than their normal counterparts (67, 123). Burlakova (16) offered a theoretical explanation of why tumor tissues have fewer free radicals by suggesting that the rate of cell division is regulated by free radicals, high concentrations inhibiting reactions necessary for cell division and low concentrations accelerating the rate. She offered some experimental evidence in support of this hypothesis but considerably more evidence is required for serious consideration of this unusual concept.

Another fairly consistent finding has been the change in the quantity and type of paramagnetic trace elements in tumor tissues (66, 80, 81). Tumors generally have more transition-metal ion signals, including many with no counterpart in normal tissues. It is tempting to speculate that these transition-metal ion signals might be of value in the early diagnosis of malignancies, but to date there are no data to support this expectation.

Another approach to early detection has been successful. Commoner's group (123) found that several different carcinogens which induce rat hepatoma result in a distinct ESR signal at $g = 2.035$ (half-width about 20 G) several weeks before any of the conventional biochemical or histological indicators of tumor transformation become positive (Fig. 4-7). This low-field signal then disappears before the onset of obvious malignancy. The carcinogen-induced signal apparently involves an unpaired spin density in a NO—Fe^{2+} complex with a thiol-containing protein. Liver slices incubated in high concentrations of NO_2^- alone also show this signal, and it appears to be related to a signal seen in anaerobic yeast in NO_3^--containing media. Increased dietary NO_2^- enhances tumor induction by the carcinogens used in these studies (see Section 7.3.12).

Several experiments have demonstrated the formation of free radicals in tissues by carcinogens. Szent-Gyorgi (104) demonstrated free-radical formation in chemical systems by carcinogens in approximate relation to their carcinogenic abilities. Rowlands and Gross (87) found that tobacco smoke led to a detectable ESR signal in isolated rabbit lungs, and Rondia

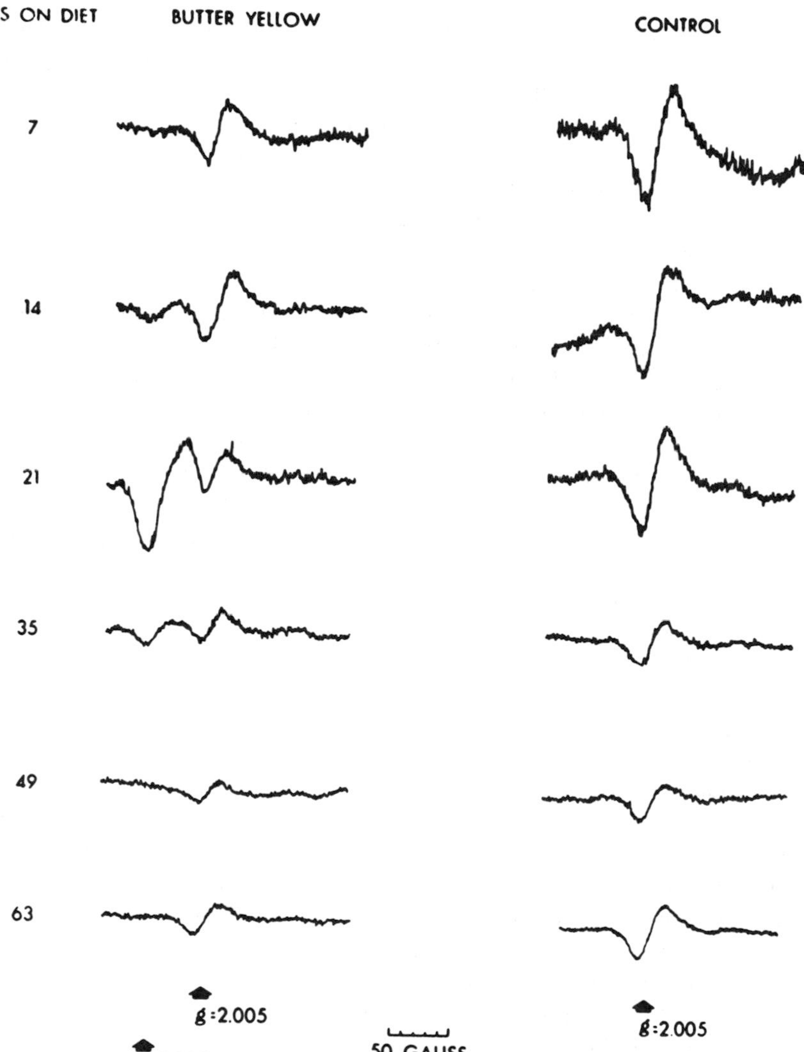

Fig. 4-7 Electron spin resonance signals from surviving liver samples from rats fed on a riboflavin-deficient diet containing 0.06 percent of *p*-dimethylamino-azobenzene (butter-yellow) and from rats fed on a control diet lacking the carcinogen. The signals shown represent averages produced by automatic summation, with a multichannel analyzer, of 50 consecutive 16-sec sweeps through a 200-G field with a modulation amplitude of 16 G; background signals due to the glass cell were automatically subtracted. Measurements were made at an ambient temperature of 15 $\pm$ 1 C, with the tissue slices suspended in a 5 percent glucose solution. Instrument gain factors and the amount of tissue examined (50–100 mg wet weight) varied somewhat from sample to sample, so that the absolute heights of the electron spin resonance signals of different samples are not comparable. (From Ref. 123, with permission of the publishers.)

(85) detected photoinduction of free radicals in skin in the presence of carcinogens, with no free-radical formation in either skin or solutions of the carcinogens alone. A Japanese group (78, 79) demonstrated free-radical production in mixtures of some carcinogenic aromatic hydrocarbons with skin homogenate without exposure to light; however, they used lyophilized preparations and the role of oxygen is not clear.

The presence of free radicals in cigarette smoke, our most prolific carcinogen, has been extensively investigated (see Section 7.6.1). These radicals have been invoked as a possible explanation of the high carcinogenicity exhibited by tobacco smoke compared with its identifiable components, with the thought that short-lived radicals might be carcinogenic or cocarcinogenic (24). A lifetime of at least 2 to 3 sec seems required if the radicals are to react with tissue. Such short- as well as long-lived radicals have been identified in tobacco smoke condensates (24, 33, 46, 62) and some of the components have been identified. Of particular interest is the apparent interaction between components of cigarette smoke which resulted in a higher free-radical content than would be expected on the basis of the individual components. These results included studies with 3,4-benzypyrene which showed radical formation on heating and a tenfold increased radical yield if certain nonradical compounds were also present (33) (see Sections 7.5.1 and 7.6.1).

B. "TRIPLET" SIGNAL

A prominent triplet noted in malignant tissues led to the suggestion that this structure may be related to some process instrinsic to carcinogenesis (12, 30). A review of the literature, however, suggests that such a spectrum has been observed under several different conditions unrelated to carcinogenesis and is probably related to the presence of an unpaired electron in a complex containing nitrogen and probably iron (see Section 7.3.12).

Brennan, Cole, and Singley (12) reported a prominent triplet signal in mouse neuroblastomas: a $g_{\parallel}$ factor of 2.01 with a 15-G splitting. Using both a 9-GHz and a 14-GHz spectrometer, they demonstrated that this structure was due to hyperfine interactions and not overlapping signals. They also concluded that the splitting developed from interaction with a nitrogen nucleus ($I = 1$) and that a heavy atom such as Fe, S, or Ca was in proximity (because of the shift of the g factor from the free spin value of $g = 2.0023$, presumably due to spin-orbit coupling). These experiments (12) are particularly noteworthy because of their application of proved physical approaches to the analysis of tissue ESR spectra (they employed two different frequency bridges and used computer averaging and computer simulation to reach their well-founded conclusions). Unfortunately they did not recognize that this triplet was not unique to this system. Several other authors reached similar conclusions (76, 88). Emanuél et al. (30) reported a similar triplet in several types of malignant tissue as well as a $g = 2.03$ signal which they felt might also be related to the triplet, but they later reported finding similar signals in nonmalignant processes (29). Maruyama et al. (75) reported similar signals in anoxic tissues, both malignant and normal.

Similar triplets have been reported in several other studies of whole tissues. Swartz et al. (102) found a prominent triplet in irradiated blood which appeared to be due to a stable paramagnetic complex. A similar structure was reported in Walker's sarcoma (30). Rowlands and Gross (87) reported the induction of a similar triplet in isolated rabbit lungs exposed to cigarette smoke (see Section 7.6.1). Kayushin and Azhipa (51) found a 45-G triplet in several tissues of animals with experimental methemoglobinemia. Unpublished studies from our laboratory indicate that a similar structure is found in red cells of animals with reticulocytosis due to phenylhydrazine-induced anemia and in the spleen of mice infected with malaria.

Addition of nitric oxide to samples containing iron also generates an apparently similar triplet (see Section 7.6.2). Azhipa et al. (4) described such a structure with a 16-G splitting and an apparent $g_{\parallel}$ value of 2.0 which they ascribed to a complex of NO and heme. Vanin and Chetverikov (119) investigated complexes of NO with whole tissue, blood, and various iron compounds. They found that both heme and nonheme iron, under the proper conditions, could form complexes with NO whose spectra included triplets similar to those already described. Spectra of nitric oxide hemoglobin preparations may also contain a triplet (59) in which the amount of hyperfine structure is related to the state of hydration. Maruyama et al. (75) believe that this triplet is due to a denatured NO-hemoprotein complex in a reducing environment; they were able to reverse its formation by adding oxygen.

C. JAUNDICE

Perhaps the most dramatic pathological variation noted was reported by Ternberg and Commoner in 1963 (109) who found that the ESR signal in liver biopsies (studied as thin slices) correlated closely with the type of jaundice present. In surgical, obstructive jaundice a large ESR signal was noted in liver biopsy samples, whereas liver from patients with nonobstructive jaundice had signals similar to those seen in samples from normal patients. This study is often cited as illustrating the possible clinical applications of ESR spectrometry. To date, however, this remains the only example and apparently it has not been applied clinically to any extent since this effect was reported.*

* In fact, one informal follow-up study failed to confirm the sharp separation of the two types of jaundice reported by Ternberg and Commoner. (H. B. Demopoulos, personal communication).

D. FREE RADICALS AND AGING

Several authors have commented on and speculated about a role for free radicals in aging processes (10, 33, 38). Many of these comments, however, are based on rather vague concepts and were offered without real experimental evidence or even detailed theory. As such, they tend to perpetuate the widespread impression that the study of free radicals in tissues is a type of pseudoscientific cultism. However, a few experimental results have been published that suggest that free radicals may indeed play a role in aging. These are principally the experiments of Harman (38, 39) in which he has demonstrated a small increase in the natural life span of some strains of mice treated with potential radical scavengers such as cysteine and MEA. These compounds, however, can have a variety of actions besides scavenging radicals, including antioxidant effects that do not involve radical reactions. Furthermore, Harman's results with diets containing radical scavengers have not been consistent, and sex and strain differences have further complicated interpretation of the findings.

Harman and Piette (40) studied free radicals in serum as possible sources of those that cause aging. They observed no free radicals in normal serum but did find detectable resonances when 10^{-2} *M* propyl gallate, epinephrine, or ascorbic acid were added (see Sections 7.3.3 and 7.3.6). Ultraviolet light also induced signals, especially in the presence of oxygen, but it is not clear what relation UV-induced free radicals in serum have with spontaneously occurring free radicals in serum.

Human collagen has been studied because of its possible role in the aging process. ESR signals were induced in collagen *in vitro* by 253.7 nm light and its response to such irradiation was found to be dependent on its age (34).

In spite of some attractive theoretical speculations on the role of free radicals in aging, we must conclude that there is no firm experimental evidence at this time to support these speculations.

E. LIPID PEROXIDATION AND FREE RADICALS

It has been suggested that lipid peroxidation plays a role in a number of deteriorative processes, including aging, oxygen toxicity, pollution damage, atherosclerosis, and chemical hepatotoxicity (105, 106). Its precise role in these processes remains to be established, but to the extent that it does participate it probably proceeds via free-radical chain pathways such as

$$R\cdot + O_2 \rightarrow ROO\cdot$$

$$ROO\cdot + RH \rightarrow ROOH + R\cdot$$

Considerable speculation and some data have been presented and it appears inevitable that ESR studies of tissue will be involved in experiments on this process. To date, however, no tissue studies appear to have been published, except for some Russian studies which used lyophilized materials that react spontaneously with oxygen, independent of lipid peroxidation, and are therefore not suitable models in any study of this problem. Current studies in this field do not employ ESR; they utilize reaction products to obtain information on peroxidation reactions.

F. OTHER STUDIES

Only a few other reports on ESR studies of pathological states have been made, with the exception of a vast Russian literature which, unfortunately, usually publishes investigations in which lyophilized material has been employed. [More recently certain Russian investigators have led the way in identifying and defining the problems involved in attempting to use lyophilized materials (e.g., 119).] By use of frozen tissue the metabolically depressive effect of nitrous oxide was investigated and it was shown to depress free-radical levels in liver but not in kidney (50). Ischemic hearts have been reported to have increased levels of free radicals which also appeared in coronary venous blood plasma (3). Epinephrine increased the release of free radicals but dipyridamole and theophylline ethylenediamine decreased it. Studies of irradiated tissue indicate that some ionizing radiation-induced radicals can be detected either by freezing post irradiation (11) or by observations during high intensity in-cavity irradiation (52). Doses within the range of biological interest appear to have little effect on normal levels of tissue free radicals.

Commoner's group has recently reported some apparently unique ESR patterns in injured nerve. They found that cutting, crushing, or otherwise mechanically damaging isolated nerves resulted in generation of a signal with a g factor varying between $g = 2.05$ and $g = 2.30$. The g factor of an individual specimen was a function of the temperature of observation and the orientation of the nerve. The signal appears to originate in a single small segment of each nerve, possibly associated with some pigmented material similiar to lipofuscin. The microscopic appearance of these regions, as well as the dependence of their ESR properties on thermal and orientational factors, suggests that they reside in a crystalline matrix. The high g factor and the chemical stability demonstrated by these resonances suggest that transition-metal trace elements are involved.

4.4 SUMMARY

Although a large number of ESR studies of tissues and tissue fragments have been reported, the validity and usefulness of many of them remain to be firmly established. ESR signals can be found in virtually all tissues and, with careful techniques, followed through a variety of manipulations. Many suggestive correlations have been reported between ESR changes and physiological and pathological processes. It seems quite possible that such studies will make important contributions in the future if they are well planned and carefully carried out. The most important current need is for more work to establish the main experimental parameters for such studies and to determine the origin of the observed ESR signals in tissue. Even without a full understanding of the origin of tissue ESR signals, some valuable correlations between these signals and cellular alterations have been obtained and many more are likely. Our present state of knowledge suggests that tissue ESR studies provide data obtainable neither by other methods nor by studies of cell fractions, but whether the tissue work will lead to significant new conclusions remains to be determined.

REFERENCES

1. G. Abagyan and P. Butyagin, *Biofizika*, **10,** 763 (1965).
2. G. Androes and M. Calvin, *Biophys.*, **2,** 217 (1962).
3. S. Aoyama, H. Matsubara, T. Wantabe, H. Yamazaki, K. Ogawa, T. Kobayashi, K. Akiyama, H. Yamamoto, and H. Sassa, *Jap. Circulation J.*, **32,** 1925 (1968).
4. Y. Azhipa, L. Kayushin, and Ye. Nikishin, *Biofizika*, **11,** 710 (1966).
5. R. Becker, *Nature*, **199,** 1304 (1963).
6. L. Bliumenfel'd, V. Benderskii, and A. Kalmanson, *Biofizika*, **6,** 631 (1961).
7. L. Bliumenfel'd, *Biofizika*, **4,** 515 (1959).
8. L. Bliumenfel'd, *Royal Acad. Belg.*, **33,** 93 (1961).
9. M. Blois, A. Zahlan, and J. Maling, *Biophys. J.*, **4,** 471 (1964).
10. H. Boenig, *J. Amer. Geront. Soc.*, **14,** 1211 (1966).
11. J. Brady, N. Aarestad, and H. Swartz, *Health Phys.*, **15,** 43 (1968).
12. J. Brennan, T. Cole, and J. Singley, *Proc. Soc. Expt. Biol. Med.*, **123,** 715, (1966).
13. A. Brues and E. Barron, *Ann. Rev. Biochem.*, **20,** 350 (1951).
14. O. Brzhevskaya, L. Kayushin, M. Kondrashova, O. Nedelina, and E. Sheksheyev, *Biofizika*, **11,** 1076 (1966).
15. O. Brzhevskaya, V. Marinov, O. Nedelina, and E. Sheksheyev, *Biofizika*, **12,** 354 (1967).
16. Ye. Burlakova, *Biofizika*, **12,** 91 (1967).
17. A. Chetverikov and A. Vanin, *Biofizika*, **13,** 255 (1968).
18. B. Commoner, J. Townsend, and G. Pake, *Nature*, **174,** 689 (1954).
19. B. Commoner and T. Hollocher, *Proc. Natl. Acad. Sci.*, **46,** 405 (1960).
20. B. Commoner and J. Ternberg, *Proc. Natl. Acad. Sci.*, **47,** 1374 (1961).
21. A. Conger and M. Randolph, *Rad. Bot.*, **8,** 193 (1968).
22. P. Cook and J. Mallard, *Nature*, **198,** 145 (1963).
23. R. Cook and L. Stoodley, *Int. J. Rad. Biol.*, **7,** 155 (1963).
24. J. Cooper, W. Forbes, and J. Robinson, *Nat. Cancer Inst. Monograph*, **28,** 191 (1969).

25. F. Cope, W. Raymond, L. Sever, and B. Polis, *Arch. Biochem. Biophys.*, **100,** 171 (1963).

26. D. DerVartanian, W. Orme-Johnson, R. Hansen, H. Beinert, R. Tsai, J. Tsibris, R. Bartholomaus, and I. Gunsalus, *Biochem. Biophys. Res. Commun.*, **26,** 569 (1967).

27. P. Duke, B. Houraine, and H. Demopoulos, *J. Nat. Cancer Inst.*, **39,** 1141 (1967).

28. A. Ehrenberg and L. Ehrenberg, *Ark. Fysik.*, **14,** 113 (1958).

29. N. Emanuél and A. Saprin, Abstracts, *3rd Intern. Biophys. Cong. Intern. Union Pure Appl. Biophys.*, p. 224, 1969.

30. N. Emanuél, A. Saprin, V. Shabalkin, L. Kozlova, and K. Krugljakova, *Nature*, **222,** 165 (1969).

31. D. Fischer, J. Downs, A. Herner, and A. Batlin, *Biochem. Biophys. Acta.*, **104,** 591 (1965).

32. A. Fitzhugh, *Science*, **118,** 783 (1953).

33. W. Forbes, L. Robinson, and G. Wright, *Can. J. Biochem.*, **45,** 1087 (1967).

34. W. Forbes and P. Sullivan, *Biochem. Biophys. Acta*, **120,** 222 (1966).

35. F. Grady and D. Borg, *J. Am. Chem. Soc.*, **90,** 2949 (1968).

36. A. Haber and M. Randolph, *Rad. Bot.*, **7,** 17 (1967).

37. D. Harman, *J. Gerontol.*, **11,** 298 (1956).

38. D. Harman, *Rad. Res.*, **16,** 753 (1962).

39. D. Harman, *The Lancet*, p. 200, (1961).

40. D. Harman and L. Piette, *J. Gerontol.*, **21,** 560 (1966).

41. Y. Hashimoto, T. Yamano, and H. Mason, *J. Biol. Chem.*, **237,** 3843 (1962).

42. T. Hollocher, *J. Biol. Chem.*, **241,** 3452 (1966).

43. T. Hollocher and B. Commoner, *Proc. Nat. Acad. Sci.*, **46,** 416 (1960).

44. D. Holmes, N. Nazhat, and J. Weiss, *J. Phys. Chem.*, **74,** 1622 (1970).

45. A. Il'Ina, I. Maktinis, Y. Moshkovskii, and L. Bliumenfel'd, *Biofizika*, **12,** 181 (1967).

46. D. Ingram, *Acta Med. Scand. Suppl.*, **369,** 43 (1960).

47. I. Isenberg, *Biochem. Biophys. Res. Commun.*, **5,** 139 (1961).

48. I. Isenberg and S. Baird, *Roy. Acad. Belg.*, **33,** 170 (1961).

49. K. Ishizu, H. Dearman, M. Huang, and J. White, *Biochim. Biophys. Acta.*, **165,** 283 (1968).

50. M. Johnson, H. Swartz, and R. Donati, *Anesthesiology*, **34,** 42 (1971).

51. L. Kayushin and Y. Azhipa, abstract, *3rd Intern. Biophys. Congr. Intern. Union Pure Appl. Biophys.*, p. 225, 1969.

52. P. Kenney and B. Commoner, *Nature*, **223,** 1229 (1969).

53. M. Kent and J. Mallard, abstract, *3rd Intern. Biophys. Congr. Intern. Union Pure Appl. Biophys.*, p. 223, 1969.

54. M. Kent and J. Mallard, *Nature*, **204,** 396 (1964).

55. G. Kerkut, M. Edwards, K. Leach, and K. Munday, *Experentia*, **17,** 496 (1961).

56. I. Kolomitseva, K. L'Vov, and L. Kayushin, *Biofizika*, **5,** 636 (1960).

57. Z. Kometiani and R. Cagan, *Biochim. Biophys. Acta.*, **135,** 1083 (1967).

58. A. Kreba and B. Benson, *Nature*, **207,** 1412 (1965).

59. M. Lion, J. Kirby-Smith, and M. Randolph, *Nature*, **192,** 34 (1961).

60. D. Lipkin, D. Paul, J. Townsend, and S. Weissman, *Science*, **117,** 534 (1953).

61. H. Longuet-Higgins, *Arch. Biochem. Biophys.*, **86,** 231 (1960).
62. M. Lyons, J. Gibson, and D. Ingram, *Nature*, **181,** 1003 (1958).
63. J. Maling, L. Taskovich, and M. Blois, *Biophys. J.*, **3,** 79 (1963).
64. A. Malinovski and D. Kafalieva, *Z. Naturforsch.*, **19,** 457 (1964).
65. J. Mallard and M. Kent, *Phys. Med. Biol.*, **14,** 373 (1969).
66. J. Mallard and M. Kent, *Nature*, **210,** 588 (1966).
67. J. Mallard and M. Kent, *Nature*, **204,** 1192 (1964).
68. A. Marino and R. Becker, *Nature*, **218,** 4667 (1968).
69. A. Marino and R. Becker, *Nature*, **221,** 661 (1969).
70. H. Mason, D. Ingram, and B. Allen, *Arch. Biochem. Biophys.*, **86,** 225 (1960).
71. H. Mason, T. Yamano, J. North, Y. Hashimoto, and P. Sakagishi, in *Oxidases and Related Redox Systems*, T. S. King, H. S. Mason, and M. Morrison, Eds., Wiley, New York, p. 879, 1965.
72. I. Miyagawa, W. Gordy, W. Norimitsu, and K. Wilbur, *Proc. Natl. Acad. Sct.*, **44,** 613 (1958).
73. A. Müller, G. Hotz, and K. Zimmer, *Roy. Acad. Belg.*, **33,** 108 (1961).
74. A. Müller, G. Hotz, and K. Zimmer, *Biochem. Biophys. Res. Commun.*, **4,** 214 (1961).
75. T. Maruyama, N. Kataoka, S. Nagase, N. Nakada, H. Sato, and H. Sasaki, *Cancer Res.*, **31,** 179 (1971).
76. J. Matsunaga, *J. Jap. Urol. Soc.*, **60,** 214 (1968).
77. C. Myttenaere, P. Bourdeau, G. Helcke, and M. Masset, *Rad. Bot.*, **5,** 443 (1965).
78. C. Nagata, Y. Tagashira, M. Kodama, and A. Imamura, *Jap. J. Cancer Res.*, **57,** 437 (1966).
79. C. Nagata, M. Kodama, and Y. Tagashira, *Jap. J. Cancer Res.*, **58,** 493 (1967).
80. D. Nebert and H. Mason, *Cancer Res.*, **23,** 833 (1963).
81. D. Nebert and H. Mason, *Biochim. Biophys. Acta.*, **86,** 415 (1964).
82. M. Randolph and A. Haber, "Effects of Ionizing Rad. on Seeds," International Atomic Energy Agency, p. 57, 1961.
83. M. Randolph, J. Heddle, and J. Hosszu, *Rad. Bot.*, **8,** 339 (1968).
84. R. Romani, *Rad. Bot.*, **6,** 371 (1966).
85. R. Rondia, *Compt. Rend.*, "D," **264,** 3053 (1967).
86. J. Rowlands and E. Gause, *Appl. Microbiol.*, **18,** 650 (1969).
87. J. Rowlands and C. Gross, *Nature*, **213,** 1256 (1967).
88. Y. Sakagishi, *Bull. Tokyo Med. Dent. Univ.*, **15,** 33 (1968).
89. Y. Shethna, P. Wilson, R. Hansen, and H. Beinert, *Proc. Natl. Acad. Sci.*, **52,** 1263 (1964).
90. H. Shields, W. Ard, and W. Gordy, *Nature*, **177,** 984 (1956).
91. R. Shulman W. Walsh, H. Williams, and J. Wright, *Biochem. Biophys. Res. Commun.*, **5,** 52 (1961)
92. B. Singh, R. Cook, and A. Charlesby, *Intern. J. Rad. Biol.*, **8,** 195 (1964).
93. D. Smith and J. Pieroni, *Can. J. Chem.*, **42,** 2209 (1964).
94. W. Snipes and W. Gordy, *Science*, **142,** 503 (1963).
95. L. Stoodley, *J. Electron. Control*, **14,** 531 (1963).

96. H. Swartz, *Rad. Res.*, **24,** 579 (1965).
97. H. Swartz, *Cryobiology*, **6,** 546 (1970).
98. H. Swartz, *Cryobiology*, **8,** 255 (1971).
99. H. Swartz, E. Copeland, and E. Larsson, *Biophys. Soc. Proc.*, 1970.
100. H. Swartz and R. Molenda, *Science*, **148,** 94 (1965).
101. H. Swartz, R. Lofberg, and J. Brady, Abstract, *3rd Intern. Rad. Res. Congr.*, 1966.
102. H. Swartz, R. Molenda, and R. Lofberg, *Biochem. Biophys. Res. Comm.*, **21,** 61 (1965).
103. H. Swartz and E. Richardson, *Int. J. Rad. Biol.*, **12,** 75 (1967).
104. A. Szent-Gyorgyi, I. Isenberg, and S. Baird, *Proc. Nat. Acad. Sci.*, **46,** 1444 (1960).
105. A. Tappel, *Federation Proc.*, **24,** 73 (1965).
106. A. Tappel, 54th FASEB Meeting, April 1970.
107. N. Tarasenko, G. Berdyshev, and V. Lopushonok, *Biofizika*, **10,** 893 (1965).
108. S. Tarusov, Y. Kozlov, S. Uostile, and C. Yungtseng, *Dokl. Akad. Nauk. SSSR.*, **163,** 752 (1965).
109. J. Ternberg and B. Commoner, *JAMA*, **183,** 339 (1963).
110. R. Treharne, T. Brown, H. Eyster and H. Tanner, *Biochem. Biophys. Res. Commun.*, **3,** 119 (1960).
111. R. Treharne and H. Eyster, *Biochem. Biophys. Res. Commun.*, **8,** 477 (1962).
112. F. Truby and J. Goldzieher, *Nature*, **188,** 1088 (1960).
113. F. Truby and J. Goldzieher, *Nature*, **182,** 1371 (1958).
114. L. Ulbert, *Nature*, **195,** 175 (1962).
115. M. VanWoert, *Proc. Soc. Exptl. Biol. Med.*, **129,** 165 (1968).
116. M. VanWoert, K. Prasad, and D. Borg, *J. Neurochem.*, **14,** 707 (1967).
117. A. Vanin, L. Bliumenfel'd, and A. Chetverikov, *Biofizika*, **12,** 829 (1967).
118. A. Vanin and A. Chetverikov, *Dokl. Akad. Nauk. SSSR.*, **178,** 249 (1968).
119. A. Vanin and A. Chetverikov, *Biofizika*, **13,** 608 (1968).
120. A. Vanin, C. Matkhanov, and Y. Belov, *Biofizika*, **12,** 1103 (1967).
121. A. Vanin and R. Nalbandyan, *Biofizika*, **10,** 167 (1965).
122. A. Vanin and R. Nalbandyan, *Biofizika*, **11,** 178 (1966).
123. A. Vithayathil, J. Ternberg, and B. Commoner, *Nature*, **207,** 1246 (1965).
124. M. Waldschmidt, H. Monig, and L. Schole, *Z. Naturforsh.*, **236,** 798 (1968).
125. W. Walsh, R. Shulman, and R. Heidenreich, *Nature*, **192,** 1041 (1961).
126. J. White and H. Dearman, *Proc. Nat. Acad. Sci.*, **54,** 887 (1965).
127. J. Windle and L. Sacks, *Biochem. Biophys. Acta*, **66,** 173 (1963).
128. J. Woolum and B. Commoner, *Biochem. Biophys. Acta*, **201,** 131 (1970).
129. S. Wyard, *Proc. Roy. Soc.* (*London*), **A-30,** 355 (1968).

CHAPTER FIVE

Free Radicals in Dry Tissues

ROBERT J. HECKLY

Naval Biomedical Research Laboratory
University of California, Berkeley

5.1 INTRODUCTION

In this chapter we consider only those free radicals that arise spontaneously, primarily in dried biological materials. Free radicals resulting from high-energy irradiation have been studied extensively and are considered in detail in Chapter 10. Free radicals can also be produced by mechanical forces (1, 34), but they are unrelated to biological functions, although they could be a possible source of confusion in certain types of preparation.

5.2 RELATION OF SIGNAL SEEN IN DRIED TO THAT IN WET SYSTEMS

Free radicals were first detected in biological materials in 1954 by Commoner et al. (9) with a variety of lyophilized samples. Lyophilization was used in these pioneering experiments because instrumental limitations prevented the examination of samples with appreciable amounts of liquid water. The assumption in the earliest studies was that lyophilization "froze in" the same free radicals that were present in wet functional tissue. Although Commoner and his co-workers abandoned lyophilized preparations as soon as they were able to develop ESR instrumentation that enabled them to examine tissue without prior drying, a large number of investigators have continued to employ lyophilized preparations, under the assumption that these preparations accurately reflect free-radical levels present in hydrated functioning cells.

Since 1954 a considerable body of evidence has grown up which indicates that the signals seen in lyophilized preparations do not ordinarily reflect free radicals in functioning tissue. Observed differences between fresh (or frozen) and lyophilized tissues have included linewidths, relative tissue free-radical concentrations and distribution of free radicals in cell components. Careful kinetic studies have indicated that during drying the original signals in tissue decrease or disappear and often a new signal appears. The rate at which the new signal is generated is a complex function of the preparation procedure as well as the type of tissue. The most important environmental factors are the physical state of the preparation (degree of fluff, etc.), moisture content and especially exposure to oxygen. The presence of different additives such as glucose, phenol, or ascorbic acid can also significantly affect the final observed free-radical content.

As early as 1958 Truby and Goldzieher (33) stated that the radicals seen in freeze-dried tissues were artifacts created during drying. Their conclusions were based primarily on the difference in linewidth and signal intensity between lyophilized and frozen liver preparations. Bliumenfel'd et al. (3) have summarized many of the published data which indicate that in general the linewidth of the absorption peak in dried animal tissue is about 8 G compared with about 14 G before drying. They also reported a shift in g factor from 2.0049 to 2.0057 in the dried samples. Malinovski and Kafalieva (24) reported that although the g factor for both fresh and dried leaves was $g = 2.0032$ there was a change in width of the absorption peak similar to that observed in animal tissue. The absorption peak in leaves was 10 to 12 G wide before drying but only 5 to 6 G after drying.

Malinovski and Kafalieva (24), in ESR studies of plant leaves, found that lyophilization destroyed the radicals demonstrable in the fresh tissue and that a different radical appeared after continued drying. They concluded that lyophilization produced free radicals because the size of the ESR signal was proportional to the length of drying at 0.01 torr. The explanation offered was that free radicals resulted from the breaking of chemical bonds, presumably due to a loss of water. They did not, however, consider the possible effect of oxygen.

Harhash et al. (12) reported that no signal was evident in moist fungal mats of *Phycomyces* and that the free radical content of the lyophilized material was the result of a reaction with oxygen. Subsequently Vanin et al. (37) noted that even a short exposure of dried liver to oxygen resulted in free radical formation. At about the same time Bliumenfel'd et al. (3) concluded that although free radicals (about 10^{16}/g) present in fresh tissue were not affected by lyophilization, another radical species, in much higher concentration (about 10^{17}/g) developed when the lyophilized material was exposed to oxygen.

Chetverikov (5) recognized the importance of technique, oxygen, and moisture content and described in great detail the procedures for obtaining reproducible results.

By freeze drying spherical pellets of homogenized liver in the cavity of an ESR spectrometer, Heckly and Dimmick (14) showed that free radicals were not demonstrable until air was admitted. The concentration of free radicals was easily measured within 5 min after admitting air and the concentration approximately doubled during the next 30 min.

The critical role of oxygen in development of the signal seen in lyophilized preparation has been quite well delineated in bacteria. Even traces of oxygen, such as are found in virtually all commercial nitrogen gases, generated free radicals in lyophilized bacteria. Only when special oxygen-scrubbing procedures (22) were used was free radical formation and bacteria toxicity prevented. This is probably the reason why some workers have failed to realize that most of the free radicals they observed in these lyophilized preparations were generated during or after drying. The rate of radical formation at low oxygen concentrations is proportional to the log of the oxygen concentration.

In fresh (or frozen) tissues liver, kidney, and heart have the highest free-radical content (about 10^{-9} mole/g), and muscle, spleen and blood have almost none (8, 25). In contrast, in lyophilized tissues spleen usually has the highest free radical content and a prominent signal is also seen in blood (3, 30).

Commoner (9) noted that the relative concentration of free radicals in fresh tissues tended to parallel the number of mitochondria in the various tissues. He also found that the development of the free radical signal in young livers paralleled the increase in functional mitochondria. He concluded that most of the free radicals seen in fresh tissue were associated with mitochondria. This was supported by Brzhevskaya et al. (4), who found that the mitochondrial fraction contained the highest free radical concentration of the various subcellular fractions of rat liver. In a similar study, but examining only lyophilized preparations, Ruuge et al. (30) concluded that the mitochondrial and nuclear fractions contributed only a minor portion of the total free radicals. They found that the particle-free supernatant fluid produced the greatest number of free radicals.

It is evident from the above considerations that the free radical species seen in lyophilized material are not representative of those found in living systems before lyophilization. Even though the free radicals in wet tissue are not necessarily destroyed by the drying procedure, their concentration is so low that their contribution to the observed ESR signal in dried tissue is negligible. The usual signal seen in lyophilized tissues is generated after drying by interaction with oxygen. Only traces of oxygen are required to generate large signals.

Although the ESR signals seen in lyophilized preparations are clearly not directly related to ESR signals present before lyophilization, they may still have some utility. This would be so if the generation of these radicals reproducibly reflect some basic properties of the living biological systems. The following sections contain a description of the characteristics of the signals generated by the interaction of oxygen with lyophilized materials, information on their possible origin, and a discussion of some of the experimental findings that suggest their possible usefulness.

5.3 CHARACTERISTICS OF THE ESR SPECTRA IN DRY MATERIALS

In general the shapes and *g* factors of the ESR spectra of most lyophilized biological materials are similar, but this does not mean that the free radicals seen in all lyophilized tissue are identical—or even similar. On the other hand, since the ESR spectra may represent the sum of absorptions by several radical species, two spectra might differ in shape only because the relative concentration of the free radical species in the two specimens differed. Qualitatively the two samples might be identical; for example, the ESR spectra of lyophilized liver and spleen usually differ as shown in Fig. 5-1, yet the radical types in these tissues may be the same and the observed differences of these spectra may be the result of the presence of different amounts of two or more free radicals differing slightly in their *g* factors. Some instances have been observed in which the ESR spectra of liver and spleen were qualitatively identical.

As shown in Fig. 5-1, the ESR spectrum of lyophilized bacteria differs from that of animal tissues. It has been suggested that the shape of the bacterial signals indicates unresolved hyperfine splitting, but, as shown in Fig. 5-2, repetitive scans made at intervals show that the absorption peak broadens because of the development of a second free radical species. The *g* factor of the free radical developing first is estimated to be about 2.0038 and that of the second, more slowly developing free radical, about 2.0057.

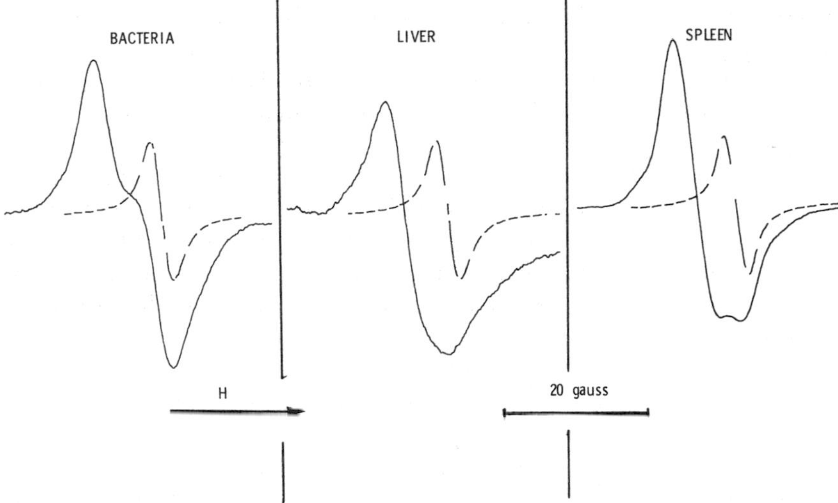

Fig. 5-1 Electron spin resonance spectra of lyophilized *Serratia marcescens*, rabbit liver, and spleen. The broken line superimposed on each is the spectrum of 0.1 percent pitch (g = 2.0028). The signal level (amplification) for recording the spleen spectrum was about one-fourth that used for the other two samples.

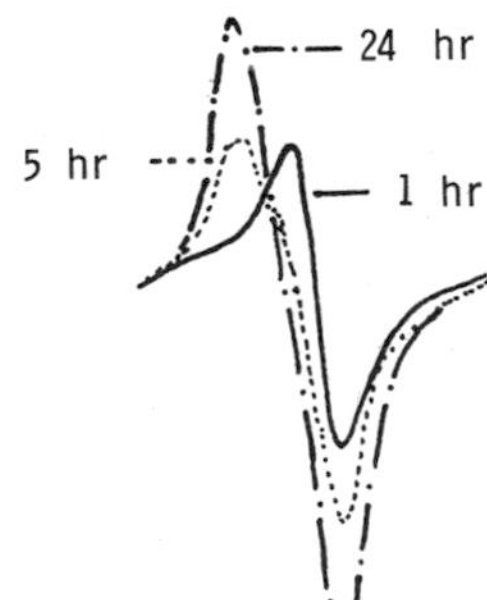

Fig. 5-2 Electron spin resonance spectra of *Serratia marcescens*. Times indicate the interval between opening the sample to air and recording the spectra.

Similar changes in the shape of the ESR spectra of animal tissues during the interval when the number of free radicals increased with time have not been reported.

Attempts to demonstrate different types of resonance in lyophilized liver and bacteria by changing the microwave power, as suggested by Swartz and Molenda (32), were not successful. There was no change in shape of ESR spectra, even of the bacterial samples, as the incident microwave power was changed from about 200 mW to less than 1 mW (25 dB attenuation).

There seems to be little disagreement that moisture increases the rate of free radical production by dry materials. However, the conclusion of Chetverikov et al. (7) that no free radicals would be produced in the absence of water (which they defined as less than 10 percent moisture) does not appear valid inasmuch as it has been shown for both bacteria (15) and liver (14) that free radical production in even the driest material eventually approached the same free radical concentration found in material at 15 and 30 percent relative humidity. Only the rate was affected by the moisture. Had Chetverikov et al. (7) extended their observations over several days, they probably would also have observed free radical production in the absence of demonstrable moisture.

Another free radical has been observed in lyophilized yeast at $g = 2.024$ (26, 35, 36) in addition to the one near 2.003. This radical at $g = 2.024$ was believed to be associated with the endogenous metabolism of the yeast. In moist yeast a slight absorption at $g = 2.03$ was demonstrable, but Vanin and Nalbandyan (36) showed that on drying this absorption was increased manyfold. The study with mascerated (cell-free) extracts indicated that the $g = 2.03$ absorption would be obtained only if the enzyme preparation were incubated with glycogen. In the presence of glucose and ATP there was no detectable absorption near $g = 2.03$.

5.4 ORIGIN AND NATURE OF THE SIGNAL

In the absence of hyperfine structure it is indeed difficult to identify the free radical from an examination of its ESR spectrum. Hence there has been considerable speculation. A number of investigators (3, 6, 18, 19, 20, 30) have suggested that the free radicals in dried biologicals involve semiquinones. Karitonenkov et al. (20) concluded that proteins in lyophilized mixtures act to stabilize free radicals. They oxidized ethyl gallate and found that no free radicals were detectable in ethyl gallate alone or in mixtures of amino acids and ethyl gallate, but a large signal was observed in mixtures of proteins and ethyl gallate. Subsequently it was shown that semiquinones (17, 18) yielded asymmetrical ESR spectra like those seen with both plant and animal tissues. They also indicated that the ESR spectra of lyophilized biological specimens may be modeled in all parameters by sorption of some free radicals (semiquinones) on protein, cellulose, and quartz powder (see also Section 7.3.1).

Kharitonenkov (17) suggested that the asymmetry of the ESR spectra of lyophilized biological specimens was not due to the summation of several lines with different g factors but rather to anisotropy. He also did not detect a progressive change in shape of the ESR spectra as observed in bacteria (Fig. 5-2). He showed that, although the shape of the ESR spectrum of spleen was markedly changed when a different spectrometer frequency was used, the spectrum of a mixture of hemoglobin and ethyl gallate was similarly affected. As shown in Fig. 5-3, however, when the spectrum of liver is superimposed on that obtained with propyl gallate plus albumin, it is evident that the spectra of the two preparations differ significantly in *g* factors. The "gallate" signal was not qualitatively influenced by the side group or the substrate. The ESR spectra obtained with any combination of ethyl, methyl, or propyl gallate and bovine serum albumin, casein, hemoglobin, or deoxyriboneucleic acid (DNA) were identical in all respects except signal intensity.

Ruuge and Bliumenfel'd (29) found that the ESR spectrum obtained with a lyophilized mixture of protein and ascorbic acid on exposure to oxygen was similar to that obtained with rat spleen. As shown in Fig. 5-3, the ESR spectrum of ascorbic acid plus albumin is qualitatively similar to that of liver, although more intense. Ruuge and Bliumenfel'd (29) believed that the free radicals they described were related to the biochemical role of ascorbic acid in enzymatic processes but we found that virtually no free radicals were detectable before exposure to air when mixtures of albumin and ascorbic acid were lyophilized. Therefore this radical produced in the dry state is probably different from that produced in the liquid state by ascorbic acid oxidase as described by Lagercrantz (21). It is quite possible

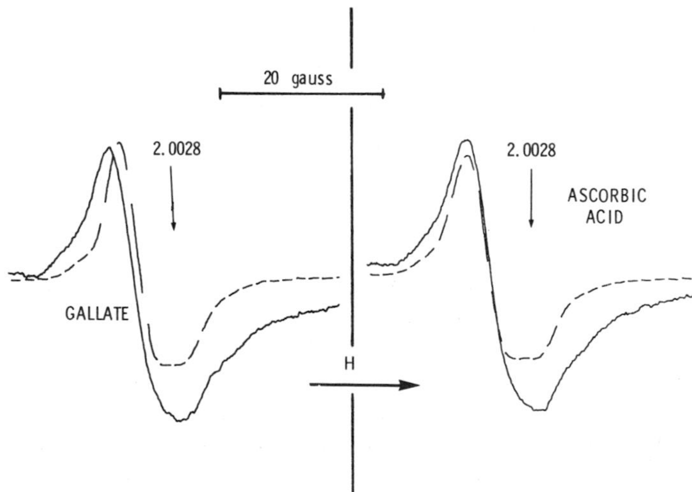

Fig. 5-3 Electron spin resonance spectra of lyophilized rabbit liver with superimposed spectra (broken lines) of propyl gallate and ascorbic acid. Both of the latter were mixed with bovine serum albumin and adjusted to about pH 7 before lyophilization. The signal level (amplification) for the liver spectra was approximately six times that used for either gallate or ascorbic acid.

that ascorbic acid or some similar substance may be involved in the spontaneously produced free radical in lyophilized animal tissues, because, as shown in Fig. 5-4, the rates of accumulation are similar in both systems. The spectra obtained from any of a number of different proteins or DNA combined with ascorbic acid has yielded spectra that are identical in shape and *g* factor. They differed only in signal intensity. There is probably more than one system that gives rise to the free radicals in lyophilized animal tissues because frequently the spectra of a given tissue are not identical in shape and *g* factor.

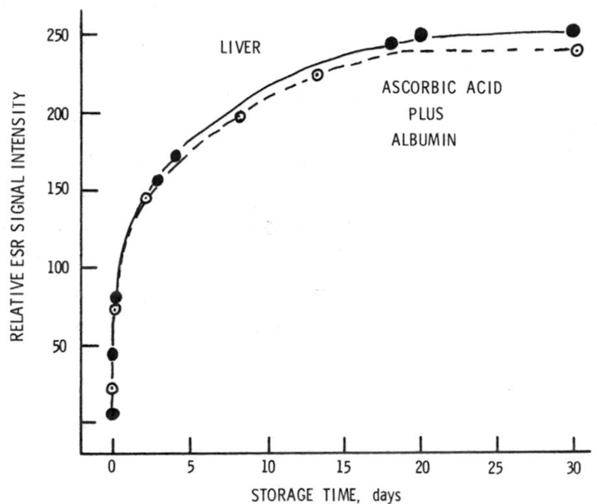

Fig. 5-4 Free radical production of liver (solid line) and ascorbic acid plus albumin (broken line). Amplification of the ESR signal from the liver sample was four times that of the sample containing ascorbic acid.

As a result of chromatographic separation of sonicated bacteria, Heckly and Dimmick (15) concluded that DNA and a polyhydroxybenzoate similar to propyl gallate (PG) or adrenalin was possibly involved in producing the free radicals in dry bacteria. This conclusion was based on the result of the following experiments: after the addition of either DNA or PG to each of the fractions obtained from the Sephadex G-50 column, samples were lyophilized and sealed in dry air. None of the fractions obtained by Sephadex G-50 separation of sonicated (solubilized) bacteria would react with oxygen to produce free radicals in a manner comparable to the whole preparation. However, a higher free-radical concentration was produced by the addition of propyl gallate to the first fraction (the high molecular-weight components) than the second fraction; and, conversely, addition of DNA to the second or (low molecular weight) fraction produced more free radical than when added to the first fraction. Furthermore, since the material in the first fraction which, in the presence of propyl gallate, produced free radicals, was heat stable and contained large amounts of deoxyribose, it was concluded that the high molecular-weight substance was DNA.

Since, as shown in Fig. 5-2, the ESR spectrum of lyophilized bacteria develops and broadens by a relative increase in concentration of the species with a higher g factor rather than simple broadening, the DNA and PG spectrum is not likely to be *the* free radical precursor in bacteria. On the other hand, it is possible that ascorbic acid or a similar material may be responsible for the more slowly developing radical species in bacteria because the low field absorption ($g = 2.0058$) nearly coincides with that of ascorbic acid, as shown in Fig. 5-5.

The $g = 2.024$ free radicals observed in lyophilized yeast (26, 35, 36) are demonstrable only under certain conditions. The ESR signal has been ascribed to an unpaired electron on a sulfur atom and has been presumed to be associated with thiol proteins. Nalbandyan and Shifman (26) concluded that the "sulfur" signal formed in the course of a phosphorylase reaction because they obtained the signal with cell-free extracts of yeast

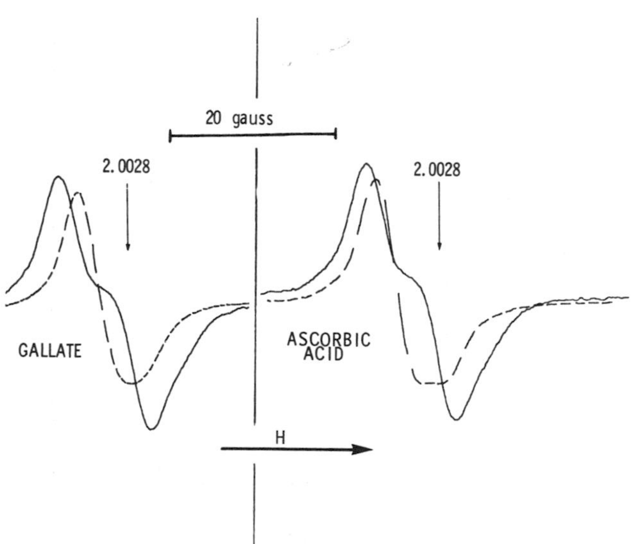

Fig. 5-5 Electron spin resonance spectra of lyophilized *Serratia marcescens* with superimposed spectra (broken lines) of propyl gallate plus deoxyribonucleic acid and ascorbic acid plus bovine serum albumin. The signal level (amplification) for the *S. marcescens* spectra was approximately five times that used for either gallate or ascorbic acid.

only if the extract were incubated with glycogen. It was not obtained when glucose was used. Heating or the presence of trace amounts of heavy metals, Ag, Hg, or Cu, in the cell-free extract prevented subsequent development of the "sulfur" free radicals in the lyophilized preparation.

Chetverikov et al. (7) concluded that the free radicals found in lyophilized tissue are not only unrepresentative of those present in living tissue but they may not even be associated with the "normal" oxidation-reduction systems. Some unpublished data indicate, however, that these radicals may be related to some metabolic product because addition of small amounts of glucose to a fresh liver homogenate increased the concentration of free radical precursor. As shown in Fig. 5-6, the precursor concentration, as measured by free radical production of the lyophilized preparation, increased as the glucose concentration was increased to about 0.06 percent. As mentioned before, addition of sugar to any of the systems before drying effectively inhibits free radical production in the lyophilized preparations. Hence it is to be expected that the higher concentration of glucose would have inhibited subsequent free radical production.

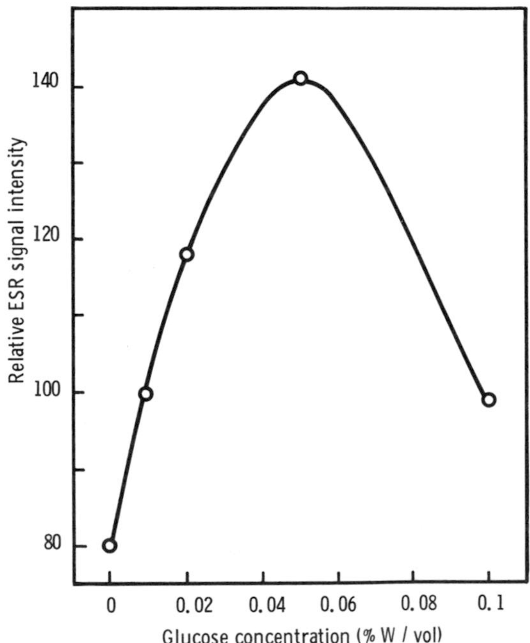

Fig. 5-6 Effect of glucose on free radical production by lyophilized rabbit liver homogenate. Glucose was added to the homogenate at room temperature about 15 min before freezing, and after lyophilization the samples were packed in dry air and sealed. The electron spin resonance was determined after 10 days' storage at room temperature.

Azhipa et al. (2) reported that when rats were asphyxiated the free radical content of lyophilized brain was reduced. They attributed this condition to a lack of oxygen interfering with the normal metabolism, hence the reduction of the free radical concentration. In view of the above discussion it is possible that the hypoxia reduced the free radical precursor content of the brain.

5.5 APPLICATIONS

Because subsequent radical generation is dependent on conditions of sample preparation, interpretation of the results of experiments in which lyophilized preparations are used must include determination that factors such as sample consistency, humidity, carbohydrate concentration, and exposure to oxygen have been held constant. *In particular, since oxygen plays such a critical role in free radical production, any study that does not explicitly consider oxygen and also allow adequate time for the reaction to approach completion cannot be reliably interpreted.* With these reservations in mind, experimental results on this kind of preparation are considered in this section. It should be noted that the results of some papers may be valid because adequate controls were done, even though the authors may have misinterpreted the origin of the observed signals (usually in terms of considering the observed spectra to reflect free radicals present before lyophilization).

Petyayev et al. (28) found significant differences in free radical precursor in carcinogenesis studies of various tissues. Of particular interest is the finding that lyophilized spleen from animals infected with SSK spontaneous sarcoma produced fewer free radicals than the spleen from normal animals and that the SSK tumor itself produced a much higher concentration of free radicals than even the normal spleen. Since they were extremely careful to standardize the method of lyophilization and exposure to oxygen and moisture, the differences were probably real.

Pavlova and Livenson (27) reported a free-radical content of lyophilized leucocytes greater than twenty-fold higher from patients with lymphoid leukemia compared with leucocytes from normal individuals. There was no significant change in leucocytes from individuals with chronic myeloid leukemia. Similarly, Saprin et al. (31) determined the free radical content of blood and various organs of mice after injection of La leukemia cells. Although the changes during the seven-day period of study were less than twofold, they indicated that the changes were statistically significant.

Valuable information may be obtained if, in addition to studying total radical production, the kinetics and factors in formation of free radicals in living systems are also studied. Seeds, eggs of certain lower animals, and microorganisms are systems that can be dried, yet considered alive or at least viable. Conger and Randolph (10) measured free radical concentrations of several kinds of seeds that had been stored for periods up to 48 years. There were fewer radicals in the older seeds and a half-life of 200 years was estimated for the free radicals. The observed changes did not correlate closely with germination (viability) but nevertheless may have been related to them.

Contrasted with the decay of free radicals in seeds is the increase in free radical concentration in lyophilized bacteria (Fig. 5-7). As is shown in this figure as well as in Fig. 5-4, free radicals initially accumulate most rapidly and the final concentration appears to be limited by some constituent of the system. The difference in kinetics shown in Fig. 5-7 for the two types of preparation indicates that the tight packing of the dried *Serratia marcescens* inhibits the diffusion of oxygen to the cell surface.

Of particular interest is the relation between free radicals and viability of microorganisms (11, 15, 16, 23, 35). The loss of viability of dried bacteria appears to be correlated with an increase in free radical concentration. As is shown in Fig. 5-8, when the dried organisms were stored under conditions favoring retention of high viability, the free radical content remained low. Conversely, when stored at 37 C the cells died rapidly, and free radical production was high. The addition of sugar or other substances before drying both reduced free radical production and increased viability of lyophilized microorganisms on storage in the presence of air (16, 23). There

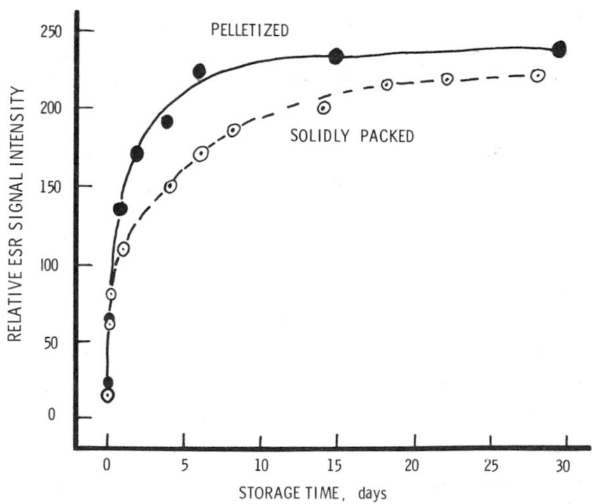

Fig. 5-7 Accumulation of free radicals produced by *Serratia marcescens*. The pelletized sample (solid line) was prepared by freezing drops of the culture in cold Freon-heptane (13) with no subsequent compression and recorded at a signal level (amplification) of eight times that used for the solidly packed sample.

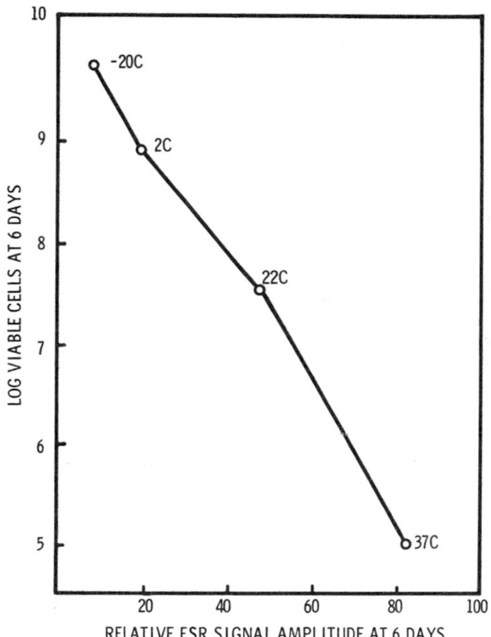

Fig. 5-8 Effect of storage temperature on survival and free radical production by lyophilized *Serratia marcescens*. (Reprinted from Ref. 15 with permission of the American Society for Microbiology.)

was a general relationship between the effectiveness of the additive in suppressing free radical production and the ability to preserve viability of cells exposed to air.

Although free radical production is associated with a change from viability to nonviability in lyophilized bacteria, it was also noted (11, 15, 23) that if cells were killed by heating, phenol, hydrogen peroxide, or mercuric chloride before lyophilization there was no detectable free radical production when air was admitted to the lyophilized cultures. A free radical precursor apparently was destroyed by the lethal agents, either directly or indirectly. As shown in Fig. 5-9, the logarithm of the number of cells surviving lyophilization after the dilute phenol treatment was proportional to free radical production. Similarly, it has been reported (15) that, after treatment with dilute hydrogen peroxide or pH adjustment of the culture before drying, free radical production was related to the log of the number of cells surviving lyophilization. The only exception to this conclusion was the observation that under certain conditions it is possible to kill bacteria by sonication without affecting the subsequent free radical production of the lyophilized sonicated material. Under these conditions the system responsible

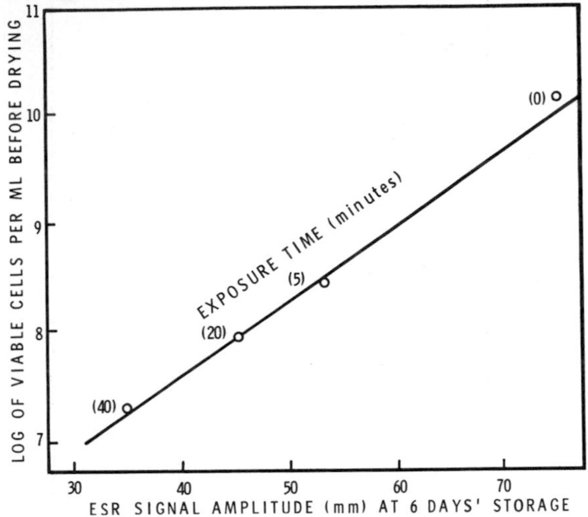

Fig. 5-9 Effect of 0.8 percent phenol on viability and free radical production by lyophilized *Serratia marcescens*. The indicated exposure times refer to the interval between adding the phenol and freezing of the sample. (Data from Ref. 15.)

for free radical production remained intact. In the whole cells (lyophilized cultures) it is not known whether the free radicals are the cause or the result of death of the organisms. It might be that the two events are merely coincident.

In interpreting free radical data of lyophilized material it is important to recognize the sensitivity of ESR; for instance, although a preparation may be "pure" DNA, the free radicals observed when it is lyophilized with ascorbic acid could be a result of ascorbic acid combining with protein or metal impurities to yield the observed spectra. Furthermore, since the radicals in a dry system are so stable, the ESR absorption represents an accumulation of free radicals rather than a steady-state condition as in an aqueous system in which the free radical is an intermediate in a chemical reaction (see Section 2.18).

The free radicals demonstrated in most dry preparations are related to living systems to the extent that they are a measure of free radical precursors. These precursors appear to be related in some manner to the ability of dry microorganisms to survive. Therefore ESR may be a useful tool in helping to understand the survival—or death—of lyophilized microorganisms. The relationship between viability and free radical accumulation in the dry preparations is intriguing. Hopefully a better understanding of the free radicals and the system producing them will permit us to control viability of lyophilized bacteria.

5.6 SUMMARY AND CONCLUSIONS

1. The free radical content of lyophilized preparations does not reflect the level of free radicals existing in the preparation before drying. The ESR spectra of free radicals in dried material are distinctly different from those in living tissues.

2. The signals seen in dry biological samples do reflect some capacity of the preparation to react with oxygen to form stable free radicals.

3. The concentration of free radicals observed in lyophilized or dryed biological preparations is dependent on oxygen concentration. Only with high vacuum pumping and sealing off under high vacuum can oxygen be excluded to prevent free radical production. Commercial gases usually have sufficient oxygen content to generate free radicals in these systems.

4. The rate of free radical formation in lyophilized materials is increased with increasing moisture content, but excess moisture leads to the disappearance of free radicals.

5. The ESR linewidth of lyophilized material is 5 to 8 G with a *g* factor of 2.0032 to 2.0058.

6. The ESR spectra of lyophilized animal tissue may be due in part to an ascorbic acid or similar radical.

7. There are probably at least two types of free radicals in most lyophilized biological systems.

8. In bacterial preparations free radical production is related to loss of viability, and in general it appears that free radical concentration is related to the numbers of cells that die after lyophilization. Substances such as sugars that preserve viability also reduce free radical production.

9. ESR study of lyophilized preparations may be useful in certain tumor or cancer studies if exposure to oxygen can be rigidly controlled.

REFERENCES

1. G. Abagyan and P. Butyagin, *Biofizika*, **9,** 180 (1964).
2. Y. Azhipa, L. Kayushin, and Y. Nikishkin, *Biofizika*, **11,** 710 (1966).
3. L. Bliumenfel'd, A. Chetverikov, D. Kefalieva, and A. Vanin, *Studia Biophys. Acta*, **10,** 101 (1968).
4. O. Brzhevskaya, V. Marinov, O. Nedelina, and E. Sheksheyev, *Biofizika*, **12,** 354 (1967).
5. A. Chetverikov, *Biofizika*, **9,** 678 (1964).
6. A. Chetverikov, A. Kalmanson, I. Kharitonenkov, and L. Bliumenfel'd, *Biofizika*, **9,** 18 (1964).
7. A. Chetverikov, L. Bliumenfel'd, and G. Fomin, *Biofizika*, **10,** 476 (1965).
8. B. Commoner and J. Ternberg, *Proc. Natl. Acad. Sci.*, **47,** 1374 (1961).

9. B. Commoner, J. Townsend, and G. Pake, *Nature*, **174,** 689 (1954).
10. A. Conger and M. Randolph, *Rad. Bot.*, **8,** 193 (1968).
11. R. Dimmick, R. Heckly, and D. Hollis, *Nature*, **192,** 776 (1961).
12. A. Harhash, W. Brucker, and G. Schoffa, *Acta biol. med. german.*, **6,** 43 (1961).
13. R. Heckly, *Cryobiology*, **2,** 139 (1965).
14. R. Heckly and R. Dimmick, *Nature*, **216,** 1003 (1967).
15. R. Heckly and R. Dimmick, *Appl. Microbiol.*, **16,** 1081 (1963).
16. R. Heckly, R. Dimmick, and J. Windle, *J. Bacteriol.*, **85,** 961 (1963).
17. I. Karitonenkov, *Biofizika*, **12,** 224 (1967).
18. I. Kharitonenkov and G. Kalichava, *Biofizika*, **11,** 708 (1966).
19. I. Kharitonenkov, A. Kalmanson, A. Chetverikov, and L. Bliumenfel'd, *Biofizika*, **9,** 172 (1964).
20. I. Kharitonenkov, G. Grigoryan, and A. Kalmanson, *Biofizika*, **10,** 1085 (1965).
21. C. Lagercrantz, *Acta. Chem. Scand.*, **18,** 562 (1964).
22. M. Lion and E. Bergmann, *J. Gen. Microbiol.*, **24,** 191 (1961).
23. M. Lion, J. Kirby-Smith, and M. Randolph, *Nature*, **192,** 34 (1961).
24. V. Malinovski and D. Kafalieva, *Z. Naturforsch.*, **19,** 457 (1964).
25. J. Mallard and M. Kent, *Nature*, **210,** 588 (1966).
26. R. Nalbandyan and L. Shifman, *Biofizika*, **11,** 359 (1966).
27. N. Pavlova and A. Livenson, *Biofizika*, **10,** 169 (1965).
28. M. Petyayev, S. Reznikov, T. Tereshchenko, I. Cherepneva, and T. Syusina, *Biofizika*, **12,** 357 (1967).
29. E. Ruuge and L. Bliumenfel'd, *Biofizika*, **10,** 689 (1965).
30. E. Ruuge, V. Timoshenkov, and L. Bliumenfel'd, *Biofizika*, **11,** 611 (1966).
31. A. Saprin, L. Nagler, Y. Koperina, K. Kruglyankova, and N. Emanuél, *Biofizika*. **11,** 706 (1966).
32. H. Swartz and R. Molenda, *Science*, **148,** 94 (1965).
33. F. Truby and J. Goldzieher, *Nature*, **182,** 1371 (1958).
34. T. Urbanski, *Nature*, **216,** 577 (1967).
35. A. Vanin and R. Nalbandyan, *Biofizika*, **10,** 167 (1965).
36. A. Vanin and R. Nalbandyan, *Biofizika*, **11,** 178 (1966).
37. A. Vanin, A. Chetverikov, and L. Bliumenfel'd, *Biofizika*, **13,** 66 (1968).

CHAPTER SIX

Photosynthesis

DANIEL H. KOHL

Biology Department
Washington University
St. Louis, Missouri

6.1 INTRODUCTION

The role assigned to single-electron transfer in photosynthesis made it natural that photosynthetic systems would come under close scrutiny early in the history of the application of ESR to the study of biological systems (1, 2, 3, 4). At the time these initial studies were undertaken van Niel's formulation of photosynthesis (5, 6)

$$CO_2 + 2H_2A \rightarrow CH_2O + 2A + H_2O,$$

where H_2A is a general oxidizable substrate, had already been demonstrated to be correct (7). In this context Michaelis's dictum that electrons are transported one at a time in a two-electron oxidation or reduction led directly to the expectation that free radical intermediates participate in the transport of electrons from the donor H_2A (H_2O in the case of green plants) to CO_2.

6.1.1 Current Model of Electron Transport in Green Plant Photosynthesis

The detailed mechanism by which electrons are transported has since that time been conceptualized into a model colloquially called the "Z scheme" (see e.g., (8) for a detailed exposition). One version of this scheme is shown in Fig. 6-1 and discussed briefly in the same manner as it is described by Boardman (8). It should be pointed out that there is controversy about the details of the scheme, particularly the relative position assigned to some of the electron carriers. For our purpose in this chapter only the broad outlines of the scheme are important, since it is this broad outline that

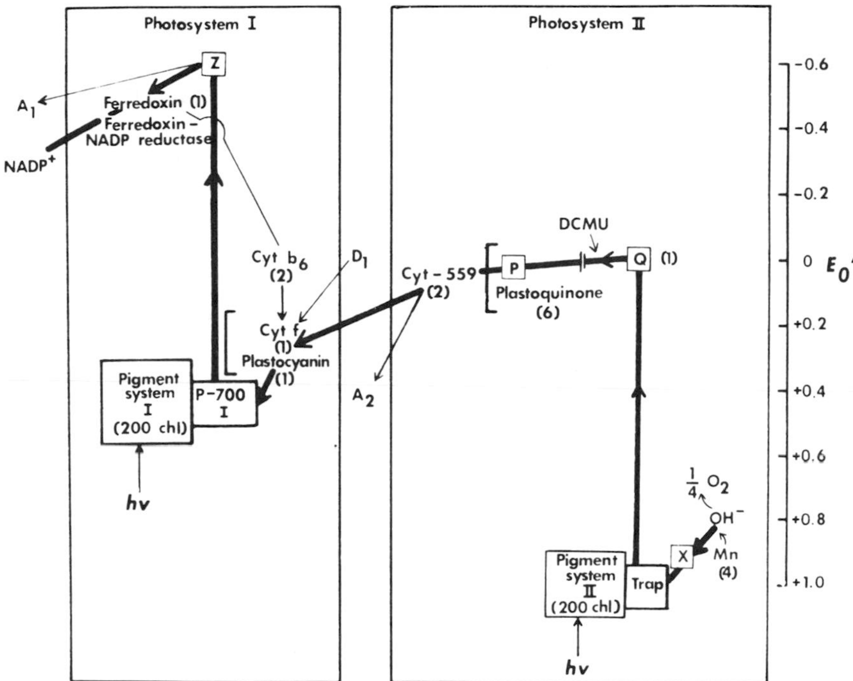

Fig. 6-1 Photoinduced electron flow in chloroplasts. Direction of flow is indicated by the heavy arrows. The pathway from OH^- to $NADP^+$ is indicated in heavier outline. The figures in parentheses indicate the moles of the electron carriers per photosynthetic unit of 400 chlorophylls. Artificial acceptors (Hill oxidants) (A_1, A_2) receive electrons after photosystem II or after photosystem I. Artificial donors (D_1) feed electrons into photosystem I. A scale of redox potentials is shown on the right. (Based on Ref. 8.)

provides the conceptual framework within which most research in photosynthesis is currently formulated.

The fixing of one carbon atom from carbon dioxide to carbohydrate requires the transfer of four electrons. The well-characterized set of dark reactions by which this carbon is fixed (Benson-Calvin cycle) requires adenosine triphosphate (ATP) and the stable reductant, reduced nicotinamide-adenine dinucleotide phosphate (NADPH), in order to operate. The diagrammatic representations (Fig. 6-1) of the mechanism by which light quanta absorbed by green plants are converted into ATP and NADPH shows water as the source of the electrons and $NADP^+$ as the stable recipient of these electrons. The *Z* scheme postulates the existence of two pigment systems, each of which contains several hundred molecules of chlorophyll *a*. Only one chlorophyll molecule in each system is directly involved in photosynthetic electron transport. The other chlorophyll *a* and auxiliary pigment molecules serve as "harvesters" of light, transferring the excitation energy of absorbed quanta to the one specially placed "reaction center" chlorophyll. This special chlorophyll *a* functioning in System I is designated P700 after the light-induced change observed at $\lambda = 700$ nm. In Fig. 6-1 the "reaction center" chlorophyll molecule of System II is given the more ambiguous name "TRAP," which reflects the fact that no specific spectrophotometric changes have been conclusively identified as corresponding to it. However, a transient at 682 nm which may arise from the System II TRAP has been observed (9). Thus the transfer of one electron requires the absorption of two quanta, one in System I and one in System II. This does not mean that one electron is transported to $NADP^+$ for every two quanta absorbed, since some electrons cycle back (cyclic photophosphorylation); the energy absorbed is sometimes re-emitted and in all probability there is some leakage.

The electron-transfer pathway diagrammatically depicted in Fig. 6-1 requires that the pigment molecule excited by the absorption of light in System II mediate the transfer of an electron from X to Q. The X^+ generated in this step extracts an electron from water, the ultimate electron donor, setting the stage for the evolution of oxygen. Electron transport then proceeds spontaneously from Q through the indicated carriers, operating in much the same manner as oxidative, terminal electron transport in the mitochondria. In the meantime the energy of a quantum absorbed anywhere within System I is transferred to the "reaction center" chlorophyll. The excited P700 reduces Z and is itself reduced by the terminal member of the intermediate electron transport chain, either plastocyanin or cytochrome f; Z^- is a strong reductant of unknown identity, strong enough to reduce CO_2 directly. The system as it has evolved, however, produces a weaker stable reductant, NADPH. The reduction of $NADP^+$ is mediated by ferredoxin and ferredoxin-NADP reductase. This stable reductant has too high a potential to accomplish the reduction of CO_2 by itself and utilizes the participation of ATP to accomplish the photosynthetic fixation of carbon.

Note that Fig. 6-1 also allows for cyclic electron flow as well as the noncyclic electron flow that leads to the production of the stable reductant. The former case is diagrammatically indicated by the "downhill" flow from ferredoxin to cytochrome b_6 (cyt b_6) and back into System I by way of cyt f or plastocyanin. Phosphorylation coupled to this cyclic flow, as well as to the transfer of electrons from Q to P700, is the source of ATP which is required for carbon fixation noted above.

Figure 6-1 also indicates that electrons may be drained out of the system by artificial electron acceptors. Among the artificial acceptors (A_1) which

Boardman (8) lists as being reduced by System I are benzoquinone, indigo-carmine, benzyl viologen, phenazine methosulfate (PMS), FMN, Vit K and, under certain conditions, ferricyanide. Chemicals that accept electrons from System II include the indophenol dyes (DCIP, TCIP), ferricyanide, methylene blue, theonine, and toluylene blue. Among the electron donors to System I are $DCIPH_2$, reduced PMS, reduced N,N,N',N'-tetramethyl-*p*-phenylene-diamine (TMPD) and diaminodural. In Fig. 6-1 DCMU (diuron) is indicated as an inhibitor of electron flow between the pigment systems (see Ref. 8 for a discussion of other inhibitors).

The *Z* scheme is generally accepted at this writing. There are, however, proposals for extensive additions to the *Z* scheme (10).

6.1.2 Current Model of Electron Transport in Bacterial Photosynthesis

Bacterial photosynthesis proceeds without the evolution of oxygen. This fact serves as the basis for the distinctions, bacterial versus O_2-evolving algal or green plant systems, that are made throughout this chapter. The absence of the evolution of O_2 may be interpreted in terms of the *Z* scheme as meaning that photosynthetic bacteria have only one system that we designate System BI, since it appears to be similar in function to System I of green plants, although recent work (11) suggests that two photosystems may operate in bacterial photosynthesis as well. The source of electrons is often reduced inorganic compounds rather than H_2O; for example, reduced sulfur compounds in the case of the thiobacillus *Chromatium*. Some active workers in the field believe that "reverse" electron flow is an important source of electrons. In a relatively early version of this conception (12) electron transport is driven from NADH by ATP which has been generated in conjunction with cyclic electron transport. One scheme of electron transport in bacterial photosynthesis is shown in Fig. 6-2. Even more than in the green-plant case the details of the participation of one or another carrier or the relative position of two electron carriers is in dispute. Again, as in the *Z* scheme, the broad outlines are what is important in providing the context for interpreting the ESR data from experiments with bacterial systems.

6.2 PHENOMENOLOGY OF STEADY-STATE ESR SIGNALS

6.2.1 Early Results

The initial experiments with photosynthetic systems provided a rich harvest of results (2, 3, 4). Although the results have been refined, they still provide

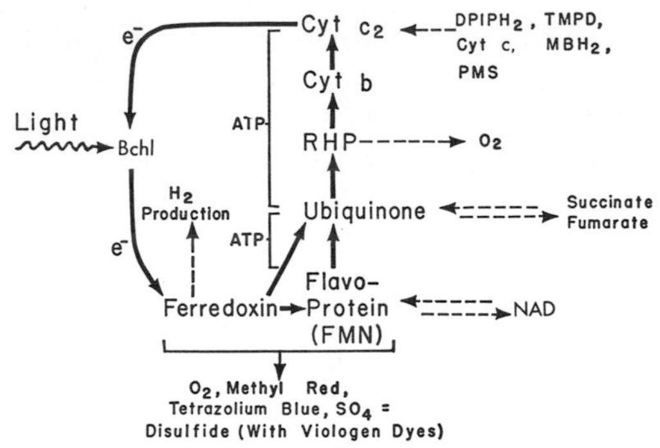

Fig. 6-2 Photosynthetic electron transport scheme for *Rhodospirillum rubrum*. This diagram indicates that light which is absorbed by bacteriochlorophyll results in the reduction of a low potential carrier, ferredoxin. This relatively reduced couple reduces the next couple, and so on, the direction of the electron flow being indicated by the arrows. Interactions of the photosynthetic electron transport system with other important cellular redox agents and with exogenous electron donors and acceptors are indicated by the dotted lines. Abbreviations used in this figure are RHP, Rhodospirillum heme protein; cyto., cytochrome; DPN, dipyridine nucleotide; ATP, adenosine triphosphate. $DPIPH_2$, TMPD, MBH_2, PMS are dyes. (Reference 86.)

the main bases for the characterization of the ESR responses of photosynthetic systems.

Two signals were distinguished when spinach chloroplasts were illuminated in the ESR cavity (see Fig. 6-3). The kinetics of signal formation and decay were often interpreted only qualitatively, since the time resolution was instrument-limited. Still the inter-relationship of the two signals was clearly perceived (14). The two signals observed in green photosynthetic material were designated Signals I and II (4). The uninitiated reader who intends to consult the early literature is warned that varied terminology has been used to refer to these signals, including I and II in the opposite sense to the original designation. The original designation, however, has now been uniformly adopted by all those working in the field and the following characterizations hopefully will be unambiguous.

Figure 6-4 illustrates an early recording from *Rhodospirillum rubrum*, a purple, nonsulfur, photosynthetic bacterium. Notice the absence of structure in the signal as compared with Fig. 6-3. This bacterial signal is designated as Signal BI, since it strongly resembles the Signal I generated by green plants. No other signal of comparable magnitude to Signal BI is seen in photosynthetic bacteria.

The early results (16, 3) also established that samples examined at temperatures low enough to exclude normal enzymatic processes (usually $\sim$ 77 K) exhibit a light-induced signal. A portion of this signal decays in the dark (3), especially in bacterial systems.

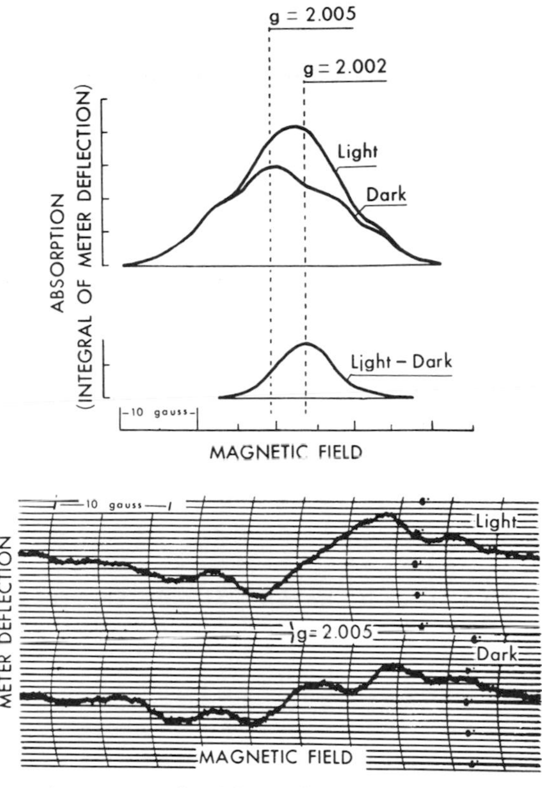

Fig. 6-3 Electron spin resonance signal from spinach chloroplasts washed twice with 0.5 M sucrose solution. The lower curves represent the actual spectrometer records, and the upper curves represent the integral curves derived from them. $T \sim 35$ C. Magnetic field increases to the right. (Reference 4.)

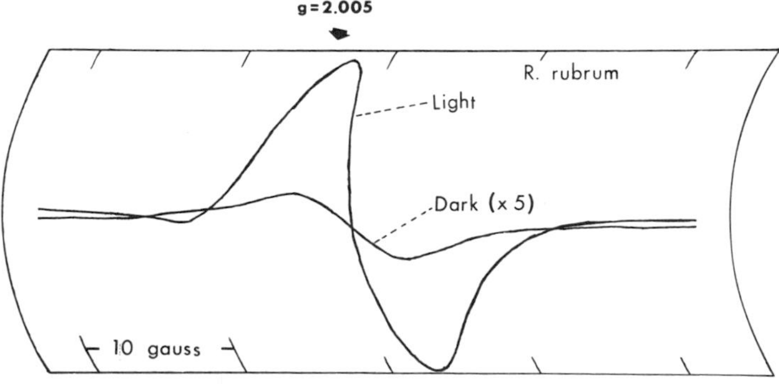

Fig. 6-4 ESR signals from *Rhodospirillum rubrum* in the light and dark. Modulation amplitudes 3 G. (Reference 14.)

6.2.2 Detailed Characterization of Signals I, II, and BI

6.2.2.1 Linewidth, Lineshape, Hyperfine Structure, and g-factors

Signals I, II, and BI are shown in Fig. 6-5. Signals I and BI are light-induced and decay rapidly in the dark. The difference between the spectra recorded in the dark immediately after illumination in the algal and bacterial samples forms the basis for asserting that the photosynthetic bacteria show no signal analogous to Signal II. The similarities in the properties of the fast-decaying signals seen in algal and bacterial samples leads to the designation of these signals as Signal I and Signal BI, respectively. This designation is meant to imply that they have a similar molecular source. The stated peak-to-peak derivative linewidths (ΔH_{pp}) for Signals I and BI vary from 7.2 to 11 G (17–21). However, much of this variation in reported values of ΔH_{pp} is probably due to overmodulation, especially in the earlier work in which low signal-to-noise ratios were a problem. The values of ΔH_{pp} given in Table 6-1 were taken from the spectra in Fig. 6-5.

Table 6-1 Characteristics of the ESR Signals Seen in Photosynthetic Systems[a]

System	Signal	ΔH_{pp} in gauss	*g* factor	Remarks
Spinach chloroplasts	I	7.4 ± 0.2	2.0025 ± 0.0001	Signal II subtracted out
Spinach chloroplasts	II	~ 19[b]	2.0047 ± 0.0002	
Subchloroplast particles				
RC–160	I	7.2 ± 0.2	2.0025 ± 0.0001	Prepared by the method of Ref. 37
RC–10	II	~ 19[b]	2.0048 ± 0.0002	
Chlamydomonas reinhardi algae	I	7.5 ± 0.2	2.0025 ± 0.0001	Signal II subtracted out
Chlamydomonas reinhardi algae	II	~ 19[b]	2.0047 ± 0.0001	
Rhodopseudomonas spheroides bacteria	BI	9.7 ± 0.2	2.0025 ± 0.0002	

[a] J. T. Warden and J. R. Bolton, unpublished results.

[b] Peak-to-peak signal width is not well defined when unresolved hyperfine structure is present. Here the width is taken to be the width at half maximum signal intensity.

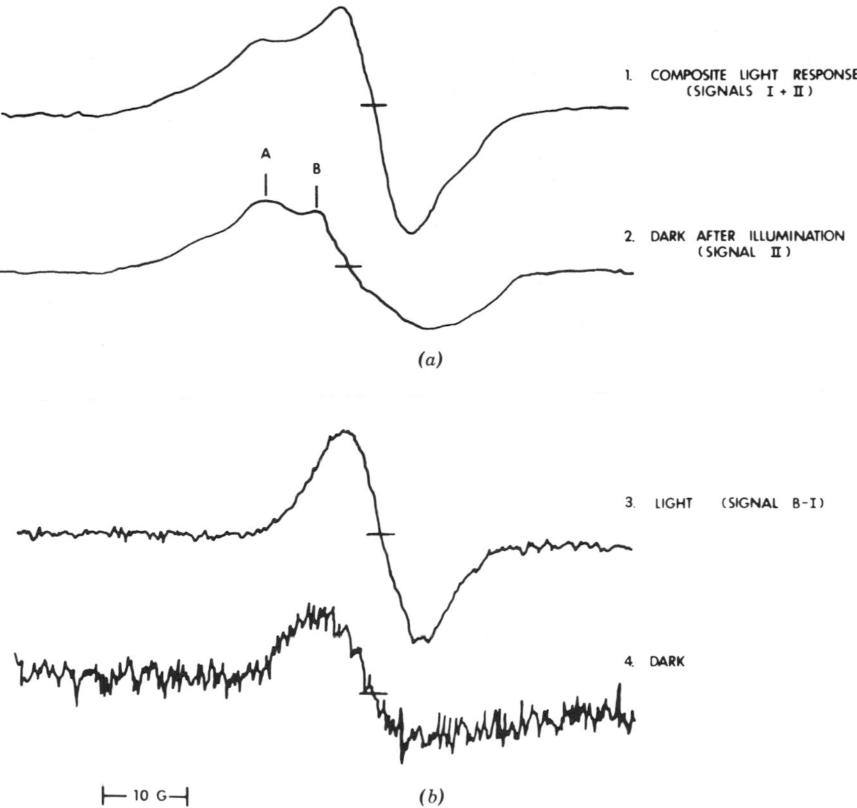

Fig. 6-5 Typical signals from O_2-evolving systems and photosynthetic bacteria. (*a*) The upper pair of spectra are typical of spectra generated when green plant systems are placed in the cavity. A composite of Signals I and II is seen in the light. Since Signal I decays rapidly in the light, only Signal II remains in the dark following illumination. The fractional decay of Signal II in the interval between the two recordings may be judged by comparing the relative signal amplitudes at the position in the magnetic field marked *A*, since there is no contribution of Signal I in that magnetic field region. Sample: *Chlamydomonas reinhardii*. Modulation amplitude, 4 G. (Bolton, unpublished results.) (*b*) The dominant signal seen in the light when photosynthetic bacteria are placed in the cavity is seen in spectrum 3. The small residual signal in spectrum 4 seen subsequently in the dark does not arise from the same molecular source as does Signal II in the green plant system. Sample: *Rhodospirillum rubrum*. Modulation amplitude, 4 G. The ordinate in the bottom spectrum is expanded five times compared with the top. (Based on Ref. 31.)

These spectra were recorded under conditions in which the modulation amplitude and microwave power do not affect the lineshape. Note that there does appear to be a small but significant difference in ΔH_{pp} between Signal I and BI. The differences between bacteriochlorophyll and chlorophyll, but more importantly between the details of the environments in which these molecules find themselves in the specific systems, is more than enough to account for the observed differences (19). [This remark, of course, anticipates the identification of Signal (B)I as a (bacterio)chlorophyll radical.]

Signal BI in photosynthetic bacteria is approximately gaussian in shape (22, 23), as shown in Fig. 6-6. Lineshapes for Signal I from O_2-evolving systems have been reported less often, presumably since it is necessary to subtract Signal II in order to observe it. Signal I in green systems also seems to be gaussian in shape, however.

No hyperfine structure is observed for Signal I or Signal BI even at very low modulation amplitude, but both Signal I, BI, and Signal II are dramatically narrowed when all the protons in the organism are replaced by deuterons (24, 19). The ratio of the peak-to-peak derivative linewidth, $\Delta H^H_{pp}/\Delta H^D_{pp}$ is of the order of 2 to 3 for a wide variety of algae and photosynthetic bacteria (19, 24). This is unambiguous proof that hyperfine interaction of the unpaired electrons with hydrogens contributes

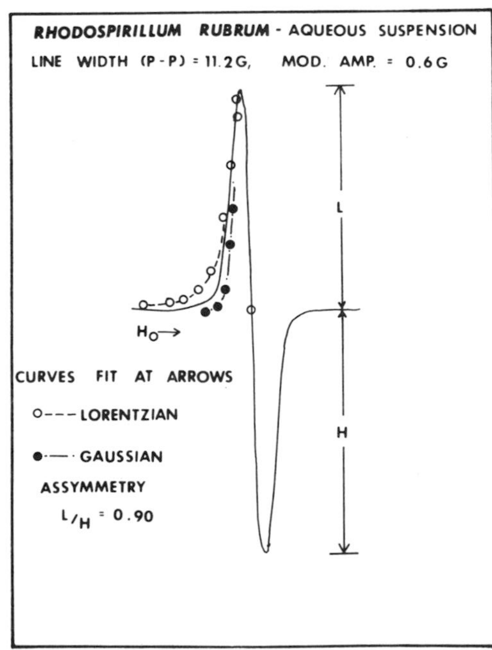

Fig. 6-6 Lineshape analysis of the ESR spectrum of *Rhodospirillum rubrum* in aqueous suspension at room temperature. (Reference 22.)

significantly to the overall linewidth of Signals I and BI. This large contribution of unresolved proton hyperfine structure to the linewidth is consistent with the observed gaussian lineshape. The ratio, $\Delta H^H_{pp}/\Delta H^D_{pp}$ would be expected to be approximately 3.8 for a gaussian line if unresolved hyperfine structure were solely responsible for the linewidth.

Careful measurements of the g factor of Signal BI from *Rhodospirillum rubrum* at 77 K (19) and "reaction-center preparations" of *Rhodopseudomonas spheriodes*, strain R-26 at room temperature (20), yielded values of 2.0026 $\pm$0.0001 and 2.0025 $\pm$0.0002, respectively. Other reported values, both for bacterial and green plant systems, fall very close, although, as with the other parameters of Signal I, in the O_2-evolving systems the reliability is lower, since the contribution of Signal II ordinarily tends to make the exact position of Signal I less certain.

The properties of Signal II have often either been misunderstood or imprecisely stated (see, e.g., p. 1110 of Ref. 24). Weaver pointed out forcefully (25) that Signal II is a light-induced signal, despite the fact that it decays only slowly in the dark. She also notes that the relatively higher maximum amplitude of Signal I compared with II has incorrectly led some to infer that the concentration of Component I exceeds that of Component II. Most often the second integral shows that [II] $\div$ [I] $\sim$ 2. Signal II may be observed by illuminating spinach chloroplasts, for example, and subsequently recording the ESR signal in the dark. The composite lineshape changes quickly with time in the dark. This is followed by a slow, proportional decrease over the whole magnetic field region. This corresponds to the rapid decay of Signal I, leaving only Signal II, which then slowly decays in the dark. The hallmark of Signal II uncontaminated by other signals is a ratio of amplitudes $B/A \sim 3/4$, as shown in Fig. 6-5. In the same authoritative review in which she so clearly enunciates the other properties of Signal II, Weaver mistakes its lineshape by not assigning the peak at B (Fig. 6-5) to Signal II. Instead she shows the amplitude monotonically decreasing from the peak at field point A to the baseline crossing. (Compare Fig. 6-5 this chapter with Fig. 1 in Ref. 25.)

The half-width at half-height of Signal II is about 19 G (4). The hyperfine peaks are separated by about 5 G, as indicated in Fig. 6-5. This hyperfine structure is largely due to interaction with hydrogen nuclei, since it disappears and the line narrows when algae grown in a totally deuterated medium are the source of the ESR signal (15, 24). The g factor for Signal II is higher than that for Signal (B)I, a typically reported value being 2.0044 (18).

6.2.2.2 *Light Saturation*

The light saturation behavior of Signals I and II has been measured. Limitations on the interpretation of data from light saturation measurements are discussed in detail by Rabinowitch (26, 27), who shows that deviations from the expected behavior at infinite dilution are of the order of 5 percent if the sample transmits 50 percent of the incident light and 10 percent if it transmits 25 percent. This is well within the experimental error associated with most ESR measurements. It is clear, however, that the centrifugally packed, essentially opaque samples sometimes used are not suitable for such studies. High light intensities must also be avoided, since radicals from the light-harvesting pigments may be generated under certain conditions (28).

In spite of the experimental difficulties, it does appear that the intensity of Signal II saturates at a lower light intensity than Signal I in green plant systems. Perhaps the best evidence is provided by Heise (15) who early reported that the apparent *g* factor (i.e., determined from the derivative zero cross-over for the composite line) for *Chlorella* preparations varied from about 2.004 to 2.002 with increasing light intensity. The shift to a lower *g* factor is consistent with a greater relative intensity of Signal I. Treharne et al. (29, 30) also report that Signal II saturates at lower light intensities for a number of algae.* The light-saturation behavior of Signal BI in bacteria appears to be similar to that of Signal I (31, 28).

It should be noted that the light-saturation behavior of the ESR signals is determined by the rate at which reaction centers are restored to their dark state. Thus we might anticipate that light saturation of Signal BI would not be achieved at -100 C at intensities more than sufficient to saturate the signal at room temperature, as was shown (31). Since these rates are highly variable from sample to sample, light saturation studies are not likely to be useful except to compare two signals in the same sample.

It may be worth noting that solutions of $CuSO_4$, which have sometimes been used in light saturation studies as a heat shield, may not be the solutions of choice, since the long wavelength cutoff is quite close to the red absorption maximum of P700. A 2.5 percent solution of copper sulfate ($CuSO_4 \cdot 5H_2O$) 1 cm thick transmits about 50 percent of the incident light at 650 nm and only 25 percent at 700 nm.

6.2.2.3 Microwave Saturation

As discussed in Section 1.3, the microwave power at which an ESR signal saturates is a function of how strongly the spin system and its surroundings interact. Fig. 2-8 shows the theoretical effect of increasing microwave power on the ESR signal amplitude. Note that the abscissa in that figure

* These conclusions hold even after correction is made for the fact that their method of measuring overestimates the amplitude of Signal I by discounting Signal II's amplitude at the magnetic field point marked *B* in Fig. 6-5.

is labeled $\sqrt{P_0}$, where P_0 is the microwave power. [Some references display saturation plots as a function of P_0 rather than $\sqrt{P_0}$ (22, 23, 32).]

Both Signals I and BI (33, 28) appear to saturate in a manner such that the signal amplitude is approximately independent of P_0 above the saturation level. (See the dotted curve in Fig. 2-8.) These results, along with the near gaussian shape (22, 31) and the fact that a large fraction of the linewidth is due to unresolved hyperfine splitting (24, 19) argue strongly that Signal I saturates by way of an inhomogeneous mechanism (34, 35).

There are no published data on the saturation behavior of Signal II, although Allen (36) mentions that it does not saturate. In our hands Signal II appears to saturate at low power and does not appear to change in lineshape or -width as it saturates (Kohl and Zide, unpublished results).

Comparison of the width of Signal II from algal cultures grown on an inorganic medium of naturally occurring isotopic content with that generated by organisms grown on a virtually totally deuterated medium reveals a considerable contribution of hyperfine interaction to the linewidth (24). This is consistent with the inhomogeneous saturation reported above.

6.2.3 Morphological Localization of Signals

Treharne, Melton, and Roppel (21) have shown that the ratio of Signals I/II induced by light in *Chlorella pyrenoidosa* was closely correlated with the chlorophyll concentration as measured by extraction and the density of chloroplast lamellae as seen in electron micrographs. The denser were the lamellae, the greater was the ratio Signal I/II (see Figs. 6-7, 6-8). Treatment for 5 min at 60 C resulted in severe damage to the cellular architecture, thus destroying Signal II but leaving Signal I intact (see Fig. 6-9). In fact, the absolute magnitude of Signal I increased under these conditions (29), presumably because photosynthetic electron transport was interrupted and the mechanism for returning Component I to its non-free radical state was destroyed. Treharne et al. (21) reported further that treatment at 80 C destroyed the lamellar structure and that Signal I disappeared.

These results show that destruction of the stroma eliminates Signal II but that Signal I survives as long as the grana are intact. The extremely plausible deduction from these results is that Signal I is associated with a component of the grana and Signal II with a component of the stroma. This conclusion is not consistent with the fact that Signal I was observed when subchloroplast particles (RC-160 particles prepared by the methods in Ref. 37) were examined (see Table 6-1). These particles which contain higher chl. *a* / chl. *b* ratios and much more P700 than do intact chloroplasts exhibit System I, but not System II activity. However, on the basis of electron microscopic evidence, Sane, Goodchild, and Park (37) conclude that these are "stroma lamallae" rather than grana lamallae.

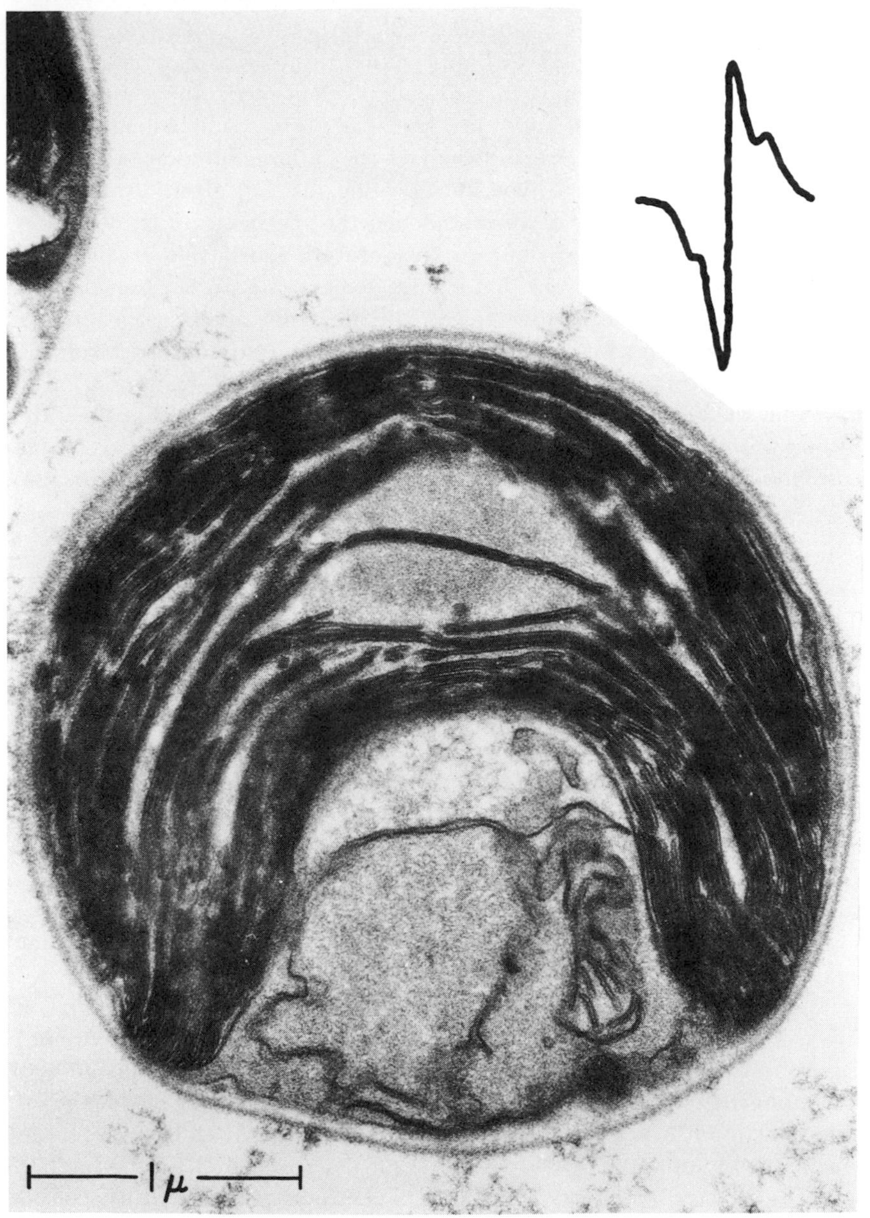

Fig. 6-7 Electron micrograph of *Chlorella pyrenoidosa* grown under 100 foot-candles and associated light-induced ESR signal. Lamellae are noticeably denser than in high-light grown cells. Insert shows corresponding light-induced ESR signal. Micrograph enlarged × 39,500. (Reference 21.)

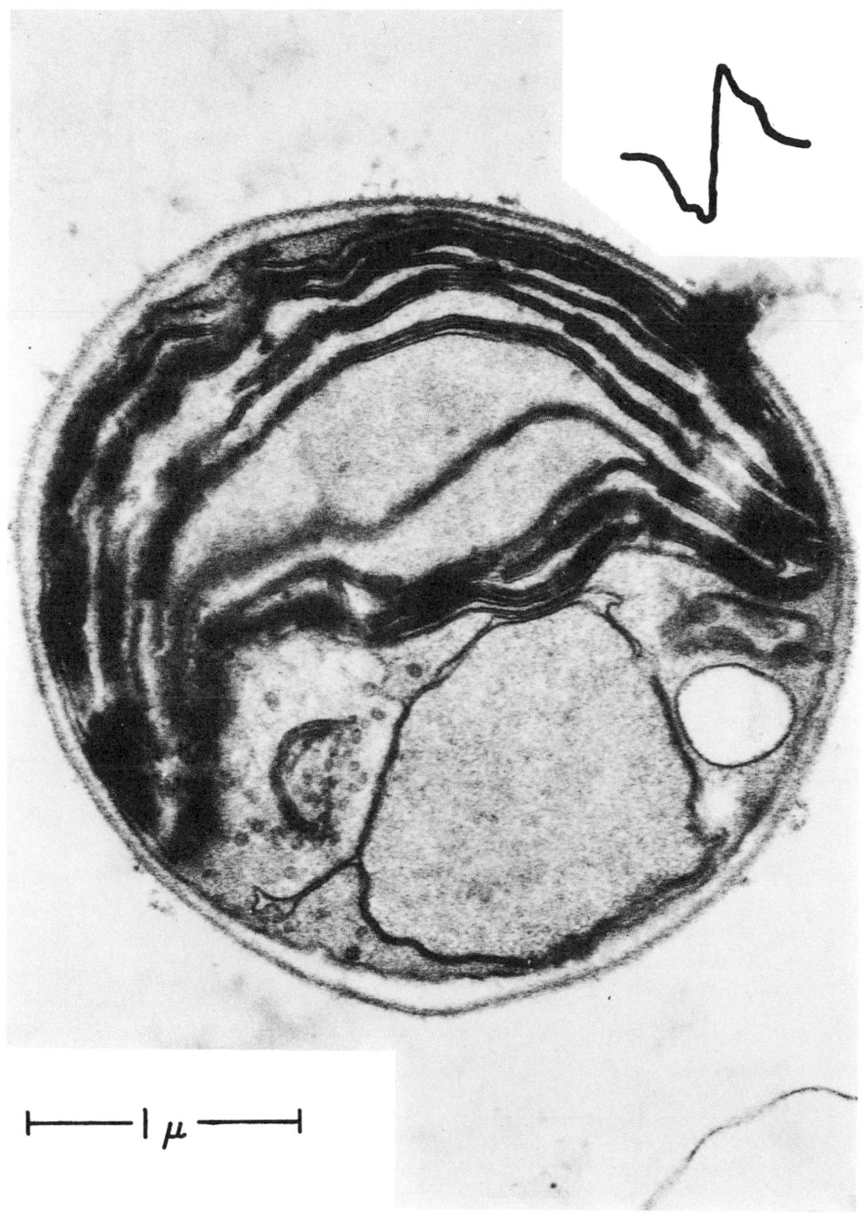

Fig. 6-8 Electron micrograph of *C. pyrenoidosa* grown under 1050 foot-candles. Lamellae, nucleus, and mitochondria are evident. Insert shows corresponding light-induced ESR signal. Micrograph enlarged $\times$ 39,500. (Reference 21.)

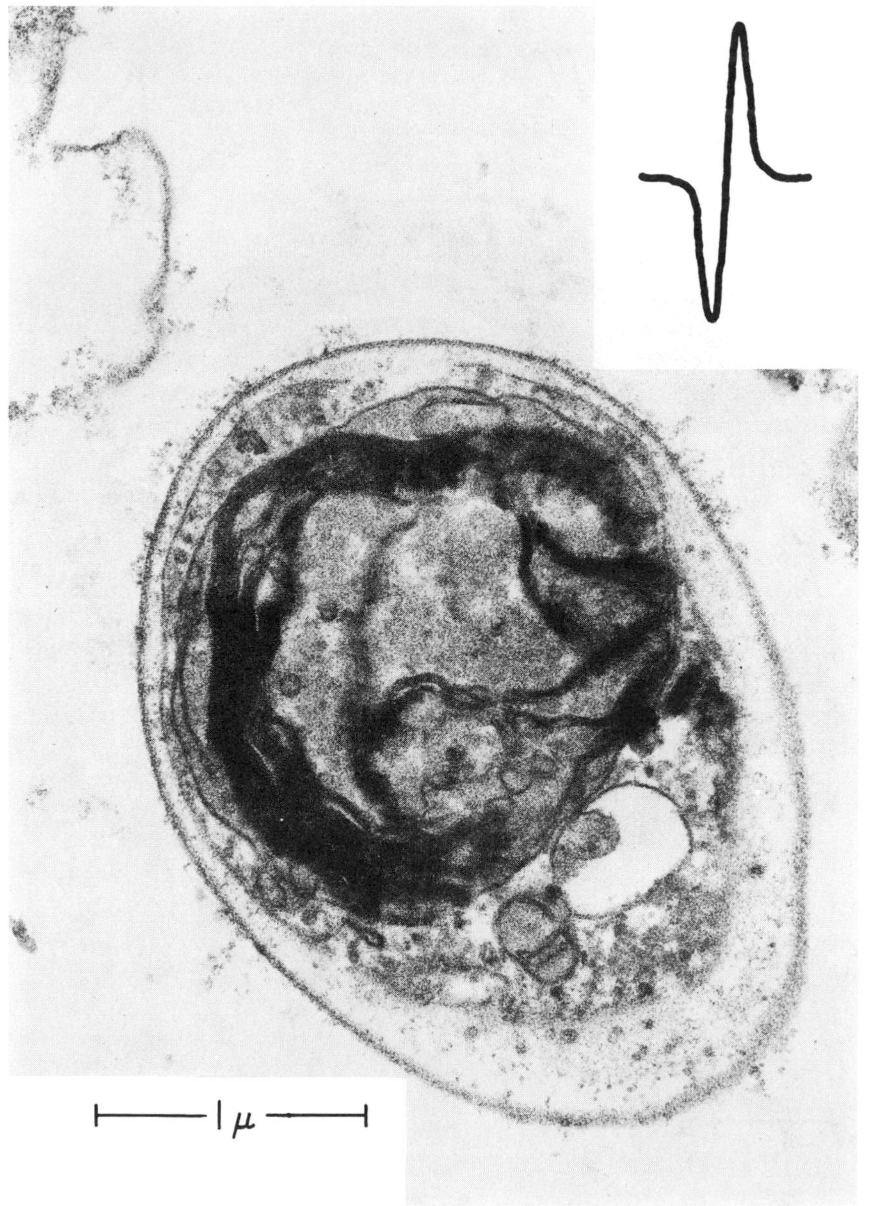

Fig. 6-9 Electron micrograph of *C. pyrenoidosa* heat-treated for 5 min at 60 C. Severe damage to the cell is evident but the lamellar structure remains relatively intact. ESR Signal II is destroyed but ESR Signal I persists under this treatment. (Reference 21.)

6.3 MOLECULAR ORIGIN OF THE SIGNALS

6.3.1 General Comments

As stated earlier, the initial experiments produced a rich yield of results. The concluding sentence of the first detailed report of ESR investigations of photosynthetic systems (2) reflected the confidence induced by the initial results: "Experiments are under way which are designed to identify the substances in question (i.e., the molecular species giving rise to the observed free radicals) and to describe their relationship to the process of photosynthesis." That the road has been rockier than anticipated is indicated by the fact that the main unanswered questions remained essentially the same for many years.

Perhaps one of the roadblocks standing in the way of obtaining the most useful information more quickly was that the system yields information so easily and there are so many experiments that can be done. Some of the variable parameters are enumerated below, the number of types of experiment, of course, being the number of meaningful permutations of these conditions.

Choice of the organism to be studied permits a large range of *genetic variability*. Such variation ranges from substitution of one strain for another to substitution across wide taxonomic gulfs. A choice must be made on each occasion between *whole cells* versus *subcellular components*. In many cases the former are preferred, but specific problems, such as permeability to a reagent, sometimes dictate the choice of the latter. Variations in *growth conditions* can result in changes ranging from pigment concentration to induction of different metabolic patterns. These conditions involve the growth medium, intensity, and spectral qualities of illumination, temperature, gas exchange, and "culture age" at harvest. Even though all of the items enumerated are controllable, batch cultures are notorious for the variable rate at which they carry out a process and it is expected, and found, that similar variations in ESR results occur. In recent years it has been possible to grow microorganisms in *isotopically altered* media. In a formal sense this could be categorized under variations in growth conditions, but the potential magnitude of the influence on the ESR response of such a change merits separate listing. Additional variation is available by selectively altering the isotopic content of certain molecules. Treatment with *inhibitors*, *electron donors* or *acceptors*, and *uncouplers* of photosynthetic phosphorylation offers further opportunity for extensive variation of the photosynthetic and other metabolic capabilities of samples. At the time of the experiment values must be chosen for *temperature*, *quantity of light* (light intensity), *quality of light* (spectral distribution), *magnetic-field position* and *sweep*, *optical density of sample* and *program of illumination*. In addition, as the experiment proceeds the *physiological state* of the organisms changes. These changes are not controllable but can probably be minimized by examining samples at an optical density and at a light intensity of the order of that in a growing culture; meeting these conditions results in a lowered signal-to-noise ratio. Low temperature may also stabilize the physiological state over time but little is known of the relation of this stabilized state to the state in which the process of interest occurs.

It is now possible to say with some certainty that Signal BI arises from the positive ion of bacteriochlorophyll *a*. It is also quite probable that Signal I arises from the positive ion of chlorophyll *a*, although the evidence in this case is not yet so conclusive as that for Signal BI. The molecular source of Signal II is less certainly identified as a plastochromanoxyl free radical. (This radical is structurally related to the more commonly discussed plastosemiquinone in the sense that the chromanoxyl may be derived formally from the semiquinone by shifting a bond to form a second ring; that is, the first isoprenoid unit on C_5 becomes part of a chroman ring.) The data on which these statements are based are the subject matter of the remainder of this section.

6.3.2 The Molecular Origin of Signals I and BI

6.3.2.1 Early Results

A chlorophyll free radical was from the beginning the favored candidate as the molecule giving rise to Signal I. The outlines of the decisive experiments were clearly deducible from a note by Beinert, Kok, and Hoch (17) which followed close on the heels of the enumeration of the properties of P700 (see, e.g., Ref. 38). They reported on the ESR response of a sample prepared from the red alga, TX27, which had been enriched in P700 by brief extraction with cold 68 percent acetone. They noted that the observed ESR signal "was affected by light, ferricyanide and PMS in a fashion identical to the absorption at 700 nm." Had this important note been accorded the significance that, in retrospect, it clearly deserved, others of us would have vigorously traveled the road it marked, and the identity of the "reaction center" (bacterio)chlorophyll positive ion as the source of Signal (B)I would almost certainly have been firmly established earlier.

6.3.2.2 Variation of Response of the Active Center Pigment and Signal I as a Function of the Reduction Potential

Another important observation made by Beinert, Kok, and Hoch (17) was the similarity among the midpoint reduction potentials* for the ESR signal

* The midpoint potential E_m of an oxidation-reduction reaction is defined by Clark (39) as $E_h = E_m + 0.06/n \log (S_0/S_r)$ at constant (H^+), where S_0 and S_r refer to the oxidized and reduced species. Thus E_m is the value of the potential when $S_0 = S_r$. To talk of midpoint potential for the appearance of the light-induced ESR signal or of the bleaching of P700

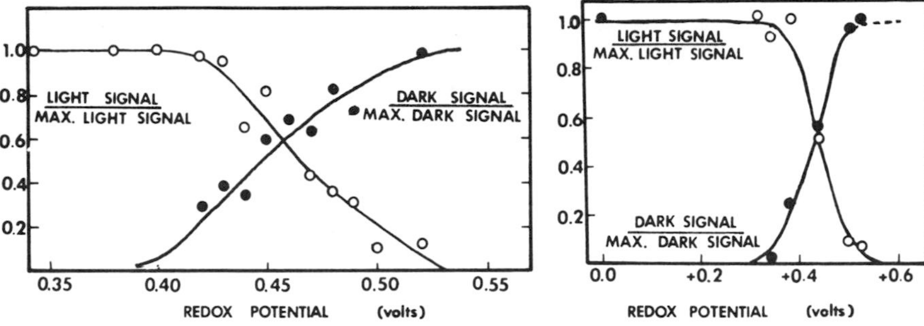

Fig. 6-10 Redox titration of the chemically induced and photoinduced ESR signal in "quantasomes" from spinach chloroplasts (left) and in chromatophores from *Rhodospirillum rubrum* (right). The light signal referred to is the additional signal observed on illumination. The dark signal referred to is produced by chemical oxidation alone. The important result is the approximate complementarity of the two methods of producing the ESR signal. (See Ref. 40 from which this figure was taken for experimental details.)

induced by light, the ESR signal produced by chemical oxidation, and the bleaching of P700. The variation of the light-induced and chemically induced ESR signals as a function of the reduction potential of the environment was reported in some detail shortly after (40) and is shown in Fig. 6-10. No correlation, however, except the similarity of midpoint potential, was made between the behavior of the ESR signal and P700 in this paper. In a subsequent elegant and thorough paper (41) the result was extended to include the observation that at low potential, between +0.05 and −0.10 V, both the ESR signal and the light-induced absorbance changes were absent. Still there is no report of an experiment in which the percentage of the maximum light-induced change at 700 nm (or 865 nm for *Rhodospirillum rubrum* chromatophores) and the percentage of maximum light-induced Signal I or BI was measured on the same sample as a function of the potential. The closest that we can come to making the comparison, which would have been convincing evidence of the molecular identity of Signal BI, is to plot the data in Fig. 6-10 of this chapter on the same scale as that of Fig. 7 of Kuntz, Loach, and Calvin (42), which shows the variation with potential of the light-induced absorption changes at 865 nm in *Rhodospirillum rubrum* chromatophores. When this is done, the observed agreement is close, although there does seem to be a difference in midpoint potential of about 10 mV.

---

seems to assume that they are the result of oxidation-reduction reactions. The spirit of the usage, however, is clearly retained and assumptions are avoided if the midpoint potential is taken to be that value of the potential at which the process has half its maximum value. Thus in Fig. 6-10 $f(E_m) = 0.5$.

The necessity for making the detailed comparison on the same sample is made clear by the result that the midpoint potential varied 40 mV in response to change in the ionic strength (Fig. 2 in Ref. 42) as well as the more general experience of variability of most parameters from sample to sample.

6.3.2.3 Long Wavelength Sensitization of Signal I

The sensitization of Signal I at a wavelength longer than 680 nm, the wavelength for the maximum absorption of bulk chlorophyll *a* in O_2-evolving systems, also implicates P700 in the production of Signal I. Of course, this result does not require the conclusion that $P700^+$ is the free radical, Component I. On this evidence alone the reaction partner of P700 would be just as plausible a candidate. The long wavelength sensitization has been reported by several laboratories (43, 44, 36, 15, 45, 46) and can be considered to be well established. Figure 6-11 shows an action spectra for ESR Signal I and P700 responses and an absorption spectrum of the sample.

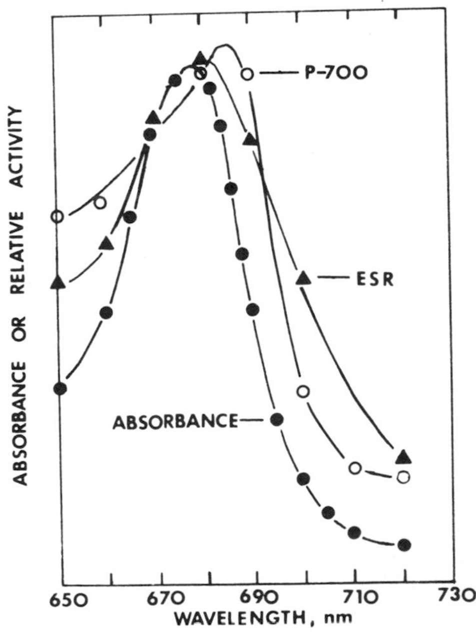

Fig. 6-11 Action spectra for the light-induced ESR (▲) and P700 responses (○) of PD10 (System I) particles. The actinic light was adjusted to give equal energy at each wavelength. ESR measurements, modulation amplitude = 4.8 G. (See Ref. 46 on which this figure is based for experimental details.)

6.3.2.4 Comparison Between the Number of Free Radicals and the Number of Active-Center Pigment Molecules

Beinert and Kok (33) reasoned that if $P700^+$ is the free radical that gives rise to Signal I then a spectrophotometric count of $P700^+$ molecules ought to give the same number as the count of free radicals by ESR spectroscopy. Table I from their paper is reproduced in part below as Table 6-2. Note that the measurements were made on three different kinds of sample (red and blue-green algae and higher plant chloroplasts), each treated in several different ways. The ratio, free radicals (spins) per P700, is higher than 1, clustering around 2. The authors, in assessing the sources of error, feel that the true number lies between 1 and 4.

Since the experiment is so important and the result surprising, possible sources of error are considered in some detail. The authors explicitly state the conditions that must be met by such an experiment, including saturation by light, in order that all the radicals that can be formed are formed and the microwave power is low enough so that the sample is not power saturated (since the standard is not). Any failure to meet these conditions, for example, by use of a too-concentrated suspension, by cutting out too much of the longer wavelength light with the 10 percent $CuSO_4$ heat filter used, or by using too high a microwave power would have led to lower, not higher, values of the number of free radicals and therefore cannot explain the surprisingly high ratio of spins per P700 measured. Such a consistently high value would seem to result from a systematic error, if indeed the value is spuriously high. The authors suggest the possibility that the extinction coefficient for P700 is too high and has thus lead them to underestimate the concentration of P700. They also assume complete bleaching of P700 by light. This assumption would seem warranted by the fact that ferricyanide oxidation yielded the same quantitative result as illumination.* In addition, they note that there is a 1 to 2 msec time lapse between the flash of light used to bleach the P700 and the time at which the measurement was made, thus allowing time for some of the bleached material to decay before the measurement was made. Although no decay kinetics were measured here, 20 to 30 msec is a typical half-time for decay, so that it seems probable that not much of the $P700^+$ is rereduced during the interval between the measurement and the flash. Signal II was subtracted out of the composite signal (I + II) seen in the light by subtracting the spectrum recorded in the dark immediately after cessation of illumination. Although Signal II will also have decayed in the interval, it seems probable that only a small fraction will have done so. (This assumption can

* Although this was reassuring when it was published, it is not so clear how it should be interpreted in view of Weaver's more recent finding (47) that the signal induced by chemical oxidation with ferricyanide is invariably smaller than that produced by light.

Table 6-2 Concentrations of Chlorophyll, *P*-700 and Detectable Light-Induced Free Radicals in various Photosynthetic Materials (based on Ref. 33)

Material[a]	Light	Additions[b]	Temperature (°C)	Chlorophyll $\times 10^5$ *M*	*P*-700 $\times 10^7$ *M*	Spins $\times 10^7$ *M*	Chlorophyll per spins[c]	Spins per *P*-700[c]
TX 27, sonicated and washed	+	ferro	25	72	38	68	108	1.8
	+	—	−53	2.5	1.3	4.3	58	3.3
TX 27, washed and extracted with 72 percent acetone	+	—	25	50	65	116	45	1.7
	+	—	−53	2.0	2.6	9	22	3.5
	+	—	−88	27	27	29	93	1.1
Anacystis, whole cells	+	—	25	120	40	120	112	2.7
	+	DCMU	25	120	40	128	104	2.9
	+	—	−53	6	2	12	55	5.5
Anacystis, sound-treated and washed	+	—	25	52	17	65	80	3.8
	+	—	−53	2.7	0.9	5.9	71	4.2
Anacystic, sound-treated	+	—	−70	90	30	125	72	4.2
Anacystis, washed and extracted with 72 percent acetone	+	—	25	11	7	20	55	2.9
	+	—	−90	11	7	12	92	1.7
Spinach chloroplasts fresh	+	—	−70	100	25	51	196	2.0
Spinach chloroplasts aged	+	—	−70	72	18	38	190	2.1
Spinach chloroplasts extracted with 72 percent acetone	+	—	−70	16	23	58	28	2.5
	+	—	−72	24	35	79	30	2.3

[a] TX 27 is a high-temperature strain of the red alga Porphorydium. Anacystis is a blue-green alga.

[b] The additions were ferrocyanide (ferro) to eliminate the light signal in materials in which the decay in the dark is slow to a final concentration of approximately 10^{-4} *M*; 3-(3,4-dichlorophenyl)-1,1-dimethylurea (DCMU) to a final concentration of 6×10^{-6} *M*.

[c] Ratios for the light-induced signals only, corrected for observed dark signals.

always be checked by comparing the magnitude at field point A in Fig. 6-5 of the signal in the light versus dark immediately after cessation of illumination.)

Thus none of the apparent systematic errors considered above can account for the surprisingly high value of the ratio; number of free radicals (spins) to number of P700.*

Results of careful experiments by Loach and Walsh (28) make it clear that they have successfully met all of conditions imposed on the investigator who undertakes such an experiment. In addition to the precautions and corrections noted previously, they also applied a correction to compensate for differences between the standard and sample in the lineshape, linewidth and modulation amplitude (48). Their calculations, however, clearly involve some of the same sorts of assumptions that Beinert and Kok (33) made and which could lead to systematic error; for example, the extinction coefficient 90 mM^{-1} cm^{-1} which they assign to the active center pigment is also close to the value generally used for the bulk pigment. They worked with unaltered chromatophores from *Rhodospirillum rubrum* and *Rhodospuedomonas spheroides*; that is, there was no treatment to enrich the chromatophores in P865 and P880, respectively. Their results are that the ratios of free radicals to active-center pigment molecules were close to 1 for both *R. rubrum* and *R. spheroides* chromatophores (see also Ref. 20). However, when Loach measured the ratio of free radicals to P700 in green algae and in green plant systems, his results (49) confirmed Beinert and Kok's (33) original report. The result is not easily interpreted, especially if one is convinced by the rest of the data that Component I is an oxidized active-center pigment.† Loach (private communication) and others feel

* In a paper that appeared after the writing of this section had been completed J. R. Norris, R. A. Uphaus, H. Crespi, J. Katz, *PNAS*, **68**: 625–628 (1971) present evidence they interpret as implicating a chlorophyll dimer as the source of Signal I. If these dimers are P700 dimers, this leads to an expectation of a value of $\frac{1}{2}$ for the ratio of spins/P700. In that case the clustering of values around 2, which Beinert and Kok report, becomes all the more unexpected.

† If systematic error is involved, a likely candidate is that too high a value of the "difference extinction coefficient" for P700 (and/or P870, P880) was used, leading to a too low apparent concentration in the computation of spins/active center pigment molecule. There are several reports of lower values. Smidt-Mende and Rumberg (50) assign $\epsilon_{(\lambda=703)} = 36\ mM^{-1}cm^{-1}$. Hiyama and Ke (to appear in *Biochem. Biophys. Acta*, 1972) report, as the result of a detailed re-examination of the problem, $\epsilon_{(\lambda=703)} = 64\ mm^{-1}cm^{-1}$. This value is only about one-half of that they had assigned previously (B.Ke, T. Ogowa, T. Hiyama, and L. P. Vernon, *Biochem. Biophys. Acta*, **226**, 53–62, 1971). Both values are substantially lower than those used by Beinert and Kok for P700 (33) and Loach and Walsh for P870 (28), 80, and 90, respectively. One might expect, however, that a downward revision of the "difference extinction coefficient" for P700 might presage such a revision for active center bacteriochlorophyll as well. If this were the case, then it would leave unexplained Loach and Walsh's results (28) of a one-to-one ratio between free radicals and active-center pigment molecules for the two species of photosynthetic bacteria reported above.

that important information may be buried in this result.

One plausible explanation for the result, free radical/P700 ~ 2, in O_2-producing systems as opposed to unity in the bacterial systems is that radicals being produced by System II in O_2-producing systems are also being observed in the ESR spectrum. If that were the case, the value of the ratio should drop to approximately 1 if the wavelength of the exciting light were greater than 700 nm. The strongest objection to this suggestion might be that the anticipated spectrophotometric changes which should accompany the production of such a System II free radical are not observed. If we pursue this line of reasoning to its conclusion, however, we may have to abandon the entire postulation of a System II chlorophyll.

One other comment may be in order about this type of experiment. In their methods section Loach and Walsh (28) warn that "the use of too much light intensity must also be guarded against because additional bacteriochlorophyll radicals can be produced from pigments other than reaction center bacteriochlorophyll." The production of these additional radicals has been demonstrated in chromatophore preparations when oxygen is present and exogenous reductants are absent (Loach, personal communication). The possibility of such an effect requires that any experiment designed to investigate the quantum yield of reaction-center chlorophyll radical production must include, as a control, a curve that clearly shows saturation at "reasonable" light intensities. The possibility of producing radicals that are unrelated to photosynthetic activity makes it highly desirable to demonstrate, in the same preparation used for the quantum yield measurement, that the radical production saturates in the same way as a parameter unequivocably associated with photosynthetic electron transport. These additional controls are required if we are to retain the principal experimental rationale; namely, that if $P700^+$ (or $P865^+$ or $P880^+$ in the bacterial systems) is the source of Signal I, the number of $P700^+$ molecules and the number of free radicals should be equal.

6.3.2.5 Comparison of the Kinetics of Oxidized Reaction-Center (Bacterio) Chlorophyll and Signal I Production and Decay

The rise and decay kinetics of the bleaching of P700 (P865 or P880 in the case of several photosynthetic bacteria) have been studied extensively since the discovery of these specialized (bacterio)chlorophyll molecules and the assignment to them of a unique role in photosynthesis. A certainty has developed that it is possible to follow their kinetics without interference from other spectral lines. Under these circumstances a number of laboratories proceeded on the assumption that if the "kinetic fingerprint" of two independent measurements (optical versus ESR kinetics) were identical the source of the two events would be identical; for example, if the kinetics of the rise and decay in the ESR signal from a sample of *R. rubrum* chromatophores are identical to that of the change at 865 nm, the radical species is $P865^+$.

It would be preferable in such an experiment for the optical and ESR measurements to be made simultaneously on the same sample. Although instrumentation that will allow this seems within reach, no results from such an experimental arrangement have been reported. Short of simultaneous measurement, it is impossible to stress too strongly the necessity for these measurements being done on the same sample without even transferring it to another cuvette. The stringency of these requirements is based on the widely experienced uncontrollable variation among bulk samples and the change of the measurable properties of a single sample with time or as the result of apparently trivial treatments, such as an additional resuspension or centrifugation. Evidence for the stability of the sample over the time period of the measurement is required to interpret the results with confidence. Thus, if the optical kinetics are recorded first, they should be repeated after the ESR kinetics. The identity of the optical kinetics in these two recordings may be taken as presumptive evidence of the constancy of the sample during the time of the experiment.

As noted earlier, almost as soon as P700 was characterized, Beinert, Kok, and Hoch (17) commented that the behavior of the ESR signal and the optical signal at 700 nm was identical, but they referred in general to steady-state rather than kinetic behavior.

The results of the first detailed study (51) based on the outlined rationale was that the ESR decay kinetics of *R. rubrum* chromatophores were identical to the changes in the optical spectrum at 433 nm and slower than the change at 865 nm. This caused the authors to conclude that "oxidized bacteriochlorophyll in the organized environment of the chromatophore is not the site of the unpaired electron producing the observed electron paramagnetic resonance signal."

Loach and Sekura (52), however, extensively reinvestigated the decay kinetics of chromatophores prepared from *R. rubrum*. They wrote that they "have not once observed the marked differences in decay kinetics (as a function of wavelength) previously reported" (42, 51). Their detailed discussion of possible sources of artifacts makes it clear that this kind of measurement must be undertaken with great care. Ruby (personal communication) now feels that his previous results were spurious. He also believes that the optical decay at 865 nm did not correspond to the decay of the ESR when the light was turned off because the measuring beam in the optical experiment was too intense.

Loach and Sekura (52) made observations at most of the principal peaks of the light-dark difference spectrum (865, 810, 790, 763, 605, 433, 385, 365 nm, as seen in Fig. 1 of Ref. 53) and at some wavelengths for which the choice is not so obvious (890, 850 nm). The consistent result is that there are no significant differences in decay kinetics of the absorbance at any of the above wavelengths (280 nm as well) under a number of experimental conditions. Although the change at 280 nm may result in part from a bacteriochlorophyll band, as Loach and Sekura (52) suggest, other authors attribute it to changes in ubiquinone absorbance (e.g., see Ref. 54). At best it would seem that only some of the change is due to bacteriochlorophyll. However, Loach et al. (55) recently demonstrated in a model system in which they used purified bacteriochlorophyll that a large fraction of the photo-induced change observed in the 280-nm region can be attributed to changes induced in the bacteriochlorophyll absorption spectrum. Loach estimates (personal communication) that, depending on the particular system being studied, 60 to 100 percent of the absorbance change at 280 nm can be attributed to bacteriochlorophyll. The ESR decay kinetics and the optical kinetics of 430, 790, 810, and 865 nm were closely correlated for the two types of sample on which the measurement was made; fresh chromatophores and deaerated chromatophores.

Vernon, Ke, and Shaw (46) have compared the kinetics of the optical and ESR changes, on turning off the light, in small, detergent-treated PD-10 particles. These particles, to a first approximation, may be considered System I particles. The ability of these authors to make comparisons was limited by the time constant of the equipment used to measure the ESR response. They state that "for the particle alone and in the presence of ascorbate the agreement between the two measurements is good." The half-times in their Figure 7, to which the statement refers, are 2.5 versus 2.6 sec and 0.4 versus 0.26 sec (ESR versus optical). Although the first two numbers are clearly in close agreement, the second two are not. The recorder response time for the ESR decay cannot be responsible for the higher value of the ESR decay time, since the next two entries in the figure for ESR decay have $t_{1/2} = 0.2$ sec.

Bolton, Clayton, and Reed (20) show that the decay kinetics of the ESR and the optical changes originally caused by an actinic beam at 800 nm are identical in preparations from *R. spheroides*. The decay of the signals is very slow under the experimental conditions, $t_{1/2} \sim 5$ sec. Using the ratio of the radical concentration (determined by ESR) with the concentration of $P870^+$ (determined spectrophotometrically) and the quantum yield for production of $P870^+$ (determined spectrophotometrically), they calculated that the quantum yield for production of the ESR signal is 15 percent less when the actinic light is at 800 nm compared with 880 nm. (This difference is attributed to the capture of quanta in the tail of the pheophytin absorption curve.) This, however, apparently does not influence the correlation between the decay of the optical changes at these wavelengths and the ESR signal which is taken to be due to $P865^+$. Loach and Sekura (52) report the same optical kinetics at 763 nm as at 865 nm, despite the fact that the quantum efficiency for 760 nm actinic light is only 50 percent of that for 880 nm, the difference being attributed to pheophytin absorption (20).

McElroy, Feher, and Mauzerall (19) report on the close correlation of the rise and decay kinetics of optical response at 795 nm of reaction center preparations of R-26 mutant of *R. spheroides* at cryogenic temperatures. Neither the choice of the wavelength at which the optical change was monitored nor its comparison with changes at other wavelengths is discussed. The fact that the rise and decay times in the optical and ESR spectra change together as the light intensity changes is particularly convincing evidence of the identity of oxidized reaction-center bacteriochlorophyll and Component I. These authors note that the rise and decay kinetics are independent measurements. Coincidence of only one or the other leaves open the possibility that what is being measured is the change in the reaction partner; coincidence of both rules out that possibility. A signal-averaging computer is used in these experiments to allow for the summation of a large number of repeated cycles. Although some have objected to this technique on the grounds that the kinetic response changes with time (in particular, the first few flashes after a long dark period give a different pattern than do subsequent flashes), this objection is not applicable here, for if the same molecule is responsible for both signals both signals will change in the same way.

Several comments may be in order concerning the results cited in this subsection. The basic rationale for the experiments implicity includes the expectation that, if optical changes resulting from illuminating or darkening the sample are due to two distinct events whereas the ESR signal changes reflect only one, the kinetics will be different. Consider the following hypothetical example:

Let

$$A \xrightarrow[X]{\text{light}} A^* \cdot X \xrightarrow{k_1} A^+ \ (+X^-) \qquad \text{(where } A^+ \text{ is an observable free radical),}$$

and

$$B \xrightarrow[U]{\text{light}} B^* \cdot U \xrightarrow{k_2} B^+ \ (+U^-) \qquad \text{(where no ESR signal is observed from } B^+\text{).}$$

Also hypothesize that the absorption bands of A and B are bleached on the transformation to A^+ and B^+, respectively. If A alone absorbs at λ_1 *and* if the optical and ESR kinetics coincide when the illumination is at λ_1

and if both A and B absorb and are *independently* bleached at λ_2 *and if* $k_1 \neq k_2$, then it follows necessarily that the ESR and optical kinetics at λ_2 will *not* coincide.

With this as background, consider the identity of the ESR and optical kinetics at 800 and 880 nm as well as at 760 and 880 nm already cited. As noted there, there is a substantial contribution of bacteriopheophytin to the absorption at these wavelengths, especially at 760 nm. The most straightforward interpretation of this result is that oxidized bacteriochlorophyll ion is the free radical and that the bacteriopheophytin band is shifted by the change in its environment resulting from BChl → $BChl^+$. It should be noted, however, that the oxidized minus reduced curve for *R. rubrum* chromatophores (53) does not have the "derivativelike" shape expected from a band shift.

In the sense of the above formulation, the bleaching of the bacteriopheophytin and bacteriochlorophyll are *not* independent. Since the bleaching of the bacteriopheophytin is caused by the bleaching of the bacteriochlorophyll, they would have the same kinetics of onset and decay. Thus the kinetics at 760 nm would be identical to those at 880 nm.

No such easy explanation is available if part of the bleaching at 280 nm is indeed due to a quinone that participates in photosynthetic electron transport and if the report of identical ESR and optical kinetics at 280 nm is confirmed. In this case clearly two pigments would be contributing to the bleaching and the two events leading to their bleaching would be mediated by separate kinetic events (see Fig. 6-2). Although experience has shown that ESR and optical kinetics may be made to differ as a result of experimental artifacts, it is hard to imagine an artifact that would make them the same. Clearly too many "facts" are being asserted. It cannot be true that the bleaching at 280 nm is due to both ubiquinone and bacteriochlorophyll *and* that both ubiquinone and bacteriochlorophyll are independently involved in photosynthetic electron transport in these particles *and* that as a result of participating in electron transport they are bleached in the light and this bleaching decays in the dark *and* that bacteriochlorophyll positive ion is the observed free radical. (An exception would require the improbable chance result that the kinetics of the independent bleaching reactions is identical.) Perhaps the most reasonable interpretation of the fact that the ESR and optical kinetics coincide at 280 nm is to suggest that there is no contribution of a quinone to the bleaching of the 280-nm band; that is, either the assignment of the band is incorrect or that quinone does not participate in photosynthetic electron transport in these particles. Of course, this result cannot be used as evidence for $BChl^+$ as the free radical, since the opposite result (i.e., difference in ESR and optical kinetics at 280 nm) could also have been interpreted as the free radical being $BChl^+$. In fact, the interpretation suggested above could be cited as evidence that the identity of the free radical as $BChl^+$ has been prejudged.

In summary, the weight of the evidence of the type of experiment considered in this subsection seems to be on the side of identifying Signal BI with oxidized reaction-center bacteriochlorophyll. There is no strong independent kinetic evidence implicating $P700^+$. The tendency, however, for optical changes at many wavelengths to display the same kinetics despite the fact that independent evidence suggests that more than one pigment is absorbing at that wavelength may be (a) disturbing, (b) taken to indicate that, in fact, only one pigment accounts for the bleaching at that wavelength, or (c) that the bleaching of the second pigment is due to a band shift induced by the influence of the newly produced free-radical positive ion.

6.3.2.6 Evidence for the Radical Produced by the Reaction Partner of Bacteriochlorophyll Positive Ion

The apparent presence of only one signal in high concentration in samples of, or derived from, photosynthetic bacteria was troublesome for many years. A second signal has recently been reported from Feher's laboratory (56). Three broad lines were observed at about 1800, 2900, and 3700 G (Klystron frequency ca. 9 GHz) in addition to the usual narrow line seen at about 3200 G (see Fig. 6-12). The extreme conditions required to observe this broad signal make it clear why it had evaded earlier detec-

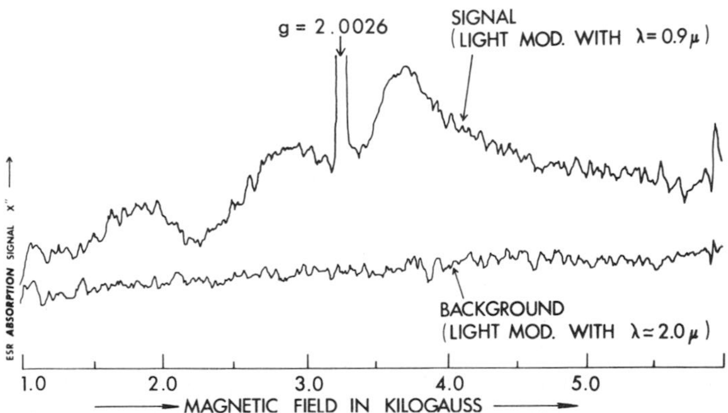

Fig. 6-12 Broad light-induced ESR signal. This signal was obtained from a reaction center preparation of *Rhodopseudomonas spheroides* at 1.3 K. Since light modulation was used, the recorded signal displays the absorption of microwave power rather than its derivative. Since the signal is so broad, it would be expected that a narrow line (as the more commonly observed signal at $g = 2.0026$) would be off scale if the same order of magnitude of free radicals were responsible for both signals. This is what is observed. Light modulation frequency, 10 Hz. (Reference 56.)

tion. The measurements were made at 1.4 K to make the line narrow enough to observe. Light modulation was employed to sort out the non-light responsive background signals due to ever-present contaminants. Since light modulation of a sample at 1.4 K invariably leads to cavity heating and higher sample temperature, it is necessary to demonstrate the absence of a "signal" when the illumination is at a wavelength which heats similarly but is photochemically inactive. The signal decay half-time forced them to modulate at a very low frequency, 10 Hz, which imposes the severe demand on the spectrometer that it be virtually noise free. The broad signals observed under these conditions had the same kinetics as the usual narrow signal in response to modulation of the light. At this writing no data have been published which unequivocably identify the broad signal(s), but Feher has proposed the tentative identification of the radical as a paramagnetic iron species with an anisotropic g factor ($g_x \neq g_y \neq g_z$) as a guiding hypothesis for further work.*

6.3.2.7 Evidence Tending to Bring into Question the Proposition that Component I is (Bacterio)Chlorophyll Positive Ion

If there is more than one population of radicals which contribute to Signal (B)I, it might be inappropriate to speak of a single Component I. In fact, there is considerable evidence that makes it certain that there are at least two populations of radicals which contribute to Signal BI in photosynthetic bacteria. Kohl (see Fig. 7-6, Ref. 31) observed that although the dark decay of radicals produced by light at low temperature (−80 C) was faster than at biological temperatures, only a fraction of the steady-state signal observed in the light at low temperature decayed in the dark (see also Ref. 57). Bolton, Cost, and Frankel (58) studied the phenomenon systematically and showed that the number of radicals stabilized by low temperature was the same as the number that decayed at the slower rate in the biphasic decay seen in *R. rubrum* chromatophores at room temperature.

The biphasic kinetics often observed in chromatophore preparations is sometimes cited as evidence that Signal BI arises from more than one source. Loach and Sekura (52) interpreted their kinetic data in a different spirit. They showed that the biphasic property of the kinetics is exaggerated by aging of the chromatophore preparations. They concluded that aging changes the chemical and/or physical conditions at the trapping site, that this aging does not take place uniformly with time at all

*J. S. Leigh and P. L. Dutton (*Biochem. Biophys. Res. Comm.* **46,** 414–421, 1972), using *Chromatium D*, have confirmed Feher's result that the primary electron acceptor can be seen by ESR at liquid helium temperature. These authors attribute the signal to an iron-sulfur protein free radical.

trapping sites, and that these changes are responsible for the biphasic decay. In fresh material a much smaller fraction of the trapping sites have "aged" and therefore the kinetics are less distinctly biphasic. In fact, they can very nearly be fitted by a pseudo-first-order model. Thus, they write, "it would seem that the biphasic decay kinetics bear witness to the inhomogeneity in the chromatophore population due primarily to aging effects and that, in fact, each kind of unit ('aged' and 'fresh', my addition) follows a pseudo-first-order decay." Although this is an intriguing interpretation, it would seem to require that the component which reduces the photo-produced oxidant be present in much larger quantity than the oxidant. The available evidence is not supportive. This objection may not be decisive, however. Loach (personal communication) argues that if the phototraps are considered to decay internally by temperature-independent processes in both "fresh and aged" units a pseudo-first-order decay would be expected without the necessity of the reductant being present at a much higher concentration than the oxidant, since, in that case, the decay of (+, −) would depend only on the probability of the electron clearing the energy barrier to return to the molecules from which the light drove it. The implicit assumption in this line of reasoning would seem to be that no electron transport takes place in these preparations and that a different kinetics should be observed in preparations that are competent, for example, to carry out photophosphorylation. The fact that whole cells show characteristically different kinctics than do chromatophores may be relevant in this regard. Perhaps of more relevance is the fact that second-order kinetics would not be anticipated when the reactants are packaged together; that is, if a bacteriochlorophyll reaction partner is absent from a subunit, that subunit is nonfunctional no matter what quantity of that molecule may be present elsewhere. In this case, if aging alters the details of the physical associations between reactants, we might anticipate an effect on the expected "first-order-like" kinetics. At any rate, if their interpretation is correct, the "aged" sites could be those that decayed at low temperature in the work already discussed.

Kohl (31) summarized the information available at that time that could be "interpreted as suggesting that (bacterio)chlorophyll is not the molecular site of Signal I." None of the objections raised seem persuasive. The reported difference in the decay of the optical changes at 865 nm and the ESR kinetics (51) was not reproducible (52) and is now felt to be an artifact probably caused by too high an intensity of the measuring beam (Ruby, private communication). The fact that Weaver and Bishop (59) observed no Signal I in a mutant whose pigment complement was apparently intact turned out to be evidence for $P700^+$ being Component I, since on closer examination the mutant was found to lack P700. Kohl et al. (24)

argued that organisms enriched in ^{13}C should have shown the effects of that isotope on the ESR line if the signal was due to chlorophyll. This same argument could be used, however, as evidence against any organic molecule and it is much more sensible to assume that the effects in that experiment were simply too small to be observed. Commoner, Kohl, and Townsend (60) reported a lag of 2 to 3 msec between the onset of illumination and the rise of the ESR signal and concluded from this that "the ESR signal observed in *R. rubrum* is not due to unpaired electrons associated with the excited state generated by the primary act of light absorption; that is, by the initial step in the photosynthetic process." Leaving aside for the moment the authenticity of the reported lag, Beinert and Kok (33) correctly pointed out that the presence of a lag does not rule out $P890^+$ as the source of Signal BI. They argue plausibly for an induction effect which results from the competition between the reaction that oxidizes P890 and that which reduces $P890^+$. They cite data that show that at low enough light intensities no $P890^+$ accumulates in intact samples (61).

6.3.2.8 Summary

The free radicals responsible for Signals I and BI clearly exist in more than one environment, but it is not clear whether this is a trivial matter or a reflection of some more fundamental process. Although criticism has been raised about one or another point in most experiments that were interpreted as providing supporting evidence for the designation of reaction-center (bacterio)chlorophyll as Signal I or BI, none of the evidence offered as counterevidence is persuasive now. The most unsettling data are those that show a ratio of two free radicals per $P700^+$ in a variety of O_2-evolving systems, despite the fact that the comparable ratio is unity when measured in photosynthetic bacteria. The fact that the ESR and optical kinetic fingerprints correspond at a number of wavelengths where more than one pigment clearly is absorbing deprives this evidence of much of its force in identifying Signal (B)I as (bacterio)chlorophyll positive ion. Nonetheless, it is my opinion that Signal (B)I can be identified as arising from a reaction-center (bacterio)chlorophyll positive ion with considerable confidence.

6.3.3 The Molecular Origin of Signal II

Weaver's (25) summary of the evidence available at the time concerning the molecular origin of Signal II led her to state: "Although conclusive correlation of electron flow through a plastoquinone pool with the EPR Signal II has not yet been demonstrated, there is no evidence to the contrary." She based her inclination to identify Signal II as arising from plastosemiquinone on the following evidence:

1. Signal II is absent in photosynthetic bacteria (14).
2. Mutants unable to evolve O_2 showed almost no Signal II (59).
3. The g factor of Signal II is consistent with the expected value for a semiquinone (62).

Treharne, Brown, and Vernon (29) concluded that "Signal II appears to be a physiological-type response because it apparently exists only in intact cells and/or systems exhibiting Hill-reaction activity." They made a distinction between the O_2-evolving system and the intermediate electron transport chain between Systems I and II with which plastoquinone is associated and interpreted the first three items enumerated above as indicating that Signal II was connected with the former. They offered no molecular candidate for the role of Component II. Although they performed a service by pointing out the possible alternative explanation, their assertion that Signal II requires a vable Hill-reaction system is clearly incorrect. The samples used in the experiments in which Signal II was first observed were prepared in such a way that Hill reactivity certainly could not have survived (2). Signal II has also been observed following heptane extraction of lyophilized chloroplasts which showed no Hill-activity (63).

Kohl and Wood (63) made a direct demonstration of the relation of Signal II and plastoquinone by taking advantage of (a) the well-known procedures (64) for organic extraction of lipids (with the consequent destruction of Hill activity) and the subsequent readdition of plastoquinone (with the consequent, at least partial, restoration of Hill activity) and (b) the collapse of the hyperfine structure and the narrowing of Signal II when deuterons are substituted for protons throughout the organism (24), including substitution in Component II, the free radical that gives rise to Signal II. When Component II was completely extracted with heptane, the readdition of purified plastoquinone resulted in the restoration of Signal II (see Fig. 6-13).

It is not possible, however, to conclude from this that Component II is derived from plastoquinone (PQ), since the removal of PQ may simply have served to disrupt the integrity of the chain of electron carriers on which Signal II depends, whereas the replacement of PQ restored the integrity of the chain, hence Signal II; that is, Component II could have survived heptane extraction and at the same time Signal II would disappear if some other electron carrier preceding it in the chain were removed. For this reason deuterated PQ was added to heptane-extracted chloroplasts as well. If Signal II is related to PQ, the observed line will be narrow (characteristic of deuterated Component II). If PQ serves only to maintain the integrity of the transport chain, the observed line will be broad, with hyperfine structure characteristic of protonated Signal II. Unfortunately the results are not so dramatic as one would like, since

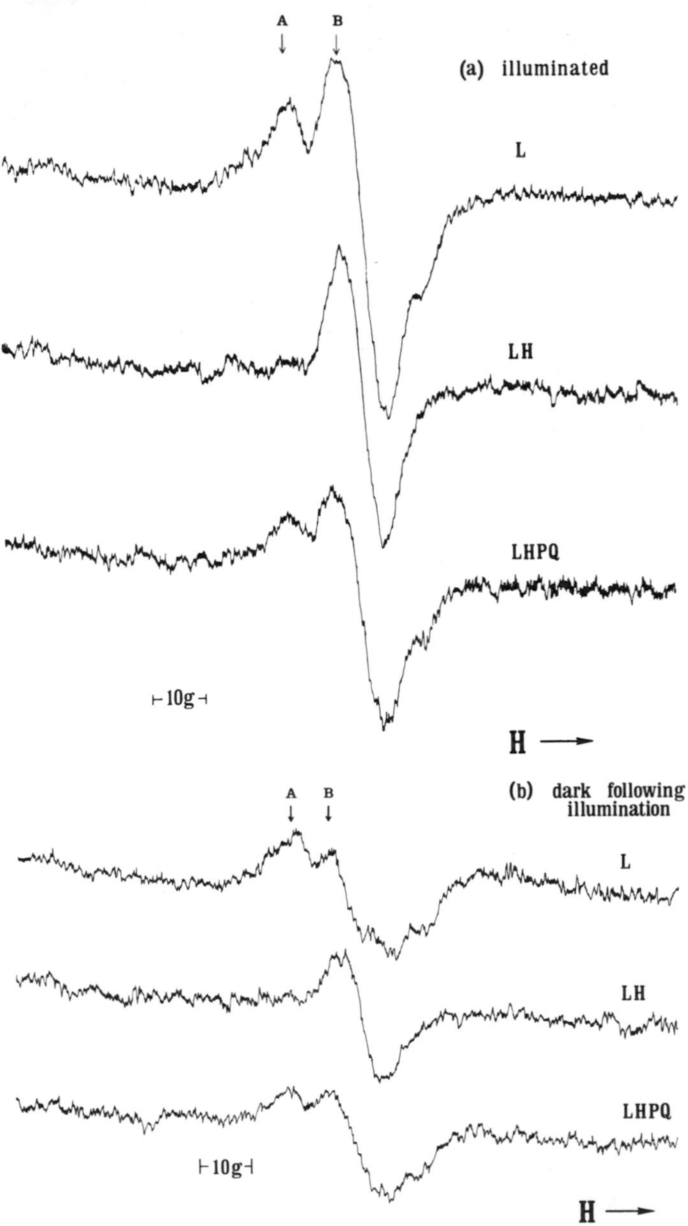

Fig. 6-13 The effect of heptane extraction and PQ readdition on Signal II. ESR signals recorded from spinach chloroplasts (*a*) in the light and (*b*) in the dark after cessation of illumination: *L* = lyophilized; LH = lyophilized and then heptane extracted; LHPQ = lyophilized, heptane extracted, and then PQ added back. Modulation amplitude = 3.0 G; T = 20 C. For experimental details see Ref. 63, especially Fig. 2. Signal II is not always extracted so completely and a small fraction of Signal I is often "frozen-in."

in those experiments a good deal of Signal II and some "frozen-in" Signal I survived the heptane extraction. Therefore the presence of the narrow line associated with deuterated Component II had to be observed against a considerable background. Nonetheless, its presence can be clearly observed (see Figs. 4, 5, 6 in Ref. 63). This shows that unpaired electrons are interacting with deuterons that are present only in PQ. The inescapable conclusion is that the free radical, Component II, is directly derived from PQ. It does not necessarily follow that Component II is plastosemiquinone. In fact, one observation argues strongly against plastosemiquinone (PSQ) being the source of Signal II; namely, the spectrum of authentic PSQ immobilized at 77 K, as well as in solution, is symmetric, whereas Signal II is decidedly asymmetric (65). Yet any anisotropy that could contribute to the asymmetry of Signal II (assuming that Component II is PSQ) would be expected to produce an asymmetric line when a sample containing authentic plastosemiquinone is frozen into a random glass.

Kohl, Wright, and Weissman (65) working with phytyl analogs of plastoquinone, observed a "tocopheroxyl" (see Fig. 6-14) radical that showed distinct asymmetry when frozen into a random glass (see Fig. 6-15). Not only was the signal from the immobilized radical asymmetric, it had all of the detailed properties of Signal II except that the amplitude of field point Z is elevated compared with Signal II. (It can be argued that this

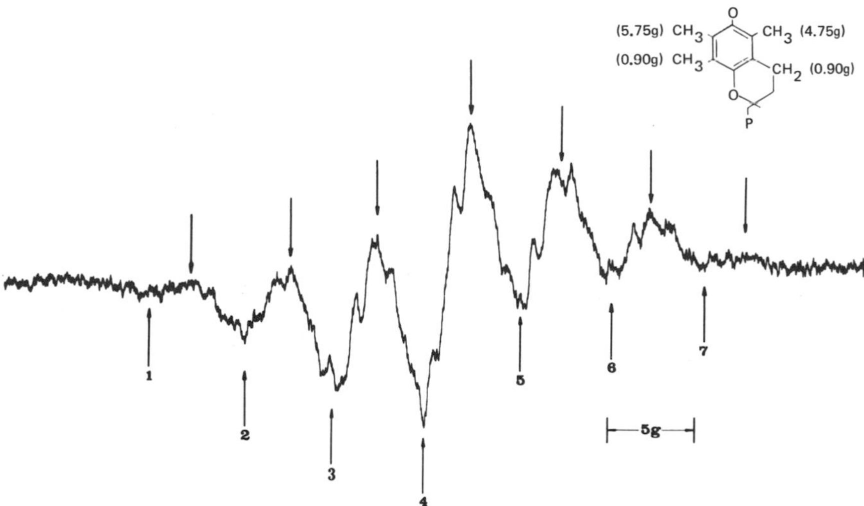

Fig. 6-14 α-Tocopheroxyl free radical. This spectrum was observed growing out of the spectrum of α-tocopherylsemiquinone as the microwave power was increased and the semiquinone was power saturated. Microwave power = 320 mW. Coupling constants used to reproduce this spectrum by computer are shown. (Reference 65.)

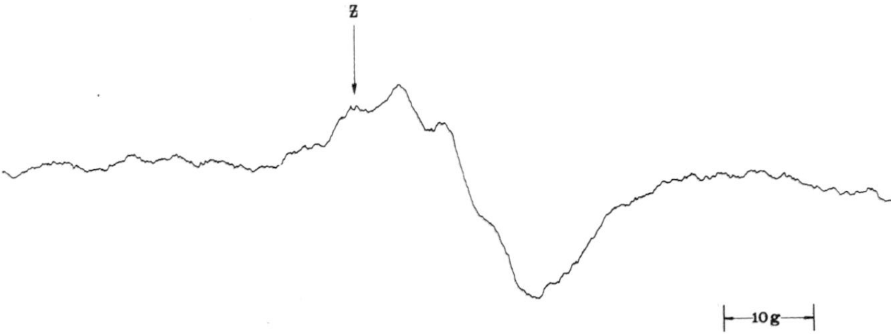

Fig. 6-15 α-Tocopheroxyl at 77 K. Modulation amplitude = 3.2 G. This high modulation amplitude was used because most photosynthetic samples, such as those shown in Fig. 6-5, are recorded at approximately that value. Microwave power = 2.0 mW. (Reference 65.)

is due to the extra methyl group at C-6 in α-tocopherol (α-T) compared with plastoquinone.) The interpretation of these spectra as being due to "tocopheroxyl" is supported by further experiments in which α- and γ-tocopherol were first taken to 77 K and then subjected to ultraviolet radiation. The resulting spectra are extremely similar to, if not identical with, the spectrum seen in Fig. 6-15.

The work reported from Kohl's laboratory is direct evidence that a free radical derived from plastoquinone contributes to Signal II. It does not, however, rule out other contributors to that signal, especially if their spectra are similar to that of the radical derived from plastoquinone. This would be the case if, for example, a radical derived from α-tocopherol were a contributor to Signal II. The inverse experiment, adding protonated α-T and α-tocopherolguinone to a deuterated photosynthetic apparatus, should shed some light on this point; γ-tocopherol cannot be a major contributor to Signal II, since it is undetectable in *Scenedesmus* down to the level of 1 per 2500 chlorophyll (N. I. Bishop, private communication), yet *Scenedesmus* gives a normal Signal II of undiminished amplitude. The work also strongly suggests that Component II is not plastosemiquinone, but rather the chroman form related to it which they have called "plastochromanoxyl" (see Fig. 6-14).

6.4 THE RELATION BETWEEN THE OBSERVED ESR SIGNALS AND PHOTOSYNTHETIC ELECTRON TRANSPORT

The first detailed work took a giant step toward characterizing the observed radicals. Much of what has followed has simply added to the certainty with which the properties, such as lineshape, hyperfine splitting parameters and *g* factor, can be characterized. The first papers on light-induced radicals in PS systems left two questions unanswered:

1. Are the radicals responsible for the observed signals active participants in the mainline of photosynthetic electron transport?
2. With what molecular species are the unpaired electrons which give the signals associated?

Much of the first part of this chapter has been addressed to the second question. The need to address the first question is less important now than it was earlier, since an affirmative answer is implicit in the case of Signal (B)I with the identification of Component I as reaction-center (bacterio)chlorophyll cation. Still it seems worthwhile to demonstrate independently its relationship to photosynthetic electron transport. The possibility that the observed signals might be unconnected with mainline photosynthetic processes arose immediately, since the chloroplast preparations which generated the free radical were photosynthetically inactive as may be deduced from the details of preparation and conditions of the experiment. The fact was further reinforced by the early demonstration that a photo-induced signal can be generated at low temperature (16) and that illuminated purified chlorophyll also produced a free radical (15). This raised the specter that perhaps Signal (B)I is merely a reflection of the fact that chlorophyll is present and has no fundamental connections with the process by which photosynthesis is carried out.

Six separate types of experimental result make it certain that Signal (B)I directly reflects events central to photosynthetic electron transport.

1. Signal I was not produced on illumination of a mutant strain of *Scenedesmus* which apparently had a full complement of pigments but was unable to fix CO_2. It was subsequently shown that although the bulk pigment was present, P700 was absent. Thus bulk chlorophyll was present and was illuminated but no ESR Signal I was observed (59).
2. The action spectrum for the production of Signal I followed that of active-center chlorophyll rather than bulk chlorophyll (46).
3. Extraction of a large fraction of the chlorophyll with cold 68 percent acetone left P700 largely intact and did not reduce the ESR signal (33). Similarly, chemical oxidation of the bulk bacteriochlorophyll left the photo-induced bleaching at 865 nm and the blue shift at 805 nm intact and the ESR signal amplitude of Signal BI unchanged (41).
4. Although many photosynthetically inactive preparations do give a light-induced ESR signal, the kinetic patterns of *Chromatium* strain D cells which are actively engaged in photosynthesis are distinctly different from cells or preparations with incomplete electron transport systems (66).

5. The quantum yield for free radical production has been measured directly and shown to be close to 1 (28). Calculations based on measurements of the quantum yield for the production of oxidized reaction-center bacteriochlorophyll gave the same qualitative result (20).

6. Perhaps the most elegant demonstration is that of Weaver and Weaver (67) who showed that the cross section for photon capture for paramagnetism in their spinach chloroplast preparations was about 150 chlorophyll molecules, which is of the order of magnitude of the size of the photosynthetic unit. If the radical arose from the simple physical presence of chlorophyll and its interaction with light, this cross section would be expected to have a value of 1.

There are many fewer data that implicate Signal II directly with photosynthetic electron transport. This is unfortunate because here the link to direct participation in photosynthetic electron transport cannot be made even if one is convinced that Component II is plastochromanoxyl free radical, unlike the case of the identification of Component I as reaction-center (bacterio)chlorophyll positive ion which makes it certain that the radical is directly involved in photosynthetic electron transport. The problem is that there is a large pool of plastoquinone that does not participate in photosynthetic electron transport (e.g., see Refs. 68 and 69). Although the same is true of chlorophyll, in the case of plastoquinone it is not possible to discriminate between the bulk material and the reaction-center molecules. Perhaps the most convincing evidence that Component II is directly involved in photosynthetic electron transport is the fact that any treatment that reduces Signal II invariably increases Signal I (e.g., see Ref. 65). A result of this kind can be interpreted conveniently in terms of the Hill-Bendall model (*Z* scheme, see Fig. 6-1), in which Signal II is associated with a component in the transport chain intermediate between pigment Systems I and II and Signal I is associated with System I reaction-center chlorophyll. In this case Signal I grows when the ability of Component II to re-reduce it is diminished, either by interrupting the transport chain, as in aging, or by reducing the concentration of Component II, as in heptane extraction. It should be noted, however, that the results can all be accommodated as well by the inverse relationship; namely, Component I feeding electrons to Component II. In this conception Signal I increases and Signal II decreases when the rate of passage of electrons to Component II is decreased or when the concentration of Component II is decreased, hence leaving fewer molecules to receive electrons from Component I. In fact, the latter relationship, I → II, was that originally proposed (4).

Preliminary experiments (Beinfeld and Kohl, unpublished results) of the effect of NH_4Cl and DCMU were also consistent with Component II lying on the mainline of photosynthetic electron transport. The addition of 10μM DCMU, an inhibitor of O_2 evolution, to a spinach chloroplast preparation virtually eliminated the light response of Signal II. The addition of NH_4Cl, an uncoupler of photosynthetic phosphorylation, resulted in a substantial decrease in the rise and decay half-time of Signal II.

To the degree that (a) the molecular identity of both radicals is established and (b) these radicals have been shown to be on the mainline of photosynthetic electron transport—to that degree, the focus in the future should shift from its former concerns of identifying the observed phenomena with molecular events to using ESR as a tool for studying photosynthesis.

6.5 KINETICS

6.5.1 General Comments

Rabinowitch (Ref. 26, p. 858) states in detail the case for the difficulty of interpreting kinetic data:

> Even when studying simple reactions *in vitro*, the physical chemist is rarely able to control all the conditions that affect the reaction rate. Consequently, seldom will two investigations of the velocity of a reaction result in agreement in more than the order of magnitude. Beside the readily controllable external factors, such as temperature, pressure and light intensity, the rate often depends on factors as elusive as the state of the walls of the vessel, or the presence of minute impurities. It is therefore easy to judge the difficulties encountered in the kinetic study of a complex chemical process in a living organism. The rate of such a process depends on many physiological factors that do not enter ostensibly into the kinetic equations. Among all life phenomena, photosynthesis is perhaps the most sensitive to slight variations in the structure and composition of the biocatalytic apparatus. No wonder that doubts have been expressed as to the very possibility of deriving significant kinetic relationships from the quantitative study of this phenomenon.

These facts lead many to the bias that kinetic data from complex systems can be more usefully used in qualitative or comparative ways (e.g., ESR kinetics in response to change in illumination compared with the kinetics of an optical spectral line or the effect on the kinetics of various treatments or temperatures) rather than as detailed evidence for or against a particular model. It is a reflection of this bias that many of the important kinetic results have been cited earlier in this chapter in a qualitative and comparative context.

The problems cited in the above quotation should not be allowed to obscure the great usefulness of kinetic experiments designed within the comparative frame. In fact, the advantage of using changes in the ESR signal compared with changes in the optical absorption spectrum (the most important difference being that in the latter case an actinic beam is required in addition to the monitoring beam) to probe the condition of the reaction-center (bacterio)chlorophyll is so great that it may well warrant relatively extreme measures in preparing the sample when this is necessary; for example, a flow system that passed the effluent of a chemostat through the sample cell would allow the summation of single flashes on dark adapted samples without requiring the experiment to continue for the unreasonably long times that readaptation to the dark between flashes would impose.

Typical kinetic results, differences observed when the sample is whole cells versus cell fractions, and induction effects are described briefly.

6.5.2 Typical Kinetic Results, Signal I

Kinetic experiments of two types have been reported. Most usually the experiments are done on bacterial systems, presumably to eliminate the contribution of Signal II kinetics. In one approach a repetitive cycle of light-dark flashes is established and the results of many cycles are averaged, usually by a small fixed program computer closely related in design to a multichannel analyzer. Typical results of such experiments are seen in Figs. 6-16 and 6-17. Notice the fact that with the whole cells the curve has not reached a zero slope, whereas the rise curve for chromatophores is well fitted by a single exponential.

The experimental design that produces data such as those seen in Figs. 6-16 and 6-17 is subject to two objections: (a) it requires the assump-

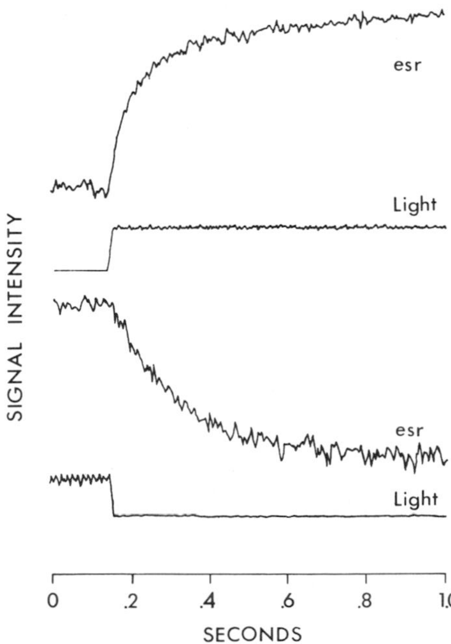

Fig. 6-16 Typical kinetic curves, whole cells *Rhodospirillum rubrum*. The upper curve shows the response to light of the ESR amplitude at the high field peak of the fast decaying light-induced signal. The curve beneath it represents the simultaneous output of a photocell which provides an exact marker for the time of transition between light and dark. Experimental conditions: summation of 400 repeated light-dark cycles, 10 C. The bottom set of curves contains the equivalent decay curves at T = 15 C. (Reference 31.)

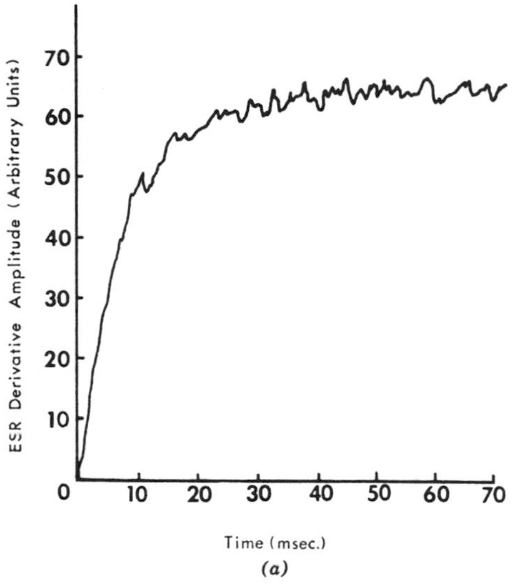

(a)

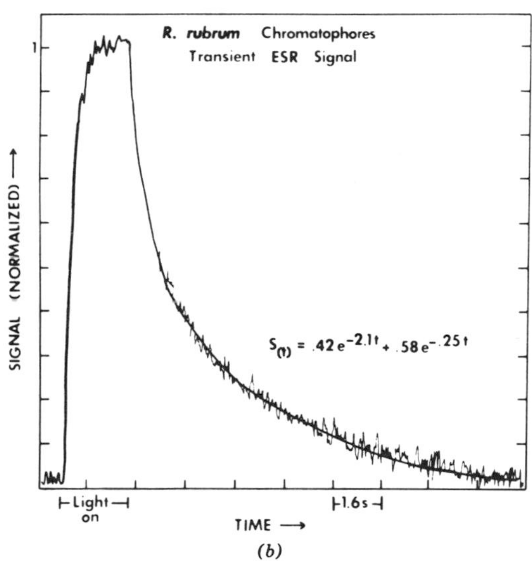

(b)

Fig. 6-17*a* Typical plot of the ESR derivative amplitude as a function of time after the opening of the shutter. This plot represents the average of 2100 individual scans. Light intensity was 3.0×10^5 ergs $cm^{-2}sec^{-1}$. The rise is a simple exponential; hence the rise kinetics are independent of the initial base line. (Reference 58.) (*b*) Decay of the light induced ESR signal in a chromatophore sample. Also shown is an exponential curve fitting the data; S_t is the normalized steady-state value of the signal. The growth of the ESR signal in response to light (not shown here) followed a simple exponential. (Reference 51.)

tion that the repeated events that are summed be exactly the same and (b) it masks the differences between the first responses to light after prolonged dark adaptation and those responses to subsequent light exposure. With respect to the first objection, the events, excluding the first few exposures to light after a substantial dark period, are substantially reproducible over long times, at least with certain systems (31, 52, 70). On the other hand, Schleyer reports considerable change with time, using a *Chromatium* preparation (66). More to the point of the objection, however, is that the shape of the kinetic curve of the first several flashes after a long dark period are different from those seen after many flashes (66, 71). This difference presumably reflects the approach of the system to a steady state. Clearly, signal averaging is inappropriate if one is investigating the type of induction effect that is observed only after prolonged equilibration in the dark. If the intention is to study deviations from the steady state, however, then signal averaging just as clearly *is* appropriate. Of course, the signal accumulation need not begin until these more transient induction effects have passed.

6.5.3 Differences Between Kinetics Observed for Whole Cells and Cell Fractions

Results of experiments in which signal averaging was employed show that rise curves for whole cells cannot be fitted by a single exponential, by the sum of an exponential with a relatively high rate constant and a slower linear function, nor, in general, by the sum of two exponentials, despite the fact that the latter provides four free parameters. On the other hand, rise curves for cell-free preparations are invariably single exponentials. Decay curves for whole cells are often nicely fitted by a single exponential, whereas those for chromatophore preparations are more complex. Rise-time constants depend on the light intensity (hence sample concentration). Both rise and decay times depend on the redox potential of the environment and even in at least one instance on the growth medium. The latter case is illustrated by the much longer decay half-times when succinate, rather than malate, was used for the carbon source in growing *Rhodospirillum rubrum* (see Ref. 31, p. 113).

6.5.4 Induction Effects

With sufficient sensitivity, usually gained by sacrificing fast-time resolution, a second type of experiment can be done; namely, observing the kinetics as the result of a single exposure to light. That important information can be garnered in this way is illustrated by the observations of rise kinetics over

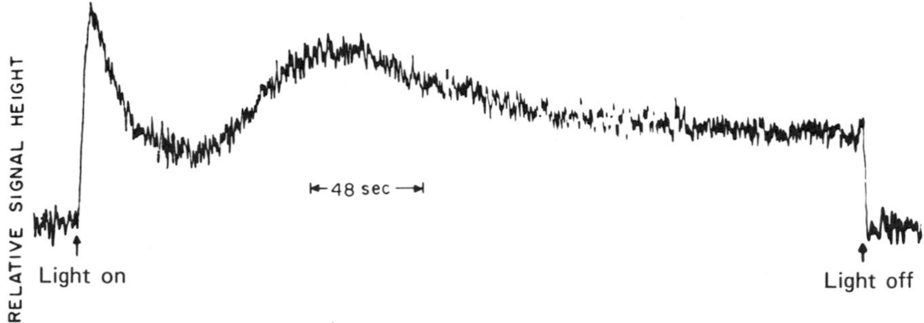

Fig. 6-18 Time course of formation and decay of ESR signal from dark-adapted whole cells of *R. rubrum*. The whole cells, suspended in modified Hunter's medium pH 6.8, were exposed to white light for 1 min, to dark for 2 min, then re-exposed for the length of time shown. EPR time constant was 0.3 sec. (Reference 70.)

a longer time course (70). These experiments revealed several transients with whole cells of *R. rubrum* (but not with chromatophores) as seen in Fig. 6-18. This behavior clearly suggests that the free radical is interacting with several other chemical species. These important observations should be extended to other photosynthetic systems.

The most likely basis for the observation of induction effects is that the number of free radicals observed is the result of competing processes that oxidize reaction-center (bacterio)chlorophyll on the one hand and re-reduce it on the other. Since the production of free radicals is assumed to depend on the light intensity, there is clearly some value of the light intensity so small that the steady-state concentration of oxidized (bacterio)-chlorophyll is undetectable. This has been observed for the bleaching of P890 (61).* This type of induction effect, or "lag", should be observable in experiments in which repetitive responses are summed. Beinert and Kok (33) invoke this as the explanation for the "lag" in the rise of the ESR signal reported by Commoner, Kohl, and Townsend (60). Several investigators have reported their inability to observe this "lag" between the time the light falls on the sample and the time at which the ESR kinetic curve begins to rise (19, 58). In one case (19) the observations were made at low temperature and one would not expect to observe the lag, since the reaction(s) that serve to re-reduce $BChl^+$ might well be seriously influenced by the low

* It is not obvious how to reconcile this result with that of Parsons (72) who shows that P870 becomes bleached in less than 1 μsec after a laser flash. The point is that it is hard to imagine processes fast enough to compete with this time. One would seem to be left with only the trivial result that at low enough intensity the number of radicals produced (or molecules bleached) is below the level of detection.

temperature. It may be relevant in this connection to recall the previously noted result that although the apparent decay kinetics at low temperature are even faster than at room temperature only a fraction of the signal decays.

In order that the apparent disagreement in the literature be resolved, it would seem worthwhile to reinvestigate the "lag" as a function of light intensity with the expectation that, if it exists, it will be most prominent at low light intensities.

6.5.5 Signal II Kinetics

There are no reliable reports of the kinetics of Signal II. Such measurements can be made on the lowfield peak (indicated as field point *A* in Fig. 6-5), since Signal I does not contribute any amplitude there. It is necessary to know the kinetic response of Signal II if the kinetic response of Signal I in O_2-evolving systems is to be measured, since the kinetics of Signal II must be subtracted from the kinetic response in the region in which Signal I contributes to the composite signal. For an investigator with an on-line computer, it might be rewarding to attempt to measure the kinetics at two field points (e.g., *A* and *B* in Fig. 6-5) in alternate intervals and subtract the contribution of Signal II from the composite seen at field point *B*. The result would be an essentially simultaneous measurement of the kinetics of Signals I and II.

6.6 OTHER OBSERVATIONS

Although this chapter has been concerned primarily with Signals I, BI, and II, a number of other ESR signals have been observed, several of which are noted, and at least one that might have been anticipated has not been reported.

6.6.1 Triplet State

It is especially worth noting that although signals assigned to the triplet state of chlorophyll have been reported (73) when that isolated pigment was the sample, there have been no reports of triplet-state chlorophyll being detected with ESR when the sample was a relatively intact photosynthetic system. The significance of the absence of a triplet signal is that the participation of a metastable triplet state of chlorophyll in photosynthesis has often been invoked on a priori grounds, since otherwise the reaction initiating photosynthetic electron transport must compete with fluorescence.

The intuitive feeling that the initiating steps in photosynthesis could not compete with the very short fluorescence lifetime, about 10^{-9} sec, has been the motivating force in the postulation of an excited triplet. The "need" for postulating the participation of a metastable triplet would seem to be reduced by Clayton's (74) calculation that the energy in the excited singlet is trapped within 10^{-11} sec. This calculation was based on measurements of the fluorescence quantum yield in reaction-center preparations and the fluorescence lifetime. The absence of reports of a triplet, along with Parsons' (72) report of the appearance of oxidized reaction-center bacteriochlorophyll in less than 1 μsec may be taken as evidence of the close physical association of the pigment and the acceptor molecules. The speed of the reaction is compatible with other known charge-transfer reactions.*

6.6.2 Paramagnetic Ions

The importance of manganese in the nutrition of green plants has long been known. More recently, however, Mn^{2+} has been assigned an important role in the dynamical, light-induced processes (75). Recent discussion has centered around the oxidation of Mn^{2+}. The higher oxidation states are also paramagnetic but their short lifetimes in aqueous solution have precluded their observation, Mn^{3+} is stable when complexed with pyrophosphate (76). No ESR signal, however, is observed when this complex is examined. (Unpublished observation, Beinfeld and Kohl.)

Manganous ions can be observed in almost any preparation from O_2-evolving photosynthetic systems. Most often the presence of the Mn^{2+} signal is an annoyance, since it provides a nonconstant base line against which Signals I and II must be observed. If the Mn^{2+} concentration is low (less than 10^{-5} M), the signal may still be observed by increasing the microwave power (there are no reports of power saturation for the Mn^{2+} resonance at the powers usually available) and/or by increasing the modulation amplitude above the values ordinarily used for observing Signals I and II. The latter is useful, since the individual Mn^{2+} lines are considerably broader than Signal I and the hyperfine structure of Signal II.

Despite the extreme sensitivity with which Mn^{2+} can be observed, there are no reports of observations that could be assigned to the oxidation of Mn^{2+} (77). The experimental difficulty of observing a small fractional change in Mn^{2+} may possibly be overcome by modulating the light used

* Samples of *Chromatium D* illuminated at liquid helium temperature have been reported to give rise to ESR signals which the authors identify as bacteriochlorophyll triplets. In these experiments the frozen samples were illuminated subsequent to the chemical reduction of the electron acceptor. P. L. Dutton, J. S. Leigh and M. Seibert, *Biochem. Biophys. Res. Comm.* **46,** 406–413 (1972).

to induce the photo-oxidation and allowing this beam to act as a reference in such a way that the signal recorded is only that induced by the modulating light beam. S. I. Weissman (private communication)* has developed such a system for the study of chemical systems.

A number of reports have been made on the effect of light on the Mn^{2+} signal over long periods of time. The Mn^{2+} signal (*Chlamydomonas reinhardi* sample) has been observed to decrease dramatically in the light and build back up in the dark (78). This signal was localized in the supernatant. Since no correlation could be made with photosynthetically related reactions, the authors (78) suggest that it is related to energy-dependent ion transport. More than this, however, must be involved, since uncomplexed Mn^{2+} would give the same ESR response, whether it was in the supernatant or in the organism. The fact that complexed Mn^{2+} (79) does not produce a signal may also be involved.

In contrast to the results with *Chlamydomonas,* Mn^{2+} signal from spinach chloroplast fragments has been observed to decrease rapidly at first to a very low level in the light and then grow back to several times its initial dark amplitude after 30 to 60 min in the light. (Unpublished results, Burton and Kohl.) On the other hand, presumably intact chloroplasts, prepared according to the prescription of Jensen and Bassham (80), did not show the initial decrease in Mn^{2+} signal, but the Mn^{2+} signal grew to about twice its original magnitude within 5 min. No change in Mn^{2+} signal was observed when *Scenedesmus obliquus* cells were the sample and very little, if any, increase was seen with *Chlorella pyrenoidosa*, in agreement with Allen (81).

Lozier, Baginsky and Butler (83) reported on a system that would seem ideal for the observation of higher oxidation states of manganese. He utilized Mn^{2+} as an electron donor to restore Hill activity in extensively tris-washed chloroplasts (82). He followed the (presumably stoichiometric) disappearance of the Mn^{2+} ESR signal as Hill activity proceeded. The fact that the ESR signal decreased with time meant that manganese was not being cycled back to aqueous Mn^{2+}. It might be suspected that this indicates an accumulation of a higher oxidation state of manganese. Although it would certainly be worthwhile to look for such a signal, the fact that complexed Mn^{2+} produces no ESR signal must also be considered (79). If, however, complexation were the final fate of the Mn^{2+} disappearing from solution, surely the Hill activity must run down, since there certainly must be a limit to the number of Mn^{2+} that can be complexed by the preparation.

In view of the very important, and little understood, role that oxida-

* Subsequently described in H. Levanon and S. I. Weissman. *J. Am. Chem. Soc.*, **93,** 4309 (1971).

tion of Mn^{2+} plays in photosynthesis, detailed ESR study of the phenomena would seem to be called for.

Signals much broader than those from Mn^{2+} are often observed. With the exception of the recent important preliminary report by McElroy, Feher, and Mauzerall (19), which links such a signal seen at 1.3 K to the primary acceptor for System I, these signals are most often acknowledged in passing as probably due to "other paramagnetic species."

An interesting nondynamical result is that *Chlorella pyrenoidosa* grown in low light accumulates considerably less Mn^{2+} than it does when grown in high light (21, 83). Electron micrographs reveal that these cells have a less extensive lamellar system in their chloroplasts.

6.6.3 Additional Light-Induced Signal from Anacystis

Weaver has recently reported (84) a new signal from cultures of *Anacystis nidulans* which she proposes to name Signal III. The signal is present in greater concentration than Signals I and II and only recently appeared in her samples of *Anacystis*. My own preference is to retain names like Signal I and II for phenomena quite generally associated with the basic mechanisms of photosynthesis. The fact that this signal is not even necessarily associated with *Anacystis* (84 and Bolton, personal communication) robs it of that generality, although its response to light certainly indicates that it is interacting with the photosynthetic electron transport system. Although the kinetics and wavelength response seem to guarantee that this signal is not Signal II, the lineshape has the properties seen in immobilized substituted phenol radicals (65).

6.6.4 Signal Observed in the Dark in Rhodospirillum rubrum

It has been clear since the earliest experiments with *Rhodospirillum rubrum* that a signal persists in the dark (e.g., see Fig. 59 in Ref. 15 or Fig. 4 in Ref. 14). The recorded intensity was so small that it was not possible to tell whether the observed signal was residual Signal I, present in small concentration even after a considerable time in the dark, or a different signal. When a signal-averaging computer was used to enhance the signal-to-noise ratio (24, 31), it became clear from both the *g* factor and lineshape that the signal was different from Signal BI (see upper trace, Fig. 6-19). However, even though the *g* factors are similar, this signal clearly is not due to the same molecular species that gives rise to Signal II, as previously characterized, despite the fact that Kohl et al. (24) unfortunately refer to it as "Signal II in *R. rubrum*." The evidence for the emphatic statement

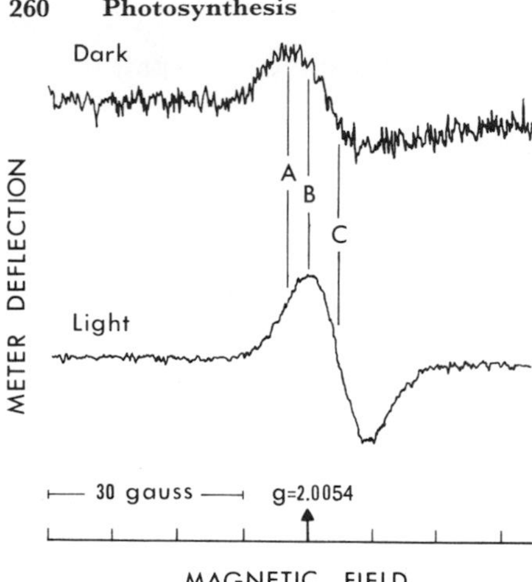

Fig. 6-19 Comparison of position in magnetic field of dark signal in *R. rubrum* and signal recorded in the light. These spectra were generated by organisms grown in protonated medium. See text for a discussion of the significance of the fact that the spectra overlap. The scale for the upper spectrum is 25 times that for the lower. (Reference 24.)

that Signal II and the small dark signal seen in *R. rubrum* have a different molecular source is that the linewidth of Signal II changes dramatically when photosynthetic green organisms are grown on a totally deuterated medium, whereas the line produced in the dark by *R. rubrum* is unchanged under those conditions. No attempt has been made to identify this signal beyond the comment (24) that it shares several properties, including the lineshape, with the flavo-protein succinic dehydrogenase free radical (85).

The fact that Signal I is significantly narrowed by deuteration, whereas the "dark" signal in *R. rubrum* is not, allows us to record the kinetics of the light response of the very much smaller "dark" signal without interference from Signal BI (24). When cultures are grown on normal protonated medium, there is no value of the magnetic field where the "dark" signal has an amplitude and Signal BI has none (see Fig. 6-19). The differential effect of deuteration on the signals suggests, however, that the kinetic responses of the "dark" signal may be observed independently of Signal BI if the measurement is made at the magnetic-field value *A* (see Fig. 6-20). Such indeed is the case (see Fig. 6-21). The signal seen in the dark decreases in response to light. Neither the magnitude of the decrease nor its detailed kinetics can be measured with confidence, for even a relatively small fractional contribution of the dominant response seen in the light (due either to the 4-G modulation amplitude or the amplitude in the wing of the dominant signal) could seriously distort the response curve of the smaller signal. The fact that the signals respond in the opposite sense guarantees that the recorded response is not predominantly due to Signal BI.

It may be that other compound spectra, which are unresolvable because of overlapping lines, may become resolvable if only one line narrows or

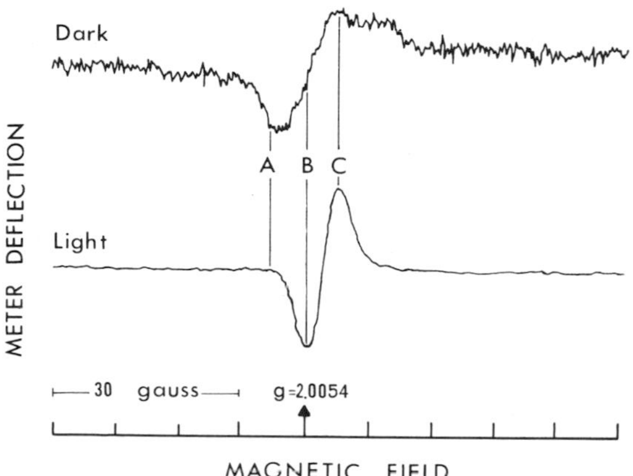

Fig. 6-20 Comparison of position in magnetic field of dark signal in deuterated *R. rubrum* and signal recorded in the light. These spectra were generated by organisms grown in deuterated medium. See text for a discussion of the significance of the fact that the spectra do not totally overlap. The scale for the upper spectrum is nine times that for the lower. (Reference 24.)

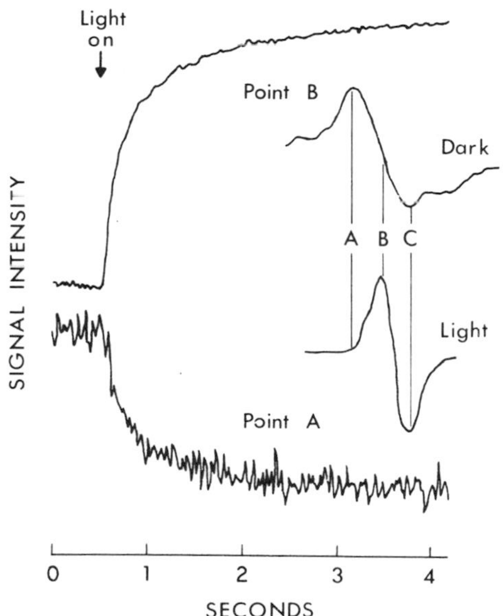

Fig. 6-21 Kinetics of dark signal seen in *R. rubrum*. When the magnetic field was held constant at the value indicated by *A* and the light was chopped, 4 sec light–4 sec dark, the concentration of unpaired electrons was seen to decrease (*lower curve*). Additional experimental conditions: 432 repeated cycles, 15 C, 4 G mod. amp. When only the magnetic field was changed and held constant at B the concentration of unpaired electrons increased in the light (upper curve). All experimental conditions the same except that only 23 repeated cycles were summed. (Reference 24.)

if there is a differential narrowing of the components of the spectrum resulting from complete or selective deuteration.

ACKNOWLEDGMENTS

Several of my colleagues were kind enough to read and comment on the manuscript. The detailed comments and suggestions of J. Bolton and P. Loach were particularly useful and the chapter is certainly better for my having often followed their advice. Since I did not invariably follow their suggestions, however, the responsibility for any faults that remain is mine alone. I am also pleased to acknowledge my special debt to Barry Commoner for his encouragement and generosity over the years.

This work was supported by a grant from the National Science Foundation, GB 12665.

REFERENCES

1. B. Commoner, J. Townsend, and G. Pake, *Nature*, **174,** 689–691 (1954).
2. B. Commoner, J. Heise, and J. Townsend, *Proc. Natl. Acad. Sci.*, **42,** 710–718 (1956).
3. P. Sogo, N. Pon, and M. Calvin, *Proc. Natl. Acad. Sci.*, **43,** 387–393 (1957).
4. B. Commoner, J. Heise, B. Lippincott, R. Norberg, J. Passonneau, and J. Townsend, *Science*, **126,** 57–63 (1957).
5. C. van Niel, *Arch. Mikrobiol.*, **3,** 1–112 (1931).
6. C. van Niel in *Photosynthesis in Plants*, J. Franck and W. Loomis, Eds., Iowa State College Press, Ames, Iowa, 1961, pp. 437–496.
7. S. Ruben, M. Randall, M. Kamen, and J. Hyde, *J. Am. Chem. Soc.*, **63,** 877–880 (1941).
8. N. K. Boardman, *Advan. Enzymol.*, **30,** 1–80 (1968).
9. G. Döring, G. Renger, J. Vater, and H. T. Witt, *Z. Naturforsh.*, **24b,** 1139–1143 (1969); R. A. Floyd, B. Chance, and D. Devault, *Biochem. Biophys. Acta*, **226,** 103–112 (1971).
10. D. Arnon, D. Knaff, B. McSwain, R. Chain, H. Tsujimoto, *Photochem. Photobiol.*, **14,** 397–426 (1971).
11. C. Fowler and C. Sybesma, *Biochim. Biophys. Acta*, **197,** 276–283 (1970); L. Rubin, A. Rubin, V. Dubrovin, E. Shrinka, *J. Mol. Biol.*, **3,** 552–558 (1969).
12. H. Gest in *Bacterial Photosynthesis*, H. Gest, A. San Pietro, and L. Vernon, Eds., Antioch, Yellow Springs, Ohio, 1963, p. 142.
13. L. P. Vernon and M. Avron, *Ann. Rev. Biochem.*, **34,** 269–296 (1965).
14. B. Commoner in *Light and Life*, W. McElroy and B. Glass, Eds., Johns Hopkins, Baltimore, 1961, pp. 356–377.
15. J. Heise, Electron Spin Resonance Studies of Free Radicals in Photosynthetic Systems, Dissertation, Washington University, St. Louis, Mo., 1962.
16. M. Calvin and P. Sogo, *Science*, **125,** 499–500 (1957).
17. H. Beinert, B. Kok, and G. Hoch, *Biophys. Boil. Res. Commun.*, **7,** 209–212 (1962).
18. E. Weaver, *Arch. Biochem. Biophys.*, **99,** 193–196 (1962).
19. J. McElroy, G. Feher, and D. Mauzerall, *Biophys. Biochem. Acta*, **172,** 180–183 (1969).
20. J. Bolton, R. Clayton, and D. Reed, *Photochem. Photobiol.*, **9,** 209–218 (1969).

21. R. Treharne, C. Melton, and R. Roppel, *J. Mol. Biol.*, **10,** 57–62 (1964).
22. G. Androes and M. Calvin, *Biophys. J.*, **2,** 217–258 (1962).
23. G. Androes, *Advan. Bot. Res.*, **1,** 327–369 (1963).
24. D. Kohl, J. Townsend, B. Commoner, H. Crespi, R. Dougherty, and J. Katz, *Nature*, **206,** 1105–1110 (1965).
25. E. Weaver, *Ann. Rev. Plant Physiol.*, **19,** 283–294 (1968).
26. E. Rabinowitch in "Photosynthesis and Related Processes," Wiley-Interscience, New York, 1951, Vol. II, 1, pp. 858–872, 965–981, 1007–1047.
27. E. Rabinowitch in "Photosynthesis and Related Processes," Wiley-Interscience, New York, 1956, Vol. II, 2, pp. 1258–1272.
28. P. Loach and K. Walsh, *Biochem.*, **8,** 1908–1912 (1969).
29. R. Treharne, T. Brown, and L. Vernon, *Biochem. Biophys. Acta*, **75,** 324–332 (1963).
30. R. Treharne and L. Vernon, *Biochem. Biophys. Res. Commun.*, **8,** 481–485 (1962).
31. D. Kohl, Studies of Photosynthesis in Intact Cells by Electron Spin Resonance, Thesis, Washington University, St. Louis, Mo., 1965.
32. J. Heise and R. Treharne, *Develop. Appl. Spectrometry*, **3,** 340–360 (1963).
33. H. Beinert and B. Kok, *Biochem. Biophys. Acta*, **88,** 278–288 (1964).
34. A. Portis, *Phys. Rev.*, **91,** 1071–1078 (1953).
35. T. Castner, *Phys. Rev.*, **115,** 1506–1515 (1959).
36. M. Allen, L. Piette, and J. Murchio, *Proc. V. Intern. Congr. Biochem.*, Moscow, I.U.B. Symposium Series, **29,** 499 (1961).
37. P. Sane, D. Goodchild, and R. Park, *Biochem. Biophys. Acta*, **216,** 162–178 (1970).
38. G. Hoch and B. Kok, *Ann. Rev. Plant Physiol.*, **12,** 155–194 (1961).
39. W. Clark, *Oxidation-Reduction Potentials of Organic Systems*, Williams & Wilkins, Baltimore, 1960.
40. M. Calvin and G. Androes, *Science*, **138,** 867–873 (1962).
41. P. Loach, G. Androes, A. Maksim, and M. Calvin, *Photochem. Photobiol.*, **2,** 443–454 (1963).
42. I. Kuntz, Jr., P. Loach, and M. Calvin, *Biophys. J.*, **4,** 227–249 (1964).
43. P. Sogo, L. Carter, and M. Calvin in *Free Radicals in Biological Systems*, M. Blois, Jr., Ed., Academic, New York, 1960.
44. M. Calvin in *Light and Life*, W. McElroy and B. Glass, Eds., Johns Hopkins, Baltimore, 1961, pp. 317–355.
45. B. Kok and H. Beinert, *Biochem. Biophys. Res. Commun.*, **9,** 349–354 (1962).
46. L. Vernon, B. Ke, and E. Shaw, *Biochem.*, **6,** 2210–2220 (1967).
47. E. Weaver, *Biochem. Biophys. Acta*, **162,** 286–289 (1968).
48. K. Poole, Jr., "Electron Spin Resonance—A Comprehensive Treatise on Experimental Techniques," Wiley-Interscience, New York, 1967, p. 554.
49. P. Loach presented at Vth International Congress on Photobiology, Hanover, New Hampshire, August 26–31, 1968.
50. P. Schmidt-Mende and B. Rumberg, *Z. Naturforsh.*, **236,** 225–228 (1968).
51. R. Ruby, I. Kuntz, Jr., and M. Calvin, *Proc. Natl. Acad. Sci.*, **51,** 515–520 (1964).
52. P. Loach and D. Sekura, *Photochem. Photobiol.*, **6,** 381–393 (1967).
53. P. Loach, *Biochem.*, **5,** 592–600 (1966).
54. D. Green and G. Brierley in *Biochemistry of Quinones*, R. Morton, Ed., Academic, New York, 1965, pp. 405–432.
55. P. Loach, R. Bambara, and F. Ryan, *Photochem. Photobiol.*, **14,** 373–388 (1971).
56. G. Feher, *Photochem. Photobiol.*, **13,** 247–258 (1971).
57. P. Sogo, M. Jost, and M. Calvin, *Rad. Res. Suppl.*, **1,** 511–518 (1959).
58. J. Bolton, K. Cost, and A. Frenkel, *Arch. Biochem. Biophys.*, **126,** 383–387 (1968).

59. E. Weaver and N. Bishop, *Science*, **140,** 1095–1097 (1963).
60. B. Commoner, D. Kohl, and J. Townsend, *Proc. Natl. Acad. Sci.*, **50,** 638–644 (1963).
61. W. Vredenberg and L. Duysens, *Nature*, **197,** 355–357 (1963).
62. M. Blois, H. Brown, and J. Maling, *Free Radicals in Biological Systems*, Academic, New York, 1961, p. 117.
63. D. Kohl and P. Wood, *Plant Physiol.*, **44,** 1439–1445 (1969).
64. N. Bishop in *Quinones in Electron Transport*, G. Wolstenholme and C. O'Connor, Eds., Little Brown, Boston, 1961, p. 385.
65. D. Kohl, J. Wright, and M. Weissman, *Biochem. Biophys. Acta*, **180,** 536–544 (1969).
66. H. Schleyer, *Biochem. Biophys. Acta*, **153,** 427–447 (1968).
67. E. Weaver and H. Weaver, *Science*, **165,** 906–907 (1969).
68. P. Wood, A Study of the Redox State of Plastoquinine A and the Importance of the Redox State in Photosynthetic Reaction, thesis, Purdue University, 1968.
69. H. Lichtenthaler, *Protoplasma*, **68,** 315–326 (1969).
70. G. Corker and W. Nicholson, *Arch. Biochem. Biophys.*, **137,** 75–83 (1970).
71. E. Weaver, *Photochem. Photobiol.*, **7,** 93–100 (1968).
72. W. Parsons, *Biochem. Biophys. Acta*, **153,** 248–259 (1968).
73. G. Rikhireva, L. Kayushin, Z. Gribova, and A. Krasnovskii, *Dokl. Adak. Nauk. SSSR*, **159,** 196–197 (1964).
74. K. L. Zenkel, D. W. Reed, and R. K. Clayton, *Proc. Natl. Acad. Sci.*, **61,** 1243–1249 (1968).
75. B. Kok and G. Cheniae, *Curr. Top. Bioenergetics*, **1,** 1 (1966).
76. R. Kenten and P. Mann, *Biochem. J.*, **61,** 279–286 (1955).
77. J. McKenna and N. Bishop, *Biochem. Biophys. Acta*, **131,** 339–349 (1967).
78. D. Teichler and R. Levine, *Plant Physiol.*, **42,** 1643–1647 (1967).
79. M. Cohn and J. Townsend, *Nature*, **173,** 1090–1091 (1954).
80. R. Jensen and J. Bassham, *Proc. Natl. Acad. Sci.*, **56,** 1095–1101 (1966).
81. M. Allen, *Biochem. Biophys. Acta*, **60,** 539–547 (1962).
82. T. Yamashita and W. Butler, *Plant Physiol.*, **44,** 435–438 (1969).
83. R. Lozier, M. Baginsky, and W. Butler, *Photochem. Photobiol.*, **14,** 323–328 (1971).
84. E. Weaver, *Nature*, **226,** 183–184 (1970).
85. T. Hollocher, Jr., and B. Commoner, *Proc. Natl. Acad. Sci.*, **47,** 1355–1374 (1961).
86. L. Vernon, *Ann. Rev. Plant Physiol.*, **15,** 73–100 (1964).

CHAPTER SEVEN

Electron Spin Resonance Applied to Free Radicals of Physiological, Pharmacological, or Biochemical Interest

DONALD C. BORG

Medical Research Center
Brookhaven National Laboratory
Upton, New York

7.1 GENERAL REMARKS

This chapter concerns itself primarily with ESR studies of free radicals of biological interest produced from various chemicals. Some of these chemicals are actually derived from biological sources, and all are of physiological, pharmacological, or biochemical interest. Nonetheless, the ESR studies have not been carried out on living systems nor on tissues or cells or their anatomically intact components. The application of ESR to intact tissues and cells is dealt with in Chapters 4 and 5.

Chapter 4 stressed that the "free radical"-type ESR signals elicited from normal tissues are generally very weak, and their isotropic hyperfine spectral components are also broadened by residual anisotropic interactions; therefore very little signal *shape* information has been obtained up to the present. Nonetheless, the ESR signal envelopes are consistent with those recorded from many organic free radicals, and a large variety would be expected to arise from many of the univalent redox steps that occur in the normal chemistry of life. Indeed, this forecast was the leitmotiv of Michaelis (166) and it remains a cogent hypothesis.

The failure of ESR to identify more biological free radicals stems in large measure from its limited sensitivity in conjunction with the generally high reactivities (hence short lifetimes) of free radicals. As pointed out in Chapter 2, the absolute concentration of free radicals required for detection in a typical ESR spectrometer is of the order of 10^{-8} *M*, and 100 to 1000 times that concentration usually are required to record a detailed ESR spectrum. On the other hand, steady-state concentrations of free radical forms of biologically occurring free radicals may represent very small fractions of the parent substances. Since some biologically active molecules, such as hormones and drugs, may be effective when their *total* concentrations are in the picomolar (10^{-12} *M*) or nanomolar (10^{-9} *M*) range, any small fractional yields of free radicals of these compounds that might exist *in vivo* would be several orders of magnitude below the concentration limits of ESR detection.

Furthermore, solution spectra of sufficiently small free radicals usually involve the averaging out of anisotropic interactions, giving rise to isotropic spectra that frequently are rich in detail and relatively straightforward to interpret (see Chapter 1). In contradistinction to the "powder spectra" obtained by ESR from tissues (see Chapter 4), these spectra may provide both identifying and descriptive information concerning the free radicals.

Although there are important exceptions to these generalizations regarding limitations of ESR sensitivity and the featureless spectral envelopes from cell preparations (see Chapters 4, 5, 6, and 8), the failure of ESR to reveal many details of the free radical milieu of living materials has led investigators to turn to model systems and to chemical reactions *in vitro* when employing ESR to study free radicals of physiological or pharmacological interest. In large measure, then, the subject matter of this chapter may be characterized as ESR studies of chemicals deemed to be of biological interest, with many of the compounds examined in the liquid state, often in solvents quite foreign to the biological environment.

In this context "biological interest" is defined in an operational sense; that is to say, it is what an investigator *declares* to be of interest. At one extreme are clear-cut cases in which the free radicals in question can be correlated with ESR signals obtained from biological or enzymic preparations. At the other, and this encompasses much of the material cited in this chapter, are studies of chemical systems proposed as models of biological reactions. Sometimes the models are claimed to be relevant on the basis of experimental evidence that suggests that free radicals—or at least one-electron oxidoreductions—are involved in the biochemistry of the substance at hand, and sometimes they are based only on open-ended speculations that free radical mechanisms are possible or plausible and have not been ruled out.

It is important to note, however, that the mere presence of ESR from a model chemical reaction involving a biochemical is insufficient proof that a free radical is of biological interest, and to substantiate the relevance of ESR evidence further correlations are desirable. Thus quantitative correlation of the spins represented by an ESR spectrum (see Chapter 3) may help to distinguish free radicals that are on the main path of a reaction from those arising from minor side paths or from adventitious impurities. Similarly, kinetic analysis of a test system in which ESR signals obey the relationships expected can support the biochemical significance of the free radicals detected. Unfortunately, with most rare biochemicals, especially when free radical products are reactive and short-lived, neither stoichiometric nor kinetic studies have been carried out, and the biological relevance of the ESR data remains correspondingly less certain. Many of the ESR investigations on molecules of physiological or pharmacological interest belong to this class, and much of the material cited in this chapter must be construed as little more than provocative speculation.

Conversely, failure to elicit ESR cannot be taken as proof that a free radical is absent in a sample or test system. Limitations of ESR detection sensitivity already have been discussed, and in Chapters 1 and 2 other factors were noted that can cause ESR to fail to detect free radicals or other paramagnets present in a sample. In cases in which free radical intermediates that serve as critical links in the overall kinetics of interrelated reactions remain undetected they may be classified as "hidden radicals," a term initially defined in a more restricted sense by Hemmerich with regard to reactions generally obeying reversible thermodynamics and involving metal-stabilized radicals, flavosemiquinones, and hydropteridenes (111). For example, after reviewing anodic oxidation pathways of aromatic compounds, Adams concluded that the overall electrode processes were cascades (or series of reactions) with strong indirect evidence of initial one-electron oxidations that produce intermediate cation radicals. These "hidden radicals" could not be measured by ESR, presumably because of their instability (3).

When attempting to correlate data from chemical model systems with the reactions to be expected within a cell or other biological milieu, the effects of biological macromolecules, especially proteins, on the model reaction system must be taken into account; for example, the isotropic hyperfine spectral resolution obtained from many small free radical molecules in solution would not be expected to be resolved from the ESR spectra of free radicals on large molecules such as proteins (see Chapter 1). Therefore, depending on the extent to which small free radical molecules were bound by proteins and thereby restricted in Brownian rotational movement, the ESR spectrum of such molecules would not be expected to be the same in free solution as when bound to protein. Additional interactions with protein or with metal sites thereon might also alter significantly the spin-lattice coupling of the free radical center, thereby affecting intrinsic ESR linewidths and altering microwave power saturation behavior.

In addition to effects on the ESR phenomenon itself, binding of small free radicals or other intermediates of a reaction system in which free radicals participate would be expected to alter the free-radical reaction paths themselves so that they might differ significantly from those seen in model systems free in solution. Thus binding to protein could stabilize one of several equilibrium forms present in a reaction system and thus alter the thermodynamics of the reaction. In the case of flavinsemiquinones, for example (111), free radical stability is strongly affected by the presence of appropriate metals and metalloproteins (see Chapter 8). The well-known effects of proteins on acidity constants of constituent moieties would also be expected to influence strongly the behavior of bound free radicals whose stability depends on proton dissociation, such as quininoid-type systems (111). Furthermore, in a manner analogous to the activating effect of protein binding during enzymic catalysis, the activation energy for bond association or formation might be altered by the binding of free radicals to proteins.

Last, and perhaps most commonly, the binding of free radicals to proteins, membranes, or other macromolecules would be expected to alter their kinetic stability. Potentially reactive free radicals bound to sites that sequester them from potential reactants are thereby trapped and either partially or completely stabilized by the binding. This is clearly demonstrated in the case of the chlorpromazine radical cation (see Section 7.4.1) when it is bound to DNA. Thus at pH 5 the chlorpromazine radical in millimolar concentrations decays away over a period of a few minutes, but on binding to DNA it is markedly stabilized (180).

Although Hemmerich (111) confined the term "free radicals of biological interest" to doublet species derived from natural products, the present use is broader. It encompasses exogenous substances that may be of pharmacological or toxicological significance and includes some nonbiochemical model compounds that are chemically related to appropriate biomolecules and whose free radical behavior and analysis thus might be of biological "interest." In the sections that follow several classes of free radical are illustrated in an attempt to include at least those subject areas that have been the subject of extensive biological or biochemical investigation, but coverage is extended from that base largely according to the enthusiasms of the author. Within each major section an example or class of free radical is selected for a more extensive discussion, whereas other representative examples are noted more briefly or are merely cited to provide the reader with a general overview of the applications of ESR to biochemical free radicals.

7.2 ENZYMIC REACTIONS

The obvious importance of free radicals in enzyme systems directed some of the earliest ESR studies on biological materials to this subject area. Within two years after the first publication of ESR applied to biological material (55) Commoner and his colleagues began investigations to detect free radical intermediates in enzyme reactions. In the first work otherwise unidentified radicals were detected by ESR and correlated with enzymic activity associated with alcohol dehydrogenase and cytochrome reductase reactions (56, 57). Subsequently ESR was used to document the presence of free radicals detected only during the course of enzymic electron transfer when five different dehydrogenases and five flavoenzymes were studied, along with the cytochrome *c*/cytochrome oxidase system (58). From that work it was concluded that the ESR observed with enzyme activity was probably associated with prosthetic groups, at least in part due to free radical forms of flavins. However, since the subject of flavins, including free radical studies, was reviewed a few years ago (12, 201) and is treated in some detail in Chapter 8 of this book, flavin free radicals, flavin coenzymes, and flavoproteins are not dealt with further here.

Because some oxidoreduction enzymes are involved with redox reactions in which the change in the redox state of the reactants is equal to one electron equivalent, enzymes of this class might be expected to exist in forms containing odd numbers of electrons. Although this is often true, the paramagnetic species of these enzymes most frequently involve unpaired electrons associated with component metal ions (e.g., iron, copper, or cobalt) or with flavin moieties. Chapters 8 and 9 of this book include discussions of such compounds. This chapter refers only to (a) a small number of additional cases in which the free radical or paramagnetic species associated with an enzyme or enzyme-substrate complex does not fall into one of these categories and (b) a class of enzyme reactions in which free radicals of the substrates themselves have been studied by ESR.

7.2.1 Free Radicals of Enzymes or Enzyme-Substrate Complexes, Excepting Flavins

7.2.1.1 Cytochrome-c Peroxidase

This enzyme, isolated from baker's yeast, is discussed in some detail as a representative of the class of enzymes shown by ESR to contain a free radical moiety in at least one of its active forms. It is a hemoprotein that contains paramagnetic ferric iron in its "native" or resting state, and to this extent it resembles the better known peroxidases from other plant and animal sources. However, although the more highly oxidized intermediate states of the latter enzymes, Compounds I and II, respectively, give evidence by magnetic susceptibility measurements of several unpaired spins, ESR has not evinced any signal from a free radical intermediate or component (53, 167, 25, 184).

However, although cytochrome-*c* peroxidase, on the addition of a stoichiometric amount of hydroperoxide, does give rise to a red enzyme-substrate complex whose optical absorption resembles that of Compound II of the more classical peroxidases, its oxidation state is then two equivalents above the ground state, like that of the green Compound I of other peroxidases (234, 247, 250). Furthermore, the red enzyme-substrate complex of cytochrome-*c* peroxidase frozen to liquid nitrogen temperature exhibits an ESR signal near $g = 2$ (248, 249, 250) that is typical of a free radical-like spin-1/2 species having nearly axial symmetry (234) (Fig. 7-1). The "free radical" ESR signal, when integrated, accounts nearly stoichiometrically for one oxidation equivalent. Although the signal shows some asymmetry at 77 K (248, 249, 250), the better resolved signal obtained at 1.5 K reveals partial resolution of parallel and perpendicular components of the signal with $g_{\perp} \simeq 2.00$ and $g_{\parallel} \simeq 2.05$ (234). Analysis of the asymmetric line and that of the related fluoride product of the cytochrome-*c* peroxidase led Wittenberg et al. to conclude that the free radical site could be assigned to an atom near the heme iron system but at least 8 Å away (234). Assuming that the porphyrin itself had not undergone an oxidation (a point to be questioned later in Section 7.3.9), they then concluded that the free radical moiety resided in an axial ligand position of the heme iron (184).

Conversely, Yonetani and his colleagues found that the narrow ESR signal of the cytochrome-*c* peroxidase enzyme-substrate complex was gradually replaced by the ferric iron signals of the free enzyme when the complex was titrated with ferrocytochrome-*c* (248, 250). They were unable to titrate preferentially one of the two oxidizing equivalents of the complex, which they

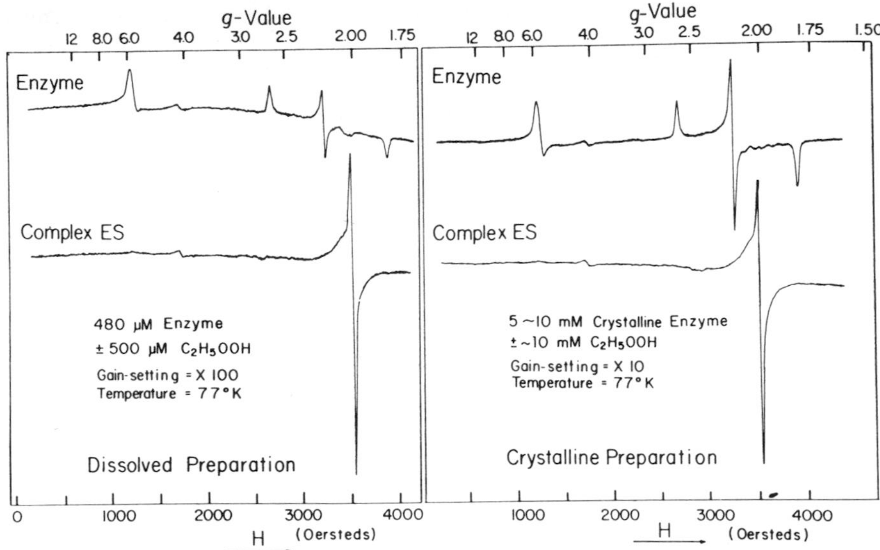

Fig. 7-1 ESR spectra from cytochrome-*c* peroxidase of baker's yeast and its 1:1 enzyme-substrate complex with H_2O_2, Complex ES. The enzyme reveals well-defined signals from high-spin and low-spin ferric iron but in Complex ES these are replaced by an intense narrow signal of the free radical type at $g = 2.0$. (From Ref. 248, with permission.)

therefore allocated to the hematin prosthetic group and to a relatively stable and reversible free radical moiety of the enzyme protein, respectively (248). On further comparison with the ESR signals produced by peroxidatic oxidation of myoglobin by King and Winfield (129) Yonetani and Schleyer concluded that one of the two oxidizing equivalents of the cytochrome-*c* peroxidase complex was separated from the iron prosthetic group in the form of a free radical, presumably of an aromatic amino acid of the apoprotein moiety (249). This is a less restrictive conclusion than that of Wittenberg et al., in which the free radical site was specifically assigned to the sixth ligand group of the heme. Yonetani and his colleagues (249, 250) described the relatively stable enzyme-substrate complex of this peroxidase as an unusual compound containing two presumably unstable and highly reactive species, namely quadrivalent iron and a free radical. They did not consider the possibility that the free radical might be situated on the porphyrin itself. Peisach and his colleagues (184) did not make an assignment of Fe(IV), but they also assumed that the porphyrin itself had not undergone an oxidation. Further consideration, however, is given to this possibility in Section 7.3.9.

7.2.1.2 *Ribonucleotide Reductase*

Another possible example of a free radical signal associated with an enzyme-substrate complex but not involving a flavin moiety has been suggested by work with ribonucleotide reductase from lactobacillus. The enzyme catalyzes a reduction of ribonucleoside triphosphates by certain dithiols in the presence of deoxyadenosyl cobalamin. Under appropriate incubation conditions the cobalamin cofactor reveals an ESR signal resembling that of divalent cobalt in cobalamin vitamin B_{12}-*r* (104) and this may involve an unidentified reactive intermediate (105). Another type of ESR signal, correlated with the rate of ribonucleotide reduction by this enzyme system, is an asymmetric doublet whose ESR behavior suggests that the signal is not due to a transition metal species (Fig. 7-2). Although full identification of the species responsible for

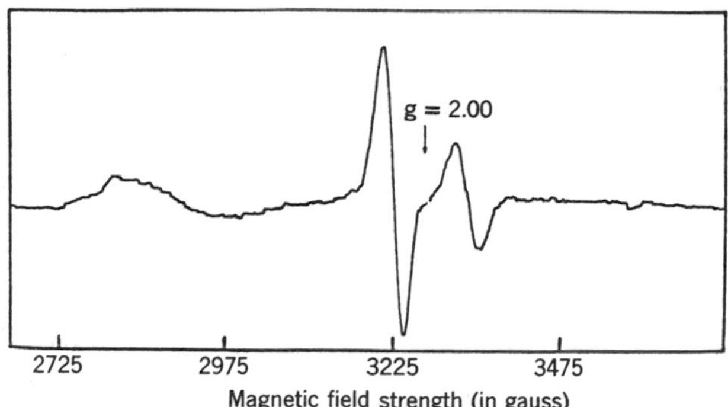

Fig. 7-2 ESR "doublet" recorded during ribonucleotide reduction when deoxyadenosyl-cobalamin is incubated with ribonucleoside reductase from *Lactobacillus*. Following 5 min of incubation, the spectrum was recorded at 77K. The broad low-field resonance is from cob(II)alamin. (From Ref. 105, with permission.)

the ESR doublet has not been achieved, its kinetics indicate that it may be a free radical intermediate directly involved in the enzymic reduction of ribonucleotides (105).

7.2.1.3 *Ethanolamine Deaminase*

An ESR signal has also been generated by the ethanolamine deaminase-coenzyme-B_{12} complex in the presence of substrate. In reactions of this type the coenzyme appears to serve as an intermediate hydrogen carrier through its cobalt-linked adenosyl group. Babior and Gould (8) reported on ESR signals whose origin was not established. Although there were resemblances to signals from transition metal paramagnetic sites, the possibility remains that the signals represent free radicals associated with an enzyme-coenzyme-substrate complex, as in the case of ribonucleotide reductase, just preceding.

7.2.2 Enzymic Reactions Involving Free Radicals of Substrates

7.2.2.1 Peroxidases

It was pointed out in Section 7.2.1.1 that with the exception of cytochrome-*c* peroxidase of yeast no free radical forms have been identified with the green Compound I or the red Compound II forms of hemoprotein peroxidases. This is so despite ample evidence (184) that Compound I is two oxidation equivalents removed from the native, or ferric, enzyme and that Compound II is an intermediate form that lies one oxidation equivalent removed from each of the preceding states (184). In the case of horseradish peroxidase, which is prototypic for this class of enzymes, it has been known for nearly 20 years that the enzyme, oxidized to the green Compound I after reaction with the acceptor substrate (usually hydrogen peroxide), then reacts with one molecule of donor substrate to form a semiquinone free radical of the latter plus the Compound II state of the enzyme (52, 96). Compound II further reacts with a second molecule of donor substrate to form the native ferric peroxidase and a second free radical molecule of the substrate (12, 52, 73, 96).

Despite the absence of ESR evidence of free radical forms of the enzyme-substrate complexes themselves (53, 167, 25, 184),* the free radical mechanism proposed for the peroxidatic oxidations of these enzymes was confirmed by the elegant ESR studies of Yamazaki, Mason, and Piette, in which free radicals associated only with the donor substrates were observed by continuous flow techniques and correlated quantitatively and kinetically with enzymic activity (239, 240). It was these quantitative analyses (in which the concentration of intermediates was found to be in great excess of the enzyme present) and the excellent correlation of the free radical signals with the kinetics expected for the peroxidase reactions (especially the dependence of free radical concentration on the square root of the total enzyme concentration) that led Yamazaki, Mason, and Piette to conclude that their ESR data supported the enzymic reaction pathway proposed earlier by Chance (73). Thus the ESR results showed that free radicals

* Actually a trace of free radical signal was noted by Chance (53) in a study of Compound I of horseradish peroxidase, and Morita and Mason (167) also found evidence of a free radical signal in ESR studies conducted at about 90 K of Compound I and Compound II of horseradish peroxidase. Quantitation of the free radical signals revealed, however, that they could represent no more than 1 to 2 percent of the enzyme, and it was concluded that the free radicals did not participate to a significant extent in the peroxidatic mechanism (167).

were formed in the peroxidase reactions *not* in combination with enzymes but as independent products existing freely in solution. The radicals decayed predominantly by dismutation reactions because there was low reactivity between the substrate free radicals and Compounds I or II of the peroxidase (239, 240, 187).

The work just discussed was performed with Japanese turnip peroxidase, and the free radicals whose hyperfine structure was seen with the ESR flow systems adapted for the biochemical work were from hydroquinone, ascorbic acid, and dihydroxyfumaric acid (239, 240). Soon thereafter the findings were extended to horseradish peroxidase itself (241) and to the additional substrates reductic acid, triose reductone, and pyrogallol (187) (Fig. 7-3). Further extension of the work to aerobic oxidase reactions catalyzed by peroxidase led Yamazaki and Piette to group donor substrates into one of two classes previously defined by Yamazaki: "redogenic" substrates, which react with Compound I of the peroxidase to form a free radical of the donor substrate which can then react further to *reduce* other reactive molecules that may be present in the reaction system, such as ferricytochrome-*c*, and "oxidogenic" substrates, which greatly accelerate the peroxidatic oxidation of donor substrates by the enzyme (243, 244).

ESR spectra were observed from the free radicals of the redogenic substrates, with the exception of indoleacetic acid, but not of oxidogenic

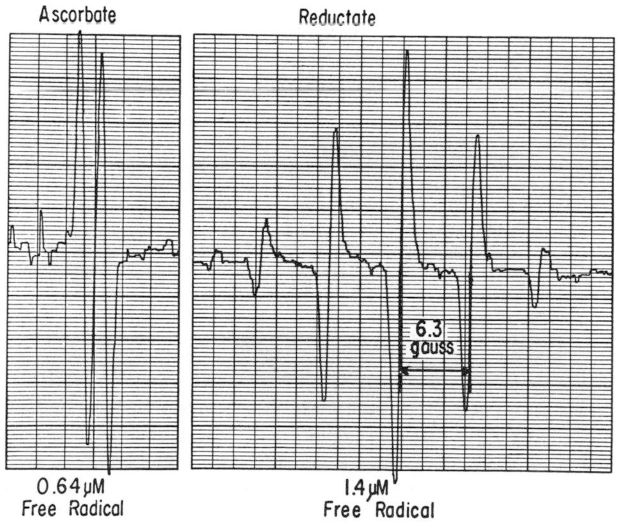

Fig. 7-3 ESR spectra from steady-state concentrations of free radicals produced enzymatically, using the continuous flow method. Ascorbate free radical produced from turnip peroxidase, reductate radical from horseradish peroxidase, using 10 mM of substrate, 0.5 mM H_2O_2, and less than $10^{-7}M$ of enzyme. (From Ref. 241, with permission.)

substrates, such as resorcinol and phenol (243). Presumably the free radicals derived from the oxidogenic substrates were very unstable and reacted rapidly with one another to form dimerized or other complex oxidation products or they reacted very rapidly with other substances in the medium—in any case, largely disappearing before ESR could be observed in the fast-flow systems (243, 244). Since, however, the same free radicals of the oxidogenic substrates are strong one-electron oxidizing agents, they may be expected to react directly with redogenic substrates present in the enzyme mixture to form the somewhat more stable free radicals of the latter, which are then detected by ESR in the actual experiments (12, 243, 244). A schematic representation of Yamazaki's analysis of the oxygen-consuming oxidation of redogenic substrates by peroxidase is given in Fig. 7-4, taken from Refs. 243, 244,and 246.

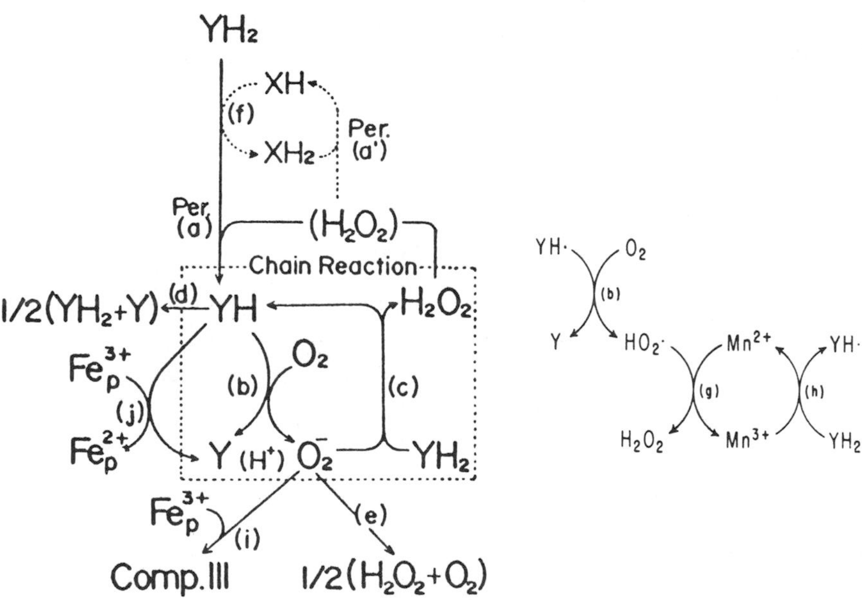

Fig. 7-4 Yamazaki's scheme for oxygen-consuming peroxidatic oxidations of substrates, YH_2, catalyzed by peroxidases. The main path consists of enzymic formation of free radical, YH or YH· (Reaction a), and a chain reaction (Reactions b and c). Chain termination may occur by Reactions d and e. Reactions g and i involve minor paths to a Compound III form of the enzyme (not discussed in the text). Mn^{2+} can promote the chain reaction by reacting with the superoxide radical $HO_2\cdot$ or its anion O_2^- (see Sec. 7.2.2.10) to reduce its dismutation via Reaction e. Certain monophenols and other substrates, XH_2, capable of being oxidized to free radical forms can facilitate or hinder the enzymic formation of free radicals by Reactions a′ and f. (From Refs. 243 and 246, with permission.)

In addition to the interactions between oxidogenic substrates of peroxidase and the oxidatic reactions with redogenic substrates just discussed, oxidogenic substrates can catalyze one-electron transfer to other biochemicals which are poor primary substrates of the enzyme itself; for example, NADH and NADPH are not donor substrates for horseradish peroxidase, but in the presence of manganese and phenol this enzyme catalyzes their aerobic oxidation (246). ESR investigations have supported this mechanism as well, and Nakamura and Yamazaki (181) were able to determine the rates of reaction with cytochrome-*c* and -b_5 of free radicals formed from naphthoquinones, ascorbic acid, hydroquinone, *p*-cresol, and chlorpromazine following their peroxidatic oxidation.

The adaptation of continuous-flow methods for ESR studies of biochemical reactions by Yamazaki and his colleagues provided explicit confirmation of reaction mechanisms whose existence had already been deduced—but only on the basis of inferences from kinetic analyses of optical absorption measurements. The isotropic hyperfine structure of the free radicals detected in the ESR work provided descriptive identification of reaction intermediates whose existence had been proposed nearly 10 years earlier (52, 96). Nevertheless, the ESR flow systems used by Yamazaki and Piette were prodigal of biochemical reactants, and it has not appeared feasible to most subsequent investigators to apply these methods to biochemical reactions in which expendable supplies of enzymes or substrates were not readily available. It is worth noting at this point, however, that the use of continuous-flow systems adapted for ESR at Q-band (35 GHz) has made it possible to record ESR spectra of transient free radicals from much smaller amounts of reactants (39) (see Section 2.18.2.2). Thus the saving of materials provided by the Q-band flow apparatus made it possible for Elmore to carry out ESR experiments that documented the presence of free radical forms of certain catecholamine hormones (see Section 7.3.6.1) in their reaction with peroxidase (73).

7.2.2.2 Ascorbic Acid Oxidase

In the preceding section a rather extensive review was made of the formation of free radicals from donor substrates of peroxidases, which are heme enzymes. These same methods were applied by Yamazaki and Piette to ascorbic acid oxidase, a copper-containing enzyme; and the ESR flow work demonstrated again that labile free radicals were formed by the enzyme from the donor substrates ascorbic acid and reductic acid (241) (Fig. 7-5). Further extending the parallelism with peroxidase behavior, it was shown that ascorbic acid oxidase could catalyze the reaction of substrates with which it did not react directly; for example, in the presence of ascorbic acid the enzyme was able to reduce cytochrome-*c*, presumably as a result of a second-

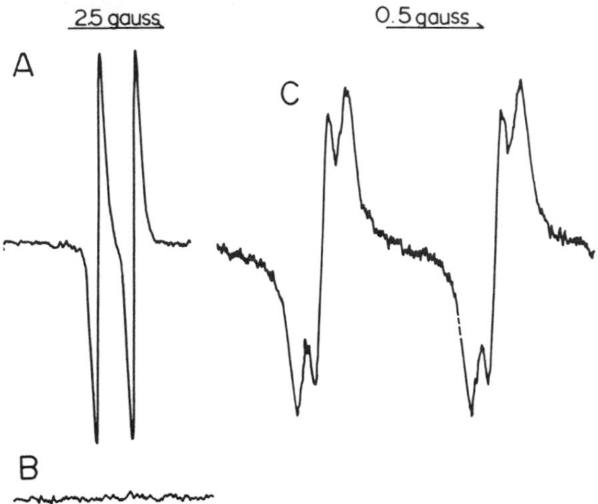

Fig. 7-5 ESR spectra of monodehydroascorbate free radical formed in the steady state of ascorbate oxidase reaction during continuous flow. A and C were taken during flow and B after flow was stopped. The modulation amplitude used was 0.1 G in A and B and 0.04 G in C. (From Ref. 181, with permission.)

ary reaction with the ascorbic free radical formed enzymically (242). As seen in the peroxidatic reaction, monodehydro free radicals formed by ascorbic acid oxidase were proposed to act not only as reductants but also as oxidants (181) (see also Section 9.13).

7.2.2.3 *Pyrocatechase*

Pyrocatechase is an iron-containing oxygenase that catalyzes the oxidative cleavage of catechol (174). Although speculations about its mechanism of action invoke intermediate free radical forms of the substrate (174) and although semiquinone free radicals of catechol have been well documented by ESR, no ESR signal of a free radical was observed with the enzyme in an equilibrium or steady-state condition (174). In this case the free radicals might have been too short-lived to be detected without a flow system or they may have remained bound to the enzyme and undetectable by ESR for reasons already discussed.

7.2.2.4 *Tyrosinase*

Tyrosinase is a copper enzyme that can catalyze the oxidation of tyrosine and of catechols, including substituted catechols such as dihydroxyphenylalanine. Using flow techniques, Mason, Spencer, and Yamazaki (161) were able to show enzymic formation of orthobenozosemiquinone free radicals from catechol, as evidenced by characteristic isotropic hyperfine structure in the ESR spectra elicited. However, a careful kinetic correlation of the ESR spectral intensity with the enzymic reaction revealed that the free radicals seen during tyrosinase catalysis at pH 7.6 were largely—if not entirely—formed by reverse dismutation from orthobenzoquinone, the primary product of the enzyme-catalyzed two-electron oxidation (161).

7.2.2.5 Dopamine β-Hydroxylase

Dopamine beta hydroxylase has been isolated and purified from the bovine adrenal medulla. It appears to be a copper-containing enzyme and it catalyzes the conversion of 3,4-dihydroxyphenylethylamine (dopamine) to norepinephrine. ESR studies of enzyme incubation media reveal signals of paramagnetic copper, which have been correlated with enzyme activity (24). A complete incubation medium shows a small monodehydroascorbate free radical signal (24). A mechanism proposed by Blumberg et al. (24) is that the ascorbate free radical, the primary product of enzyme action, then reacts with dopamine to produce a dopamine free radical, which interacts further with an oxygen-complexed form of the enzyme.

Since the dopamine free radical was not observed in these studies and the ascorbate free radical was not present in stoichiometric amounts, it cannot be said that ESR provided definitive support of a free radical mechanism. When they are produced nonenzymically, however, the dopamine free radicals detected by ESR are known to be short-lived (34, 38). Therefore it may be that the application of high-velocity flow techniques to the dopamine beta hydroxylase reactions could prove highly profitable, provided that the turnover rate of the enzyme is sufficiently fast under some achievable reaction conditions to take advantage of the continuous-flow method.

7.2.2.6 Laccase

Laccase is another copper-containing enzyme that can oxidize hydroquinones. This enzyme has been isolated from plant sources and its catalysis of hydroquinone oxidation has been followed by ESR continuous-flow techniques, which give evidence of free radicals being formed from the substrates (171), with a reaction mechanism (172) similar to that already discussed for peroxidase and ascorbic acid oxidase (see Sections 7.2.2.1 and 7.2.2.2). A laccase-type copper enzyme from mushroom was also isolated, and its catalysis of catechol oxidation used the same mechanism, according to ESR flow studies (173).

7.2.2.7 Ceruloplasmin (ferroxidase)

Ceruloplasmin is a copper-containing protein of blood plasma whose concentrations are markedly reduced in most cases of hepatolenticular disease (Wilson's disease) but whose physiological role has been suggested only recently. Frieden has concluded that ceruloplasmin is the molecular link between copper and iron metabolism (165), where it functions as an oxido-reduction enzyme linking ferrous iron with oxygen (91). Because of this function, he has proposed that ceruloplasmin be given the enzymic name ferroxidase.

From ESR work following the spectra of the copper components of the enzyme (220, 221, 223) or measuring the signals of free radical products (183) from various *p*-phenylenediamines, sometimes with continuous-flow techniques (45) or with rapid freezing methods (222), it was shown that the catalytic action of ceruloplasmin once again involved the oxidation of the electron donor substrate to its free radical form, which was released free into solution to disproportionate or to react with other substrate molecules nonenzymically. This conclusion was supported by quantitative and kinetic analyses (45).

7.2.2.8 *Microsomal Cytochrome Reductases*

Two cytochrome reductases have been isolated from liver microsomes: cytochrome-b_5 reductase and NADPH cytochrome-*c* reductase. These enzymes catalyze electron transfer from reduced pyridine nucleotides to the respective hemoproteins, but they can also reduce ferricyanide, certain phenols, and quinones (123). They are free of transition metals and both are flavoenzymes containing FAD as prosthetic groups (123).

Using an ESR spectrometer and an optical spectrometer, both equipped with flow apparatus, Iyanagi and Yamazaki were able to carry out quantitative and kinetic studies essentially comparable to those reported by Yamazaki and his associates concerning peroxidatic oxidations (see Section 7.2.2.1) (Fig. 7-6). The reductases were found to be mirror images of the peroxidases previously discussed with regard to the formation of free semiquinone radicals, the reductases catalyzing one-electron donation to quinone electron acceptors and the oxidases catalyzing one-electron oxidation of hydroquinone donors. Once they are formed, however, the semiquinones react similarly in both instances, so that in the presence of suitable electron acceptors, such as the cytochromes or molecular oxygen, single electron transfer then occurs to reduce the acceptor (123).

Although flavoenzymes may often serve as two-electron carriers (see Chapter 8), these ESR studies of the free radicals produced from acceptor substrates in any case establish a one-electron step mechanism for the flavin cytochrome reductases from microsomes.

7.2.2.9 *Lipoxidase*

Lipoxidase attacks certain unsaturated lipids in which double bonds have a *cis* configuration, in general producing products that are similar to those formed by autoxidation. The enzyme has been obtained from several plant

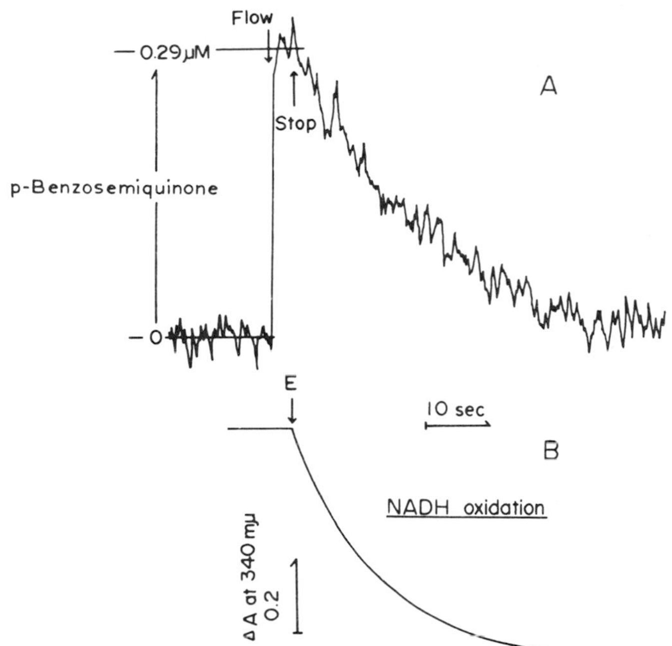

Fig. 7-6 Time courses of NADH oxidation and *p*-benzosemiquinone decay in the cytochrome-b_5 reductase system. In A the magnetic field was adjusted to obtain the maximum of the ESR signal. In B NADH oxidation was measured spectrophotometrically in a different cell under the same conditions. In the overall reaction NADH is oxidized by *p*-benzosemiquinone formed by enzymic reduction of *p*-benzoquinone: hence the parallel kinetics of A and B. (From Ref. 123, with permission.)

sources, but it is uncertain whether it exists in animals. It appears to be neither a flavoenzyme nor a metalloenzyme, but it has been suggested from ESR observations that free radical mechanisms are involved (224).

Walker (224) concluded that odd electron localization on sulfur was present in the free radicals, which would indicate that they do not derive from substrates such as linoleic acid. Nonetheless, in the absence of quantitative or kinetic work the functional role of these radicals was not clear, and a double peak observed with aerobic incubation was attributed to peroxy free radicals whose formation is in accord with postulated reaction mechanisms of lipoxidase (224).

7.2.2.10 Enzymically Formed Superoxide Radical Ions

In the discussion in Chapter 8 of the molybdenum-containing flavoenzyme, xanthine oxidase, the appearance of ESR signals typical of the superoxide radical is noted during the reoxidation of reduced flavoproteins by molecular oxygen. It is pointed out there that consideration of the steps that might produce this product, which can be considered a free radical ion of oxygen, the electron acceptor substrate, leads to the possibility that radicals of donor substrates might also be intermediates in these enzymic processes, although no evidence for the latter species has yet been obtained.

The first clear ESR evidence for the presence of the superoxide ion, also known as the perhydroxyl or hydroperoxy radical, was obtained from samples of incubation mixtures of xanthine oxidase at alkaline pH prepared by the rapid-freezing technique of Bray (133) (Fig. 7-7). Further work by Bray and his associates (176) provided additional confirmation that the asymmetric free radical ESR signal with $g_{\parallel} = 2.08$ and $g_{\perp} = 2.00$ could be attributed to the $O_2^{\dot{-}}$ or superoxide ion radical because a species with the same ESR spectrum and pH dependence was obtained by pulse radiolysis combined with the rapid-freezing technique.

A search for the ESR spectrum of the superoxide ion was extended to other iron-sulfur flavoenzymes than xanthine oxidase. Results with some

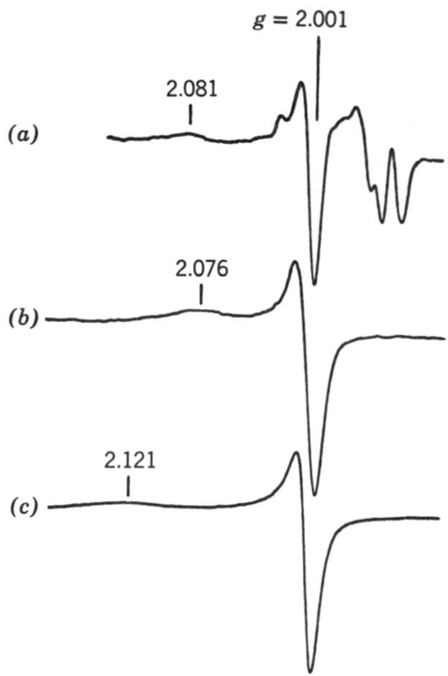

Fig. 7-7 ESR spectra from the superoxide anion $O_2^{\dot{-}}$, using the rapid-freeze technique of Bray (see Sec. 2.18.2.1). (*a*) Reaction between xanthine and O_2 catalyzed by xanthine oxidase after a reaction time of 150 msec. (*b*) Reaction between H_2O_2 and $NaIO_4$ at pH 9.9 after a reaction time of 600 msec. (*c*) As for (*b*) but at pH 13.2. In (*a*) overmodulated molybdenum signals are also present, and an iron signal underlies the sloping base line. (From Ref. 133, with permission.)

ferridoxins, such as that from spinach, were entirely negative, with only the iron ESR signal being detected; but $O_2^{\dot{-}}$ was observed in reoxidation of *Clostridium Welchi* ferridoxin. Using glucose for reduction of the flavoprotein, glucose oxidase, no superoxide ion was seen, which may be consistent with the understanding that no flavosemiquinone is involved in the overall mechanism of that enzyme's reaction (176).

Yamazaki and his associates have proposed that $O_2^{\dot{-}}$ is involved in the oxidatic activity of peroxidase toward substrates such as dihydroxyfumarate (see Section 7.2.2.1 and Fig. 7-4), in which a monodehydro free radical of the donor substrate formed enzymatically reacts with molecular oxygen to yield the superoxide ion radical (243). By using a rapid-freezing procedure, relatively weak ESR signals were observed from a peroxidase reaction that were nevertheless characteristic of the anisotropic superoxide ion spectrum (176). This did not allow the firm conclusion to be drawn that Yamazaki's proposed mechanism involving superoxide ion was clearly the main reaction path in these peroxidase reactions. The persisting uncertainty of the role of this intermediate is heightened by the recognition that the superoxide ion is generally rather unreactive, its normal fate probably being slow disproportionation, so that its presence in biochemical systems may simply signal the action of strongly reducing intermediates (176). Nevertheless it is likely that the superoxide radical ion produced by xanthine oxidase can reduce cytochrome-*c*, although this may not be biologically important (176).

7.3 FREE RADICALS FROM NATURAL SUBSTANCES

For the most part the ESR studies discussed in this section involve free radicals produced in solutions by chemical or physical means. The work noted is confined largely to ESR investigations of free radicals produced by oxidation-reduction mechanisms whose potentials are within the range encountered in cellular metabolism, or not far beyond that range, or by mechanisms to which tissues or tissue products might naturally be exposed. Nonetheless, the ESR data, by themselves, are moot regarding the question of biological interest (see Section 7.1), although other pieces of evidence treating the biological relevance of the free radicals studied by ESR are cited in particular cases.

7.3.1 Biologically Occurring Quinones, General Aspects

The existence of semiquinone free radical intermediates in thermodynamically reversible oxidation-reduction of quinone-hydroquinone couples is by now a part of "classical" chemistry (166, 190). Because many natural biochemicals, as well as many pharmacological agents, belong to this class

(166), some of the early applications of ESR to molecules deemed to be of biological interest involved quinols and quinones. Thus in 1955 Blois (20) reported on ESR studies of approximately 30 quinones undergoing nonenzymic oxidation-reduction reactions. In addition to simple benzoquinones, dihydric quinol derivatives, such as adrenalin and dopa, were examined; and not only were simple naphthoquinones included but so were biological naphthoquinols or naphthoquinones, such as Vitamin K and tocopherol (20).

The early observations did not employ steady-state regenerative techniques and only free radicals of substantial lifetimes were observed. Often these radicals were not the primary radical species formed from the initial substrates. Nonetheless, alkaline oxidation-reduction produced at least some derivative free radicals whose concentrations could be measured by ESR for hours or days. Blois (20) was able to make some generalizations regarding the apparent behavior of free radicals from biologically occurring quinones. He showed that they behave in much the same way as their nonbiological counterparts (190); namely, parasemiquinones are generally more stable than orthosemiquinones, especially in the case of the naphthoquinones, and in general free radical stability depends on pH, with hydroxy compounds frequently stabilized in alkali and amino compounds frequently stabilized in acid.

Except that natural substances were included, these ESR observations did not point to specific biological roles for the free radicals observed (20). Some indication, however, of the way in which semiquinone radicals may undergo redox reactions with biochemicals is given by the kinetic analysis of the oxidation-reduction equilibrium between quinol-quinone and ferro-ferricytochrome-*c* reported by Yamazaki and Ohnishi (245). They employed ESR continuous-flow systems to observe the one-electron transfer reactions between semiquinone formed nonenzymically from the equilibrium between the quinone and quinol (hydroquinone) and the cytochromes (245). The acceleration of the reduction of cytochrome-*c* by quinol in the presence of added quinone was ascribed to the formation of parabenzosemiquinone, produced by an equilibrium reaction in this case. Kinetic studies of the ESR data showed that the semiquinone thus formed could react with ferricytochrome-*c* to form quinone and ferrocytochrome-*c*, with the overall reaction being the reduction of two molecules of ferricytochrome-*c* by one molecule of quinol to produce quinone and two molecules of ferrocytochrome-*c* (245).

In Sections 7.2.2.1 and 7.2.2.8 references were made to the formation of parabenzosemiquinone in enzymic reactions. Sequential redox reactions between the enzymically formed semiquinones and other electron donors or acceptors were also observed, and these are entirely analogous to the reactions observed in the nonenzymic system discussed by Yamazaki and Ohnishi (245). Since a number of primary free radical species produced enzymically were also observed to undergo subsequent one-electron transfer reactions with other biochemicals (see Section 7.2.2), the ESR studies of the chemical system involving quinol and cytochromes did, indeed, provide a good model for biologically relevant reactions. In most other cases of free radical intermediates from biological substances observed by ESR, however, it is not so clear that a biochemical reaction is being modeled, and the reader is left to make his own final evaluation.

At this point it is worth reminding the reader of an observation cited in Section 7.1 because it provides some underpinning for the sweeping assumption that biomolecules which undergo free radical formation *in vitro* under conditions of pH and redox potential that are within the biological range could be expected to behave similarly *in vivo*, should they be exposed to a comparable reaction environment. Harman and Piette (106) showed that, when high concentrations of various substances were incubated aerobically in human serum in the absence of light, ESR of resulting free radicals could be observed (Fig. 7-8). The materials included epinephrine, norepinephrine, and ascorbic acid. To be sure, their concentrations were many orders of magnitude above the physiological range, and the observations did not prove the existence of free radical forms at normal physiological concentrations; but they add some weight to the generalization that the chemical behavior of natural substances observed *in vitro*, including free radical reactions, should also apply *in vivo*, unless there are specific properties of the biological environment that make the chemical reaction system studied a poor model. Thus Harman and Piette's extensive observations of additional free radicals produced by ultraviolet radiation of serum (106) would *not* appear to model the situation that obtains within the body.

7.3.2 Naphthoquinones and Tocopherols: Vitamins E, K, and Q

Vitamin E quinone, or alphatocopherol quinone, is a highly substituted parabenzoquinone with three methyl substituents and a fourth long side chain that includes the phytyl group (65, 92, 134) (Fig. 7-9*b*). Vitamin K_3, or menadione, is a 2-methyl substituted 1,4-naphthoquinone, and the natural vitamin K_1 is the same except for a phytyl group substituted in position 3 (21, 65, 92) (Fig. 7-9*a*). Vitamin Q quinone, also known as coenzyme Q_{10} or ubiquinone, resembles Vitamin E quinone in being a highly substituted parabenzosemiquinone, although its even longer side chain is partially unsaturated (21, 65).

Considering the relatively high stability of benzosemiquinone and naph-

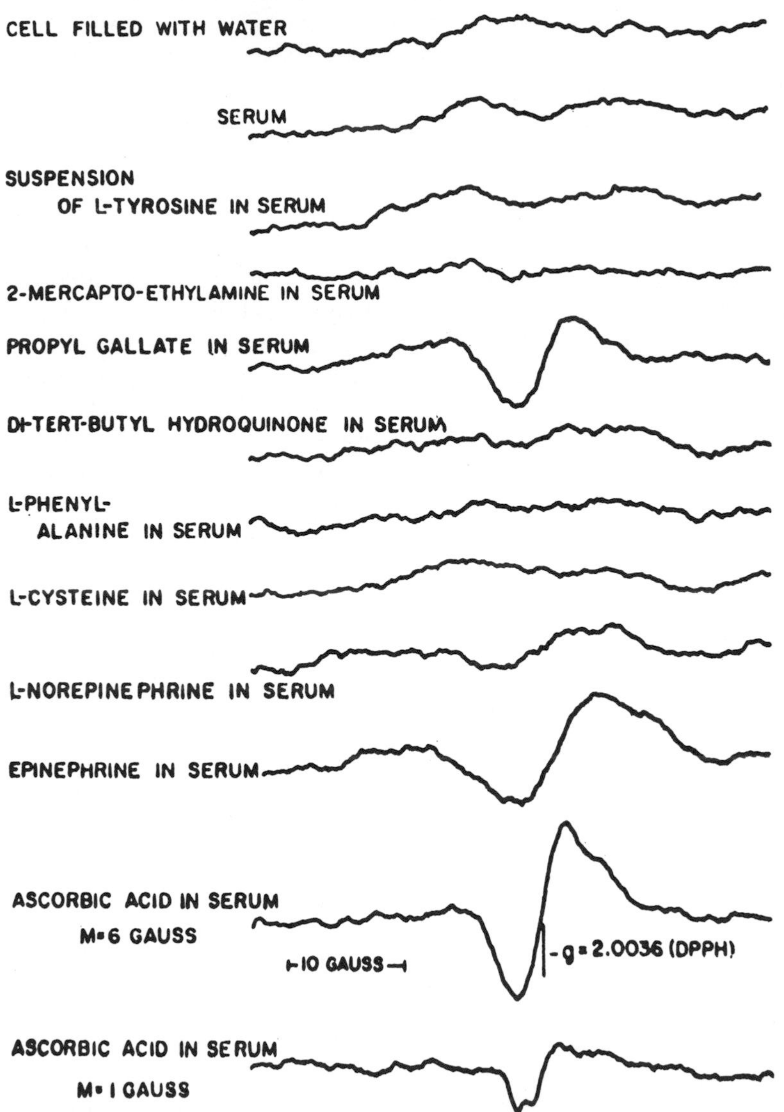

Fig. 7-8 Effect of various substances on the ESR signal of human blood serum equilibrated with air. The compounds were approximately 10 mM in concentration. (From Ref. 106, with permission.)

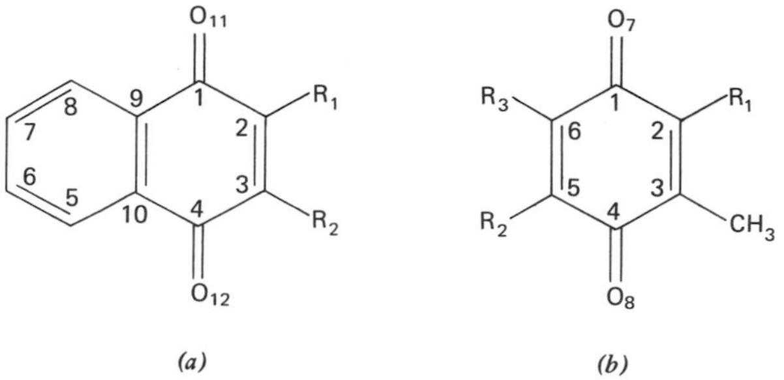

(a) (b)

Fig. 7-9 (*a*) Naphthoquinone and related vitamin quinones: (1) $R_1 = R_2 = \mathrm{H}$, 1,4-naphthosemiquinone; (2) $R_1 = \mathrm{CH_3}$, $R_2 = \mathrm{H}$, menadione (Vit. $\mathrm{K_3}$); (3) $R_1 = \mathrm{CH_3}$, $R_2 = -\mathrm{CH_2CH{=}C(CH_3)} - \mathrm{(CH_2CH_2CH_2CH(CH_3))_3CH_3}$, 2-methyl-3-phytyl-1, 4-naphthosemiquinone (Vit. $\mathrm{K_1}$). (*b*) Duroquinone and related vitamins: (1) $R_1 = R_2 = R_3 = \mathrm{CH_3}$, duroquinone; (2) $R_2 = R_3 = \mathrm{CH_3}$, $R_1 = \mathrm{CH_2CH_2C(OH)(CH_3)(CH_2} = \mathrm{CH_2CH_2CH(CH_3))_3CH_3}$, α-tocopherol quinone (Vit. E quinone); (3) $R_2 = R_3 = \mathrm{OCH_3}$, $R_1 = \mathrm{(CH_2CH{=}C(CH_3)CH_2)_{10}H}$, ubiquinone. (From Ref. 65, with permission.)

thosemiquinone anion radicals in alkali, it is not surprising that Blois and Maling (21) were able to obtain good ESR spectra of the semiquinones of coenzyme $\mathrm{Q_{10}}$ and Vitamin $\mathrm{K_1}$ in alkaline ethanol solutions. A more detailed ESR analysis, including assignment of smaller hyperfine splittings, was subsequently made of the monoanion free radicals of Vitamin $\mathrm{K_3}$ and $\mathrm{K_1}$, as well as of Vitamin E semiquinone, following their electroreduction in aprotic organic solvents (92).

An even more detailed analysis of the semiquinones of Vitamins K, E, and Q was recently reported by Freed and his associates (65) who used the ENDOR method (see Section 1.11.1), which provides vast simplification of complex isotropic hyperfine structure. In the present case additional small hyperfine splittings were resolved by ENDOR that were not observable by ESR (Fig. 7-10) because of the fact that the ENDOR linewidths were approximately one-fifth of the ESR linewidths (65). This detailed analysis (65) provided satisfactory agreement with molecular orbital calculations and confirmed Blois's earlier finding (21) that the introduction of a long side chain in the vitamin semiquinones has little effect on the spin density distribution.

There is some indication that at least two of these cofactors, vitamins E and Q, may function in such a way *in vivo* that the properties of their semiquinone intermediates may be relevant. Although the roles of Vitamin E are not clearly known, some data suggest that it functions to inhibit the autoxidation of unsaturated fatty acids (229); and since the latter process probably involves peroxy radical reactions, a competitive role for Vitamin E semiquinone is an attractive speculation.

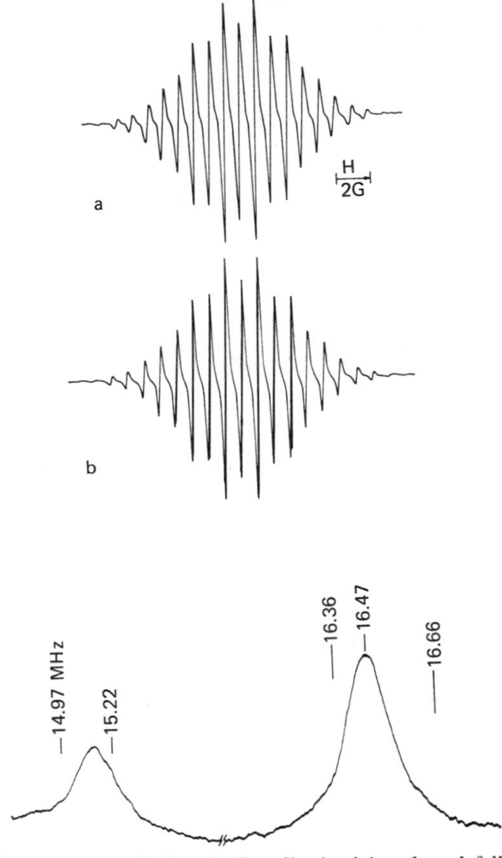

Fig. 7-10 (*a*) ESR spectrum of Vitamin E redissolved in ethanol following reduction by potassium in DME. (*b*) Computer simulation [protonic splitting constants in gauss:1.905(3) and 0.910 (1)]. *Lower:* ENDOR lines (see Sec. 1.12.1) corresponding to the methylene (*left*) and methyl (*right*) proton in Vitamin E. (From Ref. 65, with permission.)

Vitamin Q (ubiquinone) may operate as a component of the main chain of electron transfer enzymes in mitochondria and in chromatophores of photosynthetic bacteria, and for a few years there has been ESR evidence that its semiquinone form exists in the mitochondrial fractions of metabolizing tissues (54). Recent ESR measurements on ubiquinone-depleted and ubiquinone-replenished submitochondrial particles provided much more conclusive evidence that Vitamin Q semiquinone is an intermediate in normal cellular function (9). The presence of rather nonspecific ESR signals correlated with the metabolism of cellular and subcellular constituents was cited earlier in this chapter and was discussed in Chapter 4. Usually these

ESR signals of active metabolism have been attributed to flavosemiquinones associated with flavoenzyme components of mitochondrial electron transfer. In certain submitochondrial particles obtained from beef heart, however, "typical" ESR singlet spectra of metabolizing tissue were obtained, and their intensity seemed to depend importantly on the presence or absence of ubiquinone (9).

These observations of Bäckström, Norling, Ehrenberg, and Ernster (9) provide impressive evidence that vitamin Q is involved in normal electron transfer, where it functions, at least in part, by undergoing cyclic conversion to its semiquinone. Although kinetic studies to prove that this free radical species is on the main path of electron transfer were not provided by this work (9), the presence of ubisemiquinone free radicals at concentrations comparable to those of the well-accepted flavosemiquinone radicals (see Chapter 8) cannot be doubted.

Another ESR investigation of free radicals from substituted naphthoquinones (and from related naphthazerines) was carried out by Piette and his colleagues (188). Some of the compounds studied were naturally occurring pigments of sea urchins, and from the analysis of the ESR spectra of their free radicals their structures were determined. Piette concluded that ESR can be a powerful structural tool in the field of natural products when suitably stable free radicals can be formed by oxidation or reduction (188).

Another study has been reported recently regarding ESR of free chromanoxyl radicals derived from tocopherols and closely related plastoquinones in photosynthetic materials (134). This work by Kohl, Wright, and Weissmann (134) is treated in Chapter 6.

7.3.3 Vitamins C and A

It is well known that a deficiency of ascorbic acid (Vitamin C) gives rise to scurvy, but it is not clear what metabolic role it fills (229). For many years it has been assumed that the metabolic role of ascorbic acid involves its reversible oxidation and reduction, but with the exception of proline (and lysine?) hydroxylase no biological oxidation system is known in which ascorbic acid serves as a specific coenzyme. In any case, a prominent chemical property of this carbohydrate is its ready oxidation to dehydroascorbic acid, a reaction that proceeds through a semiquinone intermediate; and it has already been stressed that the monodehydroascorbate radical can be formed by the action of a number of enzymes (see Section 7.2.2). The prominent doublet ESR splitting of this free radical was noted in the earlier enzyme studies (187, 239, 240, 241, 242), and more recently greater hyperfine structure detail has been reported from both nonenzymic (84, 145) and enzymic (181) reactions (Fig. 7-5).

Despite the ready formation of monodehydroascorbate both enzymically and nonenzymically, its role in the normal function of the vitamin is not established. Nevertheless, high concentrations of Vitamin C in oxygenated blood serum *do* manifest an ESR signal (106) (Fig. 7-8) (see Section 5.4).

Another vitamin from which free radicals have been formed is retinol (Vitamin A). Within the body not only the alcohol but also the acid and aldehyde of Vitamin A, retinoic acid and retinaldehyde, are known, and it is not clear which is the active form of the vitamin. In its participation as the chromophore in visual pigments, however, Vitamin A exists as the 11-*cis* retinaldehyde (99, 229).

Although the chemical oxidation or reduction of Vitamin A to form free radicals has not been reported, exposure of either retinaldehydes or retinol to visible light produces transient free radicals which can be trapped at low temperatures (99). Preliminary indications of similar light-induced free radicals in the visual protein rhodopsin led to the postulation that they might be related to the primary photochemical steps of vision (99). The light-induced ESR signal in Vitamin A alcohol itself is extremely broad and only partially resolved (99), but some more recent work with low-temperature liquid systems has provided ESR evidence that more than one radical may be produced by visible light from both retinol and retinaldehyde (41, 196a).

7.3.4 Semiquinone Phosphates

It is not established that quinol phosphates exist in living systems; however, schemes have been suggested for the trapping of high-energy phosphates by various quinol intermediates in the important intracellular process of oxidative phosphorylation (64), and there is some evidence that links intracellular quinones directly to oxidative phosphorylation (169). Furthermore, the oxidation of quinol phosphates by peroxidase results in P-O bond cleavage, which therefore suggests that when acting as substrates for this enzyme quinol phosphates are *capable* of being oxidized to semiquinone free radical forms. Phosphorylated free radicals of another kind have also been invoked by Wang (225, 226) to propose a molecular mechanism of oxidative phosphorylation based on model reactions.

Despite the fact that the existence of quinol phosphates within living systems is uncertain and that the involvement of semiquinone phosphates in the coupling steps of oxidative phosphorylation is highly speculative, the biological importance of coupled oxidative phosphorylation is sufficient to warrant brief notice in this section of ESR evidence that semiquinone phosphates exist. Bond and Mason (26) noted the quantitative chemical oxidation of 2,3-dimethyl-1,4-naphthoquinol-1-phosphate to produce the corresponding naphthoquinone and pyrophosphate. By quickly freezing the products of the reaction small ESR signals from free radicals were obtained from these materials (26) and highly resolved ESR signals were obtained at room temperature by using a continuous-flow system. In subsequent investigations additional semiquinones from naphthoquinol phosphates and from a parabenzoquinol phosphate were examined by ESR with flow methods (7).

7.3.5 Flavins

Free radicals of flavins and flavoproteins are treated in detail in Chapter 8. The heading is included in this listing only to remind the reader that these radicals are among the most important of those from natural substancces that have been studied by ESR.

7.3.6 Hormones

Although the physiological and pharmacological actions and functions of hormones have been studied extensively, detailed understanding regarding their actions at the molecular level remains uncertain. There are some peptide and polypeptide hormones, but most hormone molecules are small chemical substances, such as catecholamines, indoles, thyronines, and steroids. In addition, there is the newly defined group of prostaglandins (13, 147), which consist of a cyclopentane ring with two hydrocarbon chains, one of which has fatty acid character. Since living processes are regulated more by the transformation of living substances than by their presence and since these classes of molecules can undergo facile oxidation and/or reduction, the possibility has been raised that the physiological effects of at least certain of these hormones in *some* of their actions might involve redox transformations of the hormone molecules. This, in turn, might involve the intervention of free radical intermediates, which could even be the reactive forms of the hormones in some instances (34).

7.3.6.1 Catecholamine Hormones

Because of the ease of oxidation of the catechol moiety at physiological pH and because catechols are orthoquinols, for which free radical semiquinone forms are well known (see Section 7.3.1), it has been proposed that free radicals exist in chemical reactions that are coupled to oxidative electron transfer and that involve catecholamine hormones such as epinephrine, norepinephrine, and dopamine. Thus electrochemical studies of catecholamine oxidation gave evidence, under certain conditions, of intial quasi-reversible reactions (34, 42), which were also seen on cyclic voltammetry (110). The oxidation pathways revealed by these *in vitro* studies were consistent with the presence of semiquinone free radicals of the catecholamine hormones as initial products of the electrode oxidations, but their steady-state concentrations were too low for direct detection (34, 110).

Other indications of the presence of free radical forms of these hormones, as well as of iodothyronine and estrogenic steroid hormones, were given by their effects on enzyme reactions *in vitro*, especially peroxidase reactions (73). Indeed, in his analysis of oxidative pathways leading from epinephrine or norepinephrine to the formation of adrenochromes Harrison (107, 108, 109) proposed a series of one-electron transfer steps which implied the existence of free radicals of the hormones themselves as well as of some of their derived products such as the adrenochromes.

Despite the many indications and suppositions that free radical forms of small hormone molecules existed, direct evidence was lacking for some time. Walaas, Lövstad, and Walaas (221) did report the presence of a small ESR singlet at $g = 2.005$ in frozen samples of an incubation mixture of dopamine with ceruloplasmin, and this was taken as a possible indication that the free radical of dopamine was present as the initial oxidation product. Firm support, however, for the existence of labile free radical forms of small hormone molecules in nature finally was provided by observations of ESR spectra from the oxidation or reduction of the hormones by inorganic reagents, for which high-velocity continuous-flow apparatus was adapted for ESR (34, 35) (see Section 2.18.2.2 and Fig. 7-11). The first studies reported on hormonal semiquinone radicals from the catecholamine hormones epinephrine, norepinephrine and dopamine as well as from the

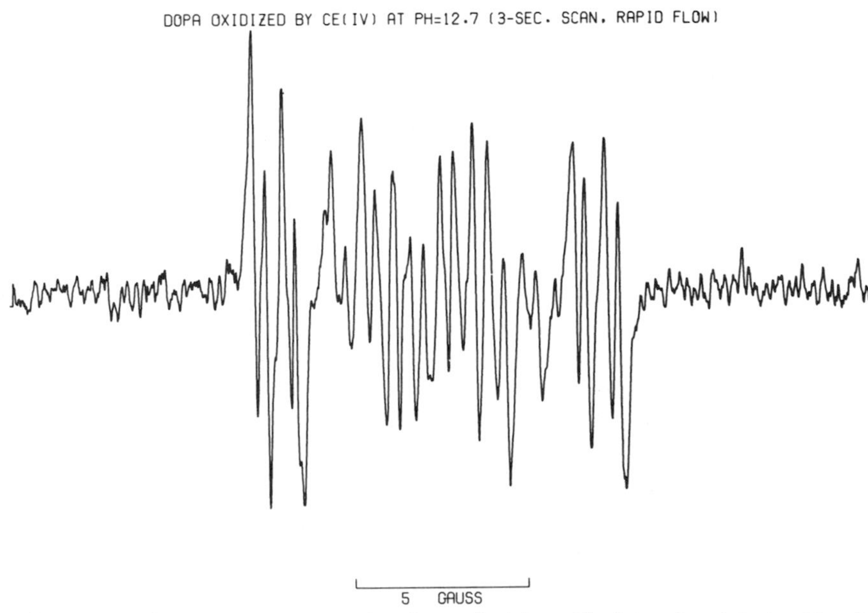

Fig. 7-11 ESR spectrum of the transient free radical from dihydroxyphenylalanine (dopa), oxidized by Ce(IV) at pH 12.7. Spectrum scanned in <3 sec.

precursor amino acid dopa and the indolized oxidation product, adrenochrome (34). These studies showed that the free radical forms of the hormones were, indeed, short-lived, especially near physiological pH's. Nonetheless, improved flow apparatus of the kind discussed in Section 2.18.2.2 did make it possible to confirm the existence of catecholamine hormone semiquinone radicals, even in enzymic reactions with peroxidase (39, 73) (see Section 7.2.2.1 and Fig. 7-12).

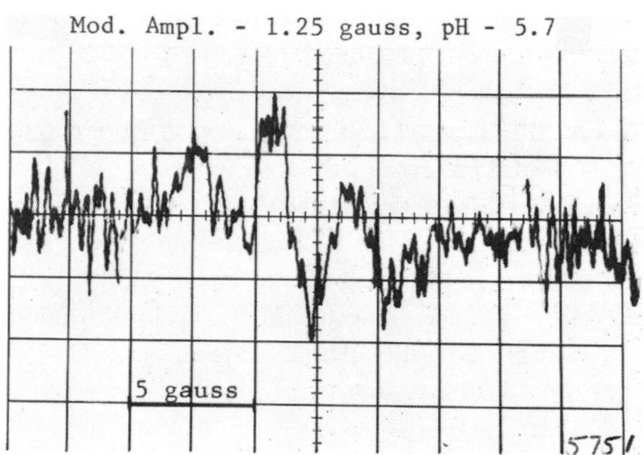

Fig. 7-12 ESR spectrum of transient free radical from norepinephrine (noradrenalin) oxidized enzymically with peroxidase, using 2,4-dichlorophenol stimulation. Spectrum obtained with continuous-flow apparatus for ESR at Q-band (35 GHz) (see Sec. 2.18.2.2). The noisy 1:2:1 triplet signal resembles that obtained from chemical oxidation of epinephrine (adrenalin) at pH 7 (Figure 7 of Ref. 34).

The ESR flow work on free radicals from hormones cited in this and the next section (34, 35) provided spectra that showed complex isotropic hyperfine structure in many instances. The resolution, however, was often incomplete, and structure analysis was not attempted at the time, although partial analyses were subsequently reported (37, 38, 73). With the improved apparatus presently available, including computerized procedures for data resolution and enhancement (see Section 2.11.4), ESR studies should be able to provide more detailed descriptions of the reactive free radical forms of various hormones, and preliminary investigations (41) suggest that this is so.

7.3.6.2 Indole and Thyronine Hormones

In addition to the free radicals from catecholamine hormones and adrenochrome, the studies of chemical oxidations of hormone molecules by ESR with continuous flow techniques were extended to other chemical classes of hormone molecules: thyroid hormones, including thyroxine and related iodothyronines; indole hormones such as 5-hydroxytryptamine (serotonin), found in animals and plants, and indoleacetic and -butyric acids, hormonally active in plants; estrogens, including both steroidal estradiol and non-steroidal diethylstilbesterol and hexesterol (see Section 7.3.6.3); and one polypeptide hormone, insulin (35) (see Section 7.3.6.4). No attempts were made to extend these studies to the prostaglandins, but their extreme instability and the presence of at least one double bond in their hydrocarbon chains (147) make it likely that free radicals of the prostaglandins can also be formed, at least *in vitro*.

In the case of free radicals obtained from iodothyronine it was reported that free radical forms were produced that were stable in alkali (35), in contradistinction to the short-lived radicals produced from other hormones. Subsequently unpublished work (42) revealed that although such stable free radical forms could be produced as a *secondary* product of the rapid oxidation of thyroxine and its derivatives there were other short-lived free radicals that were produced as the first oxidation species.

The confusion had developed because, in the presence of the heavy-atom effect of iodine, ESR hyperfine structure of the type that could be seen from the labile free radicals of unsubstituted thyronines (42) (Fig. 7-13) was smeared out and only a broad singlet resulted. This singlet spectrum was little different in shape or width from that of a longer lived species that persisted for many minutes after the initial oxidations. However, fast-flow work at room temperature and adaptations of the rapid-freezing technique of Bray (see Section 2.18.2.1) showed that with many iodinated thyronines the ESR singlet corresponding to the first free radical product has a g factor of approximately 2.019, whereas the residual singlet has a g factor of 2.006 (42) (Figs. 7-14, 7-15). This was interpreted to mean that the first free

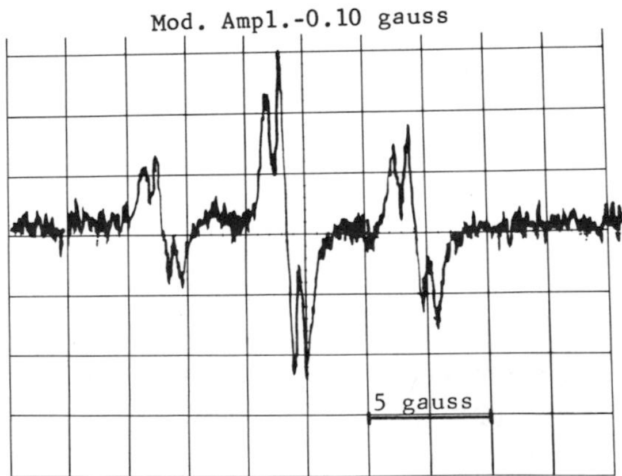

Fig. 7-13 ESR spectrum of transient free radical from oxidation of thyronine in acid, using continuous flow.

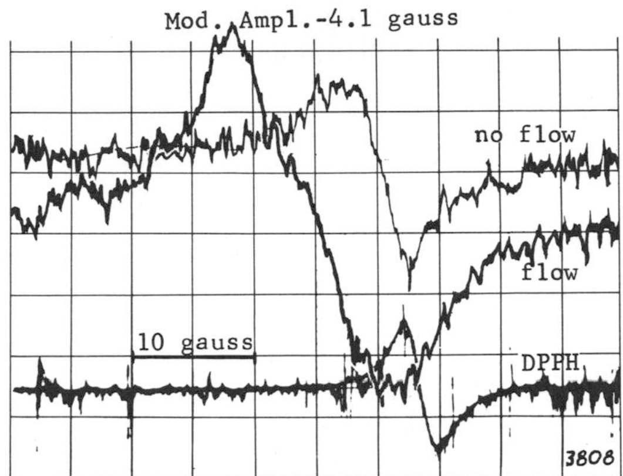

Fig. 7-14 ESR spectra of free radicals from triiodothryronine oxidized by $KMnO_4$ in alkaline solution. Spectra obtained with continuous-flow apparatus in conjunction with a dual cavity (see Sections 2.15 and 3.4) containing a reference DPPH sample in one half. Magnetic field increases left to right, so the singlet spectrum recorded from the transient radical present during rapid flow has a higher g factor ($g = 2.0186$) than the metastable radical persisting after flow has stopped ($g = 2.0059$).

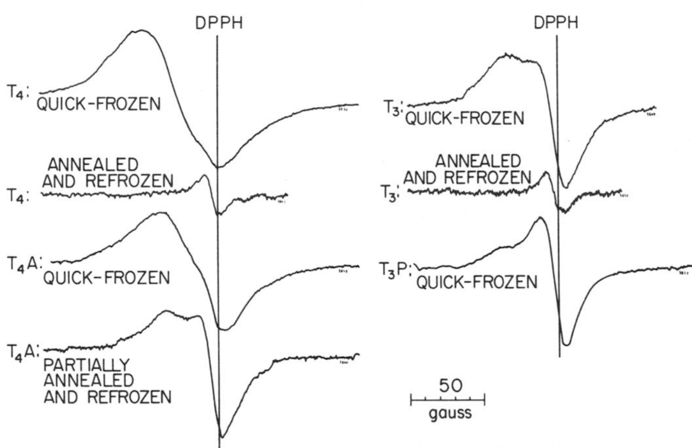

Fig. 7-15 ESR spectra of alkaline solutions of iodothyronines quick-frozen after reaction with chemical oxidants (see Section 2.18.1). Samples were annealed by thawing briefly. Magnetic field increases left to right, so the quick-frozen radical species are seen to have higher g factors than the secondary species obtained by annealing. Symbols: T_4 = thyroxine (tetraiodothyronine), T_3 = triiodothyronine, T_4A = tetraiodothyroacetic acid, T_3P = triiodothyropropionic acid.

radical formed was that of the iodinated thyronine hormone itself, with the high spin-orbit contribution of the iodine giving rise to the high *g* factor. With some of the halogen substituents labilized by the free radical formation (46), subsequent deiodination occurred to produce the more stable secondary radical. In point of fact product analysis gave evidence of iodine release (42), and the conclusion (42) that free radical formation of thyroxine derivatives produces a chain of events giving rise to deiodination is compatible with the observation that normal catabolism of thyroid hormones involves deiodination as an early step.

Another biological role may also exist for free radicals that are closely related to those that can be formed from the thyronines themselves. The biosynthetic mechanism for the formation of thyroxine is not known, but model reactions have been proposed which involve the autoxidation of 4-hydroxy-3,5-diiodophenyl-pyruvic acid or closely related compounds. In any case, in the examination of model reaction systems for thyroxine biosynthesis ESR signals of free radicals have been observed (19, 177, 178).

7.3.6.3 Estrogenic Hormones

Natural estrogens are phenolic steroids whose molecular mechanism of action remains unknown. In certain *in vitro* reactions, however, a reversible phenol-phenoxyl radical cycle has been indicated (see references cited in 35). Although the initial ESR flow work with steroidal estrogens provided insufficient spectral resolution for structural assignments (35); estradiol, estriol and estrone, nevertheless, had identical ESR hyperfine patterns. This was at least consistent with aryloxy radical formation, with unpaired electron delocalization over the phenolic *A*-ring common to the estrogenic steroids.

Furthermore, should free radicals be intermediates in at least some of the initial steps of the estrogenic response, free radicals would also be formed from structurally distinct, *non*steroidal synthetic estrogenic substitutes. This condition was met under *in vitro* conditions, in which the same chemical reactions that produced free radicals from natural estrogens were also observed to yield ESR evidence of transient free radical formation from stilbestrol, diethylstilbestrol, and hexestrol (35).

A series of investigations by Russell and his colleagues on nonhormonal steroids also suggested that extensive information on the *molecular structure* of steroids can be provided by ESR in appropriate cases. They analyzed the ESR spectra of alicyclic semiquinones derived from steroidal ketones in aprotic solvents containing potassium *t*-butoxide, in which base-catalyzed oxidations in the presence of oxygen produced the semidione forms of the steroids (194). In this way ESR studies of the derived semidione radical anions were applied to prove the structure of many organic ketones, including steroidal ketones (195, 205, 206).

7.3.6.4 Peptide Hormones (Insulin)

A number of polypeptide hormones are known, but a free radical form has been reported only from insulin (35, 37, 38). In that case, over a wide range of pH and in more than one solvent, the ESR signals from the labile free radical centers formed resemble overmodulation of spectra from tyrosine free radicals (37, 38, 39) in those instances in which rotation about tyrosine's methylene bridge is severely hindered (38). These results are not entirely surprising because electrochemical measurements indicate that the first oxidation reactions of insulin probably derive from its tyrosyl residues (35, 42).

On the other hand, comparable studies of casein, a tyrosine-rich protein in milk (35), provided more detailed ESR patterns in which some of the smaller hyperfine splitting assigned to tyrosine under conditions of hindered rotation were also observed (35, 38). These observations were explained by proposing that the reactive tyrosyl groups on insulin, a functional hormonal polypeptide with a specific conformation, were more tightly confined by the main protein chain than were the tyrosyl moieties of casein, a randomly organized linear bulk protein in milk.

This interpretation is concordant with the line of reasoning applied to the analysis of spin labels (see Chapter 11), and in the example of casein and insulin it was supported by experiments in which insulin was oxidized at pH's above 11, where there is evidence that the hormone denatures and ultimately undergoes scission (35). Under these conditions the tyrosine radical centers on insulin also gave rise to ESR spectra of high resolution. Therefore there appears to be rapid unfolding of the configuration of native insulin and/or bond breaking within a few milliseconds of insulin's exposure to a sufficiently alkaline medium (38). Under these conditions the ESR also gave evidence of further change in the insulin structure, following the initial formation of tyrosyl radicals, in that the characteristic ESR envelope of the tyrosine radical was replaced within a few milliseconds by a doublet of 10 G (42) (Fig. 7-16), which might have signaled bond rupture or other spin transfer.

7.3.6.5 Relevance of ESR Findings to Mechanisms of Hormonal Action

It is worth emphasizing once again that these demonstrations of short-lived free radical transients from various hormones prove only that the radicals can exist as distinct chemical species in nature but *not* that they occur as

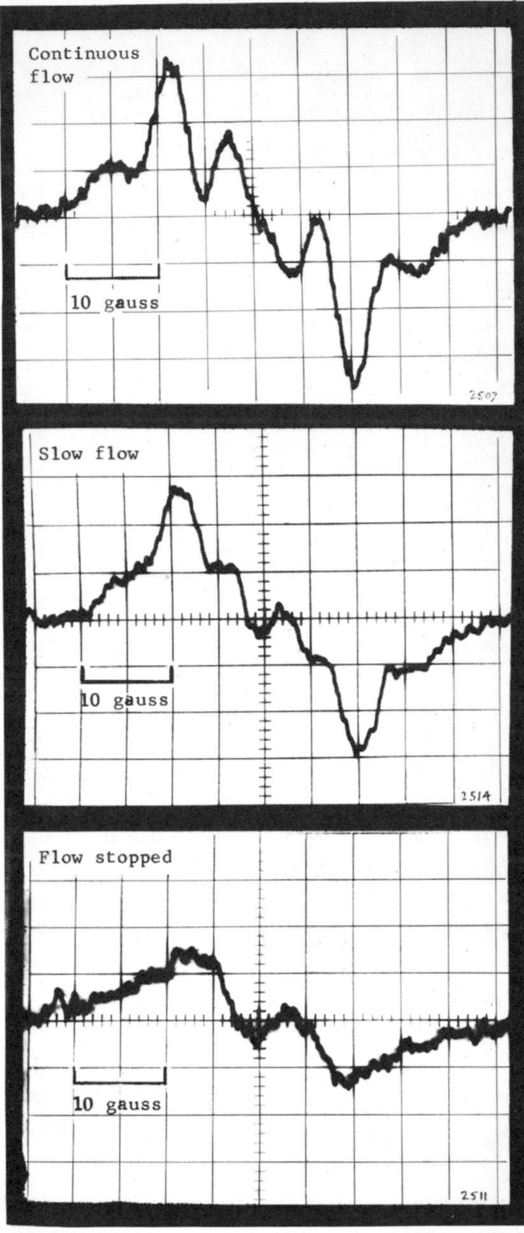

Fig. 7-16 ESR spectra of transient free radicals from insulin oxidized by Ir(IV) in 50 percent acetonitrile at pH 10.5, using continuous flow and a modulation amplitude of 2.1 G. The transient species detected during fast flow was previously identified as a tyrosyl aryloxy radical (Refs. 35 and 38), but immediately on cessation of flow it is replaced by a doublet spectrum, which can also be seen "growing in" with slow flow. The 10-G doublet is compatible with a $-CH\cdot$ fragment, such as would be expected following homolytic side-chain scission (see Chapter 10 for similar signals found in free radicals produced by ionizing irradiation).

normal intermediates in hormone function within the body. This remains an attractive speculation for reasons noted briefly above and referred to in more detail in references 34, 35, and 73; but speculation it still remains.

To be sure, Harman and Piette (106) found ESR signals from high levels of epinephrine and norepinephrine incubated in human serum (Fig. 7-8). This, however, only supports the contention that the free radical forms of these hormones are *compatible* with the biological environment and does not confirm the more meaningful speculation that they are actually *related* to hormonal function.

In any case, it is clear that even if the free radical hypothesis actually turns out to apply to some hormone reactions *in vivo*, high biological target specificity, which is a characteristic of hormones, must reside in other properties of the molecules than those leading to free radical formation. Free radical formation appears to be a nonspecific response even *if* it is intrinsically important. Furthermore, the important work of Sutherland and his colleagues (47, 48) has established a general picture of hormone action in which the hormone is viewed as a "first messenger" that travels from cells of origin to target tissues, causing therein alteration of intracellular levels of another substance, the "second messenger" of hormone action. Although this model does not apply to *all* hormone actions on *all* cell systems, it has been observed in many cases, and the "second messenger" has been identified by Butcher and Sutherland (47, 48) as adenosine 3′,5′-phosphate (cyclic AMP). Alterations of tissue levels of this substance have been seen as the result of exposure to a number of hormones, including catecholamines, prostaglandins, insulin, and other polypeptide hormones (47). What is significant about this model is that it is the "second messenger," cyclic AMP, which does the real work of the hormone in altering cellular function; and since the *same* intermediate is involved in many tissues and cell systems, the *differences* in hormone actions must reside only in their specificity for the target cell's membrane or other surface.

Actually, it is not unattractive to speculate that, since many hormones funnel their effects into the same "second messenger" within cells, a common mechanism of hormone transformation at the cell surface may apply to them all. Conceivably this transformation involves oxidoreduction reactions of the hormones, in which the production of triggering free radicals is the common feature. Whether or not this situation obtains in nature many of the delayed effects of hormone action, both the intermediate changes in intracellular cyclic AMP levels and the longer range changes in RNA and protein synthesis, cannot depend directly on short-lived hormonal free radicals. Therefore, if the latter are biologically relevant at all, it is likely that they function only in initiating reactions that have many delayed biological consequences.

With regard to a possible triggering effect of hormone free radical formation on cell surfaces, a provocative study by Polis and others (189) may be pertinent. In that work they formed stable free radicals from purified plasma proteins, peptides, and hydroxyamino acids by reacting them with the free radical, nitrosyldisulfonate, in alkaline solution. Stable, red-colored free radicals resulted, which were stable for weeks and whose ESR spectra were simply singlets of approximately 10-G peak-to-peak linewidth (189). Illumination by visible light, however, enhanced the free radical concentration, as documented by ESR signal intensity, with a subsequent slow decay in the dark.

The most significant finding in this investigation was that intravenous administration in rabbits of the free radical compounds produced sudden electroencephalographic arousal patterns, accompanied by behavioral changes indicative of brain excitation (189). The observed central nervous system effects were correlated with the free radical content of the administered material, as enhanced by light exposure and measured by ESR (Fig. 7-17), and the likelihood that the observed effects were due to other properties of the administered material was ruled out. In explaining this effect, the authors pointed out that prior interaction of the free radical compounds with serotonin to increase their ESR free radical signal and with norepinephrine to quench it suggested the plausibility that similar reactions at

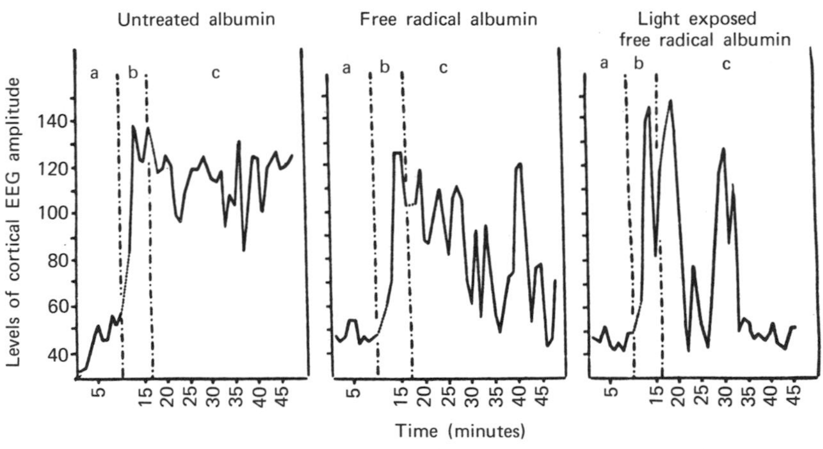

Fig. 7-17 The effects of control serum albumin and free radical serum albumin on the cortical electroencephalogram (EEG) of rabbits. Time course variations of the EEG amplitudes, measured per minute in three experiments, were determined on the same animal with normal rabbit albumin, free radical albumin, and enhanced free radical albumin (light illuminated). The protein was administered intravenously. The recordings in time sections a, b, and c represent the control period, the 5-min period following intravenous pentobarbital, and the period of 30 min following the test compound. (From Ref. 189, with permission.)

neuronal receptor sites were part of the normal action of neurohumoral agents (189). Since the documentation by ESR of free radical forms from norepinephrine (34) and serotonin (35) already has been discussed, the findings of Polis et al. (189) might be interpreted as supporting a role for these free radical forms when norepinephrine or serotonin function as neurotransmitter substances in the central nervous system.

7.3.7 Amino Acids

The effects of ionizing radiation on amino acids and proteins are dealt with in Chapter 10, and mechanical trauma, heat treatment, and other types of nonspecific bond breakage can also give rise to free radicals detectable by ESR (2, 213). Irradiation with energetic ultraviolet light can produce free radicals from amino acids, and partially resolved ESR spectra from polycrystalline samples evidence hydrogen atom abstraction from the alkyl-substituted tertiary carbon atoms or from side-chain hydroxyl, sulfhydryl, or amino groups (86).

Of greater biological interest are radicals produced by oxidoreduction mechanisms in (or close to) the range of biological redox potentials. A number of these radicals were referred to in the preceding section on hormones, but similar transient free radicals have been observed by ESR, with continuous-flow methods, from other amino acids, amino acid derivatives, and dipeptides (38, 39, 42). Comparable studies have been made on many amino acids and on some peptides (36) by using Norman's (66) titanium/hydrogen peroxide radical-generating system. In that work, however, the initiating radical is a hydroxyl radical, or a weakly complexed form of it, and the resulting free radical attacks on amino acids and other molecules are quite different from those believed to occur in the normal biological milieu. In fact, because these reactions are radiomimetic, that is to say, they are models of the oxidative chain of radical reactions involved in ionizing irradiation of oxygenated solutions, the work is discussed in Section 10.2.4.2.

In addition to the short-lived free radicals produced from some amino acids and bioamines as the initial products of one-electron oxidation and studied by continuous flow ESR apparatus, longer lived radicals from some of these substances can be observed on alkaline air oxidation (Fig. 7-18). Wertz and his co-workers who reported on ESR studies of the autoxidation of 3,4-dihydroxyphenylalanine (dopa), considered that these reactions might serve as a model for biological melanin formation (228). Although a number of intermediate free radicals were identified and several sequential reactions were noted under different reaction conditions (228), the ephemeral semiquinone radical formed on initial oxidation and observed in the flow

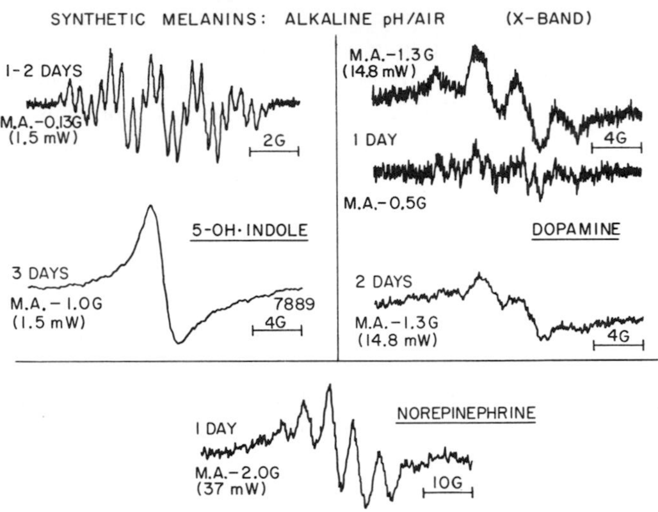

Fig. 7-18 Formation of melaninlike polymers monitored by ESR. Indole or indolizable catecholamines were allowed to autoxidize in alkaline solutions. Initial ESR spectra have partially resolved hyperfine structures which differ among precursors, betokening loosely bound monomer units. In time insoluble melaninlike precipitates form, and the ESR spectra become indistinguishable and characteristic of all melanins, as shown here only for the 5-hydroxyindole melanin.

work (34, 38, 41) was not detected. Nonetheless, the ESR characteristics of biologically formed melanins and of apparently related pigments formed by alkaline air oxidation appear to be nearly identical (23, 100), in consonance with the current picture of melanin chromophores as random or irregular polymers made up of cross-linked indole and catechol-like molecules from many biological precursor sources and containing scattered, trapped free radical forms of some of them (23) (see Section 4.3.5.2).

Although initially the radicals found by ESR along the course of alkaline air oxidation *in vitro* (42, 228) were not taken to be good models of the biological case, in which melanin formation was thought to result from tyrosinase catalysis (23, 228), recent histochemical studies of the conversion of tyrosine and dopa to melanin suggest that mammalian peroxidases may catalyze melanin formation to a far greater extent than tyrosinases (182). This is important in comparing the *in vitro* and *in vivo* studies in that tyrosinase does *not* appear to act on its donor substrates by one-electron abstraction (see Section 7.2.2.4), whereas peroxidases have been cited many times in these discussions as enzymes in which free radical formation is the primary result of the enzyme catalysis (see Section 7.2.2.1). Therefore, if melanogenesis *in vivo* involves peroxidase catalysis predominantly or to a significant degree, the nonenzymic free radical studies *in vitro* (Fig. 7-18) may serve as better models of the intermediate mechanisms of melanin formation than would be the case if most biomelanins are formed from tyrosinase action.

7.3.8 Proteins

In Section 7.2.1.1 it was noted that yeast cytochrome-*c* peroxidase differs from most other heme peroxidases in that the product formed by the interaction of a suitable electron acceptor with the ferric form of the enzyme is not the usual green Compound I (from which no stoichiometric ESR signal has ever been elicited) but rather a red complex which manifests a narrow ESR singlet near $g = 2$ and whose integrated intensity represents approximately one oxidation equivalent (249). Yonetani and Schleyer (249) attributed the signal to a free radical moiety on an aromatic amino acid residue, probably tyrosine, of the protein portion of the enzyme. The similarity of their signal to the ESR signal obtained by Winfield and his associates on oxidation of horse heart metmyoglobin (the ferric form of myoglobin) by hydrogen peroxide (129) was cited (249) as justification for this conclusion. The ESR observed by King and Winfield (129), however, pertained only to radicals examined at the temperature of liquid air and formed after several minutes of incubation at 0 C.

Since the optical absorption of the metmyoglobin/H_2O_2 product was the same as that attributed to ferryl myoglobin, the free radical was interpreted as a complex of Fe(IV) in which neither the porphyrin nor an amino acid directly linked to iron or porphyrin had an odd electron, but in which some component of the globin moiety had lost a hydrogen atom (129). In follow-up studies (130, 131) the ESR signal from the free radical formed by H_2O_2 attack on metmyoglobin was compared with spectra from individual amino acids and peptides irradiated at -100 C by ultraviolet light in the presence of H_2O_2 and then annealed. On the basis of empirical criteria (apparent linewidth, a "saturation factor," ease of formation and stability of the radicals, and an "asymmetry factor"), the ESR singlets detected during the oxidation of metmyoglobin by H_2O_2 were attributed to tyrosine radicals (131). In fact, from this work Winfield concluded that the mechanism of myoglobin autoxidation involves a chain of free radical reactions in amino acids adjacent to the heme site, and he even proposed this as a model for electron transfer within and between hemoprotein molecules (233).

When Nichol and his colleagues (175) subsequently studied the incubation of hydrogen peroxide with hemoglobin, they also found a $g = 2$ ESR signal in samples frozen at -152 C. On the basis of King and Winfield's attribution of the $g = 2$ ESR signal to a tyrosine radical they concluded that their signal was also probably due to a tyrosine residue. Yet it should be noted that in all these studies the oxidations with peroxide of cold solutions of metmyoglobin were compared with the products generated *by ultraviolet light* from frozen matrices containing amino acids or peptides. Ultraviolet light, however, can produce free radicals nonspecifically in amino acids and peptides (86), and no short-lived free radicals formed on the proteins would have been trapped by the techniques used. Thus, in any case, aryloxy radicals of short lifetime formed from tyrosine and from related monohydroxy and dihydroxy phenolic amines and amino acids (34, 35, 37, 38, 42) by one-electron oxidants (see Sections 7.3.6 and 7.3.7) could *not* have been the radicals seen by Winfield and his colleagues.

Hence, in contradistinction to the ESR/flow work's unequivocal identification of free radicals by means of their hyperfine spectral patterns, the Australian group was confined to empirical correlations based on gross descriptive properties of the spectra (131). In the last analysis, then, the nature of the free radicals produced by incubation or complex formation between hydrogen peroxide and various hemoproteins is probably not yet definitively established.

7.3.9 Porphyrins

The oxidation-reduction properties of porphyrins play key roles in their

The Metalloporphyrin Nucleus:
(metalloporphine)

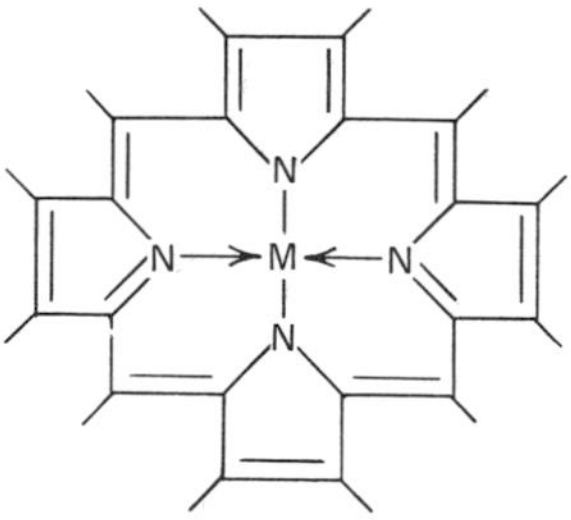

biological functions, as alluded to in Section 7.2.1 and briefly in Section 7.3.8. For some time it has been known from electrochemical studies that porphyrins undergo facile reduction. Felton and Linchitz (79) demonstrated two main reduction waves from a number of porphyrins studied in aprotic solvents, and singlet ESR spectra from the mononegative ion radicals were obtained as well. Calculations of underlying hyperfine splittings led to the conclusions that in both the formation of the mononegative radical and in the subsequent formation of the diamagnetic dianion electrons were added into orbitals belonging mainly to the porphyrins (79). A later study of porphyrin reduction in tetrahydrofuran by Hush and Rowlands (115) provided well-resolved hyperfine structure from sodium reduction of zinc tetrabenzporphyrin and etioporphyrin-I. From these data either the trinegative ion radicals of the porphyrins or chlorin dianions, in which a hydrogen atom was attached to a methine carbon of the porphyrin, could be reconciled as the paramagnetic species giving rise to the spectra observed (115). ESR studies of closely related phthalocyanines and metallophthalocyanines were also carried out following reduction by sodium in nonaqueous solvents (103). Nitrogen hyperfine structure seen with iron and chromium radicals again gave evidence of electron spin delocalization into the pi-orbitals of the porphyrinlike phthalocyanine structure.

Both porphyrin radical anions and cations may be involved in photosynthesis (Chapter 6), and Mauzerall and Feher (164) showed that solutions of uroporphyrins irradiated by visible light in the presence of different reducing agents gave rise to ESR singlets of about 5-G linewidth when observed at room temperature. Although phlorin (dihydroporphyrin) is the known product of the reaction, the authors concluded that their signal represented a porphyrin radical or radical anion (164). Hush and Rowlands (115) concluded, however, that Mauzerall and Feher probably had demonstrated the neutral phlorin radical.

Indeed, the possible role of porphyrin radical anions in photosynthesis was suggested by the analysis of a model system involving porphyrin-sensitized photoreduction of ferridoxin by glutathione (72). Spectrophotometric data and ESR studies of singlet spectra produced by photoreduction and chemical reduction from hematoporphyrin, as well as ESR monitoring of the overall reaction with the free radical DPPH as monitor, gave evidence that photoexcited hematoporphyrin first captured an electron from glutathione to form a porphyrin radical anion, which then transferred its extra electron to ferridoxin, the final electron acceptor in the system (72). In other words, in the test system thought to model the formation of chlorophyll radical anions from the natural electron donors of photosynthesis, the photoexcited hematoporphyrin (representing excited chlorophyll in photosynthesis) was first produced by an electron donor (glutathione in the case of the model system) to form the reduced hematoporphyrin radical anion (corresponding to the chlorophyll radical anion), which then reduced the final electron acceptor (72).

As discussed in Chapter 6, chlorophyll cation radicals are also invoked in current understandings of the photosynthetic process; in fact, the first chemical species produced photochemically in at least System I of photosynthesis appears to be the cation radical of chlorophyll *a* (or bacteriochlorophyll in the case of red photosynthesizing bacteria), and a recent investigation of chlorophyll oxidation *in vitro* has confirmed the presence of a pi-cation radical of chlorophyll *a* whose ESR and other properties correspond to the findings from photosynthetic organisms (40).

With the possible exception of photosynthesis, however, oxidation of porphyrins appears to be of greater biological interest than their reduction. Thus in heme enzymes catalyzing oxidation-reduction reactions in which *not* all electron equivalents are accounted for by changes in metal valence states, the reactive intermediates (whose redox nature remains unknown) are more highly oxidized than are the native or "ground state" proteins. Reference has already been made in this chapter to intermediates of this class, of which the most interesting from the point of view of oxidative biochemistry are Compounds I and II of the peroxidases.

In 1968 Fuhrhop and Mauzerall (93) reported that treatment with iodine or other mild oxidants of methanolic solutions of magnesium octaethylporphyrin (MgOEP) gave rise to a reversible reaction which produced a green product that manifested a single ESR spectrum (linewidth = 6.9 G, g = 2.0026) and, on quantitation, appeared to represent stoichiometric formation of a free radical form. Electrophoresis indicated that the species bore a positive charge, and, based on other properties, particularly comparisons of optical absorptions, the authors concluded that they had formed a cation radical of the phlorin derivative of the MgOEP (93). Shortly thereafter others (80) prepared electrochemically and by bromine oxidation cation radicals and dications of several porphyrins and of ethylchlorophyllide *a* under conditions in which the free radical formation rather clearly indicated that porphyrin cation radicals rather than phlorin radicals had been formed; for example, with zinc tetraphenylporphyrin (ZnTPP) radical cation, ESR hyperfine splittings were readily assigned to four equivalent nitrogen atoms, which would be expected with the symmetrical tetrapyrrole structure of a porphyrin free radical (80).

Oxidation of cobalt OEP showed two distinct one-electron steps, the first corresponding to metal oxidation to form the trivalent oxidation state of cobalt and the second yielding a green species formulated as the Co(III)-$OEP^{2+\cdot}$ radical dication (80). Because of the resemblance of its optical absorption spectrum to those of Compound I of catalase and of peroxidase enzymes, this product is of particular interest and is discussed further below.

Following these reports on the identification and nature of porphyrin cation radicals, there has been a growing interest in the question of their biological significance, and several recent papers on porphyrin radicals have appeared. Thus in the case of synthetic octaethylporphyrins Fuhrhop and Mauzerall (94) found that various metal complexes could be reversibly oxidized in one-electron steps, and ESR singlet spectra were obtained from the oxidized metalloporphyrin radicals. Oxidometric titrations showed that bacteriochlorophyll was more readily oxidized than any of the synthetics studied but that the chlorophyll oxidation potential was well within the range of the octaethylporphyrins (94).

Fajer and his co-workers (78) in a further description of pi-cation radicals and dications of metalloporphyrin showed that ZnTPP and MgOEP underwent reversible one- and two-electron oxidations. With the help of deuterium labeling the observed ESR hyperfine structure was assigned to interaction of the unpaired electron with *meso* protons in the case of $MgOEP^{+\cdot}$ and to interactions with the *ortho* protons of the phenyl groups in the $ZnTPP^{+\cdot}$ radical (78) (Fig. 7-19). From the experimental data and some molecular orbital calculations it was concluded that a porphyrin cation radical may occupy either one of two close-lying ground states, one of which provides for less spin density on *meso* carbon atoms and nitrogen atoms (78). Because these states are nearly degenerate, relatively small differences in the properties of the complexed metal or its other ligands may determine which of these two states is more low-lying in any given metalloporphyrin cation (78).

Complicating reactions of the porphyrin pi-cations and dications were

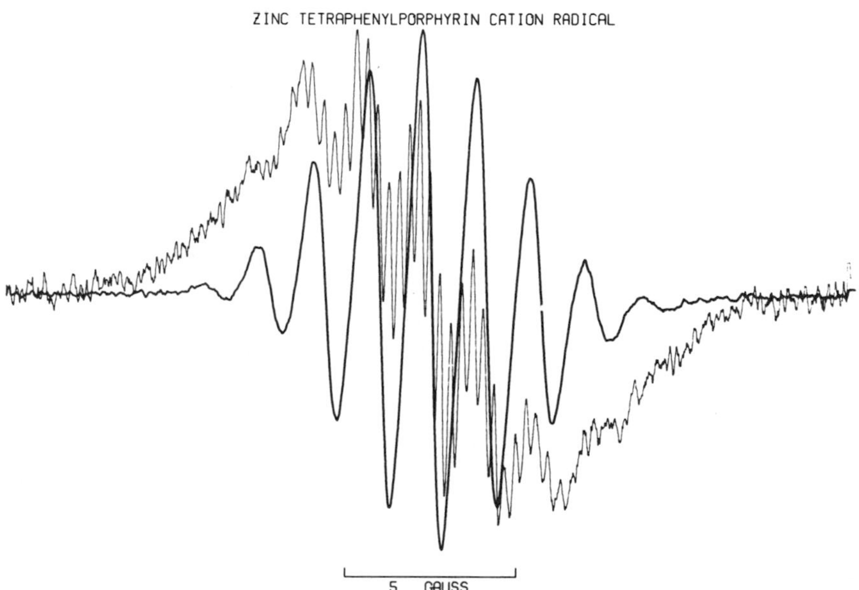

Fig. 7-19 ESR spectra of $ZnTPP^{+\cdot}$ produced by anodic electrolysis in butyronitrile. Light trace: normal compound, with proton splittings of 0.316 G partially obscuring the underlying nine-line spectrum due to 1.58-G splitting from four equivalent nitrogens (78). Heavy trace: compound with fully deuterated phenyl groups and distinct nine-line spectrum (78).

also encountered (78). Thus the ESR and electronic absorption spectra of the radicals gave evidence of interaction with salt, including dimerization of the $MgOEP^{+\cdot}$ radical cation in a manner dependent on both the solvent and the anionic species present and which was enhanced at low temperature (78). Disappearance of the ESR signal with dimerization suggested broadening due to electronic triplet formation or the creation of a new bond. Hence it is conceivable that the absence of ESR from some of the paramagnetic forms of heme enzymes studied at very low temperatures (25, 53, 167, 184) may also reflect dimer formation, and magnetic susceptibility measurements *at those low temperatures* would be valuable. The attractiveness of the dimer hypothesis is enhanced by the recent observation (251) that paramagnetic complexes of manganese protoporphyrins do not evince ESR in frozen solutions unless they are suspended in a matrix that maintains magnetic dilution in the solid state, thereby avoiding the intramolecular dipole broadening of ESR caused by the solvent-solute segregation that otherwise may occur on freezing (251).

A further complicating reaction was seen in the case of the dications in the presence of nucleophiles, such as water or methanol (78). In organic solvents the dications showed reversible and stoichiometric reduction through the stage of cation radical back to the initial porphyrin (78). However, nucleophiles attack the dications at *meso* positions to form hydroxy- or methoxyisoporphyrins, with a saturated bridging carbon atom (68). The optical absorption spectrum of the magenta dication is then replaced by that of the green isoporphyrin monocation, which suggests itself as a possible candidate for the green Compound I forms of peroxidase and catalase, which are also two-electron equivalents more oxidized than the starting enzymes (25, 53, 167, 184) (Table 7-1). However, the strong near-infrared absorption band of the isoporphyrin (68) is absent in Compound I of peroxidase (Gregory Schonbaum, personal communication).

The observation, made earlier in this section, that cobaltous porphyrins could be oxidized in successive one-electron steps to cobaltic porphyrin and thence to cobaltic porphyrin radical dication (80) also leads to speculations concerning the possible nature of Compound I of the hemoprotein redox enzymes. More extensive investigations showed that various metalloporphyrins could undergo two successive, reversible one-electron oxidations to yield (a) pi-cation radicals and dications in the manner of MgOEP and ZnTPP (78) or (b) oxidized metals followed by pi-cations in the fashion of the CoOEP and CoTPP (78, 80). Whether the complexes were initially oxidized by electron abstraction from the central metal atom or underwent ligand oxidation first, the second electron abstraction was *always* from the ligand; and in cases of initial metal oxidation a third electron transfer step to form a trication could be documented (235). In fact, magnetic suscept-

Table 7-1 Horseradish Peroxidase: Formulations of Oxidation Levels and Unpaired Electrons

		Oxidation Equivalents (P = porphyrin; Pr = protein)					Unpaired Electrons (room temperature)						
	Ref.	No. on iron	+	No. on P or Pr	=	total	Iron "d"	No. on iron	+	No. on P or Pr	=	total	Remarks
Ferric peroxidase:													
in acid	25, 184	3	+	0	=	3	5	5	+	0	=	5	High-spin form
in alkali	25, 184	3	+	0	=	3	5	1	+	0	=	1	Low-spin form
Compound II (red):													
free radical form	44	3	+	1	=	4	5	1	+	1	=	2	
Peisach *et al.*	184	2	+	2	=	4	6	0	+	2?	=	2	Ferrous iron
Fe(IV)	69	4	+	0	=	4	4 ↕	2	+	0	=	2	
							←						Unchanged even no. of d electrons consistent with Mössbauer data
Compound I (green):													
Fe(IV) + P·(green)	69	4	+	1	=	5	4	2	+	1	=	3	
Fe(III) + isoporphyrin	(68)	3	+	2	=	5	5	3	+	0	=	3	IR band of isoporphyrin not seen
Peisach *et al.*	184	3	+	2	=	5	5	3	+	0	=	3	

ibility and ESR determined that for the cobalt TPP four oxidation levels could be defined: cobaltous TPP was paramagnetic, revealing a typical cobaltous ion ESR spectrum at liquid nitrogen temperature; cobaltic TPP monocation was diamagnetic; cobaltic TPP dication showed the free radical type ESR signal with evidence of odd electron interaction with the ^{59}Co nucleus noted before (78); and cobaltic TPP trication was diamagnetic (235).

The pi-radical nature of the porphyrin cations formed was supported by the ESR observations of small splittings due to the cobalt nucleus in the case of the radical-like spectra from the cobaltic porphyrin dications (78, 235) and by the corresponding evidence of pyrrole nitrogen hyperfine splitting seen in the copper signals of cupric TPP and cupric TPP dication (78). Therefore both the oxidized metal porphyrin complex and the metalloporphyrin free cation represent hybrid or resonance forms with significant unpaired electron delocalization over both central metal atom and ligand pi-orbitals in each case.

From the values for Compounds I and II of catalase and peroxidase summarized in Table 7-1 it is clear that there is no general concensus regarding the electronic configuration of these reactive forms of the enzymes. In particular, the green Compound I forms, which are two-electron equivalents more oxidized than the native ferric enzymes, do not seem to fit the general pattern of heme compounds: their magnetic susceptibilities are difficult to reconcile with the usual spin states of ferrous or ferric iron in different ligand fields, and their visible absorption bands are unique among known hemoproteins, giving rise to their distinctive green color. Magnetic susceptibility measurements (70, 207) indicate three and two unpaired electrons in Compounds I and II, respectively, although the data for horseradish peroxidase Compound II are less convincing than those for catalase (44).

There is general agreement (44, 234) that the "formal" oxidation state of Compound I is five, that is to say, two oxidation equivalents above the native ferric enzyme, as just noted. The attempts to rationalize these findings have led many scientists to propose that the central iron atom in Compound I and Compound II is in the ferryl state, or quadrivalent, as recently reviewed by Brill (44). On the other hand, Peisach et al. (184) state that the formation of higher oxidation states of iron, such as Fe(IV), has not yet been clearly demonstrated and that such a formal oxidation state is highly improbable.

Certain findings, however, do seem compatible with the concept of quadrivalent iron's being present in the metalloporphyrin of Compounds I and II (44). Thus Mössbauer spectra, which are sensitive to the *S*-state character of the iron, should reflect altered valence states of the iron, insofar as electron density at the metal would be expected to change; and Mössbauer studies of the native and peroxide derivatives of horseradish peroxidase (170) showed major changes when the enzyme was converted from the ferric state to Compound I or II, but there was little, if any, change following the transformation from green Compound I to red Compound II. Hence the Mössbauer spectra were taken as evidence that the additional oxidizing equivalent of Compound I, compared with Compound II, is not found in the metal's valence state but must be localized at a more distant site (158, 170).*

With the quadrivalent iron model there still remains the question of identifying the site of the additional oxidation equivalent of Compound I and of explaining its green color. In this regard Maeda and Higashimura (158) raise the possibility that "one unpaired electron might be carried on porphyrin ring orbitals," and Brill (44), too, considers the possibility of porphyrin free radical components in Compounds I or II but then dismisses them as too unstable to be likely, although not absolutely ruling them out. However, in light of the new findings regarding porphyrin radical cations, especially the metalloporphyrin free radicals associated with transition metals (78, 80, 235), the possibility that porphyrin free radicals are reactive sites in Compounds I or II of heme enzymes deserves reconsideration.

It was noted in the discussion of cobaltic porphyrin dication radicals (78, 80) that their green color and free radical nature commended them for consideration as models of the porphyrin components of Compound I. Additional details are even more provocative: although both are green, the cobaltic OEP radical dibromide possesses an optical absorption spectrum somewhat different from that of the cobaltic OEP diperchlorate (which also resembles the tetrafluoroborate salt) (69). Moreover, the former closely resembles Compound I of catalase (44) in its absorption, whereas the latter resembles Compound I of peroxidase (25, 44) (Fig. 7-20). These relatively small differences in porphyrin radicals are reminiscent of the cited conclusions that certain porphyrin pi-cation radicals can exist in either of two ground states so nearly degenerate that relatively minor features of the molecule or its environment can select one over the other (78). Similar subtle changes are seen with the cobaltic porphyrin radicals: there are the optical absorption differences just mentioned; room temperature ESR is obtained only from the perchlorate or tetrafluoroborate salts, whereas the dibromide

* Indeed, the Mössbauer spectra actually suggest that the iron possesses an integral spin because no zero-field magnetic interaction is seen (158, 170). A hyperfine magnetic splitting, however, *would* be expected in the Mössbauer spectrum of a half-integral species but *not* from integral-spin iron, where electrostatic effects would separate the ground state into levels without magnetic moments in the absence of spin-orbit mixing with magnetic states, which would occur only in the presence of strong external magnetic fields. (G. Lang, personal communication.)

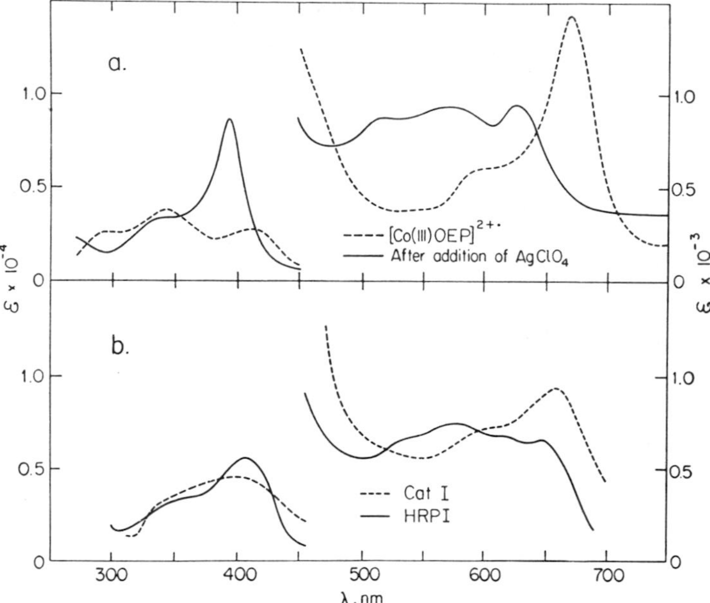

Fig. 7-20 Comparison of optical absorption spectra. *Upper:* $[Co(III)OEP]^{2+\cdot}$, $2Br^-$ and $[Co(III)OEP]^{2+\cdot}$, $2ClO_4^-$ in chloroform. *Lower:* Compounds I from catalase and horseradish peroxidase (HRP). Resemblance is seen between the bromide salt of the cobalt OEP free radical and catalase I and between the perchlorate salt and peroxidase I. (From Ref. 69, with permission.)

exhibits strong spin-lattice coupling in which ESR is detectable only at low temperature (69); and the ESR splitting due to the cobalt nucleus is greater in the TPP than in the OEP radicals (78). Relatively minor dissimilarities of this kind in the ligands bound to heme might also be expected to exist, for example, between Compounds I of catalase and peroxidase.

A major problem that must be reconciled before considering porphyrin radical models seriously concerns the absence of their detection by ESR in Compounds I and II, even at temperatures down to 1.4 K (25, 53, 167). Thus Peisach, Blumberg et al. concluded that lack of an ESR signal at 1.5 K (25) was not inconsistent with a spin of $\frac{3}{2}$ for Compound I, but their explanation that a high-lying $\pm\frac{1}{2}$ spin state might be depopulated at 1.5 K (184) would not seem to apply to the similar failure to detect ESR from Compound I at 77 K and above (53, 167). Alternatively, if interaction with a second spin system were strong enough to produce sufficient anisotropic broadening of the ESR signal, the magnetic susceptibility due to the unpaired electrons of free radicals might then be detected without observable

ESR. Some support for this conclusion is given in a paper by Wolberg and Manassen (235), who found the presence of low-spin ferric iron in a metalloporphyrin-radical complex which had no detectable ESR as a result of signal broadening due to its electronic triplet character.

At the present time low-spin quadrivalent iron with a green porphyrin pi-cation radical electronically coupled to broaden ESR resonance and prevent detection appears to be the most attractive model for Compound I (see Table 7-1). As a spin $\frac{3}{2}$ system its ESR—like that of electronic triplet states—might be anisotropically broadened beyond the limits of detection or, with sufficient zero-field splitting, it might occur at apparent g factors too low for the range of ordinary spectrometers (Chapters 1 and 2). Alternatively, as already cited in this subsection, the lack of ESR detection might indicate dimerization at low temperature. The corresponding Compound II would then retain the Fe(IV) configuration, with the magnetic moment, oxidation equivalent, and green color of the porphyrin radical omitted (see Table 7-1).

Thus, in summary, the porphyrin radical itself would turn out to be the reactive center of Compound I. It could accept an electron from the donor substrate to produce the quadrivalent Compound II described, plus a free radical product from the substrate, as reviewed at some length in Section 7.2.2.1.

7.3.10 Pteridines

Pteridines take part in some aromatic oxygenations and in hydroxymethyl and methyl group transfer (111, 229). Thus hydropteridine is a component of the vitamin folic acid, which is involved in methyl transfers; and pteridines are cofactors in microsomal hydroxylases that hydroxylate phenylalanine (229). In their biocatalysis pteridines shuttle between their dihydro- and tetrahydro-states (111), and from work with model compounds Viscontini et al. (218) were able to show the presence of relatively stable trihydro-

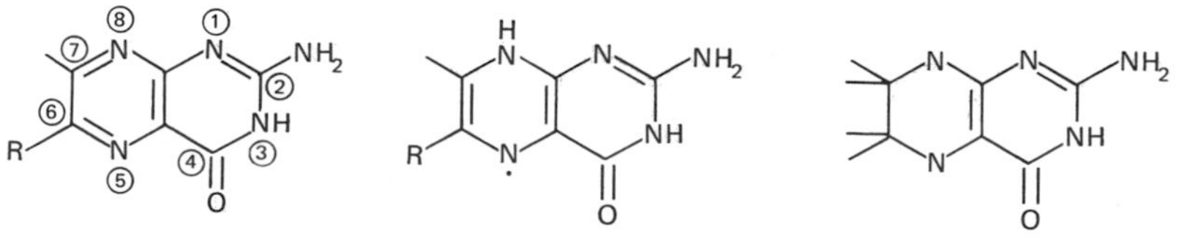

a Pterin (2-amino-4-oxopteridine)

8-Monohydropterin

5, 6, 7, 8-Tetrahydropterin

pterin free radicals. The likelihood that pterin free radical intermediates could play a role in biocatalysis led Ehrenberg and his colleagues (71) to carry out ESR studies on the relatively stable 8-monohydro- and 6,7,8-trihydropterin radical cations produced by oxidation *in vitro* of dihydro- and tetrahydropteridine derivatives (71).

From the ESR hyperfine analysis, monohydropterin radicals were seen to be analogous to flavosemiquinones (Chapter 8), in that odd electron delocalization was seen over the whole pyrazine structure but not over the pyrimidine ring: coupling was seen from N-5, N-8, and C-7 as well as from their substituent atoms (71, 111). Trihydropterin radical cations showed spin localized to nitrogen-5 and its substituent atoms, so that high metal affinity could be expected for this species, a property that might relate to iron-pteridine-dependent microsomal hydroxylation and to methyl transfer from 5-methylfolinic acid in the course of methionine synthesis (71, 111). Although the model studies on pteridine free radicals are suggestive of a biological role, no ESR or other evidence of their existence in cellular preparations or enzymic systems has yet been reported.

7.3.11 Sugars and Other Carbohydrates

Although free radicals have been formed from carbohydrates on exposure to ionizing irradiation (Chapter 10) and transient radical forms might also be expected on chemical oxidation, ESR investigations of the latter intermediates have not been reported except in radiomimetic reactions (see Section 10.2.4.2). However, after heating in strong alkali, radicals were obtained from D-glucose, D-fructose, D-mannose, D-galactose, D-glucuronic acid, D-glucosamine, L-fucose, and D-xylose (146). The results for most of the substances were similar, and the initial ESR patterns suggested that more than one radical was present. Within 20 minutes or so following the heating, each ESR spectrum became dominated by a 1:2:1 triplet of 0.81 G splitting constant (146). The residual triplet signal was stable for many days and may have been due to radicals from 1,3-dihydroxyacetone or from glyceraldehyde, which are known to be formed from carbohydrates in strong alkali (146). In support of this, alkaline solutions of dihydroxyacetone, glyceraldehyde, hydroxymethylglyoxyal, and methylglyoxal gave rise to identical ESR triplet spectra (146).

In another report multiple signals were found in the ESR spectra of sodium hydroxide-cellulose systems (10). Similar signals were obtained, however, from copper in strong alkali, which suggests that the signal-generating species are trapped more by the alkaline matrix than by the pyranoside ring of the cellulose (10). In any case, the paramagnetic species found seems different from that reported by Lagercrantz (146) and is not likely to be of great biological significance, considering the extreme conditions required for its formation.

7.3.12 Iron-Nitric Oxide Complexes with Amino Acids and Peptides

In Section 4.3.6.2 there is a discussion of asymmetric ESR signals with $g = 2.035$ which appear in some tissues during the latent period of chemical carcinogenesis (74, 219, 237). Reference to these signals is also made in Section 7.5.1 and what appear to be related ESR spectra are discussed in Section 7.6.2. Vanin (216) suggests that these signals are related to complexes of iron, nitric oxide, and sulfur moieties on protein, and Woolum, Tiezzi, and Commoner (236) studied the ESR of iron-nitric oxide complexes with amino acids, peptides, and proteins as models for the biological signals.

MacDonald, Phillips, and Mower (157) had already examined the ESR of complexes of iron, nitric oxide, and various anionic ligands. From hyperfine structure analysis of ferrous iron complexes, complemented by the use of materials isotopically enriched in ^{57}Fe or ^{15}N (Fig. 7-21), they proposed a structure for the complexes that involved tetrahedral distribution of four coordinating groups about iron, two being NO groups and two being the other anions in the system (157). In all the complexes studied the single unpaired electron of the free radical-like component appeared to be in the isotropic hyperfine splitting environment of one iron atom and four or five ligand molecules.

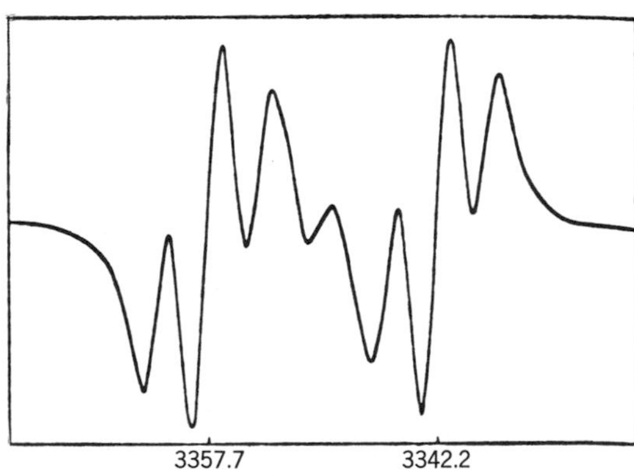

Fig. 7-21 ESR spectrum of ^{57}Fe-^{15}NO-OH^- complex at pH 11. Hyperfine splitting from both ^{57}Fe ($I = \frac{1}{2}$) and ^{15}N ($I = \frac{1}{2}$) is resolved. (From Ref. 157, with permission.)

In their investigations of similar complexes as models of the tissue signals seen in carcinogen-treated animals Woolum, Tiezzi, and Commoner (236) found that when iron and nitric oxide complexes were allowed to react in essentially neutral aqueous solutions with amino acids and peptides for a few minutes an ESR signal was observed initially at $g = 2.035$, with a 1:1:1 triplet spectrum consistent with a single nitrogen splitting. Over a few minutes the ESR spectrum evolved into a multiline one similar to those seen by MacDonald et al. (157), which indicated the formation of a more stable paramagnetic complex involving equal unpaired electron distribution over two nitrogen atoms (236). Evidence for significant odd electron density on the iron atom was provided by the nuclear hyperfine structure seen in the ESR spectra when ^{57}Fe was used.

From observations of this kind Woolum et al. (236) concluded that iron-nitric oxide complexes formed by proteins could give rise to two different types of ESR signal, depending on the amino acid composition of the protein. With a protein poor in —SH groups, the complex was associated with imidazole moieties available in the protein's histidine residues. If the protein was rich in accessible —SH groups, the free radical complex was preferentially formed with them because of the high affinity of iron for sulfhydryl, as pointed out by Vanin (216). In summary, the analyses of the ESR signals from the free radical complexes of iron, nitric oxide, and amino acid ligands —both on and off proteins—appear to provide a good model for an understanding of the biological ESR signals discussed in Sections 4.3.6.2A, 7.5.1, and 7.6.2.

7.3.13 Plant Materials: Lignins and Humic Acids

Although they may not be thought of as substances of physiological interest, at least in terms of dynamic cellular biochemistry, free radicals in some natural substances of botanical origin deserve at least passing mention in this section. For example, lignins, polymers found in wood, represent one-quarter or more of its bulk. The lignin monomer (or monomers) is incompletely known, but phenolic compounds of the guaiacol and syringol classes appear to be involved, and significant amounts of stable organic free radicals are known to exist in lignins (191, 202). Furthermore, a number of model studies on phenoxy radical intermediates related to lignin have been performed in which ESR hyperfine structure analyses have identified many unstable and long-lived phenoxysemiquinone intermediates (49, 82, 83, 202). To some extent this trapping of stable radicals within a complex polymer is similar to the situation that exists in melanin pigments, as noted in passing in Section 7.3.7.

The depolymerization of lignin by wood-rotting fungi may result from a series of similar one-electron steps catalyzed by phenol oxidase (49), and in the case of decay-resistant cedars certain fungicidal phenols may provide their protective effect by virtue of free radicals formed from them (82). ESR studies have also provided indications that the phenoxy radicals formed from the lignins of hardwoods and softwoods are different (83).

Since humic acids are the acid decomposition products of organic matter found in soil, particularly dead plants, and since some fungal degradation of lignins may produce free radical products from phenol oxidase action (49), it is not surprising that ESR shows evidence of semiquinonelike free radicals in soil humic acids (19). Aqueous alkaline extractions of humic acid contain phenoxy free radicals from which ESR hyperfine structure can be obtained (208), but humic acids themselves—like most other solid samples—give rise only to singlet ESR spectra (132), which are sometimes asymmetrical (208).

7.3.14 Charge Transfer Complexes

There has been some speculation that free radicals from certain natural substances exist in, or are formed from, charge transfer complexes (119). When the usual charge transfer complex is formed by the weak association of an electron donor and an electron acceptor, there is the transfer of only a small fraction of an electronic charge from the donor to the acceptor and the complex is not paramagnetic (119). At the other extreme is the rapid transfer of essentially one entire electronic charge on complexation, and this may be considered essentially as a one-electron redox reaction, although the "virtual" donor-acceptor intermediate stage has led some to characterize such reactions as "strong" charge transfers (119). Potentially there is a whole spectrum of intermediate stages of charge transfer, in some of which free radicals of the donor and acceptor components remain tightly enough coupled to represent an electronic triplet state whose ESR spectrum consequently is usually so broad that it is undetectable in the region of $\Delta M_s = 1$ transitions, although half-field $\Delta M_s = 2$ transitions sometimes are detectable. In other cases the donor and acceptor radicals may be weakly complexed but still electronically separate enough to give rise to distinct ESR signals.

Actually, only a few examples of charge transfer complexes have been documented in which free radicals of both the donor and acceptor component have been seen by ESR (117). However, in an example of a "strong charge transfer" complex between the electron donor, serotonin, and the electron acceptor, flavinmononucleotide, ESR spectra that clearly reflected the presence of flavin radicals, plus some indication of an overlapping spectrum taken to be that of the indole free radical (118), were recorded. Although the spectra probably did not originate from the charge transfer complex itself, dissociation of "strong charge transfer" complexes into their component free radicals can easily be obtained (118, 119).

Leterrier, Balny, and Douzou (151) also concluded that in the reaction between *p*-benzoquinone and imidazole they had evidence for the formation of a complex between two radicals whose individual ESR spectra could be observed. However, the major evidence that a true "complex" had formed —even if a weak one—was the presence of a fluorescence emission attributed to it that could not be accounted for by any other components of the system (151).

7.4 FREE RADICALS FROM DRUGS

The "biological interest" of the free radicals whose ESR studies are cited here is a matter of subjective evaluation in many cases. For some of the drugs discussed there is biological evidence that at least *some* pharmacological effects are exerted by the free radical forms themselves or under circumstances in which free radical formation from the drugs is highly likely. On the other hand, no such supporting evidence is available for many other classes of drug whose free radicals have been studied by ESR. In some instances the conditions required for free radical detection are highly unphysiological, but in any case the biological relevance of the ESR studies of such compounds must remain conjectural. Even so, the knowledge that free radicals are readily formed from a number of drugs whose active forms are not otherwise known and that in some cases the free radical forms have been definitely correlated with biological actions suggests that free radical mechanisms of pharmacological action may be more general than is commonly recognized.

7.4.1 Phenothiazines

The mechanism of action of phenothiazine drugs is of great interest because of their broad spectrum of pharmacological effects, and therefore they have been selected for a relatively extensive discussion (see Section 7.1). Some phenothiazines have been known as biological dyes or as antihelminthic agents for many years, but their more spectacular pharmacodynamic effects involve the central nervous system. Phenothiazine "tranquilizers," of which chlorpromazine was the first and the best known, have revolutionized treatment of many psychotic conditions in which hyperactivity and anxious excitement are prominent manifestations. In addition, some phenothiazines have been pharmacologically effective as anti-Parkinsonian agents: for example, ethopropazine.

As early as 1958 ESR singlet spectra were obtained from solid chlorpromazine derivatives extracted from the urine of patients receiving the drug and from an ultraviolet-irradiated product produced from it (88). Cationic and neutral free radicals from the parent compound, phenothiazine, and its nondrug derivatives had been prepared chemically and studied by ESR in many investigations (17, 18, 81, 97, 124, 141, 142, 162, 211), some of which involved detailed hyperfine structure analysis (17, 18, 81, 124, 211) and correlation with molecular orbital calculations and computer-simulated spectra (97).

Similar findings of ESR spectra from free radical forms of the drug derivatives themselves, especially chlorpromazine (27, 29, 62, 81, 142, 185, 186), led to speculations that comparable free radical forms might be produced within the body and that they might be related to some of the pharmacological effects of these drugs. The first speculations of this kind had little experimental support (142), but correlations of the optical absorption spectra of free radicals from different phenothiazine drugs (28), as well as strong similarities in the resolved ESR spectra of different congeners (42, 81, 185), led to the recognition that the redox behavior of these drugs and the relative stabilization of their free radical forms derived from the properties of the phenothiazine nucleus itself rather than from the various side groups which altered the biological distribution and metabolic fate of different derivatives. The extreme delocalization of the unpaired electron of the free radical form through the phenothiazine ring system is well demonstrated by the most detailed hyperfine structure analyses of phenothiazine (97, 124) and the chlorpromazine and promazine drug derivatives (81) (Fig. 7-22).

Thus the ready formation of free radicals with sufficient electron delocalization to be relatively stable was recognized as a property of the entire class of phenothiazine drugs; so, if free radical formation were relevant to pharmacological action, phenothiazine derivatives should show more similarities than differences. In fact, general correlations of this kind were made (30), and the pharmacological effect of a number of phenothiazine drugs on the treatment of Parkinsonism was rationalized in a similar way (62). Studies of chlorpromazine free radical formation by peroxidase enzymic action led to the suggestion that other oxidative enzymes within the body might act similarly (186), and ESR analyses of the enzymic formation and decay of the radical led Piette, Bulow, and Yamazaki (186) to propose that its stability was sufficiently great under biological conditions to permit its free radical form to be active in the central nervous system.

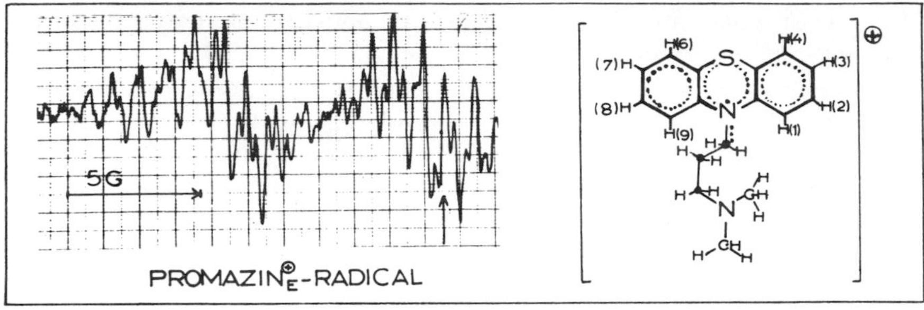

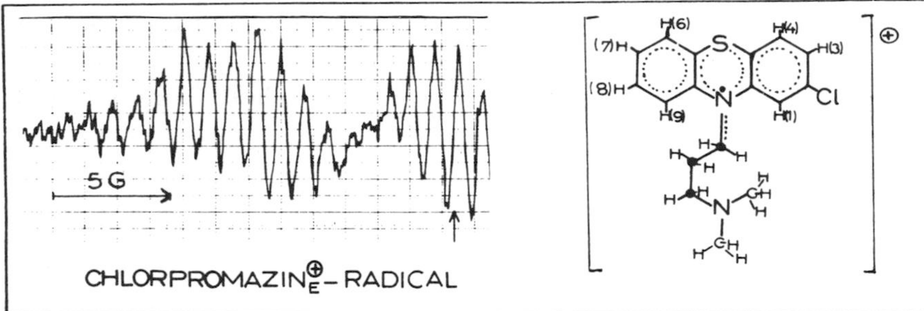

Fig. 7-22 ESR spectra and formulas for the cation radicals of promazine and chlorpromazine. Vertical arrows represent midpoints of the spectra. (From Ref. 81, with permission.)

Although unrelated to the primary pharmacological effect of phenothiazine drugs, hyperpigmentation of the skin has been observed in some individuals who received high doses of these drugs for long periods of time. ESR studies of the formation of chlorpromazine free radical by light led Blois (22) to propose that this form was related to the hyperpigmentation seen in human beings and animals. ESR studies at X band and Q band of the pigments themselves showed them to be distinctly different from melanins (217), whose production is also stimulated in the areas of hyperpigmentation. Another ESR study of chlorpromazine that is not clearly related to its central nervous system effects was cited earlier in Section 7.1 and concerns the demonstration that the chlorpromazine free radical is stabilized *in vitro* by binding to DNA, with which it intercalates (180). The biological relevance of this finding is mooted, however, by the absence of clear indications that these drugs act through nuclear effects.

In fact, the free radicals of phenothiazine studied by ESR probably *are* of biological importance, at least in certain instances; because this is one class of drug for which evidence has been accumulated that implicates the free radical form in some biological actions. Thus the inhibition *in vitro* of the enzyme, uridinediphosphate-glucose dehydrogenase, by chlorpromazine involves the free radical form of the drug, as deduced by a number of observations and as shown explicitly by the potent action of *pre*formed chlorpromazine semiquinone radical (152). Similarly, the free radical is the active inhibitor form of chlorpromazine in its action on microsomal sodium- and potassium-stimulated ATPase from rat brain (4). However, the magnesium-dependent ATPase is less sensitive to free radical inhibition but potassium-dependent paranitrophenyl phosphatase of rat brain is equally sensitive (5). The effect of chlorpromazine radical on ATPase is of particular pharmacological interest because this is a prominent enzymic activity of many biological membranes, and one of the well-documented effects of this drug has been to alter or inhibit the transport of several substances across membranes.

Chlorpromazine sulfoxide is a major metabolite of chlorpromazine in man, and it is likely that a free radical path to chlorpromazine sulfoxide exists *in vivo* (4, 30). Furthermore, it has been demonstrated that the pharmacological effects of chlorpromazine in intact mice depend, at least in part, on the free radical form of the drug. This is especially clear when *pre*formed radical is administered (98).

Finally, Craig's earlier suggestion (63) that the antihelminthic activity of certain phenothiazines seems to be related to the formation of their semiquinone radical forms has been supported by recent electrochemical studies (209). Whether the free radical form of chlorpromazine intervenes in any of its usual pharmacological actions or not, a clinical exploitation of its presence in biological fluids has been suggested by Piette (as cited in Ref. 238). Chlorpromazine in blood serum can be detected by the ESR singlet it manifests while undergoing ultraviolet photolysis within the microwave cavity (106). The signal disappears rapidly in the dark, but its level during irradiation seems to correlate with drug dosage, and thus it may provide a way of assaying serum levels of the drug. Difficulties in calibrating absolute drug levels have not yet been overcome, however, and Piette's suggestion has not been followed up in practice (238).

7.4.2 Phenothiazinelike Antidepressants

As noted above, the phenothiazine drugs represent a class of potent tranquilizers which exerts a marked calming effect without excessive sedation. Some years after their introduction into clinical practice, drugs that seem to have essentially the opposite effects were made available; that is, they act primarily as antidepressants or "psychic energizers." Paradoxically, however, a number of these antidepressant agents belong to chemical classes that strongly resemble the phenothiazines; for example, iminodibenzyls (imipramine and desipramine), thioxanthenes (chlorprothixene), or dibenzocycloheptadienes (amitriptyline). In fact, several pharmacological studies have indicated that all the drugs that possess similar reactive chemical nuclei will share similar mechanisms of biochemical action, but the site of that action will reflect the distribution of the drug at the tissue and cellular level, as determined largely by side-chain properties. Therefore within the class of such drugs there will be a spectrum of pharmacological actions (30), ranging from alerting to tranquilizing effects (32, 148). Furthermore, the simpler the biological test system, the less critical the role of the distribution-determining side chains, so that with simple *in vitro* test systems mainly quantitative differences will remain between one and another derivative. Indeed, a number of biological and biochemical comparisons between phenothiazines and antidepressant drugs of similar structural types have supported these predictions (1, 11, 15, 16, 51, 112, 148, 154, 155, 156).

However, if these classes of antidepressants resemble phenothiazines in mechanism of action and if phenothiazines act, in part, by free radical mechanisms, as proposed in the preceding section, free radicals should be obtainable under similar conditions from the antidepressants. In fact, electrochemical and ESR studies have confirmed a free radical product from imipramine, a member of the iminodibenzyl class of antidepressant (32). The requirements for free radical formation resemble those for phenothiazines, but the imipramine free-radical formation was complicated, and the failure to elicit resolved hyperfine structure did not allow a detailed comparison of free radical types to be made (32).

Recently, however, anion radicals from reduction by potassium in 1,2-dimethoxyethane were reported for a thioxanthene derivative and a thioanalog of a dibenzocycloheptadiene (210). Although the proposed pharmacological mechanism of action involving free radicals described in this and the preceding section invokes the corresponding cation radicals, the well-resolved hyperfine structure from the anion radicals was still able to support the thesis that free radicals of these classes are resonance-stabilized by delocalization of the unpaired electron over all parts of the coupled ring systems (210).

7.4.3 Sedatives

Following the conjectures of the last two sections, it might be supposed that other drugs acting on the central nervous system could be shown to form free radicals under conditions compatible with an intracellular environment. Actually, however, there is little evidence of this kind, although the findings of Polis (189), cited in Section 7.3.6, do support the hypothesis that free radicals produced on the appropriate membranes of neurons within the brain can drastically alter central nervous system activity.

There is at least one case, however, of a free radical being formed from a sedative, namely, chloral hydrate. The radical was short-lived after being formed by a strong oxidant in aqueous solution, but a seven-line ESR hyperfine structure, compatible with nuclear hyperfine interaction with two chlorine atoms, was obtained with the use of an ESR flow system (67).

7.4.4 Opium Alkaloids

Clearly, opiates have an effect on the central nervous system, but their overall biochemistry is complex and must involve various adaptive enzyme changes as well. Nonetheless, it is worth noting in passing that free radicals have been formed from morphine, apomorphine, and codeine, even though the reaction conditions were far from physiological (198). In particular, the Marquis reagent, used as a test for opium alkaloids, develops deep colors with morphine derivatives. ESR examination of these colored products revealed different free radical spectra with different alkaloids. The hyperfine resolution was incomplete and elucidation of free radical structures was not possible, but the variation of ESR patterns with different morphine derivatives suggested that the site of radical formation was in the aromatic group of the alkaloids (198).

Subsequently direct oxidation of several morphine alkaloids, including heroin, with antimony pentachloride in chloroform solution produced stable free radicals with distinctive ESR signatures (150). Once again, however, the hyperfine resolution was incomplete, and structural analyses were not made (150).

7.4.5 Salicylates

Salicylates, of course, are well known as analgesics, aspirin (sodium acetylsalicylate) being the best known form. Their mechanism of pharmacological action remains unknown, although there is some evidence that they can act by uncoupling or suppressing oxidative phosphorylation as well as biochemical sulfation. As will be noted in Section 7.5.5, some uncouplers of oxidative phosphorylation may function through their free radical forms, which shunt certain steps in the main electron transfer path of oxidative mitochondrial enzymes. Nonetheless, there are no data that actually support a biological role for free radical forms of salicylates.

Since ESR studies with flow apparatus have given evidence of transient free radicals on the oxidation of many monohydric phenols (203), the ready formation of salicylate free radicals might be expected. Indeed, a well-resolved ESR spectrum has been recorded from the aryloxy radical produced by the oxidation of salicylate (orthohydroxybenzoic acid) in acid (33, 203). The corresponding labile free-radical anion has also been produced in alkali from salicylate (33) (Fig. 7-23) as well as from salicylaldehyde (33). Although these observations of chemical oxidations do not prove biological relevance, electrochemical studies suggest that salicylate oxidizes readily within the range of biological potentials (33).

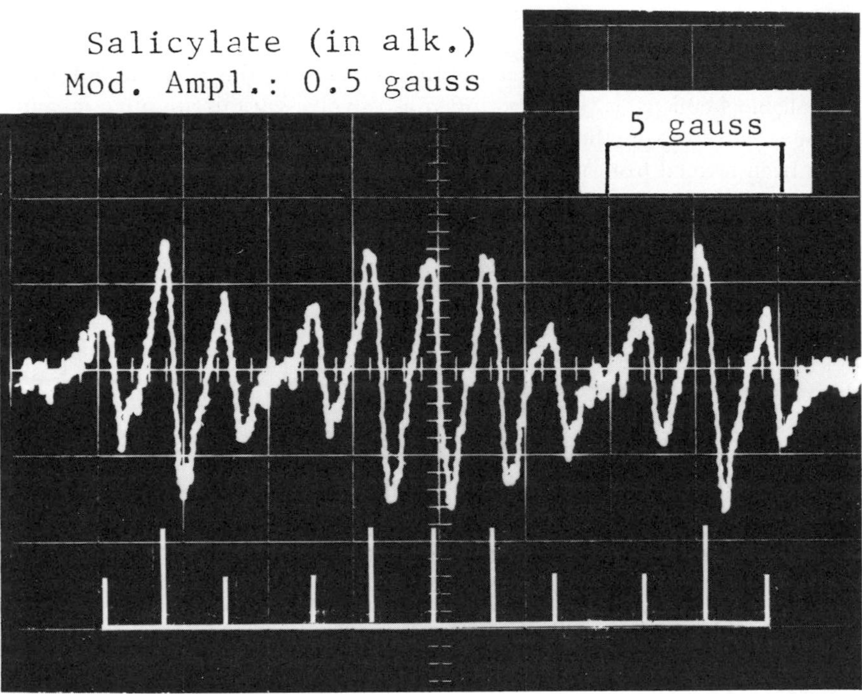

Fig. 7-23 ESR spectrum of transient free radical from sodium salicylate oxidized by $KMnO_4$ in alkaline solution, using continuous flow. The stick spectrum represents proton splittings of 10.2, 6.5, 1.9, and 1.9 G. (From Ref. 33, with permission.)

7.4.6 Tetracycline Antibiotics

The molecular mechanisms of antibiotic action are not known, but indications exist that tetracyclines can act antibiotically by virtue of inhibiting electron transport in sensitive organisms (197) (also see Section 7.5.4). From some of the preceding sections of this chapter it is clear that free radical forms of tetracyclines *could* be functional in this regard.

Nonetheless, with little real implication of free radical mechanisms in tetracycline action, it is not clear what the finding of ESR singlets in crystalline preparations of various tetracyclines (138) may mean. Furthermore, the signal intensity was increased by inactivating the tetracyclines with boiling at pH 10 (138), thus showing *no* correlation between ESR and antibiotic activity. Moreover, the ESR signals obtained appear to be associated with tetracycline breakdown products rather than with the primary antibiotic molecules, and no ESR is seen, in any case, except at alkalinity far above the biological range (144). Thus, although the polyhydroxylated nature of the tetracycline nucleus suggests that there are molecular sites for ready oxidation (possibly to semiquinone radical forms), there are no good data presently available that associate tetracycline free radicals with antibiotic action.

7.5 FREE RADICALS FROM OTHER PHARMACOLOGICALLY ACTIVE AGENTS

As in the preceding section on drugs, a miscellany of compounds is cataloged in this section, some of more biological interest than others. Once again, as well, the weight of the supporting evidence concerning the relevance to biological function of free radicals seen by ESR is highly variable within the list.

7.5.1 Polycyclic Carcinogens

Physical carcinogenic agents, such as ionizing radiations or ultraviolet light, are known to induce free radical formation in many kinds of target molecules. Hence it has been suspected for some time that carcinogenesis by chemical agents might result from their intracellular metabolic conversion into free radicals sufficiently stable to react with cellular target molecules, presumably DNA. Indeed, nearly 30 years ago Kensler, Dexter, and Rhoads (128) used electrochemical methods to determine the stability of free radicals from aminoazobenzene carcinogens, such as butter yellow. They found a correlation between free radical stability and toxicity in an enzyme assay which, in turn, was correlated with carcinogenesis in rat livers, and they concluded that the proximate carcinogens from these azo compounds were probably their free radical forms (128).

The physical chemistry of the carcinogenic hydrocarbons is entirely compatible with the suggestion that relatively stable free radicals may be formed. Electrochemical oxidations of a large number of aromatic hydrocarbons show that all of them initially undergo a one-electron abstraction step to form cation free radicals, some of which persist with sufficient stability to allow good ESR spectra to be obtained and others of which manifest rapid follow-up chemical reactions after the initial electron transfer (159). Actually, most aromatic hydrocarbons readily undergo either one-equivalent oxidation or reduction to form radical cations or radical anions, respectively, and the ESR spectra of many of these radicals have been completely interpreted (160, 215). Although the investigations that will be noted in this subsection point to oxidation reactions leading to cation radicals as being more common biologically, the first attempt to observe ESR spectra from carcinogenic hydrocarbons presupposed that their toxicity stemmed from their ability to form negative hydrocarbon free radicals with mild reducing agents, and partially resolved ESR spectra were reported from radical anions of some carcinogenic and noncarcinogenic hydrocarbons reduced by sodium in organic solvents (153).

A number of biological observations have also led to an interest in possible free radical intermediates in carcinogenesis. In Section 4.3.6.2 the observation of abnormal ESR signals from tissue during the course of chemical carcinogenesis (219, 237) or during the growth of certain animal cancers (43, 74) was noted. In Section 7.3.12 ESR studies were cited in which iron-nitric oxide complexes with amino acids and peptides were found to produce free radical signals that corresponded well to the biological ones (236). In Section 7.6.2 further reference is made to the tissue ESR signals that are associated with various nitrogen oxides, but at this juncture it is important to note that the feeding of nitrite along with carcinogen not only induces the early appearance of the abnormal nitric oxide-iron protein ESR signal in the livers of rats but it also significantly reduces the frequency of the liver tumors that result (237). This suggests that the paramagnetic complex responsible for the abnormal tissue signal may function in a process that inactivates the carcinogen, as opposed to one that itself causes the malignant changes (237). This conclusion can be reconciled with the hypothesis that the proximate forms of the carcinogens are free radicals by postulating that the paramagnetic centers responsible for the tissue signals are able to react with the toxic free radicals from carcinogens to neutralize some of them before they attack the biological target molecules.

A number of biological observations lend credence to the hypothesis that some carcinogens operate through free radical intermediates. Within this class 3,4-benzpyrene (benz[a]pyrene) is well known because it appears to be the dominant carcinogen in cigarette smoke (see Section 7.6.1), and several findings concerning the interactions of benzpyrene with DNA are pertinent in the present context; for example, the chemical linkage of benzpyrene and other hydrocarbons to DNA compounds *in vitro* (but in aqueous solutions at neutral pH and room temperature) is induced by incubation with dilute hydrogen peroxide, and free radical reactions under these mild conditions are likely (168). Other free radical-generating, mild oxidation systems (iodination or Fenton's reagent) can also form covalent linkages between carcinogenic 3,4-benzpyrene and DNA in neutral aqueous solution. Denatured DNA is even more reactive, but noncarcinogenic 1,2-benzpyrene hardly reacts with DNA under the same conditions (149, 214).

These findings suggest that relatively inert polycyclic hydrocarbons are transformed into reactive free radicals, probably cationic, under mild oxidizing conditions and that the free radicals are the proximate—or immediately reactive—intermediates that alter DNA (149, 214).* The correlation of 1,2-benzpyrene's noncarcinogenicity with its failure to react under the experimental conditions indicates that the properties of its free radical form may be responsible for its different behavior: either its radical may not form under mild conditions or, once formed, it may not react with DNA (149).

The fact that benzpyrene appears to be covalently bound to DNA following a free radical-mediated reaction and that this binding is associated with carcinogenicity is consistent with observations on other classes of carcinogens. For example, fluorescent studies show that metabolites of the hepatic carcinogen, 2-fluoranilacetamide, remain bound to DNA for weeks to months following dietary withdrawal of the agent (76). The DNA-bound metabolites are seen in cancerous tissue only and not in surrounding noncancerous tissue (76), thus suggesting that some carcinogens may, indeed, require a tight binding with DNA to be effective.

The long persistence of at least certain carcinogenic metabolites in the chromatin may relate to yet another observation about the biology of cancers. There has been much interest in recent years in the role of latent oncogenic viruses in neoplasia. It is thought that such lysogenic viruses become incorporated into the host's genome, where they remain latent until derepressed by some metabolic or environmental stimulus (116). Recently it was shown that the induction of lymphomas in mice by some chemical carcinogens was accompanied by the development of a leukemia viral antigen, suggesting

* There is some evidence that within the cell benzpyrene may first be transformed into a derivative, 3-hydroxybenzpyrene (95). At least with regard to cytotoxicity in cultured mouse, hamster, and human cells, a microsomal arylhydrocarbon hydroxylase inducible by hydrocarbons appears to be the enzyme system responsible for cell susceptibility to benzpyrene cytotoxicity; and it is the 3-hydroxy derivative of benzpyrene that is formed by the hydroxylase and acts as the immediate cellular toxin (95). However, even if this same conversion to a hydroxybenzpyrene is involved in cellular carcinogenicity, the kinds of free radical reaction just discussed with regard to 3,4-benzpyrene itself would still be expected to apply.

that unmasking of the latent virus was the immediate cause of the lymphomas (116). Since antibody determinations indicated the activation of the leukemia virus for some time before the development of overt lymphoma (116), a *prolonged* activation process consistent with the persistence of the carcinogen in the DNA was suggested. In any case, these observations may serve to link free radical theories of chemical carcinogenesis with concepts of viral etiology of certain tumors; that is, free radical reactions attach some carcinogens to DNA, whence they derepress oncogenic virus genes.

Carcinogens of the nitroquinoline class also may act through their free radicals. Thus, from a correlation of several reports on aminoquinoline carcinogenesis,* the free radical form of 4-hydroxylaminoquinoline-1-oxide appears to be the common proximate carcinogen derived from a number of related nitroquinoline compounds, and it (or a product of its reaction) remains bound to DNA (75) in the same fashion as other carcinogens (76). The free radical of HAQO implied by these mechanisms has been examined by ESR spectroscopy (Fig. 7-24). Incubation of HAQO in aerobic solutions of various organic solvents or aqueous alkali gives rise to a stable cation radical (127). The ESR hyperfine structure of deuterium- and ^{15}N-labeled derivatives has been correlated with molecular orbital calculations to give a complete analysis of the free radical structure, which is seen to be that of the parent compound from which a hydrogen atom on the nitrogen of the -NHOH group has been abstracted (127).

Free radical reactions appear to be involved in still another class of carcinogens. The formation of N-arylhydroxamic acids following N-hydroxylation has been shown to be a key step in the metabolic activation of carcin-

* 4-nitroquinoline-1-oxide (NQO) is a potent carcinogen that is converted *in vivo* (and *in vitro*) to 4-aminoquinoline-1-oxide (AQO) via the intermediate 4-hydroxylamino quinoline-1-oxide (HAQO) (127). AQO is not a carcinogen itself, but HAQO is a more powerful carcinogen than NQO, and a redox pathway between NQO and HAQO is thought to be intimately connected with carcinogenicity (127). A number of findings indicate that the reactive intermediate along this pathway is the free radical of HAQO; for example, the carcinogenicity of quinoline derivatives has been correlated with their reactivity toward sulfhydryl compounds, and glutathione and cysteine are oxidized *in vitro* at neutral pH by HAQO but not by AQO, thus implicating free radicals of the former (114). Furthermore, among five derivatives of NQO, only HAQO gave rise to marked inactivation of bacteriophage T4, and it was a metastable oxidation product of the HAQO—presumably the free radical—that was active (120). Other observations show that *in vitro* incubation of DNA with HAQO gives rise to single-strand scission, whereas NQO and AQO are inactive (204). Furthermore, a reductive pathway to produce HAQO derivatives from NQO seems to be necessary for carcinogenesis to occur with the latter, and fluorescent studies of the DNA suggest that only the carcinogenic derivatives remain bound to it (163). In this regard it is the fluorescent derivatives of HAQO that are found bound to DNA *in vivo*, and, in conformity with an oxidative free radical mechanism, diacetyl derivatives of HAQO bind to DNA and RNA *non*enzymically in aerobic incubations (75).

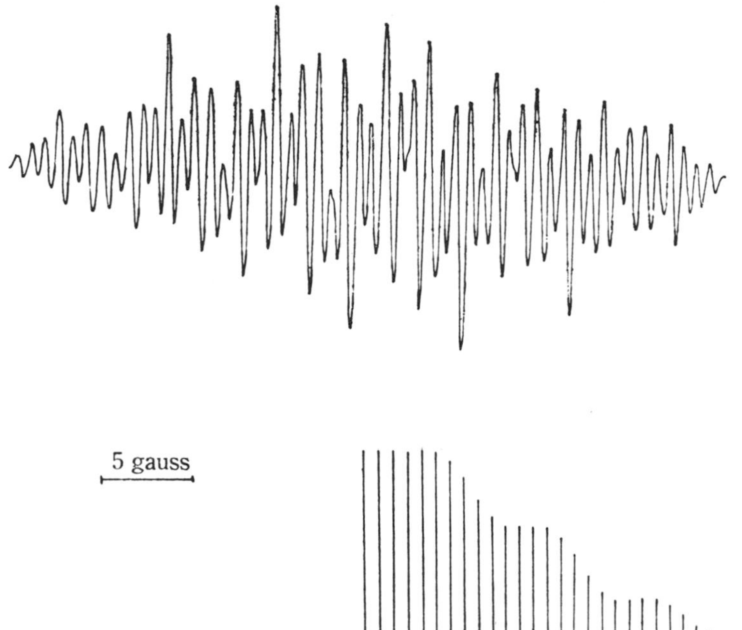

Fig. 7-24 ESR spectrum of the free radical produced from 4-hydroxyaminoquinoline-1-oxide in dioxane. The reconstruction is based on a nitrogen splitting of 5.9 G and proton splittings of 5.9, 3.0, 1.5, 1.5, and 0.74 G. (From Ref. 127, with permission.)

ogenic amides (89), whose oxidation in turn produced aryl nitroso-compounds plus an unknown acylating agent that reacts with other constituents, including, probably, DNA. ESR studies of the oxidation of N-arylhydroxamic acid *in vitro* give evidence of a pathway involving both ionic and free radical species, the latter being defined by their ESR hyperfine analyses as acyl/aryl nitroxides which may serve as the reactive acylating species capable of attacking nucleophilic sites in adenine and elsewhere *in vivo* (89).

In summary, then, although there are many classes of carcinogens and many potential chemical mechanisms for their interaction with target molecules (presumably DNA), there is a substantial body of evidence to implicate free radical forms as the proximate carcinogens, at least for several classes of cancer-producing chemicals. The inhibitory effects of some anti-oxidants on carcinogenesis (see Section 7.5.7) and on tumors themselves (see Section 7.5.3) also support this hypothesis. Moreover, there is ample ESR documentation of free radical formation *in vitro* from known carcinogens and related hydrocarbons.

7.5.2 Acridine Dyes

Acridine dyes, such as acridine orange, are known to have mutagenic and growth-inhibiting effects on organisms. These biological effects are enhanced on illumination, and since illumination of frozen complexes of DNA and acridine also produces paramagnetic species that can be observed by ESR (101) the involvement of intermediate free radicals in the reaction of acridine with DNA is implied. Quantitation of the ESR spectra and correlation with the reaction stoichiometry and with the effect of substituting polydeoxyadenine-thymidine (poly dAdT) for DNA led to the conclusion that light gives rise to free radicals which seem to originate at particular binding sites in DNA, most likely AT-rich regions (101). Further reactions of the free radicals formed by light could lead to changes in the structure of certain bases, especially thymine, to change the base-pairing properties and give rise to some of the mutations known to be induced by acridines in the presence of light (101).

Although the ESR spectra of the frozen complexes of DNA and acridine did not give rise to hyperfine structure from acridine radicals, the mononegative radical ion of acridine has been produced by electrolysis in pyridine (113). In this case a detailed hyperfine structure was obtained, which led to a complete assignment of splitting constants for the entire ring system (113).

7.5.3 Tumor Inhibitors

To complement the hypotheses of free radical mechanisms involved in cancer formation a number of Russian investigators have related free radicals to *anti*tumor activity. From the conceptual point of view this is not unreasonable, because one might argue that competition for carcinogenic free radicals can be provided most effectively by other free radicals that act as scavengers or quenchers. In fact, this was the line of reasoning invoked in Section 7.5.1 when we attempted to reconcile with the proposed free radical mechanism of carcinogenesis the observation of Woolum and Commoner (237) that an increase in the intensity of abnormal free radical signals in tissue was actually associated with a *de*crease in tumor incidence.

Soviet workers have reported that quinone and hydroquinonelike inhibitors of free radical processes (i.e., antioxidants) are effective in the treatment of malignant growths; tumor cells lose their transplantability under treatment with these preparations *in vitro* (126). Since the formation of free radicals from quininoid molecules is well known (see Section 7.3.1), it is not surprising that alkaline air incubation of so-called tumor inhibitors of the quinoid kind gave rise to mixtures of semiquinone anion radicals with characteristic ESR signatures (126). The ESR signals increased when the antioxidants were incubated with cells or with acidic plasma containing protein, from which it was concluded that semiquinone radicals were adsorbed by proteins in the form of free ion radicals, thus stabilizing them and increasing the recorded ESR spectral intensities (126).

In later studies stable free radicals derived from 4-substituted tetramethylpiperidine oxides were synthesized and administered to mice suffering from transplanted leukemias (136). Antileukemic activity correlated with dosage levels was claimed, and the data were taken to support the concept of antitumor activity due to certain free radicals (136). Another pertinent observation was a correlation between antitumor activity and the ability of dichlorodiethylarylamine compounds to give rise to free-radical type ESR signals on oxidation in weakly acid solutions. This led to the loosely supported speculation that the antitumor activity of these compounds might be related to their conversion into free radical states *in vivo* (139).

7.5.4 Inhibitors of Metabolism

N-methylphenazinium-methylsulfate (phenazine methosulfate or PMS) can function as an electron transfer agent and can catalyze photophosphorylation in some enzymic reactions and in incubation media of living cells. In acid solution phenazine and its derivatives are reduced (or oxidized) in distinct one-electron steps involving semiquinone intermediates (252), but it is not certain whether the semiquinone radical forms of PMS can serve as electron donors or acceptors within metabolizing cells.

Zaugg (252) undertook a study of the intermediate oxidation states of PMS at different pH values, using optical and ESR techniques, and found that in biological pH ranges a significant fraction of the PMS can exist in the semiquinone form, which might indicate sufficient stability to allow single-electron transfer steps in the biological redox reactions of PMS (252). Subsequently, Cost, Bolton, and Frenkel (61) investigated by ESR and optical methods the interaction of PMS with the light-induced free radical in the chromatophores of red photosynthetic bacteria. They found evidence that the N-methylphenazinium free radical interacts with light-induced chromatophore free radicals and concluded that PMS interferes with the normal transfer of electrons within the chromatophore, with the interactive form of PMS being its semiquinone free radical (61).

Streptonigrin and rubiflavin are antibiotics that can also inhibit bacterial metabolism, possibly via their pathway of antibiotic action. When these inhibitors are added to suspensions of appropriate bacteria, free radicals are produced by intracellular reduction (230). Hyperfine structure was missing in the ESR signals obtained by White and Dearman (230) from the incubation media with rubiflavin, which is to be expected if the free radicals are bound to large molecules within the cell. However, the ESR spectra of the media following incubation with PMS or streptonigrin manifested highly detailed isotropic hyperfine structure (Fig. 7-25). Since a similar intracellularly formed, resolved ESR signal from naphthoquinone is strong and persistent at pH 7.4 (121) (and this is below the pH at which the chemically generated free radical can be detected), there seems to be some residual interaction between bacterial components and even those biogenic free radicals mobile enough to manifest well-resolved ESR spectra. Nevertheless, several quinones that can be readily reduced to semiquinone intracellularly are not lethal, and therefore the biogenic formation of a free radical is not, in itself, sufficient to cause a bactericidal action (121). Possibly, then, further reactions of the semiquinones are necessary for such an outcome, and only those semiquinones capable of carrying out these secondary reactions are lethal (121).

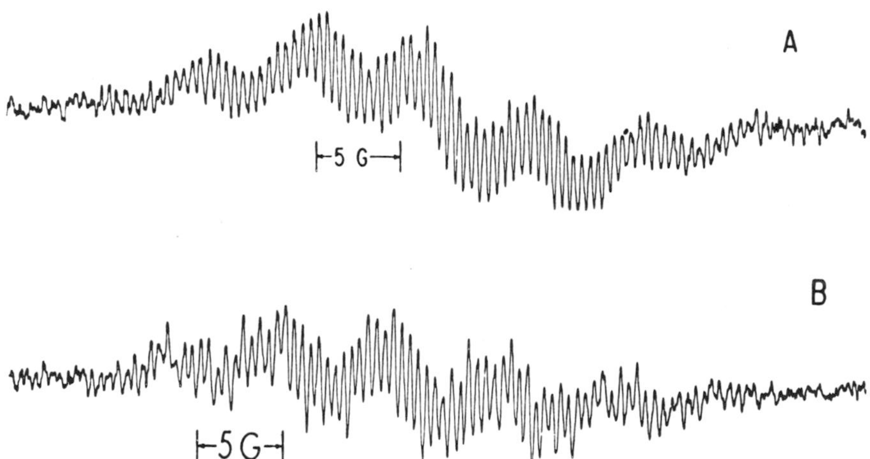

Fig. 7-25 ESR spectra of phenazine methosulfate free radicals. A. PMS reduced chemically by sodium borohydride. B. PMS biologically reduced by a suspension of *Bacillus megaterium*. (From Ref. 230, with permission.)

7.5.5 Uncouplers of Oxidative Phosphorylation

The mechanisms by which metabolic uncoupling agents dissociate phosphorylation reactions from mitochondrial electron transfer remain unknown, despite an extensive literature documenting the many sites in the respiratory enzyme chain at which different uncoupling agents seem to act. The discharge of high-energy bonds involving phosphorylated intermediates or their precursors has frequently been advanced as one way in which uncoupling agents could separate electron transfer from the synthesis of ATP. Recalling the speculations of Section 7.3.4, in which semiquinone phosphates were considered as possible intermediates of oxidative phosphorylation, we might propose that the same or similar free radical reactions operating in the reverse direction could uncouple oxidative phosphorylation. However, although free radical forms are not known for many members of the vast catalog of uncoupling agents, many uncouplers do belong to classes of chemical compounds (such as phenols and aromatic amines) for which facile formation of free radicals is well established. Other uncoupling agents are antibiotic compounds, and free radical forms of at least several antibiotics have already been cited in Sections 7.4.6, 7.5.3, and 7.5.4. Perhaps the most celebrated uncoupler of oxidative phosphorylation is 2,4-dinitrophenol, an aromatic compound containing both easily reducible and easily oxidizable substituents. The remainder of this section is devoted to consideration of free radicals that can be formed from dinitrophenols.

Despite the speculation just advanced, present concepts of dinitrophenol action do not involve it in oxidoreduction reactions. Rather its properties as a lipophilic weak acid are thought to be ruling (140). It is proposed that the dissociated uncoupler anion can enter the mitochondrion and exchange for other anions and that the uncoupler can leave as an uncharged acid by virtue of its lipophilicity. Once within the mitochondrion dinitrophenol may be able to couple in some way with one of the factors involved in oxidative phosphorylation to prevent optimal operation of the phosphorylating pathway.

Although the weakly acid and lipophilic character of the uncoupler may explain its accumulation by mitochondria, the uncoupling mechanism itself might still involve the redox properties of the reactants. As the locus of the main chain of respiratory enzymes, the intramitochondrial environment must include the full range of biological redox potentials. Although the linked chain of electron transfer enzymes is thought to be isolated from random access by unwanted redox substrates, it is clear that its insulation is imperfect; for example, the well-mapped catalog of respiratory shunts produced by various exogenous electron acceptors of different redox potentials gives evidence that many sites along the respiratory chain are accessible to redox-active agents. Moreover, as a lipophilic weak acid, dinitrophenol could reach both hydrated and hydrophobic reaction sites, much as it is supposed to pass back and forth through the mitochondrial membrane itself. Since nitrophenols are readily reducible, in both aprotic and aqueous solvents (42, 90), their reactions within the electron transfer chain or at a phosphorylating site might conceivably be determined by their redox properties, including the possibility of one-electron transfer reactions to form free radicals.

Bernal and Fraenkel (14) carried out ESR studies of electrochemical reductions of aromatic polynitro compounds in organic solvents and found different spectra corresponding to the free radicals produced by successively higher polarographic waves. Later Freed and Fraenkel (90), carrying on similar work with other nitro-substituted benzene anions, obtained a strong and completely resolved ESR spectrum of the 2,6-dinitrophenolate anion. Using similar techniques, Nordio and his associates (179) obtained excellent ESR spectra from 2,4-dinitrobenzoic acid, but they did not examine 2,4-dinitrophenol.

In fact, there are very few published data on free radicals from 2,4-dinitrophenol, although one spectrum is contained in an atlas (37) and another is offered as a casual illustration of the use of a high-velocity continuous-flow apparatus adapted for ESR (31). Nonetheless, Borg and Elmore (42) have carried out many studies on free radicals from dinitrophenols, although the work is not complete. Radicals were generated by electrolysis *in situ* within the microwave cavity and by chemical reduction with titanium trichloride, using a fast-flow apparatus (see Sections 2.18.2.1 and 2.18.2.2). Spectra were obtained from radicals in both acid and alkaline aqueous solution and in solvent mixtures of dimethylformamide/water (see Table 7-2).

For symmetrical 2,6-dinitrophenol, the same radical dianion is seen with both electrolysis and fast flow in aqueous alkali. Free radicals of the unsymmetrical 2,5- and 2,4-dinitrophenols are much less stable, being difficult to resolve with steady-state electrolysis and requiring very high flow velocities in the continuous-flow apparatus. For the 2,4- and the 2,5-dinitrophenolate dianions produced by titanium in aqueous alkali the hyperfine splittings are given in Table 7-2. In the 2,4-dinitrophenol case the spectrum obtained in aqueous acid is very nearly the same, but in acidic 50 percent dimethylformamide and also in aqueous buffers at pH of about 7 to 8 the spectrum obtained, even at fastest flow, is a 1:1:1 triplet of 1:2:1 triplets, showing rapid reduction of one nitro group to an amino group (Fig. 7-26). In fact, the same spectrum can be obtained by oxidizing 2-nitro-4-aminophenol in a flow system (37), whereas similar oxidation of 2-amino-4-nitrophenol gives a triplet of barely resolved quartets (Table 7-2), thus pointing to the 4-nitro group as the one being reduced.

The electrolysis results were generally consistent with those obtained from chemical reduction; for example, 2,4-dinitrophenol with a gold foil electrode gives rise to the 3×14 pattern as the first radical seen in aqueous

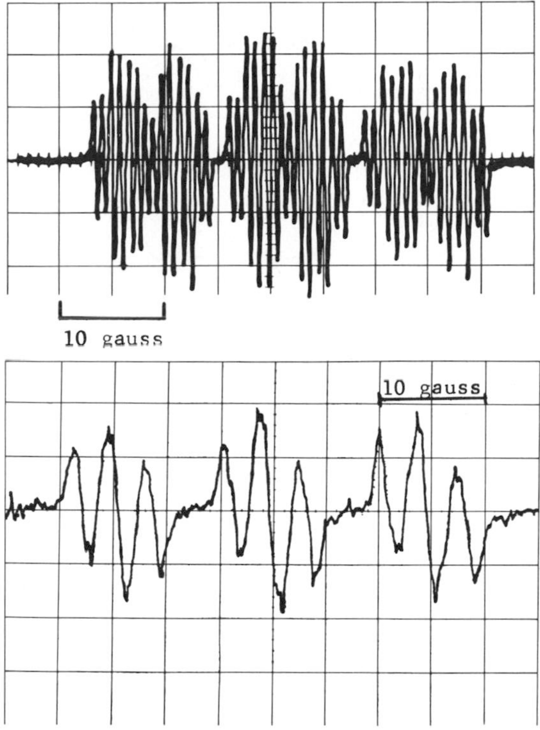

Fig. 7-26 ESR spectra of transient free radicals from 2,4-dinitrophenol reduced by Ti(III) in acid solutions, using continuous flow. *Upper:* reduction in aqueous solution. *Lower:* reduction in 50 percent dimethylformamide.

alkali (42). With mercury pool or platinum gauze electrodes, however, weaker signals are elicited, and a triplet of triplets signifying the 2-nitro-4-aminophenol radical slowly appears without prior detection of the 3 × 14 dinitrophenolate anion pattern (42).

Because they are not regularly available elsewhere, the incomplete results describing some of the free radicals from 2,4-dinitrophenol and its congeners have been reported here in some detail. Nonetheless, except for the relevance the reader chooses to give to the speculations of the first three paragraphs of this subsection, there is no biochemical evidence to support the intervention of free radical forms of 2,4-dinitrophenol in its pharmacological actions.

Table 7-2 Hyperfine Splitting Constants for Free Radicals from Dinitrophenols and Derivatives[a]

Parent compound	(O)xidation or (R)eduction	(E)lectrolysis *in situ* or (F)ast flow methods	Electrode material or Redox reagent	Solvent	Splitting Constants (in gauss)	
					Nitrogen	Proton
2,6-Dinitrophenol	R	E	Pt, Au	Aqueous (alkaline)	7.32 (2)	4.31 (2), 1.35
	R	F	Ti^{3+}	Aqueous (alkaline)		
2,5-Dinitrophenol	R	F	Ti^{3+}	Aqueous (alkaline)	11.22, 0.30	4.32, 1.54, 0.68
2,4-Dinitrophenol	R	F	Ti^{3+}	Aqueous (alkaline)	13.09, 1.73	4.83, 1.73, 0.77
	R	E	Au	Aqueous (alkaline)		
	R	F	Ti^{3+}	50% DMF/H_2O or aqueous (pH 7-8)	4.5	3.4 (2)
	R	E	Pt, Hg	Aqueous (alkaline)		
2-nitro, 4-aminophenol	O	F	Ce^{4+}	Aqueous (acid)	4.5	3.4 (2)
2-amino, 4-nitrophenol	O	F	Ce^{4+}	Aqueous (acid)	15.09	3.58, 2.87

[a] See Ref. 37.

7.5.6 Alloxan

Alloxan is a diabetogenic substance that can cause destructive lesions in the beta cells of the pancreatic islets of Langerhans. However, injection of large doses of either glutathione or cysteine before the administration of alloxan protects animals from its destructive effect. Accordingly, Lagercrantz and Yhland (143) used ESR spectroscopy to investigate the reaction of alloxan with glutathione and ascorbic acid. Radicals were detected in aqueous solutions and the identical ESR spectrum was seen following oxidation of dialuric acid by potassium ferricyanide (143). Lagercrantz concluded that the radicals seen belonged to a complex system in which several reactions occurred, including irreversible conversion of alloxan to alloxanic acid, formation and decay of dialuric acid, and formation and decay of alloxantin. None of the properties of the reactions studied indicated whether the free radicals described might be of any significance for the toxic effect produced by alloxan in animals.

A few years later Russell and Young (196) reported that radical anions were easily formed by reduction of alloxan as well as by the dissociation of alloxantin in basic solution. They obtained ESR spectra of higher resolution than those recorded by Lagercrantz (143), but the work did not cast more light on the question of biological relevance.

7.5.7 Sulfur and Selenium Antioxidants

Selenium is an essential trace element in animal nutrition, in which it appears to function as a lipid antioxidant with as much as 500 times the antioxidant activity of Vitamin E (see Section 7.3.2) (231). Thiols are known to be effective radioprotective agents, and selenoamino acids are even more potent in this regard (see Chapter 10). Although atom transfer mechanisms by which thiol groups can "repair" hydrogen abstraction defects in irradiated peptides (see Chapter 10) are known, it is likely that against the less potent oxidants produced in the course of normal physiological chemistry selenium and sulfur antioxidants act as radical scavengers, forming free radicals of their own which then disproportionate or otherwise decay without attacking essential biological target sites (59, 232).

In presenting the hypothesis in Section 7.5.1 that some polycyclic carcinogens might operate through free radical mechanisms, it was pointed out that ionizing radiation—which is known to act on tissues largely through free radical mechanisms—is a physical carcinogen. The possibility was thus brought forward that both agents might give rise to cancers in a similar way by virtue of producing free radicals as proximate carcinogens in both instances. This speculation is given added weight by the observation that radioprotective thiols also protect against the toxicity of carcinogenic alkylating agents (59). Although thiols may protect against both ionizing radiation and alkylating agents, there are indications, however, that the protective mechanism is not exactly the same in both cases. It appears likely that protection against alkylating agents requires a high concentration of the free form of the thiol, which appears to react directly *in vivo* with the administered alkylating agent, thereby diminishing the alkylation of DNA (59). Furthermore, it is not at all clear that this interaction is of a free radical nature.

Sodium selenide manifests an even greater protective effect against cancer formation by chemicals (199). Protection is seen both when selenium is given at the same time as the chemical carcinogen (200) and when tumors are first initiated with one hydrocarbon and selenium is then provided only to protect against the cocarcinogenic effect of a tumor promotor such as Croton Oil (199, 200). Some other antioxidants, such as Vitamin E, provide similar but less potent protection, suggesting that the protective effect is common to several antioxidants and therefore may represent a common mechanism, such as free radical scavenging (199, 200). On the other hand, not all antioxidants are effective (200), and there may be special requirements for protection such as sufficiently low oxidation potential.

It is also relevant (see Section 7.6.1) that the effect of cigarette smoke in inhibiting phagocytosis of bacteria by macrophages from the lung is counteracted by the addition of glutathione or cysteine to the cigarette smoke (102). The protective effect of sulfhydryl agents in this instance suggests an oxidant action of cigarette smoke on the cells, which is consistent with the roles proposed for free radicals from cigarette smoke components (see Section 7.6.1), as well as being consonant with the present hypothesis that selenium and sulfur compounds provide antioxidant protection by virtue of their own ready conversion to free radical forms.

Free radicals from selenium and sulfur antioxidants have been characterized by ESR in experiments in which frozen samples of the compounds were irradiated with ultraviolet light and examined at 77 K (231, 232). Although the samples were in the frozen state, the ESR spectra revealed some spectral shape, usually asymmetric, and the analysis showed, among other things, that the free radicals formed fell into four categories: alkyl, benzyl, sulfur, and selenium species. Furthermore, the ESR data provided some insight into the greater antioxidant protection provided by selenium compounds than by sulfur analogs in that the selenium and sulfur free radicals did not behave in the same ways in some important regards; for example, under the experimental conditions used disulfide bonds ruptured, whereas diselenide bonds didn't; in the latter case the free radical localized elsewhere on the molecule. However, protons on both thiol and selenol groups are labile when free radicals form (231, 232).

7.5.8 Viologen Herbicides

Recently a class of herbicides which appears to work by being transformed to relatively stable free radicals (6) has come into use. These compounds are 4,4′-bipyridyl derivatives, and a large number of quaternary compounds of this class are active as herbicides, the most potent of which is "paraquat," also known as the redox indicator "methyl viologen" (1,1′-dimethyl-4,4′-bypyridylium cation dichloride). Correlations of molecular structure with herbicidal activity show that when a number of these compounds are compared on the basis of the amount of free radical formed they are equipotent (6).

These herbicides kill plants rapidly, provided that light is admitted, chlorophyll is present, and oxygen is not excluded. It is likely that the production of hydrogen peroxide by atmospheric oxidation of the viologen radicals formed under these conditions gives rise, ultimately, to the creation of unstable reactive peroxy free radicals, which may be the primary toxins (6).

Paraquat and its viologen derivatives are expensive, but they are selective and nonpersistent herbicides because they are rapidly inactivated by soil so that they affect only the plants on which they are sprayed. Even then photosynthesis is required for their lethal action (6).

ESR analysis of a methyl viologen monocation free radical is complete, and some of its analogs have been analyzed as well. Spontaneous dimerization, on reduction of pyridine (50, 227) or N-methylpyridinium salts (41, 122, 137), can produce viologen radicals, but irradiation by sunlight of scrupulously deoxygenated solutions of the viologens in aqueous ethanol gives rise to monocation radicals with the best resolved hyperfine structure (125). Analysis shows delocalization of the unpaired electron throughout both ring systems, and it is the resonance stabilization that stems from this fast exchange of the odd electron between the two pyridine ring systems that underlines the stability of the free radical, which, in turn, is responsible for the herbicidal efficacy of the compounds.

7.6 FREE RADICALS FROM ENVIRONMENTAL AGENTS

This section is small, and both its subsections overlap with topics treated elsewhere. Nevertheless, to emphasize the different origin of these biologically interesting free radicals the section is given separate identity.

7.6.1 Tobacco Smoke and Its Components

Tobacco smoke is claimed to be dangerous to health, in part because of its carcinogenic propensity and in part because of its toxic effect on the mucous membranes of the upper respiratory tree. Tobacco carcinogens include many polynuclear hydrocarbons (85), of which the most prominent and best known is 3,4-benzpyrene (benz[a]pyrene), but benzanthracenes, benzperylenes, and benznaphthacenes also are known. The likelihood that free radical forms of benzpyrene may be associated with its carcinogenicity has been discussed at some length in Sections 4.3.6.2 and 7.5.1. In this section comments are confined to ESR work related to the identification of reactive constituents in tobacco smoke or to the interaction of those constituents with tissues.

When ESR studies on smoke and its condensates were carried out by Forbes and his colleagues (85), a variety of paramagnetic centers was seen, some with lifetimes of a few seconds. Furthermore, when benzpyrene itself was heated to near its melting point, it gave rise to an intense ESR absorption that indicated that more than one radical had been formed (85).

Another ESR study on the condensed vapor phase of cigarette smoke has been carried out (212). As the condensed sample was slowly annealed, a series of ESR spectra followed one on the other, showing that chemical reactions involving free radicals occurred at low temperatures. From the complexity of the spectra little could be construed about the chemical and biological properties of the species involved, although there were indications of nitrogen oxide participation (212).

ESR studies on pure polynuclear hydrocarbon preparations have also been carried out, to some extent as models for the complex situation presented by tobacco smoke. As far back as 1958 Kon and Blois (135) produced cation radicals in concentrated sulfuric acid from hydrocarbons, but only 3,4-benzpyrene displayed any hyperfine structure and that was incomplete. Subsequently Forbes (87) obtained much better spectral resolution from benzpyrene (Fig. 7-27) and from a number of cation and anion radicals formed from aromatic hydrocarbons (60).

ESR studies also have been made to determine some of the effects on tissues of the known and unknown free radicals and other reactive constituents of tobacco smoke. In the first such study Rowlands and his colleagues (192) placed the lungs and respiratory trees of rabbits on a smoking machine, following which the tissue was homogenized promptly and examined by ESR at liquid nitrogen temperature. This was followed by a much more extensive ESR study of tobacco smoke condensates and their effect on lung tissue and blood constituents which showed that tobacco smoke constituents could enter into the bloodstreams of living mice through

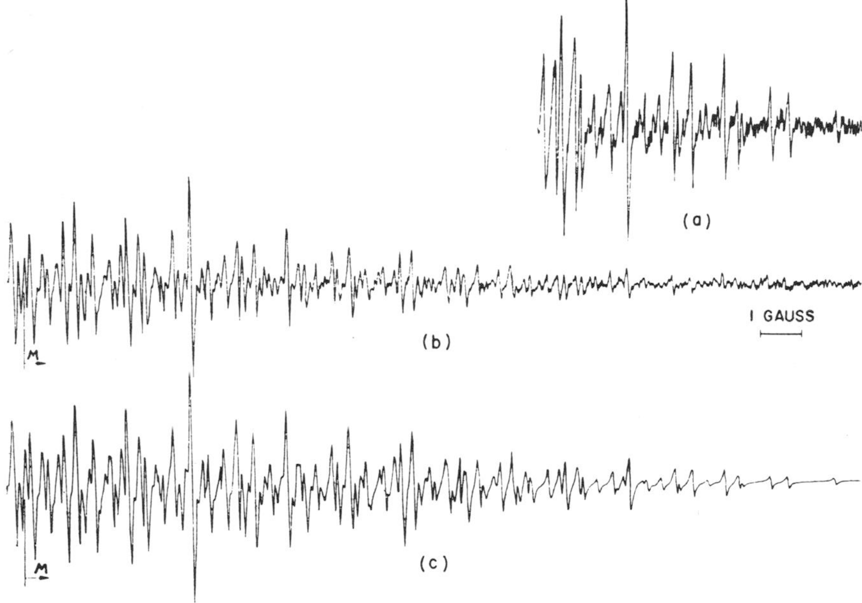

Fig. 7-27 ESR spectrum of free radical obtained on heating benz[a]pyrene: (*a*) wing of spectrum under high gain; (*b*) half-spectrum with midpoint at *M*; (*c*) computed spectrum. (From Ref. 87, with permission.)

their lung membranes to react with the cellular constituents and with the hemoglobin (193). It was established that *non*-free radical constituents of smoke and its condensate could interact with hemoglobin and with the phospholipids of lung tissue to produce stable free radical species, and nitrogen oxides were implicated as the causative agents that gave rise to the tissue ESR signals in this way (193).

7.6.2 Nitrogen Oxides

Reference has already been made several times to distinctive ESR signals from tissues that are associated with certain phases of chemical carcinogenesis (219, 237) or with some tumors in animals (43, 74) (see Section 4.3.6.2). In Section 7.3.12 ESR spectra from models of the paramagnetic centers giving rise to the signals (236) were discussed, and in Section 7.5.1 it was pointed out that the intensity of the tissue signals bore an inverse relationship to the incidence of tumor, suggesting that the signals reflect a detoxification mechanism operating on a carcinogen rather than the carcinogenic reaction itself (237). Similar, but slightly different, signals could be obtained from animal tissues following incubation with nitrate, nitrite, or hydroxylamine (Fig. 7-28). Since nitrate is readily reduced by animal tissues and identical ESR signals were obtained from the three nitrogen oxides, it was concluded that the agent responsible for the nitrogenous component of the $g = 2.035$ signal was the reduction product of nitrite, which could be nitrogen oxide, NO (237).

Woolom and Commoner (237) undertook some long-term feeding experiments and determined that the development of the ESR signal in the rat is a synergistic effect of the carcinogen and nitrite, as found in the diet. Considering the enhancement by dietary nitrite of the amplitude of the abnormal liver ESR signal concomitantly with protection against tumor in carcinogen-fed rats, it may be concluded that environmental levels of nitrates and

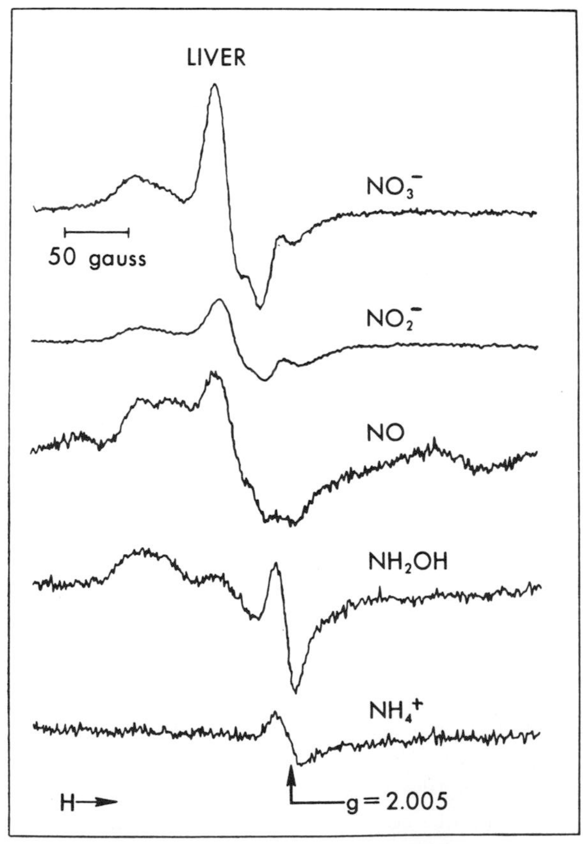

Fig. 7-28 ESR signals from rat liver slices incubated in phosphate buffer at pH 7.0 with the addition of NO_3^-, NO_2^-, NO gas, NH_2OH, or NH_4^+. (From Ref. 237, with permission.)

nitrites in the diet might possibly have a functional consequence in terms of cancer induction (237).

As a follow-up to the studies noted in Section 7.6.1, Rowlands and his associates (77) carried out investigations on the interaction between nitrogen dioxide and unsaturated lipid components. In most tissues the characteristic triplet ESR signature of the nitric oxide was seen in addition to hyperfine lines from free radicals induced in the target materials, and some of the transient and stable free radicals that were produced were identified (77).

In summary, this last section has emphasized ESR studies that elucidate the reactions of tissues with nitrogen oxides at an oxidation level of nitrate or lower, as found in the food and water components of an animal's environment and as opposed to the direct reactions with the nitric oxide which might be a constituent of an animal's respiratory environment.

REFERENCES

1. P. Abadom, K. Ahmed, and P. Scholefield, *Can. J. Biochem. Physiol.*, **39,** 551 (1961).
2. G. Abagyan and P. Butyargin, *Dokl. Biophys.*, **154,** 1444 (1964) (Eng., p. 32).
3. R. Adams, *Accounts Chem. Res.*, **2,** 175 (1969).
4. T. Akera and T. Brody, *Mol. Pharmacol.*, **4,** 600 (1968).
5. T. Akera and T. Brody, *Mol. Pharmacol.*, **5,** 605 (1969).
6. A. Albert, *Selective Toxicity*, 4th ed., Methuen, London, 1968. Chapter 13, p. 430.
7. B. Allen and A. Bond, *J. Phys. Chem.*, **68,** 2439 (1964).
8. B. Babior and D. Gould, *Biochem. Biophys. Res. Commun.*, **34,** 441 (1969).
9. D. Bäckström, B. Norling, A. Ehrenberg, and L. Ernster, *Biochim. Biophys. Acta*, **197,** 108 (1970).
10. M. Bains, O. Hinojosa, and J. Arthur, Jr., *Carbohyd. Res.*, **6,** 233 (1968).
11. G. Bartholini, A. Pletscher, and K. Gey, *Experimentia*, **17,** 541 (1961).
12. H. Beinert and G. Palmer, *Advan. Enzymol.*, **27,** 105 (1965).
13. S. Bergström, *Science*, **157,** 382 (1967).
14. I. Bernal and G. Fraenkel, *J. Am. Chem. Soc.*, **86,** 1671 (1964).
15. M. Bickel, F. Sulser, and B. Brodie, *Life Sci.*, 247 (1963).
16. M. Bickel and B. Brodie, *Intern. J. Neuropharmacol.*, **3,** 611 (1964).
17. J.-P. Billon, G. Cauquis, and J. Combrisson, *Compt. Rend.*, **253,** 1593 (1961).
18. J.-P. Billon, G. Cauquis, and J. Combrisson, *J. Chim. Phys.*, **61,** 374 (1964).
19. F. Blasi, *Biochim. Biophys. Acta*, **121,** 204 (1966).
20. M. Blois, *Biochim. Biophys. Acta*, **18,** 165 (1955).
21. M. Blois, Jr. and J. Maling, *Biochem. Biophys. Res. Commun.*, **3,** 132 (1960).
22. M. Blois, Jr., *J. Invest. Derm.*, **45,** 475 (1965).
23. M. Blois, Jr., in *Solid State Biophysics*, S. Wyard, Ed., McGraw-Hill, New York, 1969, p. 243.

24. W. Blumberg, M. Goldstein, E. Lanber, and J. Peisach, *Biochim. Biophys. Acta*, **99,** 187 (1965).
25. W. Blumberg, J. Peisach, B. Wittenberg, and J. Wittenberg, *J. Biol. Chem.*, **243,** 1854 (1968).
26. A. Bond and H. Mason, *Biochem. Biophys. Res. Commun.*, **9,** 574 (1962).
27. D. Borg, *Federation Proc.*, **20** (Suppl. 10), 104 (1961).
28. D. Borg and G. C. Cotzias, *Proc. Natl. Acad. Sci.*, **48,** 617 (1962).
29. D. Borg and G. C. Cotzias, *Proc. Natl. Acad. Sci.*, **48,** 623 (1962).
30. D. Borg and G. C. Cotzias, *Proc. Natl. Acad. Sci.*, **48,** 643 (1962).
31. D. Borg in *Rapid Mixing and Sampling Techniques in Biochemistry*, B. Chance, R. Eisenhardt, Q. Gibson, and K. Lonberg-Holm, Eds., Academic, New York, 1964, p. 135.
32. D. Borg, *Biochem. Pharmacol.*, **14,** 115 (1965).
33. D. Borg, *Biochem. Pharmacol.*, **14,** 627 (1965).
34. D. Borg, *Proc. Natl. Acad. Sci.*, **53,** 633 (1965).
35. D. Borg, *Proc. Natl. Acad. Sci.*, **53,** 829 (1965).
36. D. Borg and J. Elmore, Jr., *3rd Intern. Congr. Rad. Res.* Cortina, Italy, 1966, p. 41.
37. D. Borg and J. Elmore, Jr., in *Atlas of Electron Spin Resonance Spectra*, B. Bielski and J. Gebicki, Eds., Academic, New York, 1967.
38. D. Borg and J. Elmore, Jr., *Magnetic Resonance in Biological Systems*, A. Ehrenberg, Malmström, Vänngård, Eds., Pergamon, Oxford, 1967, p. 341.
39. D. Borg and J. Elmore, Jr., *Magnetic Resonance in Biological Systems*, A. Ehrenberg, Malmström, Vänngård, Eds., Pergamon, Oxford, 1967, p. 383.
40. D. Borg, J. Fajer, R. Felton, and D. Dolphin, *Proc. Natl. Acad. Sci.*, **67,** 813 (1970).
41. D. Borg, unpublished.
42. D. Borg and J. Elmore, Jr., unpublished.
43. M. Brennan, T. Cole, and J. Singley, *Proc. Soc. Exptl. Biol. Med.*, **123,** 715 (1966).
44. A. Brill in *Comprehensive Biochemistry*, Vol. 14, M. Florkin and E. H. Stotz, Eds., Elsevier, Amsterdam, 1966, p. 447.
45. L. Broman, B. Malmström, R. Aasa, and T. Vänngård, *Biochim. Biophys. Acta*, **75,** 365 (1963).
46. A. Buchachenko, *Stable Radicals*, Consultants Bureau, New York, 1965.
47. R. Butcher, *New Eng. J. Med.*, **279,** 1378 (1968).
48. R. Butcher, G. A. Robison, J. Hardman, and E. Sutherland, *Advances in Enzyme Regulation*, Vol. 6, Pergamon, Oxford, 1968, p. 357.
49. E. Caldwell and C. Steelink, *Biochim. Biophys. Acta*, **184,** 420 (1969).
50. A. Carrington and J. dos Santos-Veiga, *Mol. Phys.*, **5,** 21 (1962).
51. M. Carver, *Biochem. Pharmacol.*, **12,** 19 (1963).
52. B. Chance, *Arch. Biochem. Biophys.*, **41,** 416 (1952).
53. B. Chance and R. Fergusson in *The Mechanism of Enzyme Action*, W. McElroy and B. Glass, Eds., Johns Hopkins, Baltimore, 1954, p. 389.
54. V. Chumakov and A. Kalmanson, *Dokl. Biophys.*, **170,** 714 (1966) (Eng., p. 122).
55. B. Commoner, J. Townsend, and G. Pake, *Nature*, **174,** 689 (1954).
56. B. Commoner, J. Heise, and J. Townsend, *Proc. Natl. Acad. Sci.*, **42,** 711 (1956).
57. B. Commoner, J. Heise, B. Lippincott, R. Norberg, J. Passoneau, and J. Townsend, *Science*, **126,** 57 (1957).

58. B. Commoner, B. Lippincott, and J. Passoneau, *Proc. Natl. Acad. Sci.*, **44,** 1099 (1958)

59. T. Connors, *European J. Cancer*, **2,** 293 (1966).

60. J. Cooper, W. Forbes, and J. Robinson, *Can. J. Chem.*, **48,** 1942 (1970).

61. K. Cost, J. Bolton, and A. Frenkel, *Proc. Natl. Acad. Sci.*, **57,** 868 (1967).

62. G. Cotzias and D. Borg, Ultrastructure and Metabolism of the Nervous System, *Res. Pub. Assoc. Res. Nerv. Mental Dis.*, **15,** 337 (1962).

63. J. Craig, M. Tate, G. Warwick, and W. Rogers, *J. Med. Pharmacol. Chem.*, **2,** 659 (1960).

64. R. Dallam and L. Chen, *Arch. Biochem. Biophys.*, **123,** 565 (1968).

65. M. Das, H. Connor, D. Leniart, and J. Freed, *J. Am. Chem. Soc.*, **92,** 2258 (1970).

66. W. Dixon and R. Norman, *J. Chem. Soc.*, 3119 (1963).

67. W. Dixon, R. Norman, and A. Buley, *J. Chem. Soc.*, 3625 (1964).

68. D. Dolphin, R. Felton, D. Borg, and J. Fajer, *J. Am. Chem. Soc.*, **92,** 743 (1970).

69. D. Dolphin, A. Forman, D. Borg, J. Fajer, and R. Felton, *Proc. Natl. Acad. Sci.*, **68,** 614 (1971).

70. A. Ehrenberg in *Hemes and Hemoproteins*, B. Chance, R. Estabrook, and T. Yonetani, Eds., Academic, New York, 1966, p. 331.

71. A. Ehrenberg, P. Hemmerich, F. Müller, T. Okada, and M. Viscontini, *Helv. Chim. Acta*, **50,** 411 (1967).

72. K. Eisenstein and J. Wang, *J. Biol. Chem.*, **244,** 1720 (1969).

73. J. Elmore, Jr., "Electron Paramagnetic Resonance Studies of Free Radical Intermediates in Peroxidase Oxidations," M.A. Thesis, Hofstra University, 1966; also report BNL-10897.

74. N. Emanuél, A. Saprin, V. Shabalkin, L. Kozlova, and K. Kougljakova, *Nature*, **222,** 165 (1969).

75. M. Enomoto, K. Sato, E. Miller, and J. Miller, *Life Sci.*, **7** (Part II), 1025 (1968).

76. S. Epstein, J. McNary, B. Bartus, and E. Farber, *Science*, **162,** 907 (1968).

77. R. Estefan, E. Gause, and J. Rowlands, *Environ. Res.*, **3,** 62 (1970).

78. J. Fajer, D. Borg, A. Forman, D. Dolphin, and R. Felton, *J. Am. Chem. Soc.*, **92,** 3451 (1970).

79. R. Felton and H. Linchitz, *J. Am. Chem. Soc.*, **88,** 1113 (1966).

80. R. Felton, D. Dolphin, D. Borg, and J. Fajer, *J. Am. Chem. Soc.*, **91,** 196 (1969).

81. H. Fenner and H. Möckel, *Tetrahedron Letters*, 2815 (1969).

82. J. Fitzpatrick, C. Steelink, and R. Hansen, *J. Org. Chem.*, **32,** 625 (1967).

83. J. Fitzpatrick and C. Steelink, *Tetrahedron Letters*, 5041 (1969).

84. G. Foester, W. Weis, and H. Staudinger, *Ann. Chem.*, **690,** 166 (1965).

85. W. Forbes, J. Robinson, and G. Wright, *Can. J. Biochem.*, **45,** 1087 (1967).

86. W. Forbes and P. Sullivan, *Can. J. Biochem.*, **45,** 1831 (1967).

87. W. Forbes and J. Robinson, *Nature*, **217,** 550 (1968).

88. I. Forrest, F. Forrest, and M. Berger, *Biochim. Biophys. Acta*, **29,** 441 (1958).

89. A. Forrester, M. Ogilvy, and R. Thomson, *J. Chem. Soc.* (C), p. 1081 (1970).

90. J. Freed and G. Fraenkel, *J. Chem. Phys.*, **41,** 699 (1964).

91. E. Frieden, *Nutrit. Rev.*, **28,** 87 (1970).

92. J. Fritsch, S. Tatawawadi, and R. Adams, *J. Phys. Chem.*, **71,** 338 (1967).

93. J.-H. Fuhrhop and D. Mauzerall, *J. Am. Chem. Soc.*, **90,** 3875 (1968).

94. J.-H. Fuhrhop and D. Mauzerall, *J. Am. Chem. Soc.*, **91,** 4174 (1969).

95. H. Gelboin, E. Huberman, and L. Sachs, *Proc. Natl. Acad. Sci.*, **64,** 1188 (1969).

96. P. George, *Nature*, **169,** 612 (1952).

97. B. Gilbert, P. Hanson, R. Norman, and B. Sutcliffe, *Chem. Comm.*, 161 (1966).

98. C. Gooley, H. Keyzer, and F. Setchell, *Nature*, **223,** 80 (1969).

99. F. Grady and D. Borg, *Biochem.*, **7,** 675 (1968).

100. F. Grady and D. Borg, *J. Am. Chem. Soc.*, **90,** 2949 (1968).

101. A. Gräslund, R. Rigler, and A. Ehrenberg, *FEBS Letters*, **4,** 227 (1969).

102. G. Green, *Science*, **162,** 810 (1968).

103. C. Guzy, J. Raynor, L. Stodulski, and M. Symons, *J. Chem. Soc.* (A), 997 (1969).

104. J. Hamilton, R. Blakley, F. Looney, and M. Winfield, *Biochim. Biophys. Acta*, **177,** 374 (1969).

105. J. Hamilton and R. Blakley, *Biochim. Biophys. Acta*, **184,** 224 (1969).

106. D. Harman and L. Piette, *J. Gerontol.*, **21,** 560 (1966).

107. W. Harrison, *Arch. Biochem. Biophys.*, **101,** 116 (1963).

108. W. Harrison and W. Whisler, *Arch. Biochem. Biophys.*, **114,** 108 (1965).

109. W. Harrison, W. Whisler, and B. Hill, *Biochem.*, **7,** 3089 (1968).

110. M. Hawley, S. Tatawawadi, S. Piekarski, and R. Adams, *J. Am. Chem. Soc.*, **89,** 447 (1967).

111. P. Hemmerich, *Proc. Roy. Soc. (London)*, **A-302,** 335 (1968).

112. F. Herr, J. Stewart, and M.-P. Charest, *Arch. Int. Pharmacodyn.*, **134,** 328 (1961).

113. H. Hoeve and W. Yeranos, *Mol. Phys.*, **12,** 597 (1967).

114. M. Hozumi, S. Inuzuka, and T. Sugimura, *Cancer Res.*, **27,** 1378 (1967).

115. N. Hush and J. Rowlands, *J. Am. Chem. Soc.*, **89,** 2976 (1967).

116. H. Igel, R. Huebner, H. Turner, P. Kotin, and H. Falk, *Science*, **166,** 1624 (1969).

117. N. Isaacs and J. Paxton, *Photochem. Photobiol.*, **11,** 137 (1970).

118. I. Isenberg, A. Szent-Gyorgyi, and S. Baird, Jr., *Proc. Natl. Acad. Sci.*, **46,** 1307 (1960).

119. I. Isenberg, *Physiol. Rev.*, **44,** 487 (1964).

120. M. Ishizawa and H. Endo, *Biochem. Pharmacol.*, **16,** 637 (1967).

121. K. Ishizu, H. Dearman, M. Huang, and J. White, *Biochim. Biophys. Acta*, **165,** 283 (1968).

122. M. Itoh and S. Nagakura, *Bull. Chem. Soc. Japan*, **39,** 369 (1966).

123. T. Iyanagi and I. Yamazaki, *Biochim. Biophys. Acta*, **172,** 370 (1969).

124. C. Jackson and N. Patel, *Tetrahedron Letters*, 2255 (1967).

125. C. Johnson, Jr. and H. Gutowsky, *J. Chem. Phys.*, **39,** 58 (1963).

126. A. Kalmanson, L. Lipchina, and A. G. Chetverikov, *Biophysics* (trans.), **6,** 21 (1961).

127. N. Kataoka, A. Imamura, Y. Kawazoe, G. Chihara, and C. Nagata, *Bull. Chem. Soc. Japan*, **40,** 62 (1967).

128. C. Kensler, S. Dexter, and C. Rhoads, *Cancer Res.*, **2,** 1 (1942).

129. N. King and M. Winfield, *J. Biol. Chem.*, **238,** 1520 (1963).

130. N. King, F. Looney, and M. Winfield, *Biochim. Biophys. Acta*, **88,** 235 (1964).

131. N. King, F. D. Looney, and M. Winfield, *Biochim. Biophys. Acta*, **133,** 65 (1967).
132. H. Kleist and D. Mücke, *Experientia*, **22,** 136 (1966).
133. P. Knowles, J. Gibson, F. Pick, and R. Bray, *Biochem. J.*, **111,** 53 (1969).
134. D. Kohl, H. Wright, and M. Weissman, *Biochim. Biophys. Acta*, **180,** 536 (1969).
135. H. Kon and M. Blois, Jr., *J. Chem. Phys.*, **28,** 743 (1958).
136. N. Konovalova, G. Bogdanov, V. Miller, M. Nieman, E. Rozantsev, and N. Emanuél, *Dokl. Biochem.*, **157,** 707 (1964) (Eng., p. 259).
137. E. Kosower and J. Cotter, *J. Am. Chem. Soc.*, **86,** 5515 (1964).
138. Y. Kozlov, A. Tambiev, G. Taranenko, *Dokl. Biophys.*, **154,** 718 (1964) (Eng., p. 19).
139. B. Kozyrev and A. Rivkind, *Dokl. Biochem.*, **175,** 1396 (1967) (Eng., p. 246).
140. R. Kraayenhof and K. Van Dam, *Biochim. Biophys. Acta*, **172,** 189 (1969).
141. C. Lagercrantz and M. Yhland, *Acta Chem. Scand.*, **15,** 1204 (1961).
142. C. Lagercrantz, *Acta Chem. Scand.*, **15,** 1545 (1961).
143. C. Lagercrantz and M. Yhland, *Acta Chem. Scand.*, **17,** 1677 (1963).
144. C. Lagercrantz and M. Yhland, *Acta Chem. Scand.*, **17,** 2568 (1963).
145. C. Lagercrantz, *Acta Chem. Scand.*, **18,** 562 (1964).
146. C. Lagercrantz, *Acta Chem. Scand.*, **18,** 1321 (1964).
147. *Lancet*, p. 226 (1970) (editorial).
148. I. Lapin, *Psychopharmacol.*, **3,** 413 (1962).
149. S. Lesko, Jr., P. Ts'o, and R. Umans, *Biochem.*, **8,** 2291 (1969).
150. F. Leterrier and B. Viossat, *Compt. Rend.*, **265,** 410 (1967).
151. F. Leterrier, C. Balny, and P. Douzou, *Biochim. Biophys. Acta*, **154,** 444 (1968).
152. L. Levy and T. Burbridge, *Biochem. Pharm.*, **16,** 1249 (1967).
153. D. Lipkin, D. Paul, J. Townsend, and S. Weissman, *Science*, **117,** 534 (1953).
154. S. Løvtrup, *J. Neurochem.*, **10,** 471 (1963).
155. S. Løvtrup, *J. Neurochem.*, **11,** 377 (1964).
156. S. Løvtrup, *Intern. J. Neuropharmacol.*, **3,** 413 (1964).
157. C. MacDonald, W. Phillips, and H. Mower, *J. Am. Chem. Soc.*, **87,** 3319 (1965).
158. Y. Maeda and T. Higashimura, *Biochem. Biophys. Res. Commun.*, **29,** 362 (1967).
159. L. Marcoux, J. Fritsch, and R. Adams, *J. Am. Chem. Soc.*, **89,** 5766 (1967).
160. L. Marcoux, A. Lomax, and A. Bard, *J. Am. Chem. Soc.*, **92,** 243 (1970).
161. H. Mason, E. Spencer, and I. Yamazaki, *Biochem. Biophys. Res. Commun.*, **4,** 236 (1961).
162. Y. Matsunaga and C. McDowell, *Proc. Chem. Soc.*, 175 (1960).
163. T. Matsushima, I. Kobuna, and T. Sugimura, *Nature*, **216,** 508 (1967).
164. D. Mauzerall and G. Feher, *Biochim. Biophys. Acta*, **79,** 430 (1964).
165. J. McDermott, C. Huber, S. Osaki, and E. Frieden, *Biochim. Biophys. Acta*, **151,** 541 (1968).
166. L. Michaelis in *Currents in Biochemical Research*, D. Green, Ed., Wiley-Interscience, New York, 1946.
167. Y. Morita and H. Mason, *J. Biol. Chem.*, **240,** 2654 (1965).
168. C. Morreal, T. Das, K. Eskins, C. King, and J. Dienstag, *Biochim. Biophys. Acta*, **169,** 224 (1968).

169. R. Morton, Ed., *Biochemistry of Quinones*, Academic, New York, 1965.

170. T. Moss, A. Ehrenberg, and A. Bearden, *Biochem.*, **8,** 4159 (1969).

171. T. Nakamura, *Biochem. Biophys. Res. Commun.*, **2,** 111 (1960).

172. T. Nakamura, *Free Radicals in Biological Systems*, M. Blois, Jr., et al., Eds., Academic, New York, 1961, p. 169.

173. T. Nakamura and Y. Ogura, *Magnetic Resonance in Biological Systems*, A. Ehrenberg, Malmström, Vänngård, Eds., Pergamon, Oxford, 1967, p. 205.

174. T. Nakamura, Y. Kojima, H. Fujisawa, M. Nozaki, and O. Hayaishi, *J. Biol. Chem.*, **240,** PC 3225 (1965).

175. A. Nichol, I. Hendry, D. Morell, and P. Clezy, *Biochim. Biophys. Acta*, **156,** 97 (1968).

176. R. Nilsson, F. Pick, and R. Bray, *Biochim. Biophys. Acta*, **192,** 145 (1969).

177. A. Nishinaga, H. Kon, H. Cahnmann, and T. Matsuura, *J. Org. Chem.*, **33,** 157 (1968).

178. A. Nishinaga, T. Nagamachi, and T. Matsuura, *Chem. Comm.*, 888 (1969).

179. P. Nordio, M. Pavan, and C. Corvaja, *Trans. Faraday Soc.*, **60,** 1985 (1964).

180. S. Ohnishi and H. McConnell, *J. Am. Chem. Soc.*, **87,** 2293 (1965).

181. T. Ohnishi, H. Yamazaki, T. Iyanagi, T. Nakamura, and I. Yamazaki, *Biochim. Biophys. Acta*, **172,** 357 (1969).

182. M. Okun, L. Edelstein, N. Or, G. Hamada, and B. Donnellan, *Life Sci.*, **9** (Part II), 491 (1970).

183. J. Peisach and W. Levine, *Biochim. Biophys. Acta*, **77,** 615 (1963).

184. J. Peisach, W. Blumberg, B. Wittenberg, and J. Wittenberg, *J. Biol. Chem.*, **243,** 1871 (1968).

185. L. Piette and I. Forrest, *Biochim. Biophys. Acta*, **57,** 419 (1962).

186. L. Piette, G. Bulow, and I. Yamazaki, *Biochim. Biophys. Acta*, **88,** 120 (1964).

187. L. Piette, I. Yamazaki, and H. Mason, *Free Radicals in Biological Systems*, M. Blois, Jr., et al., Eds., Academic, New York, 1961, p. 195.

188. L. Piette, M. Okamura, G. Rabold, R. Ogata, R. Moore, P. Scheuer, *J. Phys. Chem.*, **71,** 29 (1967).

189. B. Polis, J. Wyeth, L. Goldstein, and J. Graedon, *Proc. Natl. Acad. Sci.*, **64,** 755 (1969).

190. W. Pryor, *Free Radicals*, McGraw-Hill, New York, 1966.

191. B. Rånby, K. Kringstad, E. Cowling, and S. Lin, *Acta Chem. Scand.*, **23,** 3257 (1969).

192. J. Rowlands, D. Cadena, Jr., and A. Gross, *Nature*, **213,** 1256 (1967).

193. J. Rowlands, R. Estefan, E. Gause, and D. Montalvo, *Environ. Res.*, **2,** 47 (1968).

194. G. Russell and E. Talaty, *J. Am. Chem. Soc.*, **86,** 5345 (1964).

195. G. Russell and E. Talaty, *Science*, **148,** 1217 (1965).

196. G. Russell and M. Young, *J. Am. Chem. Soc.*, **88,** 2007 (1966).

196a. R. Sack, D. Borg, and S. Freed, *Nature*, **235,** 224 (1972).

197. A. Saz and L. Martinez, *J. Biol. Chem.*, **233,** 1020 (1958).

198. D. Schieser, *J. Pharm. Sci.*, **53,** 909 (1964).

199. R. Shamberger and G. Rudolph, *Experientia*, **22,** 116 (1966).

200. R. Shamberger, *J. Nat. Cancer Inst.*, **44,** 931 (1970).

201. E. Slater, Ed., *Flavins and Flavoproteins*, Elsevier, Amsterdam, 1966.

202. C. Steelink, *J. Am. Chem. Soc.*, **87,** 2056 (1965).

203. T. Stone and W. A. Waters, *J. Chem. Soc.*, 213 (1964).

204. T. Sugimura, H. Otake, and T. Matsushima, *Nature*, **218,** 392 (1968).

205. E. Talaty and G. Russell, *J. Am. Chem. Soc.*, **87,** 4867 (1965).

206. E. Talaty and G. Russell, *J. Org. Chem.*, **31,** 3455 (1966).

207. H. Theorell and A. Ehrenberg, *Arch. Biochem. Biophys.*, **41,** 442 (1952).

208. G. Tollin, T. Reid, and C. Steelink, *Biochim. Biophys. Acta*, **66,** 444 (1963).

209. T. Tozer, L. Tuck, and J. Craig, *J. Med. Chem.*, **12,** 294 (1969).

210. A. Trifunac and E. Kaiser, *J. Phys. Chem.*, **74,** 2236 (1970).

211. L. Tuck and D. Schieser, *J. Phys. Chem.*, **66,** 937 (1962).

212. G. Tully, C. Briggs, and A. Horsfield, *Chem. Ind.*, 201 (1969).

213. K. Ulbert and P. Butyagin, *Dokl. Biophys.*, **149,** 1194 (1963) (Eng., p. 345).

214. R. Umans, S. Lesko, Jr., and P. Ts'o, *Nature*, **221,** 763 (1969).

215. G. Underwood, D. Jurkowitz, and S. Dickerman, *J. Phys. Chem.*, **74,** 544 (1970).

216. A. Vanin, *Biokhimiya* (English translation), **32,** 228 (1967).

217. M. Van Woert, *Nature*, **219,** 1054 (1968).

218. M. Viscontini, H. Leidner, G. Mattern, and T. Okada, *Helv. Chim. Acta*, **49,** 1911 (1966).

219. A. Vithayathil, J. Ternberg, and B. Commoner, *Nature*, **207,** 1246 (1965).

220. E. Walaas, O. Walaas, and S. Haavaldsen, *Arch. Biochem. Biophys.*, **100,** 97 (1963).

221. E. Walaas, R. Lövstad, and O. Walaas, *Biochem. J.*, **92,** 18P (1964).

222. E. Walaas, R. Lövstad, and O. Walaas, *Arch. Biochem. Biophys.*, **121,** 480 (1967).

223. O. Walaas, E. Walaas, T. Henriksen, and R. Lövstad, *Acta. Chem. Scand.*, **17,** 5263 (1963).

224. G. Walker, *Biochem. Biophys. Res. Commun.*, **13,** 431 (1963).

225. J. Wang, *Proc. Natl. Acad. Sci.*, **58,** 37 (1967).

226. J. Wang, *Science*, **167,** 25 (1970).

227. R. Ward, *J. Am. Chem. Soc.*, **83,** 3623 (1961).

228. J. Wertz, D. Reitz, and F. Dravnieks, *Free Radicals in Biological Systems*, M. Blois, Jr., et al., Eds., Academic, New York, 1961, p. 183.

229. A. White, P. Handler, and E. Smith, *Principles of Biochemistry*, 3rd ed., McGraw-Hill, New York, 1964.

230. J. White and H. Dearman, *Proc. Natl. Acad. Sci.*, **54,** 887 (1965).

231. J. Windle, A. Wiersema, and A. Tappel, *Nature*, **203,** 404 (1964).

232. J. Windle, A. Wiersema, and A. Tappel, *J. Chem. Phys.*, **41,** 1996 (1964).

233. M. Winfield, *J. Mol. Biol.*, **12,** 600 (1965).

234. B. Wittenberg, L. Kampa, J. Wittenberg, W. Blumberg, and J. Peisach, *J. Biol. Chem.*, **243,** 1863 (1968).

235. A. Wolberg and J. Manassen, *J. Am. Chem. Soc.*, **92,** 2982 (1970).

236. J. Woolum, E. Tiezzi, and B. Commoner, *Biochim. Biophys. Acta*, **160,** 311 (1968).

237. J. Woolum and B. Commoner, *Biochim. Biophys. Acta*, **201,** 131 (1970).

238. S. Wyard in *Solid State Biophysics*, S. Wyard, Ed., McGraw-Hill, New York, 1969, p. 263.

239. I. Yamazaki, H. Mason, and L. Piette, *Biochem. Biophys. Res. Commun.*, **1,** 336 (1959).

240. I. Yamazaki, H. Mason, and L. Piette, *J. Biol. Chem.*, **235,** 2444 (1960).

241. I. Yamazaki and L. Piette, *Biochim. Biophys. Acta*, **50,** 62 (1961).
242. I. Yamazaki, *J. Biol. Chem.*, **237,** 224 (1962).
243. I. Yamazaki and L. Piette, *Biochim. Biophys. Acta*, **77,** 47 (1963).
244. I. Yamazaki, K. Yokota, and R. Nakajima in *Oxidases and Related Redox Systems*, T. King, H. Mason, and M. Morrison, Eds., Wiley, New York, 1965, p. 485.
245. I. Yamazaki and T. Ohnishi, *Biochim. Biophys. Acta*, **112,** 469 (1966).
246. K. Yokota and I. Yamazaki, *Biochim. Biophys. Acta*, **105,** 301 (1965).
247. T. Yonetani and G. Ray, *J. Biol. Chem.*, **240,** 4503 (1965).
248. T. Yonetani, H. Schleyer, and A. Ehrenberg, *J. Biol. Chem.*, **241,** 3240 (1966).
249. T. Yonetani and H. Schleyer, *J. Biol. Chem.*, **242,** 1974 (1967).
250. T. Yonetani, H. Schleyer, and A. Ehrenberg, *Magnetic Resonance in Biological Systems*, A. Ehrenberg, Malmström, and T. Vänngård, Eds., Pergamon, Oxford, 1967, p. 151.
251. T. Yonetani, H. Drott, J. Leigh, Jr., G. Reed, M. Waterman, and T. Asakura, *J. Biol. Chem.*, **245,** 2998 (1970).
252. W. Zaugg, *J. Biol. Chem.*, **239,** 3964 (1964).

CHAPTER EIGHT

Flavins and Flavoproteins, Including Iron-Sulfur Proteins

HELMUT BEINERT

Institute for Enzyme Research
The University of Wisconsin, Madison

8.1 INTRODUCTION

The EPR spectroscopy of flavins and flavoproteins—including metal flavoproteins—probably represents today the most comprehensive example of the application of this technique to biological materials. The variety of approaches, the number of ancillary techniques, and subspecialties of EPR spectroscopy that are possible and indeed useful in this area span a wide range. So do the answers obtained and the lessons learned. Mastery of the experimental and instrumental problems involved, and the evaluation and interpretation of the results should equip the student of biologically applied EPR to tackle most problems in this field as a whole. We shall proceed from the consideration of simple flavin compounds and then of simple flavoproteins to increasingly complicated materials—the flavoproteins containing iron and finally those containing iron and molybdenum.

8.2 OBSERVED RESONANCES AND THEIR INTERPRETATION

8.2.1 Semiquinones

8.2.1.1 Free Flavin Compounds

The development of this field in the last 10 years is both impressive and instructive. It is probably just to say that the rapid progress in this area was possible only because of the intensive collaboration and interaction among groups of investigators with very different backgrounds and skills. The interpretation of the optical as well as EPR spectra of flavin semiquinones would have been impossible without the great number of variously substituted or modified derivatives that required the talents of chemists (1, 2); it would have been equally impossible without the skills and refined instrumental and computing techniques of the EPR spectroscopists (3–5); and, finally, decisive clues and the atmosphere of challenge were provided by those observing the behavior of protein-bound flavin (6, 7). The literature on the subject is not extensive but full of detailed information; therefore only a few aspects and the principal conclusions can be presented here. Anyone planning or attempting similar work should study the original publications in detail (3, 5, 8–14).

For an understanding of the EPR spectra of flavin semiquinones the resolution and interpretation of the hyperfine splitting (hfs) of these spectra is a prerequisite. It should be recalled that all studies on hfs of small molecules must be carried out in solution, since rapid tumbling of the molecules is essential for averaging out the anisotropic part of the hfs, which would immensely complicate and for all practical purposes prevent analysis of the hfs pattern. This consideration does not necessarily apply in the same way to protein-bound species, for in this instance the spin system may already be maximally immobilized by the binding to the protein which rotates only slowly. Thus, if hfs of protein-bound species can be resolved at all, it may be irrelevant whether spectroscopy is carried out at low or room temperature; in other words, a "powder spectrum" (see Section 1.4) is observed in either the liquid or frozen state.

As discussed in Section 2.13 isotopic substitution is the most promising approach to the unraveling of a complex hfs pattern. The electronic structure of a molecule is not substantially changed, say, by substitution of ^{15}N for ^{14}N or even of H by D. The approach of group substitution, for example, Cl for CH_3, to which one must resort when suitable isotopes are not available, is more objectionable from this viewpoint. In this case criteria must be found to test whether the compound resulting from substitution has in fact the essential properties of the compound to be studied. An example of this will be found below under metal constituents of metal-flavoproteins.

The effect of isotopic substitution is best illustrated by the example of the exchange of hydrogen for deuterium. In the simplest case of protons exchangeable in water this is readily accomplished by exposure to D_2O. Hydrogen has a nuclear spin I of $\frac{1}{2}$, resulting in two hfs lines for every line of the parent spectrum, and a nuclear magnetic moment μ of 2.79 nuclear magnetons. Deuterium has a spin of 1, resulting in three hfs lines but has a moment of only 0.86 nuclear magnetons. Thus a splitting of 4 G by a hydrogen will result, on substitution by deuterium, in a splitting of $4 \times 0.86/2.79 = 1.23$ G between the outermost lines or one half of this amount between the individual lines. A splitting of this magnitude, however, is rarely resolved with flavins, since it falls in the range of the widths of the hfs lines observed with these compounds. As a result, after deuterium substitution a single line will replace the two-line hfs of the proton.

Unfortunately riboflavin and its phosphates (FMN, FAD) are quite unsuitable for detailed study by EPR. With riboflavin itself the poor solubility is the greatest handicap, but, in addition, with all compounds having the intact ribityl side chain, a rather complicated hfs pattern develops. It was surprising at first sight that a compound such as lumiflavin, which has a methyl group with three protons in position N(10) (see Fig. 8-1), resulted in a less complicated pattern than compounds having the intact ribityl side chain, with a methylene group at N(10). It is not expected that protons attached to the 2′ carbon, that is, the second carbon of the ribityl chain attached to N(10), would bear significant unpaired spin density. The methylene group at N(10) would thus provide only two protons, compared with the three of the methyl group. The observed complication can be

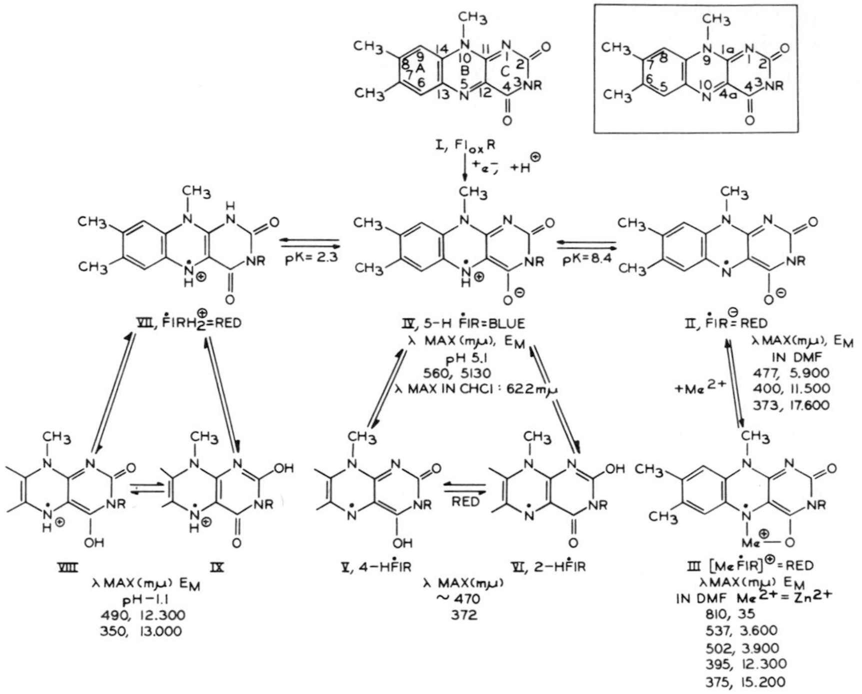

Fig. 8-1 Structures and optical characteristics of flavin semiquinones at different states of protonation, according to Müller et al. (14). Attention is drawn to the numbering systems of the flavin rings as shown in the top row. The system shown in the center corresponds to that presently recommended and used; the system shown to the right, however, is found in publications as recent as of 1968. The reader is therefore warned of potential confusion in the numbering of the positions labeled with isotopes or substituted. The numbers 1a, 4a, etc., as well as 11, 12, etc., for the carbon atoms connecting the rings are still in use today.

understood, however, if it is considered that the two 1′ protons of the ribityl side chain are not equivalent (8). If a substituent with two or more carbons is attached to N(10), the rotational freedom of this substituent may be impaired by the neighboring groups in the 1 and 9 positions. In addition, a longer complex side chain (e.g., ribityl) at N(10) may assume some rigidity by interaction (e.g., by hydrogen bonding) with other groups in the molecule.

The readily available lumiflavin derivatives were therefore the key compounds for exploring the hfs of flavin semiquinones. Lumiflavin itself is not sufficiently soluble in water in the pH range around neutrality so that satisfactory resolution of hfs could be achieved. Two approaches proved helpful, namely, substitution with an ionizable group at N(3) (e.g., lumiflavin acetic-acid) (8, 9) and, what should be more generally applicable, modification of the solvent and a temperature increase; for instance, a mixture of equal parts of 0.1 *M* acetate buffer (pH 5.7) and cellosolve (ethyleneglycol monoethylether, $CH_2OHCH_2OC_2H_5$) at 65 C gave a resolution far superior to that observed in water (8). Most recently the resolution was further improved by the use of appropriately substituted lumiflavin derivatives in nonpolar solvents such as benzene (15).

It has been known from early potentiometric titrations (16, 17) as well as from spectrophotometry (18) that flavin semiquinones can exist in cationic, neutral, and anionic forms. The p*K* values governing the equilibrium between these forms were found by EPR and spectrophotometric studies to lie at approximately 2.5 and 8.5 (5, 9, 19). They depend to a minor extent on the substituents on the flavin skeleton. The three species are readily differentiated by their light absorption spectra. The cationic form is red (λ_{max} 350 and 490 nm), the neutral form is blue (λ_{max} 350 and 560 nm), and the anionic form is again red (λ_{max} 379, 400 and 480 nm) (5, 9, 14). The most readily interpretable hfs pattern is found with the anionic semiquinone (9). This suggests that the extra proton in the neutral form [at N(5)] bears unpaired spin density and contributes to the hfs, thus complicating the pattern compared with the anion. By the same criterion the additional proton present in the cationic semiquinone [at N(1)] does not interact with the unpaired electron, since the hfs patterns of the neutral and cationic forms are not substantially different.

With the lumiflavin anion radical, for instance, 14 lines have been resolved. The interpretation of this pattern was then arrived at by the laborious substitution of isotopes with different nuclear spins in every position of the flavin molecule to which preparative routes were available. A number of group substitutions (e.g., Cl or H for CH_3) were also carried out and their effects investigated (9). The unraveling of the hfs pattern of the neutral and cationic semiquinones met with more difficulties (5). An unforeseen advantage, which could not be anticipated, accrued from the fact that a number of splittings from different atoms were almost identical in value [e.g., N(5) and its proton in the neutral semiquinone] or were simple multiples of the splitting from other atoms [e.g., N(5) and N(10)]. Otherwise an apparent 14-line pattern, found with the anionic form, could not be understood for a molecule as complex as a flavin semiquinone with so many nuclei bearing spin density. It should be noted that although such an apparent simplication of the hfs pattern is indeed an advantage in the early stages of the analytical approach it may, in the final analysis and assignment, lead to ambiguities. The final results are summarized in Table 8-1.

The calculation of unpaired spin densities from hyperfine coupling

Table 8-1 Isotropic Hyperfine Splitting Constants and Experimental and Theoretically Calculated Unpaired Spin Densities of Neutral and Anionic Flavin Semiquinones[a]

		Neutral semiquinone			Semiquinone anion		
		a	Unpaired spin density		*a*	Unpaired spin density	
Position	Atom	Gauss	Experimental	Calculated	Gauss	Experimental	Calculated
1	N		~ 0	0.020			−0.002
3	N		~ 0	−0.021			−0.036
5	N	8.7 ± 0.4	0.282–0.432	0.382	7.3 ± 0.3	0.256–0.394	0.361
	H(NH,NCH_3)	7.7 ± 0.2					
6	C		0.067–0.085	0.146		0.129–0.167	0.201
	H	1.7 ± 0.2			3.5 ± 0.5		
7	C		~ 0	−0.085			−0.117
8	C		0.089–0.115	0.120		0.148–0.190	0.140
	H(CCH_3)	2.7 ± 0.3			4.0 ± 0.5		
9	C		~ 0	−0.077		0.033–0.048	−0.060
	H				0.9 ± 0.1		
10	N	3.3 ± 0.4	0.126–0.194	0.328	3.2 ± 0.3	0.112–0.173	0.164
	H(NCH_3)	3.8 ± 0.5			3.0 ± 0.2		

[a] The values given for the neutral semiquinone refer to N(3,5) dialkylated lumiflavin radicals in chloroform according to Müller et al. (Ref. 5), those for the anion to 3 alkylated lumiflavin in dimethylformamide according to Ehrenberg et al. (Ref. 9). The values of the hyperfine splitting constants were obtained by taking differences between the total widths of pairs of EPR spectra according to Ehrenberg et al. (cf. Ref. 9). The maximal errors were estimated from the accuracy of the total width determination. The values obtained by simulation of spectra and fitting to experimental spectra were in good agreement. The value for a_6^H of the neutral semiquinone given above was obtained by the simulation technique. The range of values stated for the experimental spin densities is determined by the limits of the spin polarization parameters (Q) found in the literature. Only positions relevant for the interpretation of the EPR spectra are included. The theoretical values were calculated by the Pariser-Parr-Pople unrestricted Hartree-Fock self-consistent field method (without annihilations), according to Ref. 20 and a personal communication from Dr. P.-S. Song.

constants is ambiguous in many instances. Table 8-1 therefore shows the coupling constants themselves and in addition some values for unpaired spin densities calculated from these coupling constants. They are compared with spin densities arrived at by quantum-mechanical calculations (20). The conclusions are that the unpaired spin density in the pyrimidine ring of flavin (ring C) is negligible. Thus N(1) and N(3) may not be significantly involved in electron transfer to and from the semiquinoid level. The highest unpaired spin density resides at N(5). In decreasing order, N(10), C(8), and C(6) also stand out as loci of high spin density. Thus atoms or groups attached to these atoms of high unpaired spin density, such as the protons at N(5) and C(6) or the methyl groups at N(10) (in lumiflavin) or C(8), will have appreciable unpaired spin density. From these results it is apparent that the strongly coupled proton, which dissociates from the neutral semiquinone as the pH is raised, is at N(5) and cannot be located at N(1), as had previously been thought. A proton at N(1) or N(3) would have negligible unpaired spin density, whereas it is found that the dissociating proton has in fact high spin density. Most recently interest was also focused on the carbon atoms that join the three rings of the flavin molecule (21). Substitution at C(12) has been observed during photoreduction in the presence of phenyl acetate (22). By labeling C(12) with ^{13}C ($I = \frac{1}{2}$) hfs could be resolved and it was concluded (21) that in the neutral and anionic semiquinone this carbon atom does indeed bear unpaired spin density of a magnitude similar to that of N(10). The unpaired spin density at C(12) appears to be particularly sensitive to the state of ionization of the semiquinone.

It had been shown that only flavin semiquinones, not the oxidized or reduced forms, are capable of forming 1:1 bidentate metal chelates (see Fig. 8-1) of appreciable stability (log K $\gtrsim$ 4) (23). Semiquinone chelates with paramagnetic metals are not detectable by EPR (24), whereas chelation with a diamagnetic metal may increase the radical signal intensity by an order of magnitude indicating that a large portion ($\sim$ 30 percent) of the flavin is in the semiquinone form under these conditions (14, 25). This is explained as a result of "comproportionation" in the equilibrium,

$$\text{flavin}_{\text{ox}} + \text{flavin}_{\text{red}} \leftrightharpoons 2 \text{ semiquinone}. \tag{8-1}$$

Hfs from the chelating metals Zn and Cd has been resolved in the semiquinone spectra, indicating spin delocalization onto the chelating metal atom. The metal replaces the proton, which in the neutral form is present at N(5). The hfs pattern of the metal chelates is therefore analogous to that of the anionic semiquinone. The chelates appear red to the eye, and this light absorption is qualitatively similar to that of the semiquinone anion, except at longer wavelengths.

8.2.1.2 Metal-Free Flavoproteins

Initial attempts to study semiquinone formation of metal-free flavoproteins were quite disappointing (26). Although a number of colored intermediates were observed on reaction of flavoproteins with substrates or substrate-related compounds (7, 27–30), EPR spectroscopy failed to show the intuitively expected radical signals. With metal-containing flavoproteins, on the other hand, EPR signals typical of free radicals were easily observed. It is now thought that most of the colored intermediates seen on addition of substrate to metal-free flavoproteins are not radicals but enzyme-substrate or reduced enzyme-product complexes which may show charge-transfer interaction. In some cases, however, it is suggested that a radical pair is formed. Under such conditions a number of possibilities for mutual interaction exist that would interfere with the straightforward observation of paramagnetism by EPR (cf. 7, 27).

Briefly, the electrons of the two radicals may be coupled by an electron-exchange interaction so that either a state with $S = 1$ (triplet state, see below) or a state with $S = 0$ (singlet state) lies lower in energy (see Section 1.9). In the former case this exchange interaction can cause electron-spin relaxation leading to a broadening of the resonance. In addition, it is likely that a strong dipole-dipole interaction exists which may cause the resonance to be spread out over a wide field. The broadening that results may be such that resonance cannot be detected. On the other hand, if the two electrons are coupled antiferromagnetically (singlet state lower), the system will be diamagnetic and no resonance will be detectable. This possibility has indeed been suggested to account for the absence of EPR signals in flavo-protein-substrate complexes.

It is easy to produce semiquinones of most flavoproteins simply by partial reduction, for example, with dithionite (26). These semiquinones often show light-absorption spectra quite similar to those of the mentioned enzyme-substrate complexes, but they do show EPR signals typical of free radicals. It must be kept in mind, however, that the semiquinone yield is not necessarily 100 percent, even on chemical reduction. As with free flavins, flavoproteins may be subject to the disproportionation equilibrium (Eq. 8-1). There may be kinetic inhibition and this equilibrium may be established very sluggishly. An interesting case is a flavoprotein from *Azotobacter vinelandii* (2, 31, 32), which at neutral pH forms 100 percent semiquinone even with an excess of dithionite and this semiquinone is remarkably stable toward reoxidation by oxygen. This protein is therefore useful as a semiquinone standard in quantitative work and in any magnetic resonance experimentation in which a protein-bound semiquinone is required at a high concentration. Thus this protein has been an ideal object for ENDOR studies (see below and Section 1.11).

A small number of flavoproteins of the type of lipoate dehydrogenase (cf. 30), which apparently have a dithiol-disulfide system at their active sites, do not show EPR signals even on reduction with dithionite. The explanation of this behavior has to be found along lines similar to those mentioned above, when the absence of signals on addition of substrate was discussed.

More recently a few flavoproteins that form EPR detectable semiquinones on addition of substrate have been found. To our knowledge the substrate in these instances has always been a reduced pyridine nucleotide. Two examples of such proteins are TPNH-cytochrome *c* reductase of liver microsomes (33) and ferredoxin-TPN reductase of spinach (34, 35).

It may be apparent from the foregoing discussion of the formation of EPR-detectable semiquinones from simple flavoproteins that the study of the enzymatic function of metal-free flavoproteins by EPR spectroscopy has not been and is not likely to become an active field.

EPR spectroscopy has rather more contributed to chemical and structural work on these proteins. The facility with which semiquinones may be produced in good yield from a number of metal-free flavoproteins by illumination in the presence of EDTA (6) has contributed to their usefulness in this respect.

It had been known since the potentiometric studies of Michaelis and his colleagues (16, 17) that semiquinone formation of flavins depends strongly on pH. This was later confirmed by spectrophotometry (18) and, as pointed out above, the hyperfine structure of the EPR spectra also indicated it very clearly. The pK values of the transition that lie in the pH range between 0 and 10 are $\sim$ 2.5 and 8.5, according to more recent measurements (5, 9, 19). It was, however, not suspected initially that anything but the neutral semiquinone form might be encountered when dealing with enzymes. An earlier suggestion that the red cationic form could be stabilized by a protein, the old yellow enzyme in this instance (36), proved to be erroneous (26, 37, 38). The red intermediate of this enzyme, formed in the presence of TPN and a reducing agent, is now considered to be an enzyme-substrate complex, as discussed above. It became apparent that not all flavoproteins formed the blue semiquinone, that is, the neutral species, but the semiquinones of some flavoproteins were reddish (6, 7). Hyperfine structure could not be resolved so that it could be used to indicate the protonation state of the semiquinone present (see above). EPR spectroscopy, however, did show a consistent difference in width ($\sim$ 4 G at 9000 MHz) between the signals of the blue, neutral flavoprotein semiquinones and those that lacked the typical long wavelength absorption. A rather convincing case in favor of the suggestion that a protonation equilibrium was involved in this phenomenon was the glucose oxidase semiquinone, which could be produced at low and high pH, partly because of the stability of this enzyme (6). Thus at pH 6 the blue semiquinone with an EPR signal of 19 G width was observed, whereas at pH 9 the reddish semiquinone appeared with a signal of 15 G width. With all other flavoproteins either the neutral or the anionic form of the semiquinone is obtained within the range of pH in which the protein is stable. Examples of the proteins that form the blue semiquinone are the azotobacter flavoprotein (31, 32), the acyl CoA dehydrogenases (39), and the ferredoxin-TPN reductases (6, 38). Examples of the proteins that form the red species are oxynitrilase (6), the old yellow enzyme (6), and the amino acid oxidases (6). Although it is likely that the red form is indeed the anion, it has been shown that a tautomer of the neutral form may have a similar absorption spectrum (5, 14) (cf. Fig. 8-1). As mentioned above, a decision could be brought about if hfs of the EPR spectra could be studied. It may also be of interest here to mention that in D_2O the width of the EPR signal of the blue semiquinone is decreased from 19 to approximately 15 G (40), whereas the width of the signal of the red semiquinone remains unchanged. This again indicates that the blue semiquinone has an exchangeable proton [at N(5)], which with protein-bound flavins increases the linewidth by unresolved hfs and which is not present in the red anionic semiquinone. It also appears that the splitting contributed by this proton is quite similar to that observed in semiquinones of free flavins (40).

In this context an interesting suggestion concerning the stabilization of the two ionic forms of flavin semiquinones by the protein may be mentioned. This is schematically shown in Fig. 8-2 (5). It is thought that the neutral semiquinone may be stabilized by a strong hydrogen bond from

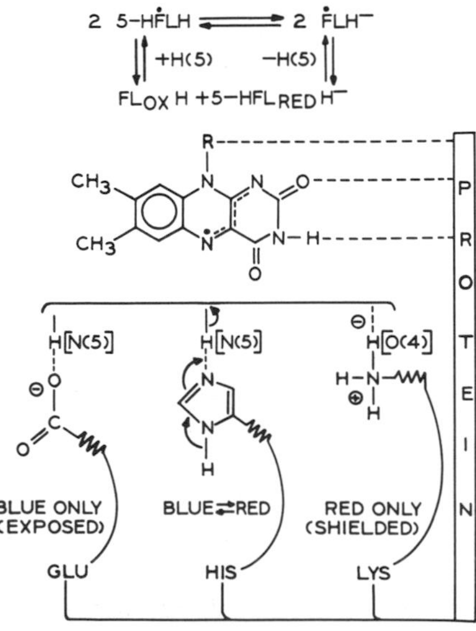

Fig. 8-2 Schematic drawing illustrating the proposed stabilization of the neutral or anionic flavoprotein semiquinone by appropriate groups on the protein; according to Müller et al. (5).

N(5) to a group from the protein, for example, a glutamic acid residue. Similarly the anionic form may be stabilized by the presence of a proton-withdrawing group, such as the ε-amino group of a lysine residue, in the vicinity of O(4). In line with this suggestion is the finding by ENDOR spectroscopy (see below) that the red semiquinone of the "old yellow enzyme" is less exposed to protons of the solvent than the blue semiquinone of the azotobacter flavoprotein. This argument concerning stabilization of different ionic forms is extended even to the one instance in which, depending on conditions, a red or a blue protein-bound semiquinone can be observed, that is, to glucose oxidase. In this case the imidazole portion of histidine is suggested as the stabilizing group.

A curious phenomenon has been discovered in the study of the semiquinone signals of glucose and *d*-amino acid oxidases and lipoate dehydrogenase (30) (signals can be obtained from lipoate dehydrogenase in the presence of DPNH and DPN). The room-temperature spectra showed structure that became much more pronounced with increasing power. It appeared as if a less readily saturable radical signal of 70 to 80 G width had been superimposed on the usual semiquinone signal of 15 to 19 G width, which is easily saturated. As the power is increased, this has the effect that the wings of the signal grow in intensity, whereas the center collapses. This behavior is seen down to $-30\,^{\circ}C$ (41) but disappears in the frozen state below this temperature. A survey then showed that this is rather generally observed with metal-free flavoproteins, whether they form the blue (neutral) or red (anionic) semiquinone on partial reduction, but this phenomenon was not observed under any conditions with the semiquinone of the simplest metalflavoprotein, that is, dihydroorotate dehydrogenase (41). However, since the semiquinone signal from this protein is much less readily saturated than those from metal-free flavoproteins, it may well be that the effect of power on the center and wings does not differ greatly in this situation. A number of explanations for this phenomenon have been advanced, none of them very convincing (41, 42). More recently it was proposed (40) that the two species, the spectra of which appear to be superimposed, are the semiquinone as such and a complex of semiquinone with water. Exchange of the water from the binding site with solvent water was thought to bring about increased linewidth and electron spin relaxation of one of the species by modulation of the anisotropic hfs and Zeeman splittings. Support for these ideas was seen in NMR measurements of the relaxation time of water protons in the presence of a flavoprotein semiquinone. These measurements showed a remarkable effect of the semiquinone on the protons of solvent water, indicating that water is close to the unpaired electron of the semiquinone and that this water does exchange with solvent water at a rapid rate.

However, another explanation for the anomalous saturation of the wings of flavin semiquinone signals involves only the intrinsic features of the "powder spectrum" of flavin semiquinones (42a) and is therefore, because of its simplicity, the most plausible yet brought forth. According to computer simulations of the expected powder EPR spectra of a flavin radical with known isotropic hfs, the two strongly coupled nitrogen atoms [N(5) and N(10)] make the principal contribution to the anisotropic hfs. The outer hfs lines due to these nitrogen atoms would be responsible for the "wings". The previously reported saturation behavior of these wings could be duplicated by a model system, that is, a lumiflavin radical in toluene.

The example just discussed emphasizes the need for careful study of the behavior of signals as a function of microwave power and temperature and illustrates the differences in appearance of relatively simple signals in the liquid and solid state. Since only one of the more plausible explanations discussed above can be correct, the example also shows the difficulty of providing unambiguous proof that a particular mechanism, reasonable as it may appear, does indeed apply.

8.2.1.3 Metalflavoproteins

Semiquinones are readily observed by EPR with all known metalflavoproteins (27) (see below) when partly reduced with substrate. The signal intensities vary widely, from less than 1 percent to approximately 50 percent, depending on the specific protein, the reducing substrate, the oxidant (if present), ratios of enzyme, reductant and oxidant concentrations, pH, temperature, and time of reaction.

Often the highest radical yields are seen in the presence of an excess over the protein of both reductant and oxidant. At X-band frequency the semiquinone signals generally overlap with the low field portions of the iron and molybdenum signals. Interference from the iron signals can be largely eliminated by working at relatively high temperature (> 120 K) and the lowest feasible power. Decrease of power may be of some help in the case of an overlapping Mo signal, since semiquinone signals generally are more readily saturated than Mo signals. There are, however, exceptions to this rule. To avoid all interference we may have to resort to EPR spectroscopy at higher frequency (see below) so that minor differences in g factors can be taken advantage of. Other interfering species, although not specific for semiquinones of metalflavoproteins, are other radical species present in the system. Recently the superoxide anion radical ($O_2^{-\cdot}$) was identified as a species occurring in flavoprotein-substrate-oxygen systems (43). The high field ($g_\perp$) portion of this signal completely obscures the semiquinone signal (Fig. 8-3). The $O_2^{-\cdot}$ signal can, however, be recognized by its anisotropy ($g_\parallel \approx 2.1$) and asymmetry of the high field line. In some instances, in which overlap with other signals is not apparent, the semiquinone signals of flavoproteins or metalflavoproteins nevertheless show

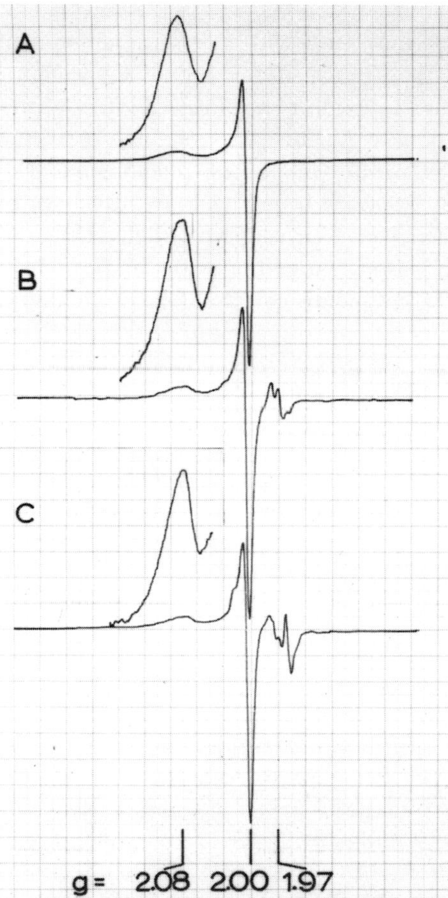

Fig. 8-3 EPR spectra of superoxide anion radical, $O_2^{-\cdot}$, produced in different ways; according to Orme-Johnson and Beinert (44). A–C, EPR spectra observed 150 msec after mixing various reducing mixtures with an equal volume of oxygenated buffer. A. 0.31 m*M* sodium dithionite in 0.01 *M* potassium phosphate of pH 7.4 was mixed with 1 *M* glycine buffer of pH 10.5. B. 0.053 m*M* xanthine oxidase in 0.01 *M* pyrophosphate of pH 8.5 was reduced anaerobically with sodium dithionite, corresponding to 14 eq per mole of enzyme, and mixed and frozen as in A. C. 0.025 m*M* xanthine oxidase, dissolved as in B, was mixed with oxygenated glycine buffer as in A, which contained 2 m*M* xanthine. The conditions of EPR spectroscopy were microwave power, 45 mwatt; modulation amplitude 2 G; and temperature, 102 K. The enlarged low-field portion at $g = 2.08$ was recorded at an amplification fourfold higher than that used for the complete spectra and at 6 G modulation amplitude. The relative amplifications used for recording spectra A to C were 1, 2, 1.25. At $g = 1.97$ signals of Mo(V) are seen with xanthine oxidase. Under the experimental conditions used the flavin and Mo signals are partly saturated. The signal at $g = 2.00$ in B and C may have a small contribution from the flavin semiquinone. All EPR spectra shown in this chapter represent the first derivative of the absorption line (except for the schematic presentation of Fig. 8-7) versus magnetic field, with the field increasing from left to right.

structure. This structure, however, is poorly resolved (45, 46). It may have an origin similar to that seen with the semiquinones of metal-free flavoproteins, although the signals of the metalflavoprotein semiquinone have so far not been found to exhibit the unusual effect of microwave power on lineshape, discussed above. The semiquinones of metalflavoproteins lend themselves to studies of spin relaxation phenomena (41), since these semiquinones are readily obtained in fair yield, relatively stable, and show easily measurable dependence of their relaxation behavior on a number of factors and conditions. This aspect, together with the possible interaction of these semiquinones with the metal components of metalflavoproteins, is discussed below. Observations on semiquinones of flavoproteins in redox titrations and studies of enzyme reaction rates will also be dealt with in subsequent sections of this chapter.

8.2.1.4 ENDOR Spectroscopy of Flavin and Flavoprotein Semiquinones (see also Section 1.11)

It is probably correct to say that the elaboration of the distribution of unpaired spin density in flavin semiquinones extends present EPR capabilities, as far as techniques, analysis, and interpretation go, to the limit.* It must be kept in mind that with an increasing number of nuclei magnetically coupled to an unpaired electron the number of lines in the EPR spectrum increases in geometrical progression, whereas the linewidth of the envelope remains essentially unchanged; that is, more lines will have to be accommodated in the same space. Analysis then requires increased resolution and thus demands decrease of the modulation amplitude. Molecular size and solubility of biologically active compounds finally set a limit to resolution by the signal-to-noise ratio achievable under such conditions.

Fortunately the technique of electron-nuclear double resonance (ENDOR) spectroscopy (47) is ideally suited to circumvent the difficulties that stem from the multiplicity of the EPR lines, at least in principle. Here the nuclei that interact with an unpaired electron can be specifically identified by their characteristic nuclear resonance frequencies; that is, we do not have to search for all nuclear couplings under a single EPR signal envelope, so to speak. Rather we have the large spectrum of nuclear resonance frequencies to choose from. In addition, since the intensity of ENDOR lines depends on the nuclear magnetic moment, the lines of certain nuclei, such as protons, will stand out in the spectrum, whereas those from other nuclei may not be detectable at all with present instrumentation. At this time the limitations of this technique appear to be more of a technical nature than inherent in its basic capability. Interesting beginnings have

* At the time this book goes to press it appears that the advent of pulsed Fourier transform EPR spectroscopy and electron spin relaxation measurements by this technique will exceed these limits in the forseeable future.

been made in the flavin and nonheme iron fields (48 to 50a, 82), both subjects with which we are concerned in this chapter.

In the study of electron-nuclear spin-spin interactions by EPR as well as ENDOR spectroscopy resolution depends critically on the degree of isotropy of these interactions. It was pointed out above that hfs cannot be resolved satisfactorily in frozen solutions of flavin semiquinones or with protein-bound semiquinones. In either situation anisotropic interactions arise by immobilization. In attempts to apply ENDOR spectroscopy to flavin semiquinones the question had to be answered whether with any electron-nuclear interaction in these systems the isotropic part would be of sufficient strength to allow resolution. Fortunately this is quite generally the case with protons attached to β carbons of π electron radicals (51) and applies particularly to methyl groups in these positions. Such methyl groups appear to rotate freely and at a velocity sufficient to average out anisotropic interactions even in the glassy state. Thus it is possible to observe ENDOR lines from the methyl group of flavin compounds, which is located in the 8 position. It should be recalled (Table 8-1) that only this methyl group and not that in position 7 bears appreciable unpaired spin density. With lumiflavin, of course, the methyl group in position 10 is also susceptible to ENDOR spectroscopy. Because of the apparently unhindered rotation of these methyl groups even at low temperature and in proteins ENDOR lines can be satisfactorily resolved even with protein-bound semiquinones at low temperature. This has been of particular interest in the study of flavin binding to succinate dehydrogenase (52–54). The FAD group of this enzyme is covalently bound, and it has been proposed that this linkage is at the 8 position. The ENDOR spectra, which are well suited for observing the substituent in this position, do indeed support this conclusion.

To date the conclusions drawn from the EPR data on the principal hyperfine couplings in flavin semiquinones have been confirmed by ENDOR spectroscopy. The resolution was not sufficient to study the weaker couplings. Eventually, however, ENDOR should be able to furnish values for the hyperfine splitting constants more accurate than those derived from the EPR spectra.

Additional information, not accessible from conventional EPR spectroscopy, can be derived from what is called the "matrix" ENDOR signal. This is generally a rather intense and broad signal centered in the spectrum around the frequency of free protons, which arises from interaction of the unpaired spin system with protons in close vicinity (6 Å). This signal therefore provides a probe for the immediate environment of the flavin.

In the case of flavoproteins the protons giving rise to the matrix signal are thought to be directly bound to the protein or as part of solvation water rather than protons of free solvent. It is then possible to probe the hydrophilic character of the site around the semiquinone by comparing the matrix ENDOR signal intensity in H_2O and D_2O. This signal will be decreased in D_2O if there are exchangeable protons, which would

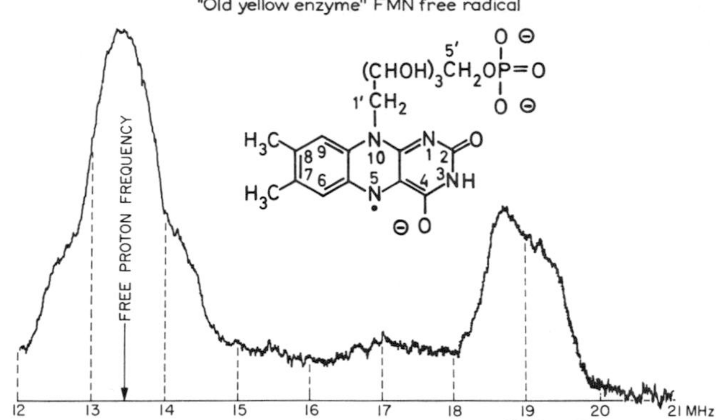

Fig. 8-4 ENDOR spectrum of the semiquinone of FMN bound to the "old yellow enzyme," recorded at 4.7 mW microwave power and 113 K. 0.5 m*M* enzyme in 20 m*M* tris buffer of pH 9.0 was photoreduced anaerobically in the presence of 10 m*M* EDTA [according to Ehrenberg et al. (48)].

indicate hydrophilic character. Thus, for instance, the matrix ENDOR signals observed with two different flavoproteins, "old yellow enzyme," a DPNH dehydrogenase (Fig. 8-4), and an azotobacter flavoprotein of unknown function, behaved in opposite ways when the proteins were dissolved in D_2O, indicating in this instance, that the flavin in the "old yellow enzyme" is in a more hydrophobic environment than that in the azotobacter flavoprotein. It may be worth mentioning that much the same information is accessible by proton relaxation studies, a pulsed NMR technique, where the nuclear spin relaxation of water protons is observed. If water protons come close to the unpaired spin system of the semiquinone, they experience a relaxation enhancement which can be measured. Indeed, both kinds of approaches have been used with flavoproteins.

8.2.2 Metal Constituents of Metalflavoproteins

To date the metalflavoproteins known are those containing flavin and iron or flavin, iron, and molybdenum (Table 8-2). The majority of the iron-flavoproteins contain nonheme iron of the ferredoxin type and may therefore also be considered as iron-sulfur proteins containing flavin. In addition, there are a few heme-flavoproteins, of which the best characterized representative is yeast L(+)lactate dehydrogenase or cytochrome b_2 (57, 58). A number of reports indicate that in microorganisms a number of heme-containing flavoproteins may exist, such as a formic dehydrogenase of *E. coli* (64). Unless they are thoroughly investigated, however, the

Table 8-2 Metal Flavoproteins

Flavoprotein	MW[a]	FAD	FMN	Components per molecule: Fe (Iron-sulfur)	Fe (heme)	Mo	Main source	Ref.
Trivial name								
Succinate dehydrogenase	200	1	—	4–8	—	—	Mammals (heart), yeast	55
DPNH dehydrogenase	500–1000	—	1	16–18	—	—	Mammals (heart)	55
Dihydroorotate dehydrogenase	100	2	2	4	—	—	Bacteria	46, 56
L(+) lactate dehydrogenase	200	—	4	—	4	—	Yeast	57, 58
Sulfite reductase	800	4	4	12	2	—	Bacteria	59
Xanthine oxidase or dehydrogenase	300	2	—	8	—	2	Mammals (milk, liver), bacteria	60, 61
Aldehyde oxidase	300	2	—	8	—	2	Mammals (liver)	62
Nitrate reductase[b]	200	+	—	?	+	+	Molds and bacteria	63

[a] Molecular weights are given to the closest 100,000 daltons merely for orientation, since in some cases the exact numbers depend on the source and type of preparation or are not yet certain.

[b] The exact composition has not been reported.

possibility must always be kept in mind that a cytochrome is merely associated with a flavoprotein and not part of the same molecule. One of the most complicated molecules belonging in the category of metal flavoproteins is bacterial sulfite reductase, which contains flavin, nonheme and heme iron (Table 8-2) (59).

It may be useful for the discussion of the EPR properties of these complex proteins if we consider separately the properties of the metal constituents involved, namely, the iron-sulfur structure of the nonheme iron component and molybdenum.

8.2.2.1 The Iron-Sulfur Group

To date no well-characterized model of low molecular weight of the iron-sulfur structure is available, so that the simplest units containing this structure remain the proteins of the plant ferredoxin type of relatively small molecular weight ($> 10{,}000$). Several of these proteins are now quite well studied. Their amino acid sequence, metal and sulfur content, EPR, light absorption, circular dichroism (CD), Mössbauer spectra, and magnetic susceptibilities are available. At this time, however, the chemical information is more definitive than what physical measurements have contributed. The reason is that the interpretation of the chemical results is intrinsically less demanding than that of physical measurements. It is likely, however, that as further progress is made it will be possible to evaluate more completely the information contained in the data obtained by the various physical techniques. Often the evaluation of data from one technique relies on results furnished by another. Thus a meaningful interpretation of the Mössbauer spectra of iron-sulfur proteins obtained in a magnetic field required information on hyperfine coupling constants which is most reliably furnished by ENDOR spectroscopy. Measurements of these values by ENDOR spectroscopy, in turn, is greatly aided by information available from EPR spectroscopy. In the history of the discovery and definition of properties of the iron-sulfur proteins, at least, EPR spectroscopy proved to be the most useful tool at the earlier, exploratory phases, whereas in the final analysis probably ENDOR and Mössbauer spectroscopy furnished more decisive information. A number of recent review articles are available on iron-sulfur proteins (65–69); therefore we can confine ourselves to the essential aspects.

The simplest of these proteins contain two iron atoms, two atoms of "labile sulfur" and in addition at least four cysteine residues. The term labile sulfur indicates that this sulfur is liberated as H_2S on acidification to pH < 3 or even on standing at room temperature at neutral pH. These are not properties typical of the sulfur of cysteine in proteins.

Magnetic susceptibility measurements in the range of 4 K to room temperature show that the paramagnetism of the oxidized forms of these simplest iron-sulfur proteins is either negligible over this whole temperature range (70) or measurable only toward room temperature, but still considerably smaller (71, 72, 72a) than what would be expected for ferric iron in the high or low spin state. Consequently no EPR signal is observed. On reduction, however, paramagnetism appears, corresponding to a spin of $\frac{1}{2}$, and the EPR signal, which is now observed (cf. Fig. 8-5), indicates the presence of one unpaired electron per molecule, that is, per two iron and two labile sulfur atoms. In agreement with this, reductive titration shows that one electron per molecule is necessary to produce the maximal EPR signal and maximal bleaching of the optical spectrum (Fig. 8-6) (74).

It is possible to exchange iron and labile sulfur in all of the simple iron-sulfur proteins. Thus proteins with various iron and sulfur isotopes and even with selenium (75, 76) instead of sulfur can be prepared simply by

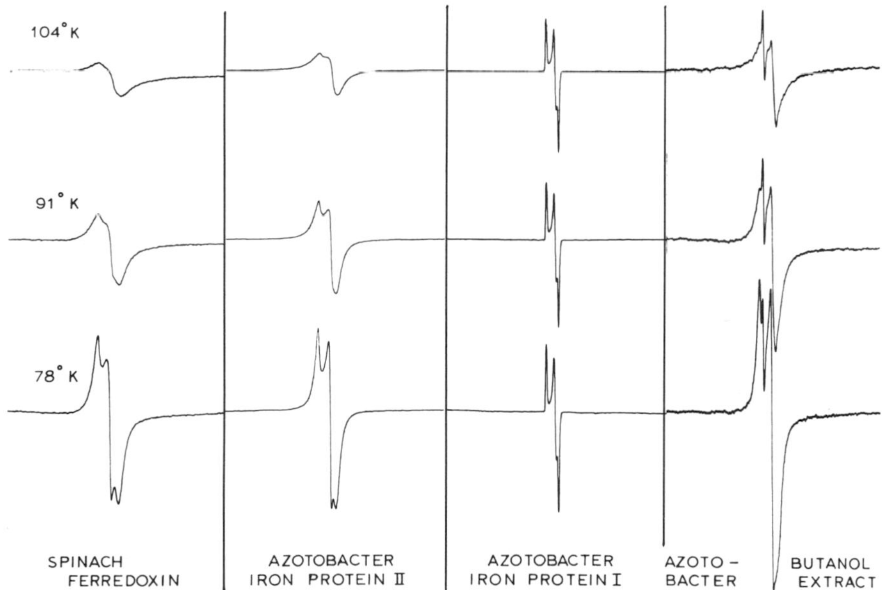

Fig. 8-5 Examples of iron-sulfur proteins with different electron spin relaxation behavior, as expressed in the temperature-dependence of their EPR signals. According to Shethna et al. (73), EPR spectra (first derivative) are shown at three different temperatures as indicated. The conditions of EPR spectroscopy were microwave power, 27 mW; modulation amplitude, 6 G; and temperature as indicated. The total scan represents approximately 2500 G, with the field increasing from left to right. The butanol extract contains both Azotobacter proteins I and II.

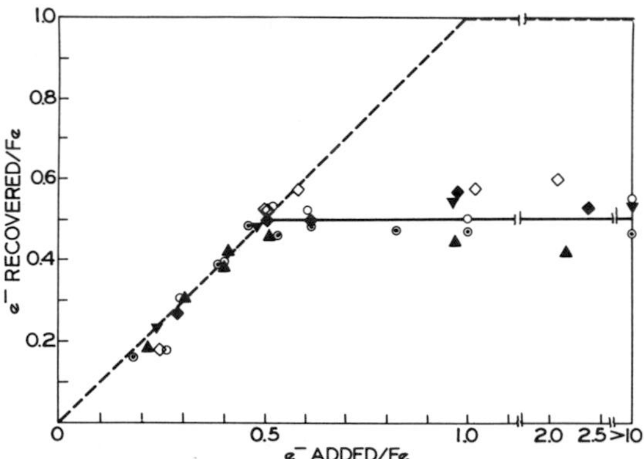

Fig. 8-6 Titration of six iron-sulfur proteins of the plant ferredoxin type with dithionite as monitored by observation of the EPR signals at $g = 1.94$, according to Orme-Johnson and Beinert (74). The symbols represent putidaredoxin (▼), spinach ferredoxin (▲), bovine (◆), and pig (⊙) adrenal iron-sulfur proteins, and *Azotobacter* iron-sulfur proteins I (O) and II (◇); methyl viologen was added to the adrenal protein. The ascending dashed line represents the theoretical curve for 1 electron recovered in the EPR spectrum per electron added; the horizontal dashed line represents the expected curve when 2 electrons are required to reduce a given protein maximally; and the horizontal full line represents the case in which 1 electron (0.5 electrons per iron atom) is needed to maximally reduce the iron proteins.

this exchange. It was thus possible to substitute ^{57}Fe for ^{56}Fe, ^{33}S for ^{32}S, and ^{77}Se for ^{80}Se in the Se-analogs. In two proteins, in which biological activity was tested, the Se analogs were found to possess catalytic activity and hfs with ^{57}Fe similar to those observed with the natural (^{32}S) materials. This showed that the analogs were not radically different structures. By observing the hfs which ensued following the mentioned substitutions it could then be demonstrated that in the reduced form the unpaired spin whose presence is indicated by the magnetic measurements, results from interactions of both iron and both labile sulfur (or Se) atoms (76, 77). From inspection of the spectra obtained with two of the simpler iron sulfur proteins, putidaredoxin and adrenodoxin, which were labeled with ^{57}Fe or ^{77}Se, one would be inclined to conclude that in the reduced state the two iron or selenium (or sulfur) atoms involved are equivalent, that is, the iron atoms among themselves and the selenium (or sulfur) atoms among themselves (the distribution of unpaired spin density between iron and sulfur cannot be derived from the EPR spectra and hfs without some arbitrary assumptions). However, recent data obtained from Mössbauer spectroscopy (78, 79) apparently cannot be reconciled with a model in which the iron atoms are equivalent. These limitations of the interpretation of EPR "powder" spectra are discussed next. Additional experiments in which bacteria were grown on ^{33}S or ^{32}S, the iron sulfur proteins isolated, and the "labile sulfur" exchanged for ^{32}S or ^{33}S, respectively, showed that cysteine sulfur from the protein also made a contribution to hfs (80). The overall splitting by the contributing cysteine sulfurs, whose exact number (≤ 5) is not known, was even higher than that from the labile sulfurs.

It may be useful at this point to digress from the main theme and consider some experiences and implications of the study and interpretation of hfs in asymmetric signals such as those of the iron-sulfur proteins. These signals, in the simplest case, are axially symmetric and show two g factors ($g_{\parallel} \approx 2.01$, $g_{\perp} \approx 1.94$). As in other transition-metal complexes, hfs can be observed at low temperature. The best resolution was obtained with putidaredoxin and "adrenodoxin." The signals of both proteins have an appearance typical of that of an axially symmetric structure. According to the known splitting scheme (Fig. 8-7) for two equivalent nuclei interacting with one unpaired electron, the shape of the resultant EPR spectrum can be predicted for various enrichments in the isotope with nuclear spin and various strengths of the splitting (width in gauss). The observed spectrum, in addition, depends on the linewidth. The most simple-minded approach, which indeed (and in retrospect surprisingly!) seemed to lead to success with putidaredoxin, was then to assume that the structure was indeed axially symmetric (i.e., $g_x = g_y$), that there was only isotropic

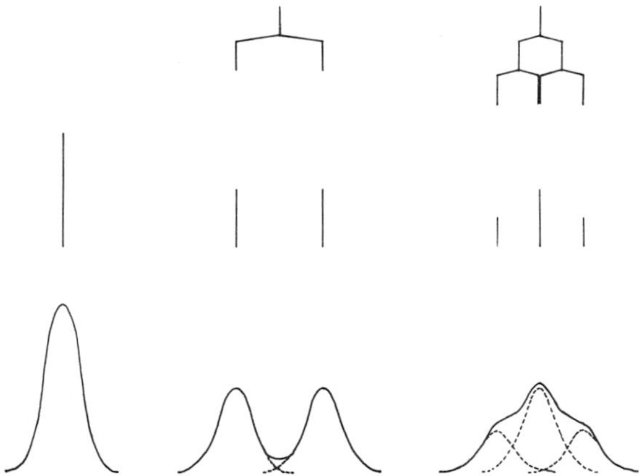

Fig. 8-7 Schematic presentation of hfs arising in an EPR absorption line (*left*) from interaction of the unpaired electron with one (*center*) or two (*right*) nuclei of $I = \frac{1}{2}$. The top row represents "stick diagrams," and in the bottom row the effect of hfs is shown when an arbitrary line width is assumed. Note that, when an EPR spectrum is presented as the first derivative of the absorption line, portions of this spectrum, which have the shape of an absorption line (e.g., low field part of Fig. 8-8) can be treated as an absorption line as shown in the example above.

hfs, and no change in linewidth of individual lines in going from the natural to the isotopically substituted protein. If these assumptions were all valid, or at least closely approximated, it should then be possible (Fig. 8-8) to reproduce the spectrum of the isotopically substituted material by superposition of the EPR spectra of the unsubstituted protein centered at different field positions and with different intensities according to the theoretical splitting scheme as represented in Fig. 8-7. The enrichment in

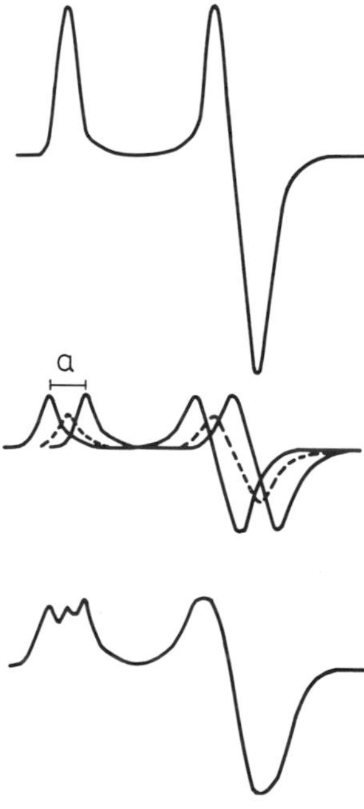

Fig. 8-8 Scheme illustrating construction of the EPR spectrum (first derivative) of an axially symmetric structure (e.g., a reduced iron-sulfur protein) for the case in which the unpaired electron interacts with one nucleus of $I = \frac{1}{2}$ and in which the enrichment of this nucleus in the molecule is 75 percent; an isotope of the same nucleus but with $I = 0$ is assumed to be present in the remaining 25 percent of the paramagnetic centers. The top line shows the original spectrum if 100 percent of the potentially interacting nuclei have $I = 0$. The center line illustrates the procedure of construction of the spectrum. The spectrum stemming from the centers containing the isotope with ($I = 0$) and representing 25 percent of the original intensity is plotted in the original field position (*dashed line*). Two spectra (cf., scheme of Fig. 8-7, *center*), each representing $\frac{1}{2} \times 75$ percent of the original intensity, are then plotted at an equal distance down- and upfield from the original position of the spectrum (*solid lines*); the distance of any point of the new spectra from the corresponding point of the original spectrum corresponds to $|\frac{a}{2}|$, i.e., one-half the hyperfine splitting. This value may be derived from observations or, if none is available, must be assumed from reasonable analogies to known spectra. To obtain the composite line of the resulting spectrum (*bottom curve*) the curves are simply added. It can be seen that hfs is resolved in some parts of the spectrum, whereas in others only broadening results.

the isotope with nuclear spin must of course be accounted for. This can be done by superimposing the original spectrum in the center (i.e., in its natural position) with the proper intensity to represent the unenriched fraction (cf. Fig. 8-8, center curve). These operations may be done by hand, which is a tedious procedure; they may be done by the computer of average transients, often available in connection with EPR or NMR instrumentation; and, of course, they are most effectively carried out by a digital computer. Although at the time these spectra were obtained and analyzed the case of putidaredoxin appeared to be quite clear-cut and the fits of the spectra by the simple model amazingly good, a warning was sounded by the fact that it was not possible to fit the spectra of any of the other simple iron-sulfur proteins nearly so well. Only the low-field portion ($g_z = 2.01$) of "adrenodoxin" allowed a similarly good fit (81); there remained a number of discrepancies with the high-field absorption. The reasons for this behavior could be one or several of the following:

1. The structure is in fact rhombic and not of perfect axial symmetry ($g_x \neq g_y$) but the separation of g_x and g_y is of the order of the linewidth.
2. The hyperfine splitting is anisotropic, that is, different in different directions of the magnetic field.
3. The axes of the anisotropic g tensor are not the same as those of the A tensor, which relates to anisotropic hfs.
4. There is hfs contributed, but unresolved, from magnetic nuclei such as the proton or nitrogen.
5. The widths of the individual lines are not the same for the substituted as for the natural material.

It appears now that the intepretation of the EPR spectra of reduced ^{57}Fe labeled putidaredoxin is still subject to ambiguities, despite the excellent fit of the spectra to those computed for a simple model of two equivalent iron atoms which interact with a single unpaired electron. According to the results of ENDOR spectroscopy (82), even in putidaredoxin $g_x \neq g_y$ and the hyperfine coupling constants A_x, A_y, and A_z are not identical so that the success in the computer simulation of the whole spectrum with a single value of A seems fortuitous. Furthermore, the most consistent interpretation of the Mössbauer spectra recorded at different temperatures and magnetic fields on a number of iron-sulfur proteins is that based on the model of Gibson et al. (83). According to this model the oxidized forms of the simple iron-sulfur proteins can be formally represented as containing two high-spin ferric ions, which are coupled by antiferromagnetic interaction, so that a spin of 0 (diamagnetism) results. In the reduced state one electron is taken up and the result is an antiferromagnetically coupled ferric-ferrous pair—both of high spin—with a resulting spin of $\frac{1}{2}$, as observed, in fact, by EPR and magnetic susceptibility measurements. When ^{56}Fe is exchanged for ^{57}Fe, the ferric as well as the ferrous ion contribute to hfs, and it so happens that the effective A values of each ion are similar. For spinach ferredoxin values of 15.2 G have been found for the ferric and 12.5 G for the ferrous ion, whereas the value that gave the best fit for the simulation of the EPR spectra of ^{57}Fe putidaredoxin was 14 G. Thus it is understandable that the two iron atoms appeared to be equivalent on the basis of hfs analysis alone, whereas in fact they may well be as different as ENDOR and Mössbauer spectra indicate. The A_x and A_y values for the ferric and ferrous ions of the reduced form differ considerably in spinach ferredoxin, which would readily explain the failure to compute the spectra for this ferredoxin or a number of other iron-sulfur proteins on the simple model of Figs. 8-7 and 8-8. It might also be mentioned that point 3 above, namely rotation of the axis system of the A tensor versus that of the g tensor, does not appear to occur to an extent that would complicate reconstruction of the spectra, whereas, according to ENDOR, point 4, namely the presence of unresolved hfs from protons and nitrogens, appears to be a source of interference. Nevertheless, the hfs analysis of the spectra of reduced putidaredoxin and adrenodoxin did furnish unambiguous proof that iron-sulfur proteins have a two-iron center, with both iron atoms interacting such that one unpaired spin results, although the further assumption that the two iron atoms may be equivalent does not seem likely now (79, 83a). In the case of the two Se atoms, which could be similarly shown to interact with the unpaired spin (76), the inference of equivalence may well be correct. The lesson to be learned from this experience is, first, that there are subtle differences between the structures of the various iron-sulfur proteins, although no doubt they are closely related, and, second, that it is probably the exception rather than the rule that analysis of complex EPR spectra on the basis of simplifying assumptions is successful. The example clearly shows the advantage of calling on a variety of physical methods for definitive characterization of complex structures.

The iron-sulfur structures of simple iron-sulfur proteins not only differ in the anisotropy of g factors and hfs but they also differ markedly in their spin relaxation behavior. Some of the proteins, such as putidaredoxin, have spectra that are readily and clearly observed at 170 K, whereas others, such as spinach ferredoxin, are barely resolved at 77 K (cf. 73, 84). The signals of proteins such as spinach ferredoxin broaden out rapidly with increasing temperature, the separation of g_x and g_y is lost, and integrations are bound to fail as the intensity moves from the center of the spectrum to the wings. This is illustrated in Fig. 8-5 by the example of two iron-sulfur proteins of *Azotobacter vinelandii.* They differ widely in their spin relaxation behavior and therefore in the temperature sensitivity of their EPR signals. All iron flavoproteins studied to date (cf. Table 8-2) show a spin relaxation behavior more akin to spinach ferredoxin or azotobacter protein II of

Fig. 8-5 than to the less relaxed species, such as putidaredoxin, adrenodoxin, or azotobacter protein I. In view of this wide variation in spin relaxation of iron-sulfur proteins, which has been observed, it becomes mandatory to check temperature and power dependence of the EPR signals of new members of this class carefully before drawing conclusions on the quantity of unpaired spins represented in the signals and on the splitting and exact location of the derivative maxima and minima. This will be appreciated by inspection of the various spectra shown in Fig. 8-5.

Another difficulty has been encountered with iron-molybdenum flavoproteins. In the EPR spectra of these proteins hfs from molybdenum signals may overlap with the signal of the iron-sulfur group (85) and the contribution from molybdenum may be mistaken for *g*-factor anisotropy in the iron signal. Again observation at different powers and temperatures will be helpful in resolving uncertainties in such instances.

For some years there has been a debate of doubtful usefulness about the valence state of the iron in the iron-sulfur structure of simple and complex iron sulfur proteins (86). Although in the formalism of the model systems mentioned the true situation is approximated by using the terms ferric and ferrous, the analysis of hyperfine interactions has shown (see above) that after reduction the resulting unpaired spin is related or interacts with a number of atoms. A valency change by an integral number of any individual atom involved can therefore obviously not occur. The initial state of the complex before reduction is diamagnetic. It is therefore ambiguous to assign a valency to the iron in this state (cf. 78). Although the idea of antiferromagnetic interaction of two ferric iron atoms provides an appealing explanation (cf. 69, 83) for a number of observations, it must be kept in mind that the metal complex has been shown by EPR (hfs), ENDOR, and Mössbauer spectroscopy to have considerable covalent character. The conclusion to be drawn at this time is probably best summarized in the words of Dunham et al. (83a) in their detailed analysis of the physical measurements so far available: "Although the assignment of definite valencies to the iron atoms in the active site is presumptuous in view of the covalent bonding present, any assignment of electron configuration other than two high-spin d^5 ions in the oxidized proteins and one each of high-spin d^5 and d^6 in the reduced proteins is much more misleading, since the electric field gradient tensor at the reduced protein ferrous iron is characteristic of the high-spin ferrous ion" [according to Mössbauer spectroscopy (79)].

Although in the reduced forms of the plant-type ferredoxins the EPR signal accounts for one unpaired electron for every two iron atoms (74), in the bacterial ferredoxins there are even more iron atoms present per unpaired electron detected by EPR (87), obviously indicating additional complexity. Of the metalflavoproteins, so far only dihydroorotate dehydrogenase appears to follow the simpler pattern of the plant-type ferredoxins inasmuch as two unpaired electrons are accounted for in the EPR signal of the molecule, which contains four iron atoms and four flavin groups, that is, 2 FAD and 2 FMN. With succinate and DPNH dehydrogenases the ratio of iron atoms present to unpaired electrons accounted for in the signal at $g = 1.94$ is between 6:1 and 8:1 (88) and ~ 4:1 (88a) respectively. It must be emphasized, though, that these ratios depend on the type of preparation considered. The ratios given are valid for the preparations most frequently used today.

A number of DPNH dehydrogenase preparations are known which on reduction do not show a significant EPR signal indicative of a metal. These are the preparations of lower molecular weight, and it is likely that a protein component, which contains all or part of the nonheme iron portion of the original complex DPNH dehydrogenase, has been separated or destroyed. Such a separation has in fact been reported (89), but the fact that it is possible does not prove that a flavoprotein and a nonheme iron protein pre-existed as discrete units.

If we assume, in keeping with the behavior of the plant-type ferredoxins, that one unpaired electron in the EPR spectrum accounts in fact for two iron atoms, there are then four to six iron atoms of succinate dehydrogenase unaccounted for by EPR spectroscopy. It appears, however, from comparisons of light absorption and EPR spectra obtained during kinetic investigations and reductive titrations that the EPR undetectable iron atoms are represented in the light absorption spectra with absorptivities not radically different from the EPR detectable ones (90). The same seems to hold for the iron-molybdenum flavoproteins (85). The example of these latter proteins has, however, taught that it is wise at this time to reserve final judgment on the detectability of iron atoms by EPR until spectra have been obtained at very low temperatures (1 to 4 K). Thus until relatively recently it was thought that, according to the results of EPR spectroscopy at temperatures of about 30 K and higher and on the basis of the one electron per two iron atoms model, four iron atoms are detectable out of the eight present per molecule in xanthine and aldehyde oxidases. These two iron-molybdenum flavoproteins have been most thoroughly studied by EPR spectroscopy. EPR spectroscopy at temperatures between 10 and 20 K has shown, however, that there is an additional absorption which must probably be attributed to iron (91, 92). This absorption occurs at $g = 2.11$. It is likely that parts of the same signal with one ($g_\perp$) or two (g_x, g_y) other g values are hidden under the main absorption of the $g = 1.94$ signal, which is simultaneously present.

It has been shown that the usual $g = 1.94$ signals of metalflavoproteins are saturated at very low temperatures. A saturation curve at 4 K for succinate dehydrogenase, for instance, is reported in Ref. 88. Nevertheless, even if additional EPR absorptions are found for these complex proteins, so that the iron present can be completely accounted for, the fact remains that there are different species of iron present. As elaborated below, these species differ not only in their EPR signals, or by the fact that one is and the other is not detectable by EPR, but also in their redox potential and kinetic behavior.

In some succinate and DPNH dehydrogenase preparations, particularly in those of low molecular weight, a significant signal may be found at $g = 4.3$ (27, 93). This signal is typical of high-spin ferric iron in a rhombic environment (cf. 94). This type of signal, however, is found in a wide variety of organic and inorganic materials and, if not present at a significant intensity, may merely indicate contaminating iron. In DPNH dehydrogenases of low molecular weight this signal may be derived from nonheme iron originally associated with these proteins, which has undergone a change in environment during enzyme preparation. This suggestion is supported by the finding that the intensity of the signal at $g = 4.3$ in many proteins depends on the presence of chelators, such as EDTA, during preparation. The EPR signal of the Fe(III)-EDTA complex is at $g = 4.3$.

8.2.2.2 Molybdenum

There are only three iron-molybdenum-flavoproteins known: xanthine and aldehyde oxidases and nitrate reductase, each of which occurs in some variant forms, depending on the organism or organ from which it is isolated. Nitrate reductase is not so well characterized as the two oxidases. The enzyme appears to contain molybdenum in all organisms in which it is found, but it seems uncertain at this time whether iron occurs in some species as heme and in others as noneheme iron or whether there are organisms in which it occurs in both forms. By far the best studied iron-molybdenum-flavoprotein is xanthine oxidase from milk. The story of the exploration of the properties of xanthine oxidase is an excellent example not only of the power and versatility of EPR spectroscopy but also of the power of man's persistence and imagination when applied to discouragingly complex problems. The progress in our understanding of the molybdenum signals of the iron-molybdenum-flavoproteins was also directly coupled to technical advances. In many respects, therefore, this development is rather instructive.

Naturally occurring molybdenum is a mixture of the seven isotopes ^{92,94,95,96,97,98,100}Mo, five of which have no nuclear spin. Twenty-five percent of the mass of Mo, however, is contributed by the isotopes ^{95}Mo and ^{97}Mo. These isotopes have a nuclear spin of 5/2. We would thus expect an EPR signal from paramagnetic ions of Mo that would mainly represent the isotopes devoid of nuclear spin, and each line of this signal

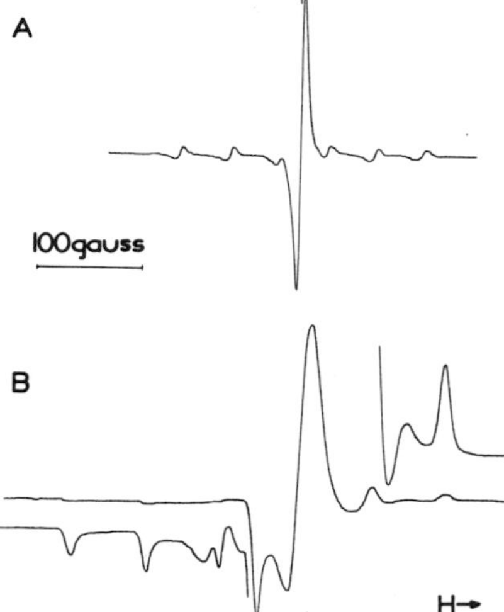

Fig. 8-9 Isotropic and anisotropic EPR spectra typical of Mo(V) compounds. Two mg Mo(V)Cl_5 were dissolved in 1 ml of concentrated HCl: A, observation at room temperature; B, at 100 K. The microwave power was 25 mW, the modulation amplitude, 0.6 G for A and 0.08 G for B. In order to show the weaker hfs lines in B, parts of the spectrum are shown at a modulation amplitude of 1 G, below or above the main line.

should be in the center of a weak symmetrical six-line pattern representing the isotopes with spin 5/2 (Fig. 8-9). This characteristic pattern is not found in any other metal ion of biological significance.

The more readily accessible forms of Mo in which unpaired electrons can be expected to be present are Mo(V) and Mo(III). Of these Mo(V) is by far the most likely one to be found in biological materials. It is also likely, however, that Mo is not a priori present as Mo(V) but rather as Mo(VI) and that Mo(V) may become apparent only under reducing conditions. Additional complications exist in that Mo(V) may play the role of a transient intermediate, similar to a flavin semiquinone, since it might be further reduced to Mo(IV) which is not detectable by EPR. Mo(V) is also known for its strong tendency to form dimeric diamagnetic compounds (95). It has, however, never been conclusively shown that either Mo(IV) or $[Mo(V)]_2$ dimers are indeed formed in biological materials. There are reasons to doubt that dimerization of protein-bound species might occur. All these properties of Mo(V) may contribute to the fact that it is one of the most difficult and evasive species to deal with in biologically oriented EPR spectroscopy.

The first signals of what is almost certainly Mo(V) and not Mo(III) were obtained before 100 kHz modulation frequency was available (Fig. 8-10, top row) (96). With biological materials such as xanthine oxidase, in which there are at best two atoms of Mo(V) to be found in a mass of MW 300,000, sufficient sensitivity could be obtained only by relatively high power and

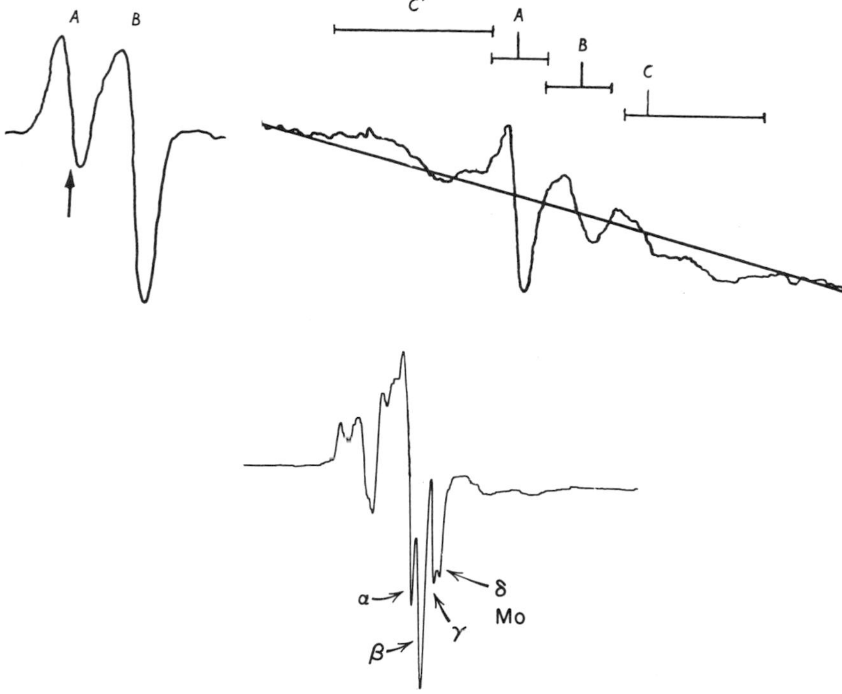

Fig. 8-10 (Part 1) EPR spectra of the Mo component of milk xanthine oxidase illustrating the role of technical advances in the resolution and interpretation of these spectra: Top row (*left*) spectrum of 0.2 m*M* xanthine oxidase aerobically reduced with xanthine (1959) at ~9500 MHz, 15-G modulation amplitude, 400 Hz modulation frequency, and 100 K according to Bray et al. (96). A indicates the field position of the flavin semiquinone signal, B that of the molybdenum signal, and the arrow, the *g* factor of the free electron. Top row (*center*) spectrum of approximately 0.1 m*M* xanthine oxidase (initial concentration), 100 msec after mixing with oxygenated xanthine (1961) at ~9500 MHz approximately 12-G modulation amplitude (modulation frequency not indicated), and 77 K according to Bray (97). It should be kept in mind that during rapid mixing and freezing an effective dilution of the sample by a factor of 4.6 (98) results. A and B indicate signals as above, C and possibly also C′ signals of the iron-sulfur group. Top row (*right*) spectrum of 0.24 m*M* xanthine oxidase (initial concentration) 26 msec after mixing with oxygenated xanthine (1964) at ~9100 MHz, a modulation amplitude of 5 G, 100 kHz modulation frequency, and 100 K according to Palmer et al. (98). The greek letter designations are those used for the various molybdenum components until recently (cf. 99).

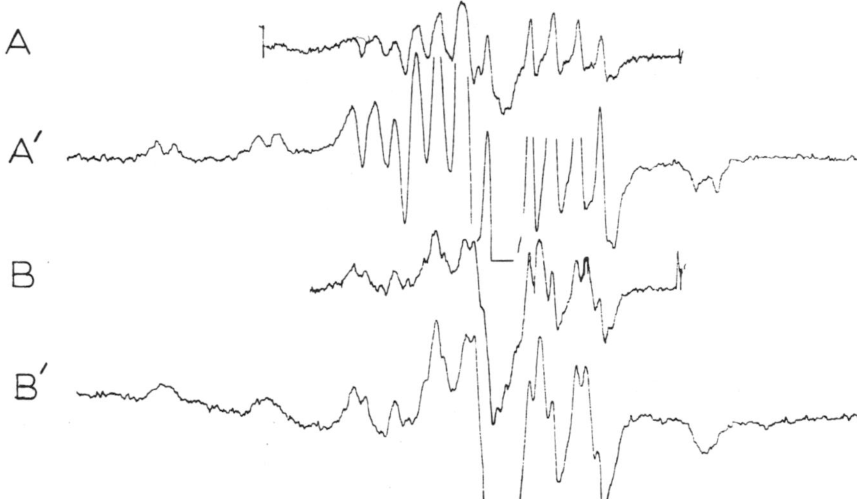

Fig. 8-10 (Part 2) Spectra of approximately 0.1 m*M* xanthine oxidase labeled with ^{95}Mo (100) and reduced with purine for 1 min in H_2O (A and A′) and 70 percent D_2O (B and B′), (1966) at ~9500 MHz, a modulation amplitude of approximately ~1 G, (H_2O) or ~2 G (D_2O), modulation frequency of 100 kHz and a temperature of 123 K. The wings of the spectra were recorded at ~4 G modulation amplitude in A′ and B′ and are shown below the main spectra A and B according to Bray et al. (101). The center portions of A′ and B′ outrun the scale of the figure.

modulation. As a consequence resolution was poor and in most of the early published spectra the Mo(V) signal appeared as a single asymmetric peak at $g \sim 1.97$. (In retrospect it is interesting that what we now know to be proton hfs in the Mo(V) signal can indeed be seen in some spectra recorded even under these conditions.) With the advent of 100 kHz modulation frequency it was then possible to resolve the signals partially, which immediately indicated a considerable complexity in the behavior of the molybdenum (98). First, the principal signal occurring on reduction of xanthine as well as aldehyde oxidase showed two peaks with additional poorly resolved structure, and, second, an entirely different signal appeared and disappeared in the early phases of reduction of xanthine oxidase by xanthine (Fig. 8-10, top row). A similar signal was present even in what was assumed to be the oxidized form of aldehyde oxidase (85), and, third, still another signal, different from the other two, gradually replaced these signals several minutes after reduction (85, 102). The fact that neither of these signals accounted for more than 1/3 of the total Mo in the enzymes added to the difficulties of interpretation. Nevertheless it was also possible at this stage to resolve the hfs contributed by the nuclei of ^{95}Mo and ^{97}Mo (see above) (85, 98). The low-field portion of the typical six-line pattern due to these isotopes was clearly seen with xanthine and aldehyde oxidases. The theoretical ratio of the intensities of the hyperfine lines to that of the main lines can be calculated from the known isotope composition of natural molybdenum. (If the linewidths are not significantly different, the amplitudes of the lines may simply be compared (see Section 8.3), but it must be kept in mind that the intensity of the signal of the isotopes with nuclear spin 5/2 is spread out over six lines.) The intensity ratios experimentally observed were indeed, within experimental error, the same as those calculated from

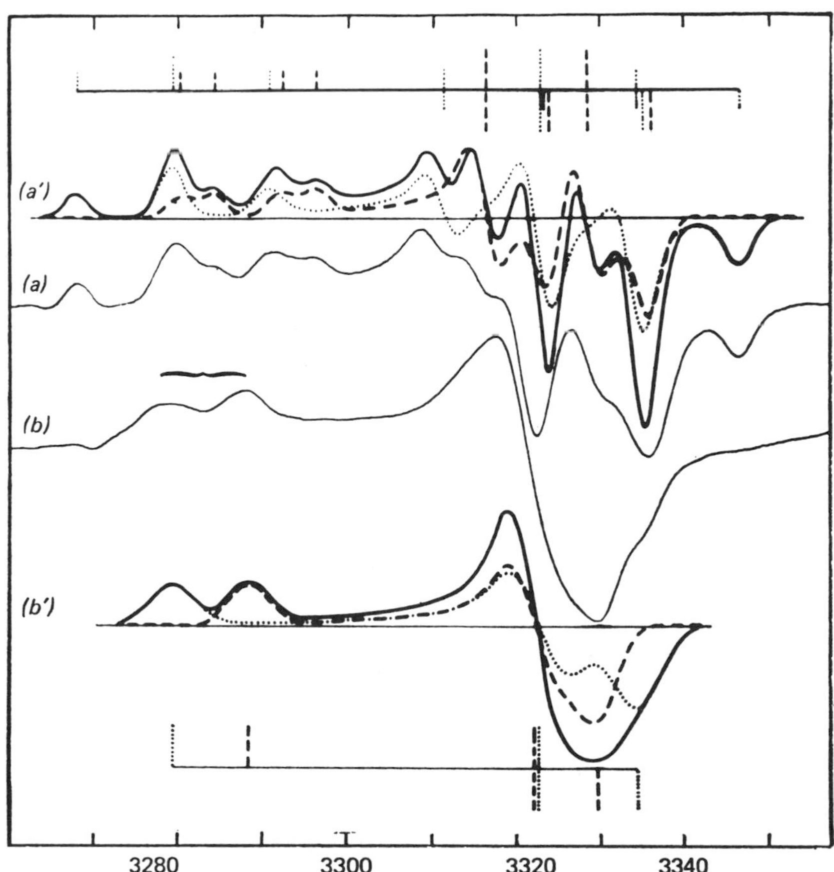

Fig. 8-10 (Part 3) Spectra of 0.3 mM xanthine oxidase reduced with xanthine for 1 min in H_2O (*a*) or 95 percent D_2O (*b*) (1969), at ~9150 MHz, modulation amplitude of 2.9 G, modulation frequency of 100 kHz, and temperature of 150–170 K, according to Bray and Vänngård (99). The spectra a′ and b′ of this row represent a computer simulation of the component spectra (*dotted* or *dashed*) and of the composite spectrum obtained by addition of the components (*full line*), using the experimentally obtained parameters (cf. Table 8-4).

the isotope composition. These spectra thus removed any doubt left that the species observed here was molybdenum.

It may be of interest to point out here what has been a general feature in discussions of the identity of EPR signals seen in biological materials. The assignment of signals was rarely doubted in biological circles—which is probably understandable because of the general lack of experience in EPR spectroscopy and possibly also from the intuition that certain assign-

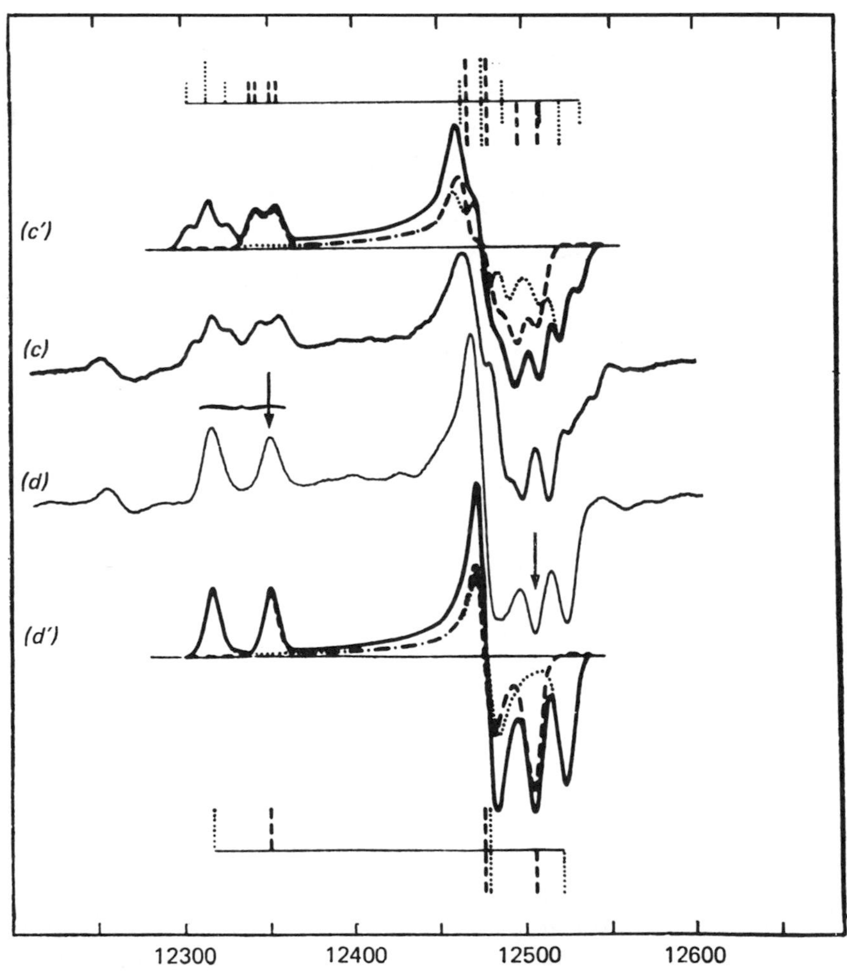

Fig. 8-10 (Part 4) The same samples as Part 3 observed at ~34,400 MHz, 3.7-G modulation amplitude, 100 kHz modulation frequency and 150–170 K. Simulated spectra (c′, d′) and curves for H_2O (c) and D_2O (d) samples as in Part 3.

ments made good sense—but most often outspoken resistance came from experienced solid-state physicists. This probably has been a healthy situation, since it forced the biologically oriented intruders into the field of EPR spectroscopy to exercise at least some of the rigor that is taken for granted in the more exact sciences.

At the state of the art at which it became feasible to resolve the various Mo(V) signals it was also realized that these signals varied widely in their spin relaxation behavior (41, 85, 103). Experiments on the kinetics of the appearance and disappearance of these signals may lead to considerable error if the saturation behavior of every Mo(V) species, which is involved, is not known. To complicate the picture even further it was observed that the spin relaxation of a certain species, or at least what appeared to be a single species at that time, could vary with the time during which the reaction had progressed and with the overall redox state of the electron carriers in the enzyme (41, 85, 103). It is therefore advisable in such (as indeed in most) experiments to use the lowest power at which an acceptable signal-to-noise ratio and sufficient resolution can be obtained. The power chosen may still have to be such that some saturation will occur if the concentration of material is not sufficient. It is then necessary to introduce a correction that can be calculated from a complete saturation curve. In such instances it is often helpful—although more costly in time—to record the spectra under different conditions for different purposes: for example, at higher and partly saturating power for resolution of overlapping signals and at low power for total amplitude under nonsaturating conditions.

At the state of knowledge, experience, and technology at which the work just discussed was carried out there was still little progress possible in the interpretation of the various signals of Mo(V) that had been observed. The next significant step came when ^{95}Mo was incorporated into xanthine oxidase (100). A cow was injected with a solution of ^{95}Mo sodium molybdate of 97 percent enrichment and from the milk obtained for three days after this injection an enzyme that contained 74 percent of the isotopes with nuclear spin 5/2 could be isolated. These experiments allowed an unambiguous assignment of g factors for two Mo(V) signals of xanthine oxidase (100, 101). It also became clearly apparent from the ^{95}Mo spectra that in one of these signals there was additional hfs present from a nucleus of spin $\frac{1}{2}$: All lines including the six of ^{95}Mo appeared in duplicate (Fig. 8-10, center row). It had already been observed (see above) that the principal signal appearing on reduction consisted of two closely spaced lines. This could also have been due to the superposition of lines from two different Mo(V) species. Although the splitting, by an equal amount, of every ^{95}Mo line into two lines could in principle also be explained in this way, it is extremely unlikely that two superimposed patterns stemming from different

Mo(V) species would show the same line separation all the way across the spectrum. The question thus emerged, what nucleus of spin $\frac{1}{2}$ might be sufficiently close to molybdenum so that its magnetic moment could interact with that of the unpaired electron of Mo(V). Since in proteins the proton is the most abundant nucleus with spin $\frac{1}{2}$, an answer was sought in experiments with deuterated compounds. Although the deuteron has a spin of 1, in practice, because of the small nuclear moment of this isotope (see above), one line is usually observed, instead of the two produced by proton hfs. Simple substitution of D_2O for H_2O as a solvent lead to the answer: the duplication of lines in the Mo spectra of xanthine oxidase and, by inference, of aldehyde oxidase is indeed due to the interaction of a proton with the unpaired electron of Mo(V), and it is evident from this experiment that the proton so involved is a readily exchangeable proton (100, 101).

Since xanthine oxidase catalyses a hydrogen transfer reaction, it was logical to ask the question whether the hydrogen, which must be in the vicinity of Mo(V), is one of those that is transferred from the substrate. This question was answered by oxidizing deuterium labeled xanthine (8-deutero xanthine) by xanthine oxidase and observing the ensuing EPR spectra (104). Since it was known that the proton involved could be exchanged against deuterium from the solvent, the only hope to see a deuteron, originating from the substrate, close to the molybdenum, was that it could be trapped there by rapid freezing. Experiments to this effect were carried out by the rapid-freezing technique with the reactants held at 2 C to slow down reaction rates. They showed that indeed up to approximately 100 msec, after mixing the enzyme with 8-deuteroxanthine, the proton splitting in the Mo(V) signal so generated was largely absent. This demonstrates that the 8-hydrogen (in the experiment mentioned, of course, the 8-deuteron) of xanthine finds its way into or close to the coordination sphere of the molybdenum of the enzyme. It was originally suggested that flavin with the hydrogen abstracted from the substrate may be, or may become during the reaction, a ligand of Mo(V). This suggestion, however, was recognized as invalid when flavin-depleted xanthine oxidase became available and it could be shown that even with this protein xanthine is still able to produce a Mo(V) signal with proton hfs (44, 105).

In this interplay of technical advances in EPR, exploitation of these by clever experimentation, and preparative advances in enzyme chemistry—the combination of circumstances most conducive to success—the next step was again one of EPR technique. Originally the Mo(V) signals had been difficult to resolve because the main lines (not hfs of isotopes) occur within a narrow range of *g* factors and have a sufficient width so that overlap is considerable. Although the use of low modulation and power contributed much to improved resolution, the situation was clearly one that suggested the use of higher microwave frequencies. As pointed out in Section 2.10, the magnetic field at which resonance is obtained increases with increasing frequency so that *g* factors remain constant, at least in uncomplicated cases. Thus the separation of resonant fields is enhanced at higher frequencies. It cannot however always be predicted whether high frequency spectra will have the expected higher resolution because unfavorable changes in linewidths may occur to offset the advantages of resonant-field separation. In the case of xanthine oxidase high frequency (35 GHz) spectra were indeed able to provide useful answers (99). Although the resonant fields for each Mo(V) species become separated by a factor of almost 4, as compared with the X-band spectra, the increase in linewidth was roughly twofold with most of the signals. It must also be kept in mind that, with anisotropic signals, intensity is lost at high frequency because the spectra are spread out over a larger field. It is therefore only in favorable combinations of circumstances that an advantage accrues from working at high frequencies, particularly since the spectrometers working at higher frequency are by no means so convenient and troublefree as the X-band instruments.

The conclusions concerning the properties and interpretation of the various Mo signals of xanthine oxidase, which could be drawn from the 35-GHz spectra (Fig. 8-10, bottom row), are sufficiently numerous and detailed that the interested reader is advised to consult the original publications on this subject (99, 106). It is possible to present only in summary form the most important conclusions in two tables (Tables 8-3 and 8-4) as

Table 8-3 Classification of Molybdenum EPR Signals from Reduced Forms of Xanthine Oxidase[a]

Signal	Appearance rate: approximately $t_{1/2}$ (sec) at 20 C and 0.1 m*M*-enzyme	Signal-producing substrates	Proton interaction
"Slow"	10^3	Dithionite, purine, salicylaldehyde	yes
"Rapid" ($\alpha\beta$, $\alpha\beta\gamma$)	10^{-1}	Salicylaldehyde, purine, xanthine	yes
"Very rapid" ($\gamma\delta$)	10^{-2}	Xanthine, 6-methylpurine	no

[a] Reprinted here with permission of R. C. Bray and T. Vänngård (99).

Table 8-4 EPR Parameters of Rapid Signals Occurring on Reduction of Xanthine Oxidase with Substrates[a]
(g factors are believed to be correct to ± 0.0005)

			2.0023 g			Proton hyperfine couplings (gauss)		
Substrate	Signal designation	Relative intensity	x	y	z	$[a_x(H)]$	$[a_y(H)]$	$[a_z(H)]$
Salicylaldehyde	No complex detected, type A	0.5	0.0397	0.0340	0.0116	14	14	14, 3(?)
	No complex detected, type B	0.5	0.0397	0.0361	0.0116	14	14	14, 3(?)
Purine	Complex formed, type 1	1	0.0379	0.0331	0.0129	14, 0	14, 0	12.0, 3.0
	—	Small	—	0.034–0.036	—	—	—	—
Xanthine	Complex formed, type 1	0.4	0.0380	0.0335	0.0134	12, 0	12, 0	12, 4
	Complex formed, type 2	0.6	0.0409	0.0338	0.0079	12, 12	12, 12	12, 12

[a] Reprinted here with permission of R. C. Bray and T. Vänngård (99).

they have been assembled by the authors and to mention examples of the kind of detail that eventually can be derived from evaluation of these spectra.

Kinetic studies have shown that the Mo signals of xanthine oxidase may be subdivided into three basic groups, as shown in Table 8-3. Those that are considered significant in the catalytic mechanism are the "very rapid" and "rapid" signals. Those that are "very rapid" are seen with only two substrates, so that the rapid signals, which are seen with all substrates within the turnover time, are most generally the more important. These "rapid" signals show hfs with exchangeable protons and each substrate leads to the appearance of two superimposed spectra with similar but distinguishable parameters, as shown in Table 8-4. The authors explain the origin of the two different spectra on the basis of the following observations: rapid reduction with dithionite and salicylaldehyde lead to one type of spectrum, which, when xanthine is then added, changes to a second type. Dithionite can hardly be considered as a "substrate" and salicylaldehyde is a substrate of rather low affinity, whereas xanthine has a high affinity for the enzyme. Since electron transfer had already taken place when xanthine was added after dithionite, its effect on the spectrum is most plausibly explained as being due to complex formation of xanthine with the enzyme. Similar observations were made with purine as substrate, which is also a substrate of an affinity much higher than that of aldehydes, although inferior to xanthine in this respect. The dependence of the shapes of the spectra on the concentration of the complexing substrates further indicates that different types of complex can be formed. The authors suggest that the substrate molecules, which are responsible for the appearance of the "complexed" spectra, are bound to the reduced enzyme at the active site "waiting for their turn to react when the enzyme has been reoxidized via some other site."

From parameters of the EPR spectra the authors were also able to draw useful conclusions on the nature of the protons that produce the hfs. First, they are all exchangeable in D_2O, which indicates that no stable covalent bonds (e.g., C—H) can be involved. Second, the proton hfs appears to be all isotropic, indicating that dipole-dipole interaction makes a minor contribution compared with contact interaction. Third, the absence of dipole-dipole coupling in turn suggests that the Mo—H distance must be greater than approximately 3 Å and, fourth, when the distance is indeed of this magnitude or larger, a direct Mo—H bond is very unlikely, since bond lengths exceeding 1.7 Å are unknown for hydrides of transition metals. Finally, if no direct Mo—H bond exists and there is an intervening atom, this intervening atom cannot be nitrogen, since no nitrogen hfs has been observed. This leaves oxygen or sulfur as possibilities.

The authors also point out that it is not clear whether the protons observed by their hfs are located on the substrate or the protein.

Replacement of H_2O by D_2O also decreased the width of the flavin semiquinone signal in xanthine oxidase. This shows that at least one of the protons in the flavin that interact with the unpaired electron is exchangeable. It follows that the semiquinone is not in the anionic form under these conditions, since this form has no exchangeable protons that would give hfs (see above). It is also apparent from these observations that if the flavin semiquinone does interact with one of the metal components this interaction will not be the type discussed above (cf. Fig. 8-1 and Refs. 14, 24, and 25) in which the metal replaces the dissociable proton at N(5), the source of a strong hfs.

No doubt xanthine oxidase is to date the outstanding example of the multiple facets of EPR as applied to the study of enzymes, and these have recently even been extended. Two groups succeeded in removing the flavin from xanthine oxidase reversibly (105), which opened the possibility of learning what functions or pathways of electron transfer of the enzyme were dependent on the presence of flavin, a subject discussed below under kinetics. Suffice it to say here that with flavin-free xanthine oxidase the EPR signals of both the molybdenum and iron-sulfur groups are still observed as they are in the presence of flavin (cf. 44, 105).

The appearance of EPR signals typical of the O_2^- radical (43, 44) during reoxidation of reduced flavoproteins by O_2 has been mentioned above (cf. Fig. 8-3). It may be pointed out here that historically these signals were first observed during reduction of xanthine oxidase by xanthine (98). Originally they were not recognized as such, although their asymmetry and, for radicals, relatively strong spin relaxation was noted. It was only when their $g_{\|}$ portion was clearly recognized (43) that attention was drawn to this unusual radical signal. A consideration of the steps that must occur during electron transfer from substrate via the xanthine oxidase molecule to oxygen points to the possibility that substrate radicals may also be intermediates in this process. No indications for such species have so far been obtained by EPR (or any other method) and it is of course not certain whether such radicals, if they exist, would be detectable by EPR. The experience with peroxidase may be recalled here (107). In this instance radical signals from substrate (hydroquinone) were not detected at low temperature but were fortunately well resolved at room temperature.

8.2.3 Triplet State of Flavin Compounds

The triplet state is an important intermediate state in photochemical reactions of flavins (cf. 108). As discussed in Section 1.9, in the triplet state two unpaired electrons with parallel spins are present in a molecule.

Furthermore, the two spins are not completely isolated but are coupled by dipole-dipole interaction which is anisotropic. Potentially, therefore, EPR signals may be detected, but the presence of two unpaired electrons with anisotropic spin-spin interaction makes EPR spectroscopy of molecules in the triplet state a specialized endeavor. Two features are significant for EPR spectroscopy of triplet state molecules:

1. Because of the presence of the neighboring paramagnets and the ensuing spin-spin interaction, there is a zero-field splitting, that is, EPR signals should be detectable in the absence of a magnetic field if the proper frequency is chosen.
2. The three spin states (triplet state!) of the system, that is, with $M_S = -1, 0, +1$ are no longer pure quantum states so that transitions with $\Delta M_S = 2$ become allowed.

Thus signals may be observed from transitions corresponding to $\Delta M_S = 1$ as well as $\Delta M_S = 2$. Unfortunately the $\Delta M_S = 1$ transitions are generally highly anisotropic so that very broad signals (several thousand gauss) are expected. There is a much better chance (100:1) to observe the more isotropic $\Delta M_S = 2$ transitions, which occur at half-field, that is, $g \simeq 4$. Both $\Delta M_S = 1$ and $\Delta M_S = 2$ transitions have been observed with the oxidized forms of a number of flavin compounds (109–111), which were irradiated in glasses at liquid nitrogen temperature. The spectra observed with the cationic form of FMN are shown in Fig. 8-11. The EPR and phosphorescence spectra of the cationic form were different from those of the neutral and anionic forms, whereas the latter two forms could not be distinguished from each other. It could thus be ascertained that the pK value (cation/neutral form) of the triplet state is not essentially different from that of the ground state. The zero-field splitting energies of the *lowest* triplet state of flavins—the only state observed to date—are among the smallest ones found among bi- or tricyclic molecules that show phos-

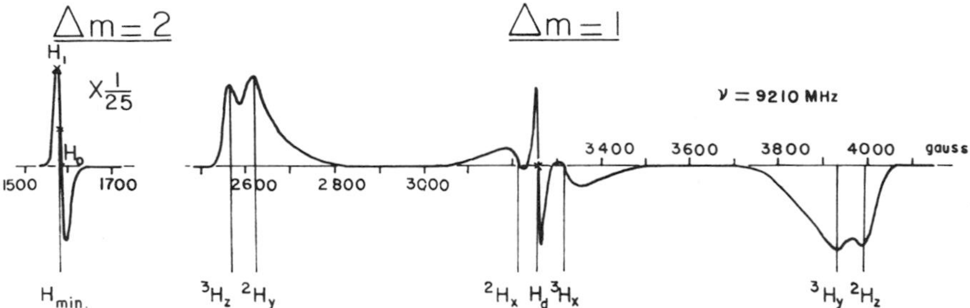

Fig. 8-11 EPR spectrum of the lowest triplet state of FMN, according to Lhoste et al., (109). FMN in a rigid solution of water-propylene glycol-6N HCl at 77 K was irradiated by a mercury arc lamp. Note that under these conditions FMN is in the cationic form.

phorescence. This is thought to be due to extensive delocalization of the two electrons involved. The radiative lifetime of the phosphorescent triplet state of riboflavin is of the order of 20 msec.

Qualitatively, the distribution of the unpaired spins in the lowest triplet state of the oxidized form of flavins is similar to that of the semiquinone (109, 112), as discussed above, and indicates a close correspondence of the electronic structures of the two species. Thus the parameters measurable from the EPR and phosphorescence spectra of the triplet state are sensitive to substitutions in the benzenoid (A) and pyrazine (B) rings rather than the pyrimidine (C) ring. The N(5) and C(8) positions are particularly sensitive.

No EPR signal of the triplet state of *reduced* flavin could be detected, although phosphorescence was observed with an intensity similar to that of the oxidized form. It is thought (109) that in the reduced form, because of the nonplanar configuration, spin-orbit coupling is higher than in the oxidized form. This may decrease the lifetime of the triplet state and may increase the zero-field splitting to an extent that the energy of the transitions is beyond the 9000 MHz frequency range.

8.3 OXIDOREDUCTIVE TITRATIONS

In the preceding sections we considered the EPR signals that may be observed with flavins, flavoproteins, and complex metalproteins containing flavin and the conclusions concerning the structure of the active sites of these compounds that can be derived from an analysis of these signals. In this section we discuss some of the most straightforward applications of EPR spectroscopy, namely, the simple use of EPR as an indicator of the oxidation-reduction state of an enzyme. This application is analogous to that practiced in other types of spectroscopy, notably spectrophotometry, in which an absorption band is followed with relation to time or some other quantity. As in spectrophotometry and in other spectroscopies it is of course necessary to make sure that the observed band or signal undergoes changes in intensity but not in shape.

Two main approaches are applicable to the area of oxidoreductive enzymes. First, that of following a band or signal as a function of reductant or—after previous reduction—of oxidant, with sufficient time allowed for attainment of equilibrium; in other words, a titration. The second is that of following a band or signal with time, generally with an excess of reductant or oxidant present; namely, a kinetic study.

Titrations will give information on the total number of electrons taken up per molecule (or other unit) and on the redox potentials of the electron carriers in the enzyme. Absolute numbers for the redox potential can of course only be derived when the system under study can be related to a redox system of known redox potential. When EPR signals can be observed only in the frozen state, it must be considered that there may be shifts in the equilibria on freezing and that a certain state established in a liquid mixture may not be exactly preserved and expressed in signals obtained from the frozen state. In most instances we may have to be satisfied with information on the relative magnitudes of the redox potentials of the electron carriers present. Thus, during a reductive titration, the first electrons entering a multicarrier enzyme will be found in the component of highest potential, or, in other commonly used phraseology, the "deepest electron sink." These electrons may, however, have passed through other carriers on their way. A titration, in which an equilibrium situation is observed, will not be able to give information on this point. The question of the pathway may, however, be answered by kinetic studies, in which the time is limiting and electrons are, so to speak, intercepted and observed on their way to the deepest sink. This is discussed in the section on kinetics.

It needs no elaboration that only well-controlled anaerobic procedures can give quantitative results in oxidoreduction titrations. In the author's own work (cf. 74) the ability of determining small quantities of oxygen has been the key step toward quantitative titration methods of these compounds. With a knowledge of the amount of oxygen to be reckoned with in a particular situation, either remedies may be found (such as decreasing gas or liquid volumes) or the concentration of the compound to be titrated may be raised to such a level that the error introduced by oxygen contamination assumes the desired value.

Two additional points deserve attention in titration experiments, although after the lesson has been learned they may in retrospect appear rather obvious. First, the oxidation-reduction potential of a number of flavoproteins or iron-sulfur proteins is sufficiently low that one has to make sure that the reducing agent used is indeed a stoichiometric titrant. With dithionite as reductant, this difficulty is not expected, but it has developed during the use of pyridine nucleotides. Second, and this is a difficulty particularly encountered with dithionite, the rate of reduction may be very slow so that equilibrium may not be reached before some hours, in which case secondary reactions or denaturation may blur the picture. Examples of the first case are the attempted titrations of adrenodoxin and putidaredoxin with pyridine nucleotides, mediated by the respective reductase flavoproteins, which appeared to indicate that one electron was taken up per iron atom, whereas in fact one electron is taken up for every two iron atoms. Examples of the second case are titrations of the azotobacter flavoprotein (2, 31), xanthine oxidase (113) or adrenodoxin (74) with dithionite or of succinate dehydrogenase with DPNH, mediated by PMS (88). The rate of reduction by dithionite can in most cases be increased so that the reaction is for practical purposes instantaneous when one of the viologens (see Section 7.5.3) is added as mediator. Experiments to establish the optimal level are necessary, since an excessive amount of viologen may inhibit, lead to side reactions, or interfere by adding the EPR signal of its reduced form, which is itself a radical in equilibrium with its diamagnetic dimer.

8.3.1 Free Flavin Compounds

A thorough study of the species present in mixtures of oxidized and reduced flavin nucleotides is available, which utilizes titration techniques and spectrophotometric as well as EPR spectroscopic observation (114). When percent reduction is plotted (on the abscissa) versus a characteristic quantity of an intermediate (on the ordinate), such as $A_{900\ nm}$ for the quinhydrone type FMN-$FMNH_2$ complex or $A_{570\ nm}$ or EPR signal intensity for the $FMNH^{\cdot}$ radical, the curve describing the formation of the complex of FMN with $FMNH_2$ is bellshaped, as expected. The curve describing semiquinone formation is, however, definitely skewed, which indicates maximal semiquinone formation at ~ 70 percent reduction, not at 50 percent as expected. This was found irrespective of whether EPR or optical criteria were used to monitor $FMNH^{\cdot}$ formation. It was then observed that not only were the radical signals in the range between 50 and 100 percent reduction larger than their counterparts in the 0 to 50 percent range but they also differed in shape (Fig. 8-12). There was less

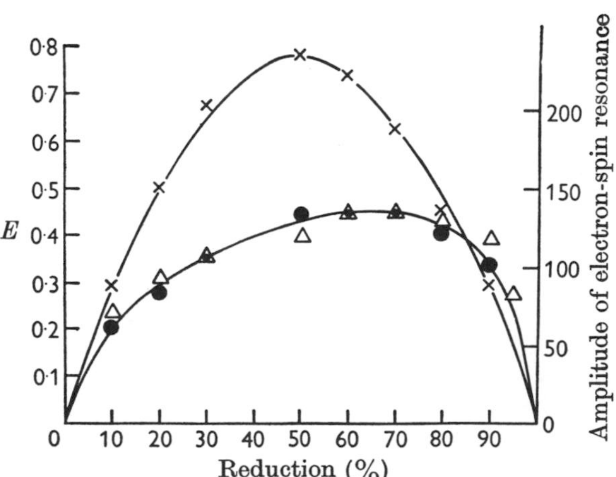

Fig. 8-12 Relation of absorbance at 900 and 570 nm to percentage reduction of FMN and EPR semiquinone signal amplitude, according to Gibson et al., (114). FMN was dissolved in a 4 m*M* solution in 0.12 *M* phosphate of pH 6.3 at 23–25C. x, $A_{900\ nm}$; ●, $A_{570\ nm}$; △, EPR signal amplitude.

resolution of hfs in the range of more extensive reduction. Since this effect was absent in the presence of certain organic solvents such as methanol or formamide or of agents that form complexes with flavin such as caffeine, it became likely that the loss in resolution of hfs was due to complex formation between flavin species. In view of the range of oxidation-reduction states in which these complexes were apparently formed, it was most likely that $FMNH_2$ might be one of the complexing partners. Indeed, the titration curve as shown in Fig. 8-13 could be simulated on the assumption that in

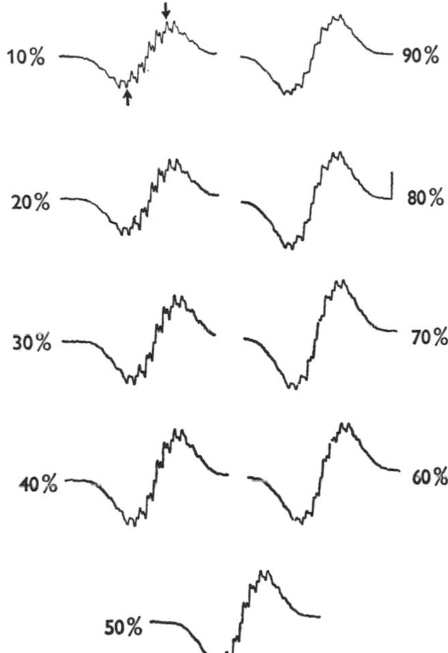

Fig. 8-13 EPR spectra of FMN as in Fig. 8-12 at various states of reduction shown as percentages, according to Gibson et al. (114). All spectra were recorded at the same instrument settings, chosen so that overmodulation or saturation effects were excluded.

addition to FMN, $FMNH_2$, $FMNH^{\cdot}$, and $FMN\text{-}FMNH_2$ a species $FMNH_2\text{-}FMNH^{\cdot}$ was involved. This work is a useful example of the combined use of EPR and optical techniques and it shows that even in an apparently simple system we may not be spared complicating events. It is also apparent that even in such a system we cannot rely on simply measuring signal amplitude without having made certain that not even minor changes in shape occur.

8.3.2 Flavoproteins

In the reductive titration of simple flavoproteins bellshaped curves of semiquinone formation and disappearance with progressing reduction have been found (cf. 30). Although the number of measured points is generally insufficient to be completely certain, it does not appear that these curves are skewed. This is another example adding to the general experience that many phenomena are simpler when studied with proteins bearing the compound to be investigated than with the free compounds, and that often what is considered a "model" may in fact behave in a more complicated way than the natural compound for which a model is sought. This was also obvious in studies of spin relaxation of flavin compounds (41), in which mutual interactions are particularly troublesome and complicating. Such interactions are of course either entirely ruled out or minimized by having the compound in question—flavin in our case—held firmly on the scaffolding of the protein and by having some of its reactive groups or areas, which are susceptible to association reactions, occupied by groups of the protein.

As far as quantitative information is available, at the midpoint of the titration of flavoproteins with dithionite a large fraction of the total flavin is accounted for in the EPR signal of the semiquinone form. A recovery of 82 percent has been reported for glucose oxidase (30), which is probably within the limits of error of a 100 percent yield.

With metalflavoproteins, however, generally only a fraction of the flavin can be accounted for in the semiquinone signal. Two reasons for this behavior have been suggested. It may be assumed that within, if not between, molecules with multiple electron acceptors of different redox potentials a disproportionation equilibrium may exist in principle analogous to that of Eq. 8-1. Another possibility is that part of the flavin, which at 50 percent reduction is not accounted for in the semiquinone signal, may be present as semiquinone metal chelate or may otherwise interact with the metal, with the consequence that no EPR signal is observed. It is known that semiquinone chelates of paramagnetic metals are devoid of EPR signals (24).

The titration behavior of metalflavoproteins obviously becomes increasingly complex as the number of communicating electron carriers rises. In the same direction there is the uncertainty of the number of titratable and, in any particular instance, titrated groups. The results obtained on titrations of these proteins are therefore in some respects still ambiguous. It has been observed with milk xanthine oxidase and rabbit liver aldehyde oxidase that the flavin and the iron-sulfur group are titrated simultaneously, whereas molybdenum is reduced only after these two sets of groups have been reduced (85, 113) in the majority of molecules. In xanthine dehydrogenase from chicken liver, on the other hand, all three types of carrier are reduced with little distinction.

It may be useful in this context to digress and point out an aspect that, by experience, is not always obvious to the newcomer to this kind of experimentation. This aspect concerns the consideration of events as they occur in individual molecules versus those that are indicated by the overall statistical average. We must realize that in EPR spectroscopy we have a tool to probe into events in much more detail than conventional methods have generally enabled us to do; for instance, in the titration of a flavoprotein that contains one flavin group per molecule, when the balance indicates that "80 percent of the flavin is reduced" this is only the overall but not a precise picture of the situation. The correct picture is that in 80 percent of the molecules these groups are reduced but not in the remaining 20 percent. In this simple example this may seem trivial, but when there are two flavin groups per molecule the situation may become complicated. In the simplest case, in which the two flavins are exactly equivalent and operate completely independently, at "80 percent reduction" the populations (calculated from the binomial theorem) of molecules are the following: 64 percent of the molecules have *both* flavins reduced, 32 percent of the molecules have one flavin oxidized and one reduced, and only 4 percent of the molecules have both flavins oxidized. It will be apparent that chemical inequivalences of the flavins, arising either from intrinsic differences in oxidoreduction potential or from cooperativity or allosteric effects, may vastly complicate this picture. The presence of other electron-transferring groups in the molecule adds further variables to the problem. The reader will appreciate that the simplest cases can seldom be expected to occur, but the problem must be considered nonetheless; for instance, it becomes important to distinguish—at approximately half-reduction—whether we are dealing with a mixture of molecules in which all carriers are reduced, with molecules in which all carriers are oxidized, or with molecules in which some carriers are and some are not reduced. In the two different situations different properties (and, as a consequence, different EPR signals) may be encountered. An example of such a situation is found in the titration of cytochrome *c* oxidase (115), in which signals occur in partly reduced molecules that are absent in the fully oxidized as well as in the fully reduced enzyme. Complicated situations of the kind alluded to here could not of course develop if there were a rapid oxidation-reduction equilibrium of all electron carriers between individual molecules as it is usually attained between the carriers within individual molecules. It has been found, however, that it cannot be taken for granted that such an equilibrium will be reached within the times usually allowed in experimentation. This refers to the time allowed in the liquid state. No instance is known of electron transfer between individual electron carriers within molecules or between molecules when solutions of enzymes, as discussed here, are frozen at temperatures of $\leq$ 150 K. Phenomena of this kind, however, have been observed in photosynthetic materials (cf. 116).

Complications have also been observed in titrations of multicarrier enzymes, when changes occur within the molecule—possibly falling into the category generally referred to as conformational changes—as reduction proceeds. After reduction of one carrier, for instance, other carriers may change their properties. This has again been observed with cytochrome *c* oxidase (115).

For the novice in the field of multicarrier enzymes it is helpful to write out in tabular form all the possible redox states such an enzyme could be found in, and it will be surprising how many possibilities may exist—at least on paper. A number of these possibilities can, of course, usually be ruled out on the basis of additional information, for example, about redox potentials. These considerations are taken up again when the interactions among electron carriers are discussed.

8.4 KINETIC STUDIES OF OXIDOREDUCTION

Up to this point situations were considered in which equilibrium between the components of a system, at least within individual molecules, was established. The described approaches are useful and necessary for establishing some structural and organizational aspects of the components of active centers and the total capacity for electron uptake, but they cannot give information on the question whether the detected components are indeed catalytically active components of an enzyme. Such information has to come from kinetic studies, which must cover the time range within which the enzyme is known to turn over according to conventional assay procedures, for example, measuring substrate disappearance or product appearance.

Consideration of the kinetic approach involving EPR spectroscopy naturally falls into two categories which demand quite different expertise and instrumentation, namely kinetics with observation in the liquid or in the frozen state. It is not the purpose of this chapter to deal with technical aspects. They are discussed elsewhere in this book. A successful study of the reduction by pyridine nucleotides of flavin and flavin-iron model systems, by combined optical and EPR spectroscopy, has been reported (117, 118), but there is probably general agreement that in work on proteins, particularly on the more complex ones, the possibilities of observation in the liquid state are limited. The components that can be observed in the liquid state are flavin semiquinone and molybdenum in metalflavoproteins but not the iron. From our discussion of the behavior of the molybdenum component it is obvious that it is not sufficient to set the instrument on a certain point of the signal and observe rise or decline, as it is to some extent feasible with the radical signal (unless there is $O_2^{\dot{-}}$ formed; see above), but that the major portion of the molybdenum signal must be scanned repeatedly as time progresses. Such attempts have been made, but resolution is understandably poor (119). Observation in the frozen state, made possible by the rapid-freezing technique (97, 98, 120–122), has been the more generally useful approach and a good deal of our progress in recent years in understanding complex metalflavoproteins and other multicarrier enzymes has been achieved by the application of this approach (cf. 27, 43, 44, 61, 88, 90, 97, 101, 103–106, 115, 123–127). It must be kept in mind, however, that changes may occur on freezing and that the species and states observed, although reproducibly related to their counterparts in solution, may not be the exact images of those present in solution. Despite this objection it is agreed by most investigators that in many instances the approach that employs the rapid-freezing technique is the best presently available. In a number of instances in which a comparison was feasible the reaction rates found by the rapid-freezing technique agreed very well with those observed in conventional rate assays in liquid solution (88, 103, 123, 124, 126). In the reactions that can be successfully studied by this technique a lower time limit is given by the freezing time, which usually lines in the range of 5 to 10 msec. Most reaction rates of flavoproteins are such that they can be studied by this technique.

A few basic kinetic experiments give the most useful information:

1. That colloquially called "single turnover." An amount of substrate is added to the enzyme, insufficient to reduce all electron carriers, and an excess of oxidant is present. In this instance the carriers in a number of enzyme molecules will be reduced and thereafter reoxidized without further turnover. The sequence of signal appearance and disappearance may in favorable instances give a clear indication of the path of electrons through the enzyme.

2. Half-reactions such as reduction and reoxidation after previous reduction. It must be kept in mind that the completely reduced and, in some instances also, the completely oxidized species may not be involved in the catalytic turnover and that under normal conditions of turnover all electron carriers in all molecules will neither be completely oxidized nor completely reduced at any one time. It is therefore more informative to observe reduction to the steady state or reoxidation from the steady state. This, however, is not always possible, since the steady-state oxidation-reduction level may lie at an unfavorable position, say 90 percent oxidized, and any changes observed would lie within the limits of the cumulative error of the procedures involved. The solubility of substrate or oxygen or the turnover rate of the enzyme may set limits to the possibility of establishing anything close to a steady state in the sense that it is implied in the usual studies in dilute solutions.

8.4.1 Free Flavin Compounds

In a study of the model system DPNH-FMN by combined optical and EPR spectroscopy (117) the kinetics clearly showed that the semiquinone $FMNH^{\cdot}$ is not the primary reduction product but is formed in a secondary reaction of $FMNH_2$ with FMN according to the following scheme:

$$FMN + DPNH + H^+ \rightleftharpoons FMNH_2 + DPN^+ \tag{8-2}$$

$$FMNH_2 + FMN \rightleftharpoons FMNH_2 - FMN \tag{8-3}$$

$$FMNH_2 - FMN \rightleftharpoons 2FMNH^{\cdot} \tag{8-4}$$

The $FMNH_2 - FMN$ complex is the species with a light absorption maximum at ~ 900 nm, whereas at neutral pH $FMNH^{\cdot}$ has a characteristic absorption at ~ 570 nm. The authors extended this system to include a model for nonheme iron, that is, nitrosopentacyano ferrate (nitroprusside) (118). In this instance the initial rates of appearance of the species absorbing at 900 nm and of the semiquinone were depressed. The course of the reaction, subsequent to the step of Eq. 8-2, is thought to be

$$FMNH_2 + Fe(III) \rightarrow FMNH^{\cdot} + Fe(II) + H^+ \tag{8-5}$$

$$2FMNH^{\cdot} \rightleftharpoons FMNH_2 + FMN \tag{8-6}$$

It cannot, however, be concluded with certainty that either the mechanism of Eqs. 8-2 to 8-4 or that of Eqs. 8-2 to 8-5 also applies to simple flavoproteins or metalflavoproteins, which are reduced by pyridine nucleotides.

The kinetics of the production of the superoxide anion radical by oxidation of reduced tetraacetylriboflavin with oxygen have been studied by the rapid-freezing technique (127).

8.4.2 Flavoproteins

A number of kinetic studies on flavoproteins which utilized combined EPR and rapid-freezing techniques—and in some instances reflectance spectroscopy of frozen samples as well—have been published (27, 43, 44, 61, 88, 97, 101, 103, 104, 106, 123, 124, 126), generally on the more challenging metalflavoproteins. For details the reader is referred to the original publications. Some more general conclusions may be summarized here. As already pointed out, when metal-free flavoproteins are reduced with substrate, no signals of flavin semiquinone are observed, with very few exceptions. Exceptions seem to be TPNH-cytochrome *c* reductase of microsomes, and TPNH ferredoxin reductases, which are both pyridine-nucleotide-linked flavoproteins. With all metalflavoproteins, however, radical signals typical of flavin semiquinone are readily observed on reduction with substrate. In no instance has it been observed, that more than a fraction of the flavin present is in the semiquinone form. This fraction varies from less than 1 percent up to approximately 20 percent. Higher yields have been obtained during titrations and with dithionite as reductant. Yet there is no reason why 100 percent of the flavin should be found in the semiquinone form in kinetic studies.

To the author's knowledge the rate of reduction of flavin in iron flavoproteins has never been clearly separated kinetically from the reduction of the iron-sulfur component. This might be taken to indicate that these two electron carriers react in some kind of obligatorily coordinated fashion or exchange electrons in the frozen state. Observations that are not compatible with such a conclusion have been made, however. With succinate dehydrogenase, for instance, it was observed that the quantity of flavin semiquinone formed depended on the substrate concentration, whereas this was not the case for the amount of iron-sulfur component reduced (88). Also, a situation was observed in titrations in which flavin was not reduced, whereas the iron-sulfur group was. The fact that the $g = 1.94$ signal appears rapidly on reduction of flavin-free xanthine oxidase by xanthine, just as it does in the intact enzyme, also speaks against a concerted reaction of flavin and the iron-sulfur group with incoming electrons.

In xanthine oxidase from milk and aldehyde oxidase from liver, iron flavoproteins which contain molybdenum, the first component to receive electrons from substrates appears to be molybdenum. (Only the reduction of milk xanthine oxidase by DPNH apparently proceeds by a different pathway.) This is in agreement with the results from anaerobic titrations which showed that molybdenum was the component with the lowest oxidation-reduction potential. The most extensive kinetic studies were done on milk xanthine oxidase. As mentioned above (cf. Table 8-3), the signals of a number of reduced molybdenum species appear in sequence, some at a sufficiently rapid rate so that the corresponding species qualify as intermediates in the catalytic process, whereas others seem to be due to species arising in slow secondary processes (cf. 106). The molybdenum and iron-sulfur components of xanthine oxidase are reduced by substrates (except by DPNH) at an undiminished rate even when flavin has been removed. The reaction with oxygen, however, is blocked. This observation indicates that flavin is involved in this reaction step. It is premature, however, to conclude that in metal flavoproteins the iron component may not also be needed for this reaction.

When pyridine nucleotides are substrates of flavoproteins, they are found to reduce the flavoproteins very rapidly ($t_{\frac{1}{2}} \lesssim 20$ msec) so that the rapid-freezing technique is at the limits of applicability. Artificial electron acceptors, such as ferricyanide, in general oxidize flavoproteins even more rapidly and resolution of the rate profile with the rapid-freezing technique, as presently practiced, is no longer possible.

8.5 ELECTRON SPIN RELAXATION OF FLAVIN AND FLAVOPROTEIN SEMIQUINONES AND INTRAMOLECULAR INTERACTIONS OF ELECTRON CARRIERS IN METALFLAVOPROTEINS

Spin-relaxation phenomena are being increasingly exploited as technical advances are made. The theory developed concerning these phenomena is extensive and complex and the nonspecialist can only be cautioned against expecting quick, easy, and unambiguous interpretations. He should also be wary of grasping for simplified presentations that often enough are at best half-truths. Since nuclear-spin relaxation rates are in general some orders of magnitude lower than those of electron-spin relaxation, the field of nuclear-spin relaxation has been technically easier to approach and is very well developed. Examples are studies on Cl nuclear resonance (128), when this atom is attached in some fashion to proteins (via Zn or Hg), and of proton resonances under a number of conditions that influence spin relaxation. A method which in a way measures electronic magnetism via its effects on nuclear relaxation is the PRR (proton relaxation rate) technique, which has found numerous successful applications to enzyme chemistry (129–131). Compared with the mentioned methods, the application of straightforward electron-spin relaxation techniques in biochemistry finds itself still in a relatively crude state. The most refined of such applications is probably implicit in the spin-labeling technique (Chapter 11) (132), although this technique obviously suffers from the indirectness of the approach. The nitroxide derivatives, which have rather generally been chosen as spin labels, have a simple EPR spectrum in which homogeneously broadened lines can be expected when the spin relaxation increases. This is not so for most endogenous paramagnetic species in biological materials, and line-broadening effects are rarely useful in spin-relaxation studies of such species. Techniques for direct measurement of relaxation times are available (cf. 133) but are still in the hands of a few experts and to our knowledge have not yet found successful application to biological materials at the time of this writing.* There remains the relatively simple approach of observing the signal intensity at different microwave power levels. If there is no significant broadening of the observed signal with increasing power, it is convenient simply to measure signal amplitude. In a first approximation this is permissible with flavin radicals, since they are inhomogeneously broadened with increasing power, that is, the individual narrow lines under the envelope, which is observed in practice, broaden with the effect that the envelope itself shows very little broadening. This method of gathering data on the relaxation properties of spin systems

* See footnote on p. 364.

does not lend itself to more than a very crude interpretation in physical terms, but it conveys practically useful information. First, it is necessary in any quantitative EPR work to operate at powers below the range of saturation or to correct the data for saturation accurately. The saturation behavior must therefore be known. Second, changes in the environment of a spin system are indicated by a change in spin relaxation. As in the application of proton-spin relaxation, electron-spin relaxation is indeed a sensitive indicator of such changes. The effects observed extend over orders of magnitude. Unfortunately most commercial equipment is unsuitable for measuring at low powers (< 1 mW) with reasonable accuracy. At 100 K radicals of free flavins as well as those of metal-free flavoproteins begin to show saturation in the range of 1 to 10 μW. In most instances the signal-to-noise ratio at this power level is poor. Examples of this application are found in Ref. 41. It should be emphasized that it is not sufficient to "check for saturation" by finding the power at which no increase in signal size occurs and then operate at a power lying lower by a factor of 2 or 3. It is always advisable to plot out the saturation data. From such a plot it will usually be observed that saturation in fact becomes noticeable at powers one or two orders of magnitude below that power at which no more increase of signal size occurs.

Because of extensive electron delocalization and small spin-orbit coupling, the semiquinones of flavin compounds, unless associated with paramagnetic metals, usually have relatively long relaxation times and the signals are therefore readily saturated with microwave power.

In model systems containing free flavins it could be clearly shown that electron-spin relaxation was enhanced by the presence of paramagnetic metal ions, but effects of the ionic environment were superimposed which complicated the picture and made quantitative evaluations difficult (Fig. 8-14).

Although intramolecular interactions of electron carriers in complex metalflavoproteins have been alluded to in the sections on titration and kinetics, it may be useful to summarize here, in connection with our consideration of electron-spin relaxation, what the present state of knowledge and thinking is on this subject.

The finding that flavin, as well as iron and molybdenum, when present, takes or gives up electrons in an ordered fashion during turnover of these enzymes suggests that the electron carriers are located in proximity to one another within or on the protein. In drawing this conclusion we neglect the possibility that there could be efficient electron transfer over long distances along polypeptide chains or that each electron carrier in a metalflavoprotein reacts with reductant and oxidant independent of the other carriers. We consider such possibilities unlikely. (For a review of semiconduction in proteins, see Ref. 134.) Location in proximity, however, does not mean that there must be direct metal-flavin or metal-metal contact. Electron transfer in such systems would be expected to be extremely rapid, whereas according to kinetic studies on metalflavoproteins with the rapid-freezing technique, the rates of electron transfer within these proteins are relatively slow. We also know that this intramolecular electron transfer is slowed down with decreasing temperature and is effectively stopped at $\lesssim$ 150 K. It is therefore likely that molecular motions are necessary to bring the electron carriers close enough so that electron

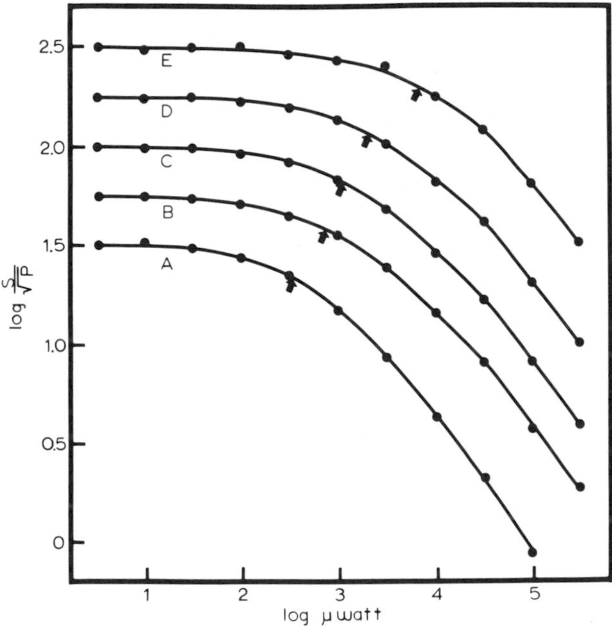

Fig. 8-14 Effect of chloride concentration on nickel-induced relaxation of 3-methyl-5-benzyl-lumiflavin semiquinone, pH 6, according to Beinert and Orme-Johnson (41). The radical was produced by air-oxidizing a 10^{-2}-*M* suspension of the leucoflavin in 2 *M* lutidinium fluoroborate, pH 6, for 5 min before addition of the indicated solutions to a final concentration of 10^{-3} *M*. A: flavin semiquinone in either 1 *M* lutidinium chloride or 1 *M* lutidinium fluoroborate, pH 6. B: flavin semiquinone in 1 *M* lutidinium fluoroborate, plus 0.1 *M* nickel fluoroborate. C: same as B plus 6×10^{-2} *M* Cl^- added as lutidinium chloride. D: same as B plus 0.2 *M* Cl^- added as lutidinium chloride. E: flavin semiquinone in 1 *M* lutidinium chloride plus 0.1 *M* nickel fluoroborate. The modulation amplitude was 3 G and the temperature 113 K. Radical concentrations were estimated to be $\sim 10^{-4}$ *M*. The arrows indicate the estimated position of $P_{1/2}$, the power at half saturation. On the ordinate is plotted the logarithm of the ratio of the observed signal height at standardized amplification to the square root of the microwave power incident on the cavity; on the abscissa, the logarithm of the microwave power. In this type of plot horizontal lines are obtained when no saturation occurs. Note that in such logarithmic plots apparently small changes may represent considerable and easily measurable differences.

transfer can occur. This transfer may then take place via ligands of the metals. The very fact that hfs from ligands is observed in the EPR spectra of flavins, molybdenum, or nonheme iron shows that electrons are delocalized in these systems and are not, as in the classical picture, strictly localized on the metal or on an assumed oxidation-reduction center of the flavin molecule. Thus electron transfer from a heme group may proceed from the periphery of the porphyrin ring as well as via the axial ligands (135).

The oxidoreductive titrations as well as the kinetic studies have indicated that the carriers within the enzymes may differ in their apparent redox potentials and react in an ordered sequence. Measurements of electron-spin relaxation have provided an even more subtle probe for interactions of paramagnetic species within macromolecules, and it may be useful at this point to reassess our knowledge on this aspect. The semiquinones of metalflavoproteins, as a group, show a definitely higher electron-spin relaxation rate than those of metal-free flavoproteins and this has in general been a reliable diagnostic. More recent work has shown, however, that the spread of these relaxation rates is wide, with the metalflavoproteins occupying the upper range and the metal-free flavoproteins, the lower one (41). There is an area of contact of these ranges in which we find the relaxation rates of the most relaxed metal-free and the most poorly relaxed metalflavoproteins. With representatives of this range the decision whether a metal is present may not be safe. Another example that calls for caution deserves mention. The electron-spin relaxation rate of the semiquinone of yeast lactate dehydrogenase (or cytochrome b_2), for instance, falls in the range of that of metal-free flavoproteins, although it is well known that a heme group is present. Measurements of the heme spectra by spectrophotometry or EPR show that when flavin semiquinone is present in this molecule the heme iron is in the reduced state. This state is presumably low-spin ferrous, which is diamagnetic, and no effect on spin relaxation would be expected. With the nonheme iron and molybdenum containing flavoproteins the iron is at least always in a paramagnetic state when semiquinone is formed.

If we accept that the increased spin-relaxation rate of the semiquinones of metalflavoproteins is due to the interaction of the paramagnetic metal and the semiquinone, it is obvious that the semiquinone and the reduced iron-sulfur complex, which are manifest in the EPR signals, occur within the same molecules. This is not trivial, since in general not all the flavin nor all the nonheme iron is accounted for in the signals and spin-spin interaction of carriers in different molecules is highly unlikely. It should also be recalled that the iron-sulfur group in its oxidized form is diamagnetic, at least in the simpler iron-sulfur proteins.

In addition to the dependence of spin relaxation on the presence of a paramagnetic metal species, changes of spin relaxation with time of reaction, with pH, and with addition of substrates or inhibitors have been observed. Similar observations were made on the molybdenum components of aldehyde and xanthine oxidases. A rational explanation of all these observations could not and cannot now be given. However, as our knowledge of the reaction mechanism of these enzymes, particularly xanthine oxidase, increases, a few observations may be better understood. Thus the apparent large spin relaxation of the radical signal observed within milliseconds after adding reductant may be due, with xanthine and aldehyde oxidases and possibly also dihydroorotate dehydrogenase, to superposition of an oxygen radical signal on the flavin semiquinone signals. At the time of the spin-relaxation studies it was not known that oxygen radicals were formed in these reactions. Similarly, the variability of relaxation rates observed with the molybdenum components of xanthine and aldehyde oxidases under different conditions is probably not so much due to a change in spin relaxation of a single species but largely to a change in the species that occur. The reader is reminded of the considerable number of molybdenum species which have recently been found in the reduction of xanthine oxidase by xanthine (99) (Fig. 8-10). Although it had previously been concluded from the shape of the spin-relaxation curves that different species of molybdenum were involved, maybe much of what was considered a change in the relaxation behavior of individual species due to interaction with neighboring paramagnets should be attributed to the replacement of certain species by others with different relaxation behavior; that is to say, in the work on molybdenum the potential of spin-relaxation measurements for providing unambiguous information on the interaction of electron carriers may initially have been overestimated. Yet, no matter what the exact explanation is, spin-relaxation measurements have clearly indicated the presence of species of molybdenum or flavin semiquinones with different spin-relaxation behavior and the occurrence of intramolecular changes during reduction of metalflavoproteins. In the early phases of this work spin-relaxation measurements have therefore been a more sensitive probe for such changes than observation of shape and intensity of the EPR spectra. They may be still more sensitive for a number of subtle changes that are not expressed in resolvable features of the spectra.

It is not known what kind of magnetic interactions between paramagnetic states of the electron carriers are the basis for the observed changes of electron-spin relaxation. We might visualize what we could call specific interactions between certain carriers or, rather, nonspecific ones among any carriers that happen to be within a minimal distance of one another. As specific interactions we would designate those that are due to partial orbital overlap. On the other hand, the observed interactions may result merely from dipole interactions between paramagnets. Changes in intramolecular geometry or in the paramagnetism of individual carriers accompanying electron transfer could then modulate these interactions, whether or not they were specific. Such modulation would lead to the observed changes in spin-relaxation rates. The rates that have been observed set an approximate upper limit to the distance at which the interacting species are located. This distance should not exceed 10 Å.

We may thus conclude that the electron carriers occur in the protein in close vicinity of one another in groups, a picture that would of course be intuitively derived from their very function in electron transfer between donor and acceptor substrates.

8.6 SUMMARY

In closing it may be useful to summarize the special features of EPR spectroscopy and the auxiliary techniques that have been brought to bear in the field of flavins and flavoproteins. They are for flavin compounds of small molecular weight: studies of hfs, particularly after substitution of ^{2}H and ^{15}N for the natural isotopes in a number of positions in the molecule; a similar purpose was served by replacing certain groups, for example, $—CH_3$ with Cl or H, or by introducing altogether new ones, for example, forming the Zn^{2+} or Cd^{2+} chelates. The peculiar enhancement of hfs resolution by certain solvents or solvent mixtures also deserves mention here. Finally, studies of electron-spin relaxation and the application of ENDOR showed great promise. For flavoproteins and metalflavoproteins hfs analysis was useful only in the study of the Mo constituent. Here spectroscopy at 35 GHz proved to be of great value. Measurements of electron-spin relaxation appear to provide a sensitive tool for studies of the flavin and Mo components of metalflavoproteins. With the wide range of relaxation rates involved—very slow for simple flavoproteins and very rapid for the iron constituents—the whole range of attainable microwave powers and temperatures can be brought into play for optimal results. Rapid reaction techniques, rapid-freezing, and anaerobic techniques, such as anaerobic reductive titrations, were of great value, and finally optical spectroscopy on the same samples used for EPR spectroscopy proved useful.

It would appear that progress toward an understanding of the chemistry of flavins and flavoproteins, which proved to be so important in previous EPR applications in this area, combined with approaches by EPR and particularly ENDOR techniques, hold the greatest promise for immediate advances in the field of endeavors that is the subject of this chapter.

ACKNOWLEDGMENTS

I am grateful to a number of colleagues for their help in assembling and presenting the material covered here: to Dr. R. C. Bray and Dr. F. Müller for letting me see manuscripts in advance of publication and their critical review of parts of this chapter, to Dr. P.-S. Song for communication of unpublished results, to Dr. W. H. Orme-Johnson and Dr. C. R. Hartzell for their helpful discussions and suggestions. I am also indebted to the Institute of General Medical Sciences for support of the research on EPR of flavin compounds in my own laboratory (GM-12394) and for a Research Career Award (5-KO6-GM-18,442).

REFERENCES

1. K. Dudley, A. Ehrenberg, P. Hemmerich, and F. Müller, *Helv. Chim. Acta*, **47,** 1354 (1964).
2. P. Hemmerich, C. Veeger, and H. Wood, *Angew. Chem.*, Internat. Edit., **4,** 671 (1965).
3. L. Eriksson and A. Ehrenberg, *Acta Chem. Scand.*, **18,** 1437 (1964).
4. A. Hedberg, in *Magnetic Resonance in Biological Systems*, A. Ehrenberg, B. Malmström, and T. Vänngård, Eds., Pergamon, Oxford, 1967, p. 389.
5. F. Müller, P. Hemmerich, A. Ehrenberg, G. Palmer, and V. Massey, *European J. Biochem.*, **14,** 185 (1970).
6. V. Massey and G. Palmer, *Biochem.*, **5,** 3181 (1966).
7. G. Palmer and V. Massey, in *Biological Oxidations*, T. P. Singer, Ed., Wiley, New York, 1968, p. 263.
8. A. Ehrenberg, L. Eriksson, and F. Müller, in *Flavins and Flavoproteins*, E. Slater, Ed., Elsevier, Amsterdam, 1966, p. 37.
9. A. Ehrenberg, F. Müller, and P. Hemmerich, *European J. Biochem.*, **2,** 286 (1967).
10. F. Müller, L. Eriksson, and A. Ehrenberg, *European J. Biochem.*, **12,** 93 (1970).
11. A. Ehrenberg, in *Electronic Aspects of Biochemistry*, B. Pullman, Ed., Academic, New York, 1964, p. 379.
12. A. Ehrenberg, L. Eriksson, and P. Hemmerich, in *Oxidases and Related Redox Systems*, T. King, H. Mason, and M. Morrison, Eds., Wiley, New York, 1965, p. 179.
13. L. Eriksson and A. Ehrenberg, *Arch. Biochem. Biophys.*, **110,** 628 (1965).
14. F. Müller, P. Hemmerich, and A. Ehrenberg, in *3rd Intern. Symp. Flavins Flavoproteins*, H. Kamin, Ed., University Park Press, Baltimore, Maryland, 1971, pg. 107.
15. W. Walker and A. Ehrenberg, *FEBS Letters*, **3,** 315 (1969).
16. L. Michaelis, M. Schubert, and C. Smythe, *J. Biol. Chem.*, **116,** 587 (1936).
17. L. Michaelis and G. Schwarzenbach, *J. Biol. Chem.*, **123,** 527 (1938).
18. H. Beinert, *J. Am. Chem. Soc.*, **78,** 5323 (1956).
19. E. Land and A. Swallow, *Biochem.*, **8,** 2117 (1969).
20. P.-S. Song, *Ann. N.Y. Acad. Sci.*, **158,** 410 (1969).

21. W. Walker, A. Ehrenberg, and J. Lhoste, *Biochim. Biophys. Acta*, **215,** 166 (1970).
22. W. Walker, P. Hemmerich, and V. Massey, *Helv. Chim. Acta*, **50,** 2269 (1967).
23. P. Hemmerich, *Helv. Chim. Acta*, **47,** 464 (1964).
24. P. Hemmerich, D. DerVartanian, C. Veeger, and J. Van Voorst, *Biochim. Biophys. Acta*, **77,** 504 (1963).
25. F. Müller, A. Ehrenberg, and L. Eriksson, in *Magnetic Resonance in Biological Systems*, A. Ehrenberg, B. Malmström, and T. Vänngård, Eds., Pergamon, Oxford, 1967, p. 281.
26. H. Beinert and R. Sands, in *Free Radicals in Biological Systems*, M. Blois, Jr., W. Brown, R. Lemmon, R. Lindblom, and M. Weissbluth, Eds., Academic, New York, 1961, p. 17.
27. H. Beinert and G. Palmer, in *Advances in Enzymology and Related Subjects of Biochemistry*, F. Nord, Ed., Wiley-Interscience, New York, 1965, p. 105.
28. V. Massey, Q. Gibson, B. Curti, and N. Atherton, *Biochem. J.*, **89,** 54P (1963).
29. T. Nakamura, S. Nakamura, and Y. Ogura, *J. Biochem.*, **54,** 512 (1963).
30. V. Massey, G. Palmer, C. Williams, Jr., B. Swoboda, and R. Sands, in *Flavins and Flavoproteins*, E. Slater, Ed., Elsevier, Amsterdam, 1966, p. 133.
31. Y. Shethna, P. Wilson, and H. Beinert, *Biochim. Biophys. Acta*, **113,** 225 (1966).
32. J. Hinkson and W. Bulen, *J. Biol. Chem.*, **242,** 3345 (1967).
33. B. Masters, H. Kamin, Q. Gibson, and C. Williams, Jr., *J. Biol. Chem.*, **240,** 921 (1965).
34. G. Foust and V. Massey, in *Flavins and Flavoproteins*, K. Yagi, Ed., University of Tokyo Press, Tokyo, 1968, p. 7.
35. K. Huang, S.-I. Tu, and J. Wang, *Biochem. Biophys. Res. Commun.*, **34,** 48 (1969).
36. E. Haas, *Biochem. Z.*, **290,** 291 (1937).
37. A. Ehrenberg and G. Ludwig, *Science*, **127,** 1177 (1958).
38. V. Massey, R. Matthews, G. Foust, L. Howell, C. Williams, Jr., G. Zanetti, and S. Ronchi in *Advanced Study Institute on Pyridine Nucleotide-Dependent Dehydrogenases*, H. Sund, Ed., Springer-Verlag, Heidelberg, Germany, 1970, p. 393.
39. H. Beinert, *J. Biol. Chem.*, **225,** 465 (1967).
40. G. Palmer, F. Müller, and V. Massey in *3rd Intern. Symp. Flavins Flavoproteins*, H. Kamin, Ed., University Park Press, Baltimore, Maryland, 1971, p. 123.
41. H. Beinert and W. Orme-Johnson in *Magnetic Resonance in Biological Systems*, A. Ehrenberg, B. Malmström, and T. Vänngård, Eds., Pergamon, Oxford, 1967, p. 221.
42. J. Van Voorst, discussion in *Flavins and Flavoproteins*, E. Slater, Ed., Elsevier, Amsterdam, 1966, p. 155.
42a. J. S. Hyde, L. E. G. Eriksson, and A. Ehrenberg, *Biochim. Biophys. Acta*, **222,** 688 (1970).
43. P. Knowles, J. Gibson, F. Pick, and R. Bray, *Biochem. J.*, **111,** 53 (1969).
44. W. Orme-Johnson and H. Beinert, *Biochem. Biophys. Res. Commun.*, **36,** 905 (1969).
45. A. Ehrenberg, *Arkiv Kemi*, **17,** 97 (1962).
46. V. Aleman, P. Handler, G. Palmer, and H. Beinert, *J. Biol. Chem.*, **243,** 2560 (1968).
47. J. Hyde, in *Magnetic Resonance in Biological Systems*, A. Ehrenberg, B. Malmström, and T. Vänngård, Eds., Pergamon, Oxford, 1967, p. 63.
48. A. Ehrenberg, L. Eriksson, and J. Hyde, *Biochim. Biophys. Acta*, **167,** 482 (1968).

49. L. Eriksson, J. Hyde, and A. Ehrenberg, *Biochim. Biophys. Acta*, **192,** 211 (1969).

50. A. Ehrenberg, L. Eriksson, and J. Hyde in *3rd Intern. Symp. Flavins Flavoproteins*, H. Kamin, Ed., University Park Press, Baltimore, Maryland, 1971, p. 141.

50a. L. Eriksson, A. Ehrenberg, and J. Hyde, *European J. Biochem.*, **17,** 539 (1970).

51. J. Hyde, G. Rist, and L. Eriksson, *J. Phys. Chem.*, **72,** 4269 (1968).

52. T. Singer, J. Salach, W. Walker, M. Gutman, P. Hemmerich, and A. Ehrenberg in *3rd Intern. Symp. Flavins Flavoproteins*, H. Kamin, Ed., University Park Press, Baltimore, Maryland, 1971, p. 607.

53. W. Walker, J. Salach, M. Gutman, T. Singer, J. Hyde, and A. Ehrenberg, *FEBS Letters*, **5,** 237 (1969).

54. P. Hemmerich, A. Ehrenberg, W. Walker, L. Eriksson, J. Salach, P. Bader, and T. Singer, *FEBS Letters*, **3,** 37 (1969).

55. T. Singer in *Biological Oxidations*, T. Singer, Ed., Wiley, New York, 1968, p. 339.

56. R. Miller and V. Massey, *J. Biol. Chem.*, **240,** 1453 (1965).

57. M. Iwatsubo, A. Baudras, A. Di Franco, C. Capeillère, and F. Labeyrie in *Flavins and Flavoproteins*, K. Yagi, Ed., University of Tokyo Press, Tokyo, 1968, p. 41.

58. O. Groudinsky, C. Jacq, F. Labeyrie, F. Lederer, C. Monteilhet, M. Ninio, P. Pajot, and J. Risler in *3rd Intern. Symp. Flavins Flavoproteins*, H. Kamin, Ed., University Park Press, Baltimore, Maryland, 1971, p. 581.

59. L. Siegel and H. Kamin in *Flavins and Flavoproteins*, K. Yagi, Ed., University of Tokyo Press, Tokyo, 1968, p. 15.

60. R. Bray in *The Enzymes*, P. Boyer, H. Lardy and K. Myrbäck, Eds., Vol. 7, Academic, New York, 1963, p. 533.

61. R. Bray, A. Chisholm, L. Hart, L. Meriwether, and D. Watts in *Flavins and Flavoproteins*, E. C. Slater, Ed., Elsevier, Amsterdam, 1966, p. 117.

62. K. Rajagopalan, I. Fridovich, and P. Handler, *J. Biol. Chem.*, **237,** 922 (1962).

63. R. Garrett and A. Nason, *J. Biol. Chem.*, **244,** 2870 (1969).

64. A. Linnane and C. Wrigley, *Biochim. Biophys. Acta*, **77,** 408 (1963).

65. B. Buchanan, *Structure and Bonding*, **1,** 109 (1966).

66. R. Malkin and J. Rabinowitz, *Ann. Rev. Biochem.*, **36,** 113 (1967).

67. T. Kimura, *Structure and Bonding*, **5,** 1 (1968).

68. D. Hall and M. Evans, *Nature*, **223,** 1342 (1969).

69. J. Tsibris and R. Woody, *Coordination Chemistry Reviews*, **5,** 417 (1970).

70. T. Kimura, H. Watari, and A. Tasaki, *J. Biol. Chem.*, **245,** 4450 (1970).

71. T. Moss, D. Petering, and G. Palmer, *J. Biol. Chem.*, **244,** 2275 (1969).

72. A. Ehrenberg, referred to in T. Moss, D. Petering, and G. Palmer, *J. Biol. Chem.*, **244,** 2275 (1969) and referred to in J. Thornley, J. Gibson, F. Whatley, and D. Hall, *Biochem. Biophys. Res. Commun.*, **24,** 877 (1966).

72a. G. Palmer, W. Dunham, J. Fee, R. Sands, T. Iizuka, and T. Yonetani, *Biochim. Biophys. Acta*, **245,** 201 (1971).

73. Y. Shethna, D. DerVartanian, and H. Beinert, *Biochem. Biophys. Res. Commun.*, **31,** 862 (1968).

74. W. Orme-Johnson and H. Beinert, *J. Biol. Chem.*, **244,** 6143 (1969).

75. J. Tsibris, M. Namtvedt, and I. Gunsalus, *Biochem. Biophys. Res. Commun.*, **30,** 323 (1968).

76. W. Orme-Johnson, R. Hansen, H. Beinert, J. Tsibris, R. Bartholomaus, and I. C. Gunsalus, *Proc. Natl. Acad. Sci.*, **60,** 368 (1968).

77. J. Tsibris, R. Tsai, I. Gunsalus, W. Orme-Johnson, R. Hansen, and H. Beinert, *Proc. Natl. Acad. Sci.*, **59,** 959 (1968).

78. C. Johnson, R. Bray, R. Cammack, and D. Hall, *Proc. Natl. Acad. Sci.*, **63,** 1234 (1969).

79. R. Dunham, A. Bearden, I. Salmeen, G. Palmer, R. Sands, W. Orme-Johnson, and H. Beinert, *Biochim. Biophys. Acta*, **253,** 134 (1971).

80. R. Tsai, J. Tsibris, I. Gunsalus, W. Orme-Johnson, R. Hansen, and H. Beinert, quoted in Ref. 69.

81. H. Beinert and W. Orme-Johnson, *Ann. N.Y. Acad. Sci.*, **158,** 336 (1969).

82. J. Fritz, R. Anderson, J. Fee, G. Palmer, R. Sands, W. Orme-Johnson, H. Beinert, J. Tsibris, and I. C. Gunsalus, *Biochim. Biophys. Acta*, **253,** 110 (1971).

83. J. Gibson, D. Hall, J. Thornley, and F. Whatley, *Proc. Natl. Acad. Sci.*, **56,** 987 (1966).

83a. W. Dunham, G. Palmer, R. Sands, and A. Bearden, *Biochim. Biophys. Acta*, **253,** 373 (1971).

84. D. Hall, J. Gibson, and F. Whatley, *Biochem. Biophys. Res. Commun.*, **23,** 81 (1966).

85. K. Rajagopalan, P. Handler, G. Palmer, and H. Beinert, *J. Biol. Chem.*, **243,** 3784 (1968).

86. P. Handler et al., discussion in *Oxidases and Related Redox Systems*, Vol. 1, T. King, H. Mason, and M. Morrison, Eds., Wiley, New York, 1965, Discussions, p. 399.

87. G. Palmer, R. Sands, and L. Mortenson, *Biochem. Biophys. Res. Commun.*, **23,** 357 (1966).

88. D. DerVartanian, C. Veeger, W. Orme-Johnson, and H. Beinert, *Biochim. Biophys. Acta*, **191,** 22 (1969).

88a. N. Orme-Johnson, W. Orme-Johnson, R. Hansen, H. Beinert, and Y. Hatefi, *Biochem. Biophys. Res. Commun.*, **44,** 446 (1971).

89. Y. Hatefi, *Proc. Natl. Acad. Sci.*, **60,** 733 (1968).

90. D. DerVartanian, C. Veeger, W. Orme-Johnson, and H. Beinert, *Federation Proc.*, **26,** 732 (1967).

91. J. Gibson and R. Bray, *Biochim. Biophys. Acta*, **153,** 721 (1968).

92. G. Palmer and V. Massey, *J. Biol. Chem.*, **244,** 2614 (1969).

93. H. Beinert and R. Sands, *Biochem. Biophys. Res. Commun.*, **3,** 41 (1960).

94. W. Blumberg in *Magnetic Resonance in Biological Systems*, A. Ehrenberg, B. Malmström, and T. Vänngård, Eds., Pergamon, Oxford, 1967, p. 119.

95. C. Hare, I. Bernal, and H. Gray, *Inorg. Chem.*, **1,** 831 (1962).

96. R. Bray, B. Malmström, and T. Vänngård, *Biochem. J.*, **73,** 193 (1959).

97. R. Bray, *Biochem. J.*, **196,** 196 (1961).

98. G. Palmer, R. Bray, and H. Beinert, *J. Biol. Chem.*, **239,** 2657 (1964).

99. R. Bray and T. Vänngård, *Biochem. J.*, **114,** 725 (1969).

100. R. Bray and L. Meriwether, *Nature*, **212,** 467 (1966).

101. R. Bray, P. Knowles, and L. Meriwether in *Magnetic Resonance in Biological Systems*, A. Ehrenberg, B. Malmström, and T. Vänngård, Eds., Pergamon, Oxford, 1967, p. 249.

102. R. Bray, P. Knowles, F. Pick, and T. Vänngård, *Biochem. J.*, **107,** 601 (1968).

103. K. Rajagopalan, P. Handler, G. Palmer, and H. Beinert, *J. Biol. Chem.*, **243,** 3797 (1968).
104. R. Bray and P. Knowles, *Proc. Roy. Soc. (London)*, **A-302,** 351 (1968).
105. H. Komai, V. Massey, and G. Palmer, *J. Biol. Chem.*, **244,** 1692 (1969).
106. F. Pick and R. Bray, *Biochem. J.*, **114,** 735 (1969).
107. I. Yamazaki, H. Mason, and L. Piette, *J. Biol. Chem.*, **235,** 2444 (1960).
108. L. Tegnér and B. Holmström, *Photochem. Photobiol.*, **5,** 223 (1966).
109. J. Lhoste, A. Haug, and P. Hemmerich, *Biochem.*, **5,** 3290 (1966).
110. T. Shiga and L. Piette, *Photochem. Photobiol.*, **3,** 213 (1964) and **4,** 769 (1965).
111. B. Smaller, *Advan. Biol. Med. Phys.*, **9,** 225 (1963).
112. P.-S. Song, *J. Phys. Chem.*, **72,** 536 (1968).
113. H. Beinert in *3rd Intern. Symp. Flavins Flavoproteins*, University Park Press, Baltimore, Maryland, 1971, p. 416.
114. Q. Gibson, V. Massey, and N. Atherton, *Biochem. J.*, **85,** 369 (1962).
115. B. Van Gelder and H. Beinert, *Biochim. Biophys. Acta*, **189,** 1 (1969).
116. D. DeVault and B. Chance, *Biophys. J.*, **6,** 826 (1966).
117. J. Fox and G. Tollin, *Biochem.*, **5,** 3865 (1966).
118. J. Fox and G. Tollin, *Biochem.*, **5,** 3873 (1966).
119. M. Uozumi, *J. Physiol. Soc. Japan*, **27,** 243 (1965).
120. R. Bray, *Biochem. J.*, **81,** 189 (1961).
121. R. Bray in *Rapid Mixing and Sampling Techniques in Biochemistry*, B. Chance, R. Eisenhardt, Q. Gibson, and K. Lonberg-Holm, Eds., Academic, New York, 1964, p. 195.
122. G. Palmer, and H. Beinert in *Rapid Mixing and Sampling Techniques in Biochemistry*, B. Chance, R. Eisenhardt, Q. Gibson, and K. Lonberg-Holm, Eds., Academic, New York, 1964, p. 205.
123. V. Aleman, P. Handler, G. Palmer, and H. Beinert, *J. Biol. Chem.*, **243,** 2560 (1968).
124. H. Beinert, G. Palmer, T. Cremona, and T. Singer, *J. Biol. Chem.*, **240,** 475 (1965).
125. H. Beinert and G. Palmer, *J. Biol. Chem.*, **239,** 1221 (1964).
126. R. Bray, G. Palmer, and H. Beinert, *J. Biol. Chem.*, **239,** 2667 (1964).
127. D. Ballou, G. Palmer, and V. Massey, *Biochem. Biophys. Res. Commun.*, **36,** 898 (1969).
128. R. Haugland, L. Stryer, T. Stengle, and J. Baldeschwieler, *Biochem.*, **6,** 498 (1967).
129. M. Cohn, *Biochem.*, **2,** 623 (1963).
130. M. Cohn in *Magnetic Resonance in Biological Systems*, A. Ehrenberg, B. Malmström, and T. Vänngård, Eds., Pergamon, Oxford, 1967, p. 101.
131. S. Koenig and W. Schillinger, *J. Biol. Chem..*, **244,** 3283 (1969).
132. C. Hamilton and H. McConnell in *Structural Chemistry and Molecular Biology*, A. Rich and N. Davidson, Eds., Freeman, San Francisco, 1968, p. 115.
133. D. Bozanic, K. Krikorian, D. Mergerian, and R. Minarik, *J. Chem. Phys.*, **50,** 3606 (1969).
134. B. Rosenberg and E. Postow, *Ann. N.Y. Acad. Sci.*, **158,** 161 (1969).
135. C. Castro and H. Davis, *J. Amer. Chem. Soc.*, **91,** 5405 (1969).

CHAPTER NINE

Copper Proteins

TORE VÄNNGÅRD

Department of Biochemistry
Chalmers Institute of Technology and University of Göteborg
Göteborg, Sweden

9.1 INTRODUCTION

In almost all copper complexes studied by EPR techniques the valence state of the copper ion is +2. The three-valent state has been observed in EPR, but only in a few cases (1), and is not likely to be of any importance in biological systems. The Cu^{1+} ion may well exist in proteins, but since this ion has no partially filled shell all compounds of Cu^{1+} are diamagnetic and cannot be studied by EPR techniques.

Cu^{2+} has in its outermost shell nine *d*-electrons, a configuration that can be considered equivalent to one unpaired "hole." The electronic structure is particularly simple and comparatively easy to study by EPR. Since copper and ligand hyperfine structure can often be observed, Cu^{2+} is one of the best characterized ions with respect to its EPR properties. Early studies concentrated on Cu^{2+} as an impurity in inorganic crystals. In recent years the interest has centered around copper in organic complexes. The reader is referred to compilations of experimental data in Refs. 2 and 3.

Studies of copper in biological systems began in the late fifties (4) and were concerned with the direct establishment of the valence state of the copper in proteins. Earlier this had to be done by indirect chemical methods. It soon became apparent from measurements of the EPR intensity (5, 6) that in some proteins not all copper was detected. This observation led to the suggestion that part of the copper was present as Cu^{1+}. As discussed fully below, however, the absence of an EPR signal can have several reasons, and a rather complicated picture of the state and function of copper in copper proteins has emerged during the last few years.

The EPR and optical properties of a complex are quite intimately connected with one another. Therefore in this chapter optical absorption and activity are also discussed. In particular, the "blue" copper proteins, with their unusually high extinction in the visible, are dealt with at some length. We will try to classify the proteins according to their spectral properties and relate these to the function of the proteins. For further discussions of some of the aspects covered in this chapter earlier review articles should be consulted (7).

GENERAL CONSIDERATIONS

9.2 OPTICAL SPECTRA AND *g* FACTORS OF Cu^{2+}

For an understanding of the qualitative features of the EPR of copper it is essential to have some knowledge of the bonding situation normally encountered in copper complexes and its consequences for the optical and magnetic properties. An elementary account of the theory is given here, but for a full description the reader is referred to textbooks on ligand-field theory (8a) and coordination compounds (8b) and to the books cited in Chapter 1.

For many copper complexes the ligand atoms will, to a first approximation, form an octahedron around the central ion. As discussed in Chapter 1, in the simple crystal-field picture the field from a regular octahedral environment splits the five *d*-orbitals into two sets with different energy, one lower set (t_{2g}) consisting of the orbitals d_{xy}, d_{xz}, and d_{yz} and one upper set (e_g) comprised by the two orbitals $d_{x^2-y^2}$ and d_{z^2} (Fig. 9-1). For Cu^{2+} with its nine *d*-electrons the lowest total energy is obtained with the unpaired "hole" in the upper set. Such a configuration, however, is not stable against distortions according to the Jahn-Teller theorem (see Ref. 8b, p. 109). The distortions may be small, even having a time average equal to zero (9), but in most cases, in particular for Cu^{2+} bound to proteins, the ligands cause large deviations from the octahedral symmetry. The coordination normally is distorted so that two opposing ligands are farther away from the metal ion than the remaining four ligands. This symmetry is called tetragonal, and of the two orbitals in the e_g set the $d_{x^2-y^2}$ will now be highest in energy, since its lobes are closer to the negative charge of the ligands than are the lobes of d_{z^2} (see Fig. 9-1). Therefore $d_{x^2-y^2}$ will contain the unpaired hole.

Thus one effect of the crystal field is to bring the unpaired hole into an orbital, well separated in energy from other orbitals. The orbital motion can

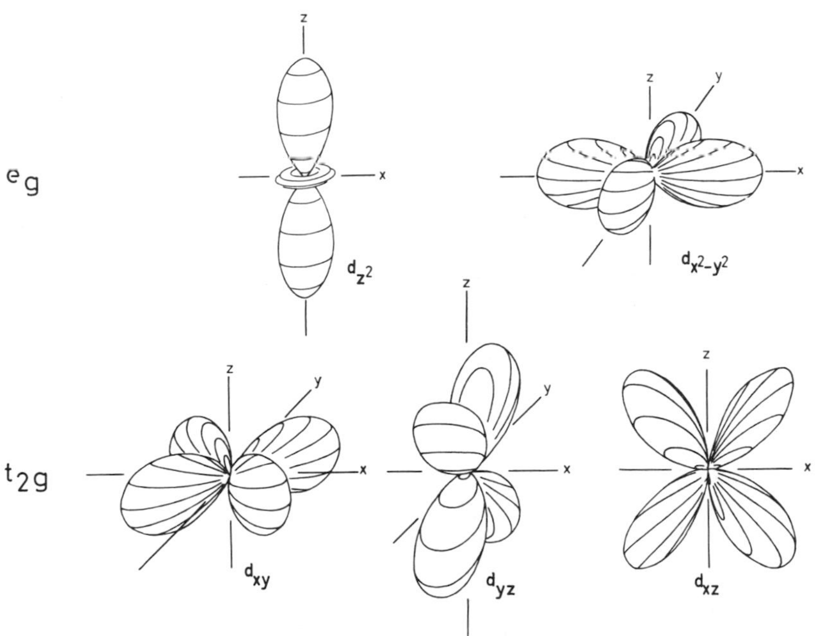

Fig. 9-1 The five 3*d*-orbitals. In an octahedral crystal field they split into a lower set (t_{2g}) consisting of three orbitals and an upper set (e_g) made up of two orbitals. The 9 *d*-electrons of Cu^{2+} fill up the lower set and leave a hole in one of the upper orbitals. In tetragonal symmetry this is usually the $d_{x^2-y^2}$ orbital.

contribute to the energy differences measured in EPR only if the "hole" can move from one orbital to another. Since this is not possible, the orbital contribution to the magnetism is "quenched." Therefore the g factors observed for Cu^{2+} are close to that of a free electron with spin motion only, that is, 2.0023. The deviations from this value are caused by the spin-orbit coupling, which is an interaction between the magnetic moments associated with the spin and orbital motions. This causes the unpaired hole to spend part of its time in other orbitals than $d_{x^2-y^2}$, and thereby some of the orbital motion is reintroduced to an extent that depends on the ratio of the spin-orbit coupling to the strength of the crystal field. Thus we have approximately

$$g = 2.0023\left(1 + \frac{r\lambda}{\Delta}\right), \tag{9-1}$$

where λ is the spin-orbit coupling constant and Δ is the splitting between the two sets of orbitals illustrated in Fig. 1-21. The constant r depends on the system under consideration and on the direction of the applied magnetic field. For Cu^{2+} in a tetragonal coordination with the unpaired hole in $d_{x^2-y^2}$, r is -4 and -1 with the magnetic field parallel and perpendicular to the fourfold symmetry axis, respectively. The basic reason why $g_{\parallel}$ departs more than $g_{\perp}$ from 2.0023 lies in the shape of the orbitals. It might be appreciated from Fig. 9-1 that a "hole" in $d_{x^2-y^2}$ can acquire angular motion around the z axis by spending part of its time in the d_{xy} orbital. To get an orbital motion around the axes perpendicular to the z axis the "mixing" of $d_{x^2-y^2}$ with d_{xz} or d_{yz} is important, but this is not so efficient as the mixing with d_{xy}.

The spin-orbit coupling constant can be obtained from optical spectra of the free gaseous Cu^{2+} ion and is about -830 K.* As a consequence of the negative value of λ, the g factors of Cu^{2+} are larger than 2.0023 with very few exceptions. The value for Δ must be obtained from the complex under study, but optical absorption spectra of copper compounds usually are poorly resolved so that no complete analysis of the spectrum is possible. Often we identify the transition frequently found in the visible region around 600 nm as an excitation of an electron from one of the orbitals in the lower set (Fig. 1-21) to the $d_{x^2-y^2}$ orbital in the upper set. Thus a typical value for Δ is 16 kK which gives $g_{\parallel} = 2.4$ and $g_{\perp} = 2.1$.

The observed values of $g_{\parallel}$ in tetragonal symmetry range from about 2.4 in complexes with water to less than 2.1 in complexes in which the metal ion is surrounded by sulfur atoms (10) and a similar variation exists in $g_{\perp}$. In part this is due to variation in Δ from one complex to another,

* Throughout this chapter K (kaiser) and the derived units kK and mK will be used for cm^{-1}, $10^3 cm^{-1}$, and $10^{-3} cm^{-1}$, respectively.

but the observed values of $(g - 2.0023)$ are always smaller than those predicted on the basis of Eq. 9-1. In part, at least, this is caused by a spreading of the unpaired electron out to the ligands. Sometimes this delocalization is described by the use of an effective spin-orbit coupling constant that is smaller than in the free ion (for an example see Ref. 11). In more elaborate treatments of covalency effects molecular orbitals are formed from linear combinations of metal and ligand orbitals. To a first approximation the coefficient α of $d_{x^2-y^2}$ in the molecular orbital containing the unpaired hole enters the expressions for the g factors in the following way

$$g_{\parallel} = 2.0023\left(1 - \frac{4\alpha^2\lambda}{\Delta}\right),$$
$$g_{\perp} = 2.0023\left(1 - \frac{\alpha^2\lambda}{\Delta}\right). \tag{9-2}$$

Since α is smaller than unity, the departure of the g factors from the free-electron value is decreased. Thus by measurements of the optical energies and the g factors the delocalization of the unpaired electron can be quantitatively estimated. Typical values of α^2 are 0.6 to 0.9. In the complete treatments coefficients of other molecular orbitals also enter into the expressions. A detailed discussion can be found in Ref. 12.

Care should be exercised in the interpretation of the molecular orbital coefficients, since the actual values obtained in some cases may have rather limited physical significance; for example, the "nephelauxetic" effect (13) does reduce the g factors without any introduction of electron delocalization onto the ligands.

On the whole, because of the combined effects of the crystal field splittings and the delocalization of the unpaired electron, there is an empirical correlation between the kind of atoms coordinating and the g factors (14). The largest g factors are obtained with oxygen as ligand, smaller ones result from coordination to nitrogen, and still smaller from sulfur coordination.

When the coordination of a copper complex differs from that of the elongated octahedron discussed above, rather different EPR results may be obtained, and the correlation mentioned breaks down completely; for example, cases are known (15) in which the symmetry is tetragonal but in which the axial ligands are closer than the four in-plane ligands. The unpaired hole will enter into the d_{z^2} orbital and the orbital contribution to the g factor is small when the magnetic field is along the z axis. As a consequence $g_{\parallel}$ is smaller than $g_{\perp}$. Admittedly, this is an unusual bonding situation, but proteins may force the metal ion into rather unique coordinations (see below).

EPR of Cu^{2+} in more or less tetrahedral coordination has been studied in several cases. The energy level diagram of Fig. 1-21 is then applicable where now the t_{2g} set is highest. As in the octahedral arrangement, a regular tetrahedral coordination of Cu^{2+} is not stable but will be distorted. With small distortions EPR can be observed only at low temperatures and the g factors differ very much from those discussed above (16). With larger distortions, however, which involve a flattening of the tetrahedron toward an arrangement with four ligands in a plane, the g factors turn out to be similar to those resulting from an ordinary tetragonal coordination (17, 18).

In general, from the g factors alone and their orientation dependence, no direct conclusions can be drawn regarding the arrangement of the ligands; for example, any coordination with an axis with a symmetry that is threefold or higher will give an axial EPR spectrum with no variation in the g factor and the copper hyperfine splitting if the applied magnetic field is turned around in a plane perpendicular to this axis. Indeed, most EPR spectra of Cu^{2+} have near axial symmetry even if the four close ligands are different, for example, in cases with two oxygen and two nitrogen atoms. Large deviations from axial symmetry of the EPR spectrum have been observed in some proteins, however. This might reflect the ability of the protein ligand to force the copper ion into unique environments.

9.3 HYPERFINE COUPLING TO THE COPPER NUCLEUS

The spins, magnetic moments and natural abundances of the relevant nuclei are given in Table A-1 (p. 61). It is seen that the two copper isotopes ^{63}Cu and ^{65}Cu have the same spin and nearly the same magnetic moment. Therefore the isotopes give closely spaced lines (see Fig. 9-2a) and, as most EPR signals from copper proteins have fairly large linewidths (about 50 G), the two isotopes usually do not give separated peaks. However, whenever ligand nitrogen hyperfine structure is observed and discussed (see below), isotopically pure copper should, if possible, be used.

The sources of copper hyperfine structure in Cu^{2+} compounds are illustrated by the following simplified theoretical expressions for the hyperfine coupling constants $A_{\parallel}$ and $A_{\perp}$. The symmetry is assumed to be tetragonal with the unpaired hole in the $d_{x^2-y^2}$ orbital (19).

$$\begin{aligned} A_{\parallel} &= P\left[-\kappa - \frac{4\alpha^2}{7} + (g_{\parallel} - 2.0023) + \frac{3(g_{\perp} - 2.0023)}{7}\right], \\ A_{\perp} &= P\left[-\kappa + \frac{2\alpha^2}{7} + \frac{11(g_{\perp} - 2.0023)}{14}\right]. \end{aligned} \tag{9-3}$$

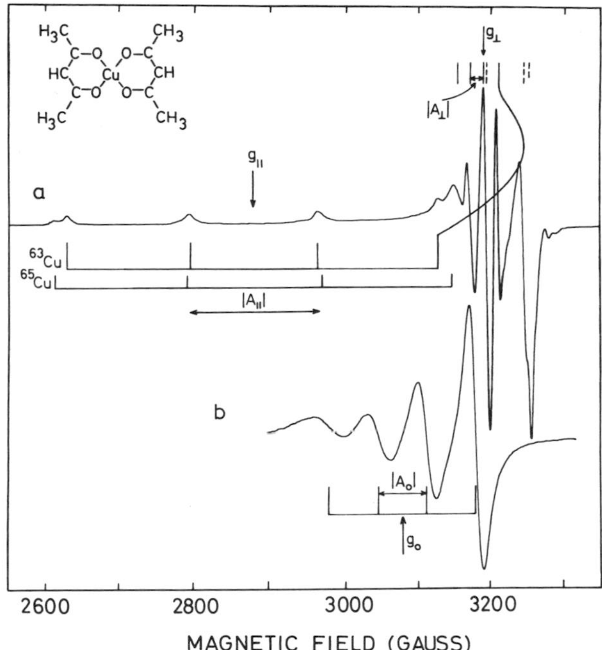

Fig. 9-2 EPR spectra of a solution of a Cu^{2+} complex, in (*a*) frozen at 77 K and in (*b*) at room temperature. The *g*-factors and hyperfine constants are measured as described in the text, and their values are $g_{\parallel} = 2.285$, $g_{\perp} = 2.060$, $g_0 = 2.135$, $|A_{\parallel}| = 167$ G. $|A_{\perp}| = 17$ G and $|A_0| = 67$ G. In (*a*) the dashed bars indicate the position of the "overshoot" lines which occur from the particular angular dependence of the copper hyperfine lines as shown for one of them (the full curved line to the right in the figure). The small peaks at the highest field in (*a*) arise from a second complex existing in low concentration (cf. Fig. 3 in Ref. 34). The sample is 5 m*M* in Cu^{2+} and 40 m*M* in acetylacetonate ($CH_3COCH_2COCH_3$) in a 1:1 water:dioxan solvent at alkaline pH. The same tube was used for both spectra with five times higher spectrometer gain in (*b*). Other settings were microwave power 2 mW, frequency 9199 MHz, field modulation 7 G, time constant 0.3 sec, and sweep time 4 min.

The constant P is taken from experimental data or calculations on gaseous ions and is about 35 mK. The terms containing the factor α^2 arise from the dipole-dipole interaction between the magnetic moments associated with the spin motion of the electron and the nucleus. If the unpaired electron is delocalized to the neighboring atoms, this contribution is reduced as α^2 decreases from unity. The terms containing the g factors are due to a similar coupling between the orbital motion and the nucleus. Of course, when the orbital contribution to the paramagnetism is quenched, that is, $g = 2.0023$, these terms vanish. Finally, the terms in κ arise from the Fermi contact interaction which has its origin in a nonvanishing probability of finding the unpaired electron at the site of the nucleus. As discussed in Chapter 1 and seen from Eq. 9-3, this term is independent of the direction of the magnetic field; that is, it is isotropic. It is quite difficult to make good theoretical estimations of the contact term and frequently κ is taken as an empirical parameter that is varied to fit the experimental data. Its numerical value is 0.3 to 0.4 and it shows a considerable variation from one complex to another (20). With $\kappa = 0.35$, $\alpha^2 = 0.8$, $g_{\parallel} = 2.30$, and $g_{\perp} = 2.07$, Eq. 9-3 yields the values for the hyperfine couplings $A_{\parallel} = -17$ mK and $A_{\perp} = -2.5$ mK. Thus we obtain $A_{\parallel} = -160$ and $A_{\perp} = -26$ G,* and these values are close to observed values. Also, in most cases in which the signs have been determined both couplings have turned out to be negative, but it should be pointed out that spectra as shown in this chapter only give the magnitude of the coupling constants.

In addition to the interactions with the magnetic dipole of the nucleus that have been discussed above there is a coupling to the electric quadrupole moment of the nucleus. This is smaller than the magnetic interaction and can usually be studied only in single crystals. However, its effect on the spectrum from powdered samples has been discussed (21).

9.4 HYPERFINE COUPLING TO THE LIGAND NUCLEI

As already pointed out, the delocalization of the unpaired electron onto the ligands affects the *g* factors and copper hyperfine coupling constants. The most direct information on such delocalization may be obtained if the ligand atoms have nuclei with magnetic moments (see Table A-1, p. 61). In such cases a splitting of the EPR lines into several components corresponding to different orientations of the spins of the ligand nuclei is often observed. With Cu^{2+} most studies have been concerned with the ^{14}N isotope, in some cases complemented with investigations on samples enriched in ^{15}N (22). The natural abundance of the stable oxygen isotope with a non-zero magnetic moment is so small that an enriched sample is almost an absolute requirement for the observation of oxygen hyperfine couplings. With sulfur the hyperfine interaction has been observed from ^{33}S in natural abundance (10), although enrichment would simplify the EPR work considerably.

As with the copper hyperfine structure, the ligand hyperfine coupling originates from dipole-dipole and Fermi contact interactions. For nitrogen the latter term is dominant and is normally considered to arise from the

* To convert from the energy unit K to magnetic field in G we multiply with 21,418 and divide by the corresponding *g* factor.

delocalization of the unpaired hole into the s-part of a σ-bonding sp^2-hybrid on the nitrogen. Thus nitrogen hyperfine couplings are quite isotropic. For Cu^{2+} complexes with the unpaired hole in the $d_{x^2-y^2}$ orbital, couplings are expected to occur to the ligand atoms in the plane only and not to the axial ligands. This is confirmed by experimental data (23).

The patterns obtained with a coupling to one, two, three, or four equivalent nitrogen atoms can be obtained by an extension of the arguments presented in Chapter 1 and are, respectively, 1:1:1, 1:2:3:2:1, 1:3:6:7:6:3:1, and 1:4:10:16:19:16:10:4:1. Thus, with many interacting nitrogen atoms, it becomes increasingly difficult to detect all the superhyperfine lines.

When nitrogen splittings are detected by EPR, they frequently have a value of 10 to 15 G. Smaller splittings are difficult to resolve but may contribute to the linewidth. Thus it seems to be a fairly general observation that the linewidth is greater with the metal coordinating to nitrogen than to oxygen atoms.

Recently it has been demonstrated that hyperfine couplings which are unresolved in ordinary EPR spectra can be detected by the use of the electron-nuclear double-resonance technique (ENDOR). Ligand hyperfine splittings from nitrogen and hydrogen have been observed in a number of organic complexes, not only in single crystals but also in powdered samples (24). Superhyperfine structure has also been detected from a frozen solution of the copper protein stellacyanin (Ref. 25a, see also below). In addition to the interaction with the magnetic moment of the ligand nuclei, ENDOR provides information on the interaction with the quadrupole moment (24). This information may turn out to be useful for the characterization of the bonding in metal complexes.

9.5 PAIRS OF COPPER IONS

An EPR signal from a copper protein that shows effects due to the proximity of two copper ions has not yet been reported.* However, a large number of studies on small complexes in which copper-copper interaction is important has been performed. Since one of these complexes involves amino acids (26), a short account of the EPR of copper pairs is given here.

Two entirely different situations are encountered. In the first case the system formally consists of one Cu^{2+} and one Cu^{+} ion and in the second we have two Cu^{2+} ions. In the former the pair contains only one unpaired

* *Note added in proof:* Evidence for dipole-dipole interaction has been found in a modified form of hemocyanin (25b).

electron and such a system has been studied by EPR (27). The spectrum differed from its normal appearance in that the number of copper hyperfine lines was increased from four to seven with unequal intensity. These results can be understood in terms of an interaction of the unpaired electron with two equivalent copper nuclei.

The second case, a Cu^{2+}—Cu^{2+} pair, is considerably more complicated, with two unpaired electrons to consider. There are two mechanisms by which the ions can interact. The dipole-dipole interaction depends on the distance between the ions and their relative orientation, whereas the exchange mechanism requires an overlap between the wavefunctions of the two ions. Depending on the size of these couplings in relation to the Zeeman and hyperfine interactions, rather different EPR spectra may result. In a number of cases studied in recent years the distance between the ions has been obtained from an estimate of the dipolar term (26, 28). The $\Delta M = 2$ transitions occurring at about half the magnetic field of the normal transitions (cf. Section 1.9) have been used for this purpose.

EXPERIMENTAL CONSIDERATIONS

9.6 SAMPLE STATE AND LINESHAPES

The most detailed information from an EPR experiment is obtained if the sample is a single crystal which has had its structure determined by crystallographic methods. This allows a rather detailed characterization of the bonding in a complex. The experimental aspects of EPR single crystal work on proteins have been discussed by Brill and Venable (29–31). The only copper protein studied in this way, however, is copper insulin, a "synthetic" copper protein (see below). In the future we would expect such studies to become more frequent as the number of protein structures determined by X-ray methods increases rapidly.

Almost all studies on copper proteins have been performed with the sample in powder form or in a frozen solution. In this case almost as much information can be obtained on the magnitudes of the g factors and hyperfine couplings as can be obtained with single crystal work, but the information on the directional properties of these parameters in relation to the molecular structure is, of course, lost.

The shape of a 9-GHz spectrum of a frozen solution or a powder of a copper complex is typically that of Fig. 9-2*a*. The spectrum resembles that of Fig. 1-3*b*, with the additional structure caused by the copper hyperfine splitting. Since the linewidth is rather small, a large number of peaks is resolved but it is fairly obvious how $g_{\|}$ and $A_{\|}$ should be measured. The copper hyperfine structure around $g_{\perp}$ is also resolved. Because of the second-order effects the field at $g_{\perp}$ is slightly off the center of the hyperfine quartet. In addition to the powder lines obtained with the applied magnetic field parallel or perpendicular to the symmetry axis, peaks will appear whenever the magnetic field of a given transition reaches a maximum or minimum at intermediate directions. In copper spectra recorded at 9 GHz this effect often produces an "extra" or "overshoot" (32) peak at the high-field end of the spectrum. Fig. 9-2*a* shows this peak split by the presence of the two isotopes indicated by two dashed bars. Another hyperfine transition also gives an "overshoot" line, although it is not resolved from the perpendicular part of the spectrum.

Fairly often the EPR spectrum of a copper protein or a low-molecular-weight complex in a frozen solution shows extra structure that can be attributed to hyperfine coupling to ligand atoms as shown in Fig. 9-3*a*. This structure is most clearly seen close to the $g_{\perp}$ field region. However, we should be very careful in trying to deduce the number of nitrogen atoms contributing

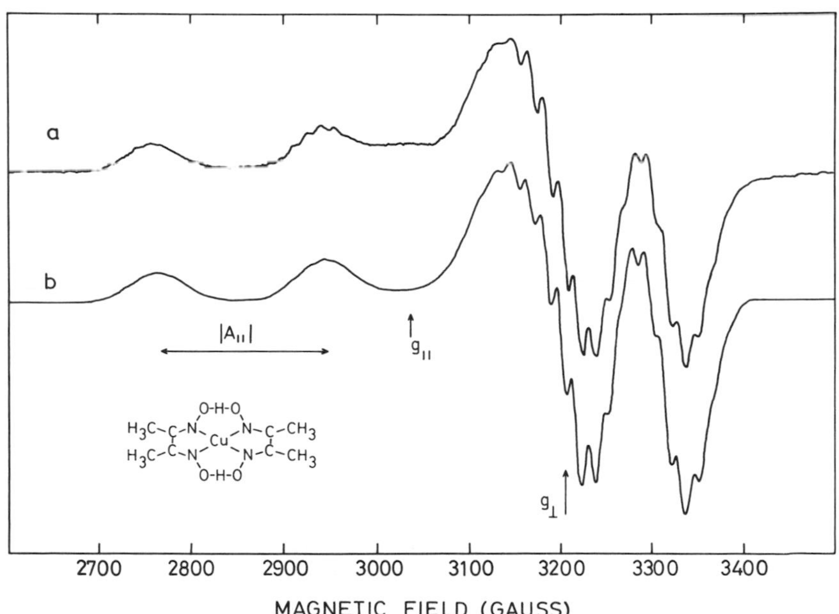

Fig. 9-3 Experimental (*a*) and simulated (*b*) spectra of a frozen solution of a Cu^{2+} complex exhibiting nitrogen hyperfine structure (23). The absorption above 3300 G is mostly due to an overshoot line (cf. Fig. 9-2*a*). The sample is Cu^{2+}-dimethylglyoxim dissolved in chloroform containing 0.2 M pyridine.

to this structure. Even without nitrogen splitting the spectra may be rather complicated because of the presence of copper hyperfine coupling, deviation from axial symmetry, and extra absorption peaks described above (see Fig. 9-2*a* and Refs. 33, 34). In addition, the presence of two copper isotopes with slightly different magnetic moments can cause further splitting (35). Whenever possible, studies on nitrogen hyperfine structure should be made with samples enriched in one of the isotopes (cf. Figs. 9-3 and 9-11). Even when the study is limited to the less complicated room-temperature spectra, isotopically pure samples should be used. The interpretation of the nitrogen hyperfine couplings and the values of the EPR parameters in Fig. 9-3*a* have been checked through a comparison with a spectrum simulated with a computer (Fig. 9-3*b*). The techniques used for such simulations have been described by many authors, see, for example, Refs. 30 to 32.

Room-temperature EPR spectra of solutions of small copper complexes look rather different from those obtained from the frozen solutions (see Fig. 9-2*b*). As discussed in Chapter 1, the reason for this is that the molecules rotate so fast at room temperature that the anisotropic couplings are averaged out and only the isotropic ones remain. Thus, instead of giving information on both $g_{\|}$ and $g_{\perp}$, room temperature spectra give only their average $g_0 = (g_x + g_y + g_z)/3$, or, in the axial case, $g_0 = (g_{\|} + 2g_{\perp})/3$. Similarly, the hyperfine coupling is $A_0 = (A_x + A_y + A_z)/3$ or $(A_{\|} + 2A_{\perp})/3$. For copper complexes, however, the averaging of the anisotropy usually is not quite complete even at room temperature. This leads to a variation in the linewidth of the copper hyperfine lines as seen in Fig. 9-2*b* (see Ref. 4 of Chapter 1, p. 97). In general, a transition with large anisotropy in frozen solution has a larger room-temperature width than a transition with smaller anisotropy.

It should be noticed that the isotropic copper hyperfine splitting, measured in a solution, has contributions not only from the Fermi contact interaction but also from the coupling between the orbital motion and the nucleus. Taking the proper average of Eq. 9-3, we obtain $A_0 = P(-\kappa + \delta g_0)$, where $\delta g_0 = g_0 - 2.0023$. The second term in A_0 is often comparable in magnitude to the first one.

With copper proteins the room-temperature spectra look almost the same as in the frozen state (36) (see Fig. 9-4). This is because the tumbling rate of proteins is not large enough at room temperature to average out the anisotropy. The spectra, however, are usually less well resolved at room temperature than at low temperatures.

It should be noticed that chemical systems may change when a solution is frozen and that some difficulties may develop when EPR results from low temperatures are to be correlated with other properties measured at room temperature; for example, small modifications in the coordination

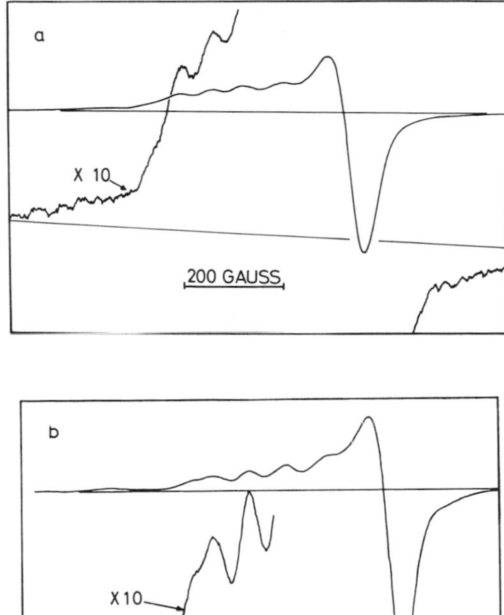

Fig. 9-4 EPR spectra of a solution of the copper protein ceruloplasmin recorded at 4C(*a*) and at about 100 K(*b*) (36). Essentially the same spectra are obtained, the main difference being the resolution of the various components.

may occur so that the energies of the optical transitions change, making determinations of bonding parameters uncertain. For low molecular complexes a difference between g_0 obtained from room-temperature work and the average of the low-temperature g factors indicates that such a change has occurred (cf. Ref. 37). Also, if several species are present in some equilibrium, their relative abundance may change in the freezing (37).

A rather serious problem in the low-temperature study of low-molecular copper complexes is the aggregation of solute molecules that frequently occurs when water solutions are frozen (23, 37, 38). In such cases the EPR spectra become quite broad and unresolved because of the interaction between neighboring copper ions. In several studies (23, 37) this aggregation has been diminished by the addition of large concentrations (about 2 M) of a perchlorate salt. This presumably causes the water to crystallize in a somewhat different fashion. With proteins this aggregation problem appears to be less serious.

9.7 QUANTITATIVE MEASUREMENTS

In many applications of EPR to copper proteins the quantitative aspects are essential. The unknown concentration is usually determined by a comparison to a standard sample. A standard should have a resonance line with well-defined peaks without long tails. A water solution of copper EDTA has been used (5) but under certain conditions this contains more than one complex. Alternatively, a 1-mM water solution of Cu^{2+} containing 2 *M* $NaClO_4$ and 0.01 *M* HCl has been suggested (40). If the standard and the unknown sample have different *g* factors, a correction factor for the difference in the transition probability should be applied. In most cases a sufficiently accurate correction is obtained if the integrated area is divided by the square of the average of the *g* factors $(g_x + g_y + g_z)^2/9 = (g_\parallel + 2g_\perp)^2/9$ (41). In cases in which the low-temperature signal consists of two components, originating from different copper species, an estimate of their relative intensity can be obtained from the lowest field hyperfine line of one of the components, provided this is sufficiently well resolved from the rest of the spectrum (36).

9.8 RELAXATION AND SATURATION

The relaxation times of copper signals are relatively long and permit an easy study of the signal at the temperature of liquid nitrogen. Some saturation experiments have been performed and have proved to be particularly useful for the differentiation between copper signals in cytochrome oxidase (see Section 9.14). It would seem that in most cases a power up to about 5 mW at 77 K can be used without any appreciable saturation of the signal from a copper complex or protein (cf. Ref. 42).

9.9 SENSITIVITY

The amount of copper needed to give an acceptable signal intensity of course depends on the sharpness of the spectrum and on the information wanted. As illustrated by the spectra shown below, a concentration of about 0.2 mM normally permits an accurate evaluation of the 9-GHz EPR spectrum obtained at 77 K from a copper protein. The sample volume is about 200 μl. At 35 GHz the concentration must be higher, up to 1mM, in part because the spectrum is now spread over a much larger field interval. However, the sample volume is in this case only about 50 μl so that the amount of protein needed is not much higher. For low-molecular weight complexes that are to be studied at room temperature a concentration of about 5 mM is convenient.

9.10 CLASSIFICATION OF Cu^{2+} COMPONENTS IN PROTEINS

Table 9-1 gives the EPR parameters and some optical properties of most of the copper proteins studied so far. For comparison some low-molecular weight complexes are listed in the same table. The EPR parameters $g_{\parallel}$ and $A_{\parallel}$, contained in Table 9-1, are plotted in Fig. 9-5, where open and closed symbols represent proteins and small complexes, respectively. Some proteins that contain different kinds of Cu^{2+} are represented by more than one symbol in Fig. 9-5. It is clear from this figure that Cu^{2+} ions in proteins can be classified according to their $A_{\parallel}$ values (36, 56, 57). One class (designated Type 2 Cu^{2+}) has $A_{\parallel}$ larger than 14 mK and the other class (Type 1 Cu^{2+}) has $A_{\parallel}$ smaller than 10 mK. In addition, if the variation of the $g_{\parallel}$ value among the ions with small $A_{\parallel}$ is considered, it appears that cytochrome oxidase falls in a class by itself and consequently the EPR-detectable Cu^{2+} ion in this protein is not included among the Type 1 ions in this chapter.

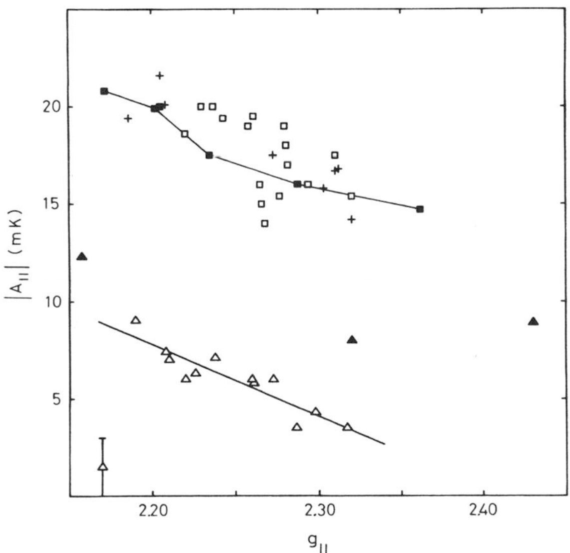

Fig. 9-5 The values of $|A_{\parallel}|$ versus $g_{\parallel}$ for the species listed in Table 9-1. The open and closed symbols denote Cu^{2+} in proteins and low-molecular weight complexes, respectively. △ indicates the Type 1 ions except for the symbol at the lower left which represents cytochrome oxidase ($|A_{\parallel}| \leq 3$ mK). Small complexes with near-tetrahedral coordination are denoted by ▲, two of which have been suggested as models for the Type 1 Cu^{2+}. Type 2 Cu^{2+} ions are indicated by □ and peptide complexes by ■, and those connected by a line represent the complexes observed in the Cu^{2+}-triglycylglycine system. The "synthetic" copper proteins are represented by +.

Table 9-1 EPR and Optical Absorption Data of Cu^{2+} in Proteins and Some Selected Small Complexes[a]

Protein	Source	Number of EPR-detectable ions	$g_\perp$	$g_\parallel$	$\lvert A_\parallel \rvert$ (mK)	N-hfs	Optical absorption: Energy (kK)	Optical absorption: Extinction coefficient $(M^{-1}cm^{-1})$	Ref.
Azurin (1)	*Pseudomonas fluorescens*		2.052	2.261	5.8		21.8	0.29	43
							16	3.5	
							12.8[s]	0.32	
Azurin (1)	*Pseudomonas aeruginosa*		2.052	2.260	6.0		21.4	0.27	43
							16	3.5	
							12.2[s]	0.39	
Azurin (1)	*Bordetella*	0.9	2.049	2.273	6		16	3.5	44
Stellacyanin (1)	*Rhus vernicifera*								
pH 1–9		1	2.025	2.287	3.5[b]		22.2	0.96	40
			2.077				16.6	4.08	
							11.8	0.79	
pH 10–11.5			2.025	2.312	<1.7[c]		~ 17	~ 4	40
			2.089						
Umecyanin (1)	Horseradish	0.7	2.05	2.317	3.5		16.4	3.5	45
Plastocyanin (2)	*Chenopodium album*	2	2.053	2.226	6.3		22		46a, b
							16.5	4.9	
							12.5		
Monoamine oxidase (3.7)	Bovine plasma	2.7	2.053[m]		16				47
Monoamine oxidase (3)	*Aspergillus niger*	1.9	2.07[m]	2.31	17.5				48
Diamine oxidase	Pig kidney	73%	2.063[m]	2.294	16	+ (?)			49

Benzylamine oxidase (2.3)	Pig plasma	1.9	2.060	2.266	15				50
Galactose oxidase (1)	*Dactylium dendroides*	0.7	2.04	2.28	19				51
Dopamine β-hydroxylase (3.6)	Bovine adrenal glands	100% (2[d])	2.056	2.282	17				52, 53
Ribulose diphosphate carboxylase (1)	Spinach	0.8	2.09	2.32	15.4				54
Superoxide dismutase (2)	Human red blood cells		2.06[m]	2.265	16				39
Superoxide dismutase (2)	Bovine red blood cells		2.029 2.108	2.265	14.2	+			55
Laccase, fungal (4)	*Polyporus versicolor*								
Type 1		1	2.033[e] 2.051[e]	2.190	9.0		16.4 13.5	4.9 [s]	56, 90
Type 2		1	2.036	2.243	19.4				56, 57
Type 2—F^-				2.261	19.5				57
Type 2—$2F^-$				2.281	18.0				57
Type 2—H_2O_2				2.22	18.6		25	≥ 1	58
Laccase, tree (4)	*Rhus vernicifera*								
Type 1 pH 3–8		1	2.047	2.298	4.3		16.3 12.5	5.7 1.1[s]	40
Type 1 pH 10–12			2.04	2.238	7.1		~ 17	~ 6	40
Type 2		1	2.053	2.237	20.0				40
Laccase, tree (5–6)	*Rhus succedanea*		2.06[m]	2.21	7		16.4 13.5	[B] [s]	59, 60
Ceruloplasmin (6–8)	Human serum								61, 62
Type 1		2	2.05	2.208	7.4		21.8 16.4 12.6	0.6[f] 5.4[f] 1.1[f]	6, 63

Table 9-1—*continued.*

Protein	Source	Number of EPR-detectable ions	$g_\perp$	$g_\parallel$	$\lvert A_\parallel \rvert$ (mK)	N-hfs	Optical absorption: Energy (kK)	Optical absorption: Extinction coefficient $(M^{-1}cm^{-1})$	Ref.
Type 2		1	2.04	2.258	19.0				63
		1	2.04	2.277	15.4				63
Ascorbate oxidase (8)	*Cucumus sativus*						16.5	B	64
							13	s	
Type 1				2.22	6[e]				64
Type 2				2.23[e]	20[e]				64
Cytochrome oxidase (2)	Beef heart	0.8	2.03[m]	2.17	≤ 3				65
Cu^{2+}-myoglobin									
pH 6.4		1	2.054	2.273	17.5				66
pH 10.4		1	2.046	2.186	19.4	+			66
Cu^{2+}-hemoglobin pH 5–9		2	2.054	2.208	20.1	+			67
Cu^{2+}-insulin			2.0	2.303	15.8	2 *N*			68
			2.1						
Cu^{2+}-transferrin			2.05	2.205	21.6	4 *N*			69
Cu^{2+}-transferrin-bicarbonate		2	2.05	2.312	16.8	1 *N*			69
Cu^{2+}-alkaline phosphatase		2		2.31	16.7				70a
Cu^{2+}-alkaline phosphatase + phosphate				2.32	14.2				70a
Cu^{2+}-triglycylglycine									
pH <4			2.078	2.362	14.7				37

pH 5	2.072	2.288	16.0		37
pH 6	2.062	2.235	17.5	2 *N*	37
pH 7	2.047	2.202	19.9	3 *N*	37
pH 10	2.041	2.172	20.8	4 *N*	37
Cu^{2+}-glycylhistidine pH 11	2.066	2.205	20.0	3 *N*	71
$Cu(NCS)_4^{2-}$	2.07	2.43	8.9	+	72
$Cu(NCCH_3)_4^{2+}$		2.32	8	+	73
$Cu(BFNA^{g})_2$	2.041	2.158	12.3		18

[a] The numbers in parentheses indicate the total number of copper ions in the protein molecule. When two values are given for $g_{\perp}$, they refer to g_x and g_y of a rhombic signal. Values for $A_{\perp}(A_x, A_y)$ are not given because the corresponding splitting is unresolved or difficult to measure (except in the case of stellacyanin). Conversion factors for hyperfine couplings: 1 mK = 21.42/g gauss = 30.0 MHz (1 K = 1 cm^{-1}). The optical extinction coefficients are based on the concentration of the copper species giving rise to the band. When this concentration is difficult to estimate, the symbol B indicates that the protein is strongly "blue."

[b] $|A_x| = 5.7$ mK, $|A_y| \leq 3$ mK.

[c] $|A_x| = 7.3$ mK.

[d] Based on chemical analysis (53).

[e] From analysis of published spectra.

[f] Based on optical data in Ref. 6 and content of Type 1 Cu^{2+} in Ref. 63.

[g] BFNA = 1-benzene-azo-*N*-phenyl-2-naphtylamine.

[m] g factor at zero absorption derivative (g_m).

[s] Shoulder.

[B] "Blue."

The $A_{\|}$ values found for the Type 2 Cu^{2+} are similar to those of small copper complexes, whereas the small values for the Type 1 ions are quite unique. Furthermore, because of a strong optical absorption band at around 600 nm, the Type 1 Cu^{2+} ions have a strong blue color compared with most low-molecular weight complexes. The Type 2 ions, on the other hand, are colorless or only faintly colored. However, the "nonblue" proteins most likely have absorption bands in the optical region as well, although they may be difficult to detect because of their weakness. Also, it should be stressed that the classification into Types 1 and 2 Cu^{2+}, as used in this chapter, is based only on the optical and EPR absorption properties and that important differences in bonding and function might exist between ions belonging to the same type. The presence of Cu^{2+} in proteins with properties intermediate to those of the Types 1 and 2 Cu^{2+} is of course not excluded either, although no good example of such a situation has yet been found.

Not much is known about the coordination of copper in proteins and no crystal structure has been determined for a native copper protein. For Type 2 Cu^{2+} ligand hyperfine structure has in a few cases been observed in EPR, indicating that the metal ion is coordinated to nitrogen atoms. This seems quite reasonable since all proteins contain a large number of nitrogen atoms that could act as ligands. The EPR spectra of Type 2 Cu^{2+} are rather similar to those obtained from copper complexes with amino acids or small peptides. A large number of these complexes has been studied (see examples in Table 9-1). Figure 9-5 includes data from an investigation of the Cu^{2+}-triglycylglycine system (37). As the pH is raised from acid values, more nitrogen atoms coordinate to the metal ion and the EPR parameters pass through the range encountered for Type 2 Cu^{2+} with a concomitant shift of the optical absorption to higher energies. Thus it seems possible to consider copper-peptide complexes as models for Type 2 Cu^{2+}. As discussed below, however, some Type 2 Cu^{2+} ions show a specific affinity for certain anions, and this has no counterpart for the smaller complexes.

The Type 1 Cu^{2+} has attracted much interest because of its unique spectral properties. In the analysis of the first EPR results (39) the optical transitions were considered to occur between different *d*-orbitals (*d-d* transitions), but it was suggested that electron delocalization might play an important role. Later Williams and co-workers (74) argued that the color was so strong that the transitions must occur between orbitals essentially centered on the ligands and on the metal ion, respectively. Such charge-transfer transitions often have a very high intensity. The same authors also pointed out that a low symmetry of the complex was likely to be important. If the symmetry is sufficiently low and lacking an inversion center, $4s$ and $4p$ orbitals can become mixed into the $3d$ orbitals. This leads to an increase in the intensities of the optical transitions between the metal orbitals. In addition, the contribution to $A_{\parallel}$ from $4p$ is opposite to that from $3d$ (75) which reduces the magnitude of $A_{\parallel}$. Small values of $|A_{\parallel}|$ have in fact been observed in some distorted low-molecular weight complexes (72, 73, 75, 76). A further consequence of the low symmetry is that optical activity is expected and this has been found in all examined proteins containing Type 1 Cu^{2+} (11, 43, 46a, 77–80). As pointed out by Williams and co-workers (74) and by Wüthrich (81), the high oxidation-reduction potential observed for some Type 1 Cu^{2+} ions (0.3–0.8 V, Ref. 7b) is also understandable in terms of a tetrahedrally distorted coordination which stabilizes the univalent state of copper.

In a quantitative model Blumberg (11) introduced distortions from the usual square-planar symmetry. However, he considered the optical transitions to be of essentially *d-d* character. By a suitable choice of certain crystal-field parameters he could account for the energies of the observed optical transitions, their intensities and activities, and for the g factors. In a related model, but with complete neglect of covalency, Brill and Bryce (82) adjusted certain coefficients describing the mixing of $3d$, $4s$, and $4p$ orbitals so that the intensities and activities of the observed optical transitions and the g factors and hyperfine constants in EPR could be reproduced.

Although the two theoretical models described above support the idea that distortions of the copper coordination are important, they are by necessity quite approximate. Recent studies of the circular dichroism of blue proteins (80, cf. Ref. 78) have revealed that there are as many as five different optical transitions in the range 10 to 30 kK. This makes the assignment of some of them to certain *d-d* transitions rather ambiguous.

The Type 1 Cu^{2+} ions all have very similar optical properties (Table 9-1 and Ref. 80), whereas their EPR parameters show a considerable variation (Fig. 9-5). There is a strong linear correlation, however, between the $g_{\parallel}$ and $A_{\parallel}$ values as shown by the line drawn in Fig. 9-5. The slope of this line is almost the same as that of the line connecting the various Cu^{2+}-triglycylglycine complexes. In the case of the peptide complexes the variation of the EPR parameters is mainly due to a change in the crystal field splitting Δ. This affects $g_{\parallel}$ according to Eq. 9-2 and, provided κ and α are constant, Eq. 9-3 predicts the observed behavior. As there seems to be no correlation between optical and EPR properties among the Type 1 Cu^{2+} ions (80), this explanation does not hold in the case of the proteins. However, the observed correlation between the EPR parameters and the similarities in the optical properties of the Type 1 Cu^{2+} ions found in the various proteins do suggest that a close structural relationship exists between these ions.

As models for the Type 1 Cu^{2+} the peptide complexes or copper added to noncopper proteins do not serve at all. The low-molecular weight complex suggested as a model by Harris and Ritchie (83) does not seem to be any more successful. In all these cases the ion supposedly acquires the preferred square-planar coordination with more or less normal spectral properties. In view of the discussion above it is not surprising that better models are obtained when the Cu^{2+} ion is forced into a distorted environment (72–73). A good example is the complex studied by Gould and Ehrenberg (73) which was produced by γ-irradiation at low temperatures of a single crystal of $Cu(I)(CH_3CN)_4ClO_4$. The Cu^+ ion is tetrahedrally coordinated and the divalent ion, produced by the irradiation, presumably has a similar coordination. Although the optical spectra were not studied in detail, the EPR parameters resemble those of Type 1 Cu^{2+}, as shown in Table 9-1 and Fig. 9-5.

9.11 PROTEINS CONTAINING TYPE 1 Cu^{2+} ONLY

The blue proteins from *Pseudomonas* and *Bordetella* (azurins) and from *Rhus vernicifera* (stellacyanin) all have only one Type 1 Cu^{2+} in the molecule. The first study on such a protein was reported by Mason (84). It illustrated that copper-copper interaction (cf. Ref. 65) was not necessary for the occurrence of the unique spectral properties of the Type 1 Cu^{2+}. Later this was confirmed by experiments on the *Bordetella* azurin (44a). A detailed examination of the optical and magnetic properties of *Pseudomonas* azurin was performed by Brill and co-workers (43) and the theoretical analysis by Brill and Bryce (82), mentioned above, was applied to these proteins in particular. These authors even gave a quantitative measure of the distortion from the planarity of the copper coordination. The values should probably not be taken too literally but it will be interesting to see how they compare with the results of the X-ray work, which has been started (85). The pH-dependence of the spectral properties was also studied by Brill et al. (43) and is discussed below in connection with similar studies on laccase.

The EPR spectrum of stellacyanin shows a large deviation from axial symmetry both in the g factors and in the hyperfine couplings (Fig. 9-6*a* and Table 9-1), but the highest g factor is associated with a small hyperfine constant as with the other Type 1 Cu^{2+} ions. The spectral properties of this protein show an interesting dependence on pH, as first studied by Peisach, Levine, and Blumberg (77). At very high pH the spectral properties become quite similar to those of the copper-biuret complex with four nitrogen atoms coordinated to the metal ion (see Fig. 9-6*d*). Peisach et al. (77) also observed an intermediate state at pH 8–11 with a strong color but with a normal EPR spectrum having a large $|A_{\|}|$ and interpreted the

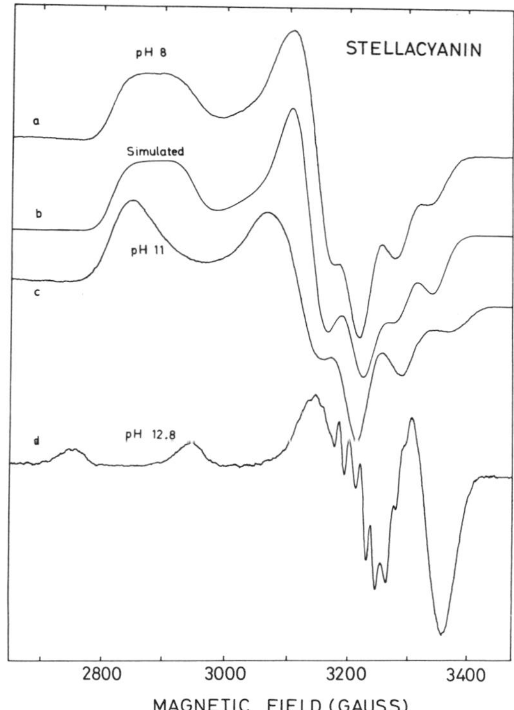

Fig. 9-6 EPR spectra at 77 K and 9.213 GHz of stellacyanin (40). (*a*), (*c*), and (*d*) are experimental spectra at various pH's and spectrum (*b*) was simulated to fit spectrum (*a*) with the parameters given in Table 1. The sample tube had an inner diameter of 1 mm and the protein concentration was 2 m*M*.

changes with pH in terms of the successive release of certain constraints on the coordination. However, later studies on stellacyanin in this laboratory (40) have shown that the intermediate state has both the narrow hyperfine splitting and the strong color characteristic of a Type 1 Cu^{2+} (see Fig. 9-6*c* and Table 9-1).

Plastocyanin from *Chenopodium album* has two copper atoms per molecule. Blumberg and Peisach (46a) found that both ions have the same EPR spectrum and probably Type 1 character.

The nature of the ligands of copper in the proteins containing Type 1 Cu^{2+} has been discussed by several authors. A recent fluorometric study (86) indicates that tryptophan and sulfhydryl are involved in the binding in azurins. For stellacyanin it was suggested from EPR data that four nitrogen atoms coordinate to copper (77). This conclusion, however, was based on the examination of the protein irreversibly modified as in Fig. 9-6*d*.

In a recent study, applying for the first time the ENDOR technique to a copper protein, Hyde and co-workers (25a) showed that at least one nitrogen atom does coordinate to copper in native stellacyanin. Another conclusion from this work was that the metal ion is at least 6 Å away from exchangeable water molecules. Thus the Type 1 Cu^{2+} seems to be buried inside the protein molecule. This conclusion was also reached in protein relaxation studies on plastocyanin (46a) and in other studies (43, 86).

The function of all the proteins containing only Type 1 Cu^{2+} is not yet established, but some at least take part in electron transport. The metal ion can be reduced, probably with an outersphere mechanism (77), but the reoxidation by molecular oxygen is slow (87). The rapid reduction of oxygen requires a more elaborate machinery, at least when the final product is water. This is discussed in Section 9.14.

9.12 PROTEINS CONTAINING TYPE 2 Cu^{2+} ONLY

The amine oxidases (monoamine, benzylamine, and diamine) and galactose oxidase are found in this category. The EPR parameters are given in

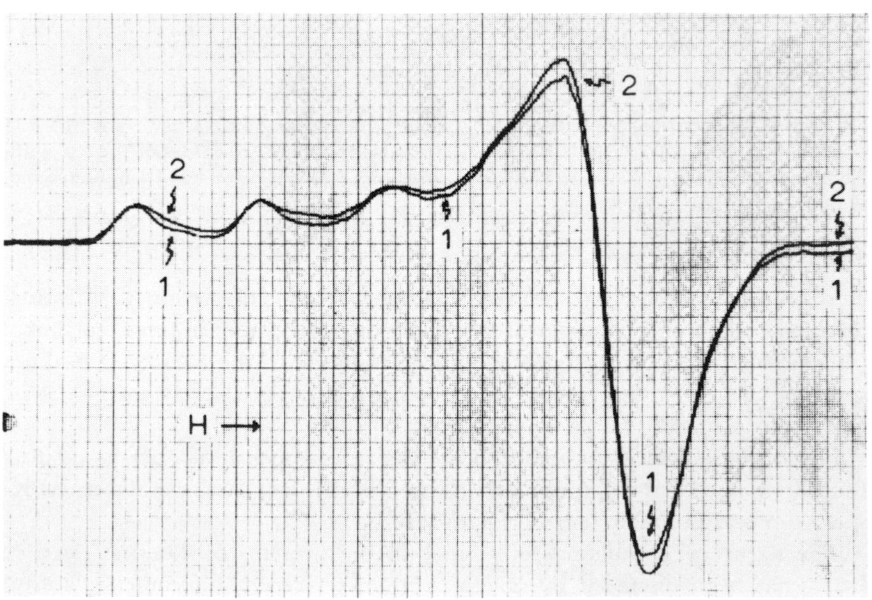

Fig. 9-7 EPR spectra of diamine oxidase from pig kidney in the absence (1) and presence (2) of the substrate putrescine (49). Curve 2 was obtained 1 min after addition of the substrate in an anaerobic cell.

Table 9-1 and a representative EPR spectrum is shown in Fig. 9-7. Most workers find that the copper ion stays divalent even in the presence of the reducing substrate, although small changes in the EPR signal are observed (see Fig. 9-7 and Refs. 47–51), and conclude that the metal ion does not change its valence during the catalytic process. For diamine oxidase this statement has been questioned (88).

The reaction catalyzed by dopamine β-hydroxylase is quite complicated and the copper ion, it has been claimed, changes its valence during this reaction (52, 53). Friedman and Kaufman (53) suggest that ascorbate reduces two Cu^{2+} ions and that the univalent ions formed are so close that both can bind to the same oxygen molecule. This would require large conformational changes on reduction because otherwise we would see interactions between the neighboring divalent ions in the EPR spectrum of the oxidized protein.

Superoxide dismutase (also known as erythrocuprein, hemocuprein, cytocuprein, etc.) was earlier thought to be a copper storage protein but recently it has been directly demonstrated, by the observation of the EPR of O_2^-, that this protein catalyzes the decomposition of the superoxide ion (89). The role of the copper ion in this reaction has not been established. According to Table 9-1 there is a difference between the EPR parameters of the human and bovine protein. Its significance has yet to be established.

9.13 PROTEINS CONTAINING BOTH TYPE 1 AND TYPE 2 Cu^{2+}

In this class of proteins the laccase from the fungus *Polyporus versicolor* probably is the best characterized. It contains four copper atoms per molecule, one each of Type 1 and Type 2 Cu^{2+} (56) and two ions that are nondetectable by EPR (5, 56). The two types of Cu^{2+} are clearly seen in the EPR spectrum as shown in Fig. 9-8. The Type 1 Cu^{2+} shows no ligand hyperfine structure and nothing is known about the ligands of this ion in laccase. Proton relaxation data, however, again indicate (56) that it is not situated on the surface of the protein. The Type 2 Cu^{2+} must be separated from the Type 1 Cu^{2+} by more than 8 Å, since there is no evidence of copper-copper interaction in the EPR spectrum. Furthermore, the Type 2 Cu^{2+} can be removed without any observable effect on the spectroscopic properties of the Type 1 ion (90). Although the Type 2 Cu^{2+} does not relax water protons effectively either (56), it is much more available for chemical modifications than the Type 1 copper; for example, cyanide binds to the Type 2 Cu^{2+} as shown by ligand hyperfine coupling (57) to the carbon nucleus in CN^- enriched in ^{13}C. On the addition of cyanide, ligand hyper-

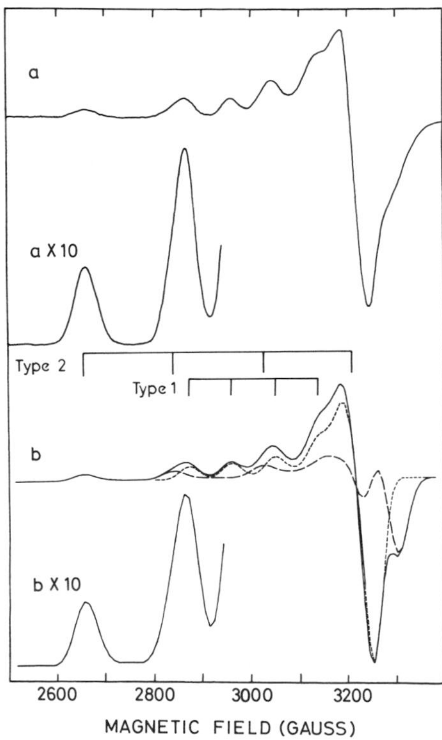

Fig. 9-8 Experimental (*a*) and simulated (*b*) EPR spectra of laccase from the fungus *Polyporus versicolor*. The simulated spectrum shows how the spectrum can be decomposed into two components, one with a narrow copper hyperfine splitting (-----, Type 1) and one with a broader splitting (- - - - -, Type 2). The simulations were performed on a HP 9100B-9125A desk calculator and the values of the parameters are given in Table 9-1. The microwave frequency was 9.20 GHz.

fine coupling to nitrogen atoms also becomes apparent (56, 57), and it was suggested that the protein provides these ligands (57). The reaction with cyanide is completely reversible, which indicates that nitrogen atoms coordinate to the Type 2 Cu^{2+} also in the native enzyme. An exceptional feature of the Type 2 Cu^{2+} is its strong affinity for fluoride ions (57, 91, 92) as illustrated in Fig. 9-9. On the addition of equimolar amounts of F^- each hyperfine line of the Type 2 Cu^{2+} signal splits up into a doublet due to the coupling to the $I = \frac{1}{2}$ fluorine nucleus (Fig. 9-9*b*). If more F^- is added, an additional fluoride ion binds with the same coupling constant (Fig. 9-9*c*). The binding of the first F^- is so strong that it was found difficult to remove it from the protein (91), and only recently this has been made possible (58) by the dialysis of the completely reduced laccase.

The two EPR-nondetectable ions were first assumed to be univalent, in particular because they show no paramagnetism even at room temperature (93). However, oxidation-reduction titrations (91) have shown that about four electrons can be accepted by each molecule, that is, two more than can be accounted for by the Types 1 and 2 Cu^{2+}. These acceptors must have a

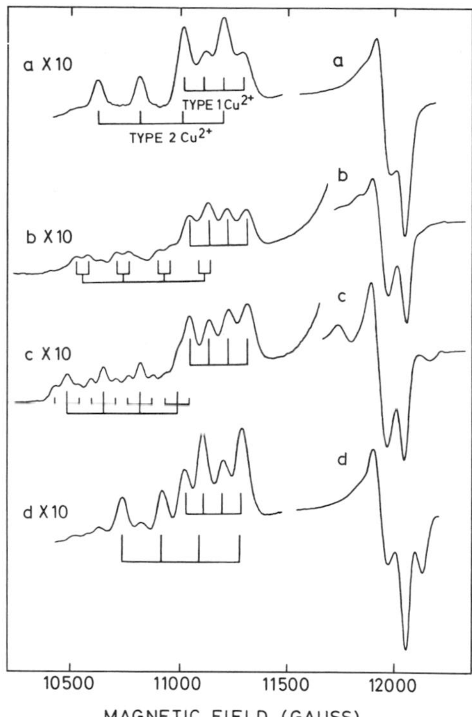

Fig. 9-9 EPR spectra at 34.5 GHz of frozen solutions of native and modified fungal laccase (57, 58). Spectrum (*a*) is obtained from the native protein (0.3 m*M*) and clearly shows the two types of Cu^{2+} better separated than in Fig. 9-8. In (*b*) 0.7 m*M* NaF has been added to 0.7 m*M* protein, resulting in a splitting of the Type 2 copper hyperfine lines into doublets due to interaction with the fluorine nucleus. When 14 m*M* NaF is added (*c*), equal coupling to two F occurs, giving a splitting into 1:2:1 triplets. The magnitude of the fluorine splitting is about 55 G. In (*d*) 10 m*M* H_2O_2 has been added to 0.3 m*M* protein, again changing the Type 2 signal. No change in the Type 1 signal can be observed on the addition of F^- or H_2O_2. For all spectra the low-field part is recorded with 10 times higher spectrometer gain. compared with the high-field part.

high oxidation-reduction potential, since they are reduced concomitantly with the Type 1 ion which has a potential of about 0.8 V (94). It has also been shown that they are associated with a strong absorption band in the near-ultraviolet region centered at 330 nm (92). The course of this band in the titrations and the fact that no EPR signal appears on partial reduction (91, 92) indicate that these two electron acceptors receive their electrons in pairs. The structure of this unit is not known, but it has been suggested (91) that the EPR-nondetectable copper ions are involved and that they might exist as a strongly coupled Cu^{2+}—Cu^{2+} pair.* Such pair formation is not uncommon in organic complexes of Cu^{2+}, but the coupling is usually not strong enough to make the unit diamagnetic, as observed for the protein.

If the pH of a laccase solution is raised above 7, the blue color and the EPR signal intensity decrease (98). This is due to a selective reduction of the Type 1 Cu^{2+} (99). Since this ion has a very high oxidation-reduction potential (94), it was first thought that water was the reducing agent (100). Later it was shown (99) that no stoichiometric amounts of oxygen were produced when the pH was raised. This means that the reduction must occur through some other reducing agent. Azurin is also reduced at elevated pH (43), and in this case the proposed oxidation of water (or hydroxyl ions) (43) is even less likely, since the oxidation-reduction potential of azurin is too low to allow this reaction to proceed.

Several laccases are obtained from the latex of lacquer trees, grown in Japan and other countries in Asia. EPR studies on the *Rhus vernicifera* laccase have been performed by Nakamura (59, 101) and by Blumberg et al. (102) with varying results. Work in our laboratory (40) has revealed a close analogy between this laccase and the fungal enzyme. Thus the *Rhus vernicifera* laccase contains four Cu/molecule, one each of Types 1 and 2 Cu^{2+} and two EPR-nondetectable ions. The EPR spectra of the protein at neutral pH is shown in Fig. 9-10, together with a simulated spectrum. Also, in addition to the Types 1 and 2 copper ions, there are two electron acceptors that are associated with a 330-nm band and they seem to accept electrons in pairs (103). The *Rhus succedanea* laccase has also been examined by EPR but not extensively. The published spectrum (59) indicates the presence of both types of Cu^{2+}, although parameters were presented only for the Type 1 ion (see Table 9-1).

Ceruloplasmin has attracted much interest, in part because it constitutes the main copper component of human serum. The number of copper atoms per molecule has in most studies been considered to be eight (5, 6, 61), but recent work indicates that it could be as low as six (62). This uncertainty makes a detailed interpretation of the EPR spectrum difficult. Ceruloplasmin, however, was the first protein for which the presence of two types

* Hemocyanin also has two EPR-nondetectable copper ions (95) in the functional unit, and the small EPR signal that is sometimes observed (96) is likely to be due to denatured protein molecules. One might think that these two copper ions would be similar to the pair suggested for laccase, but it is only the oxygenated form of hemocyanin that has absorption bands at wavelengths above 300 nm (97), whereas no oxygen binding seems to be required for the appearance of the 330-nm band in laccase (92). Also it should be noted that although oxyhemocyanin is blue the corresponding absorption band is about 10 times weaker than for the "blue" proteins discussed in this chapter (Ref. 97, Table 1).

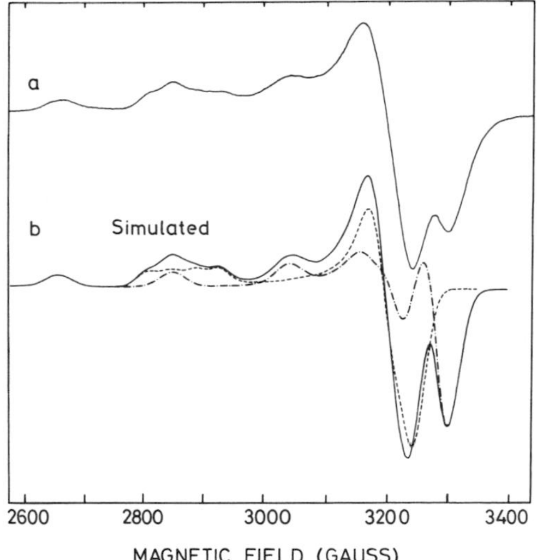

Fig. 9-10 EPR spectra at 9.21 GHz and 77 K of tree (*Rhus vernicifera*) laccase (40). An experimental spectrum of a solution, 0.3 m*M* in protein at pH 7.5, is shown in (*a*) and a simulated spectrum is given in (*b*) (-----, Type 1; —· —· —· —· —·, Type 2 Cu^{2+}). The values of the EPR parameters are listed in Table 1.

of Cu^{2+} was recognized (36) (see Fig. 9-4), and on the basis of eight Cu/molecule we find approximately two of each (63) of Types 1 and 2 Cu^{2+} and four EPR-nondetectable ions. As seen in Table 9-1, the two Type 2 ions have been assigned different EPR parameters (63), although the 35 GHz spectrum is difficult to reproduce in detail (63). Again EPR studies have shown that Type 2 Cu^{2+} is a binding site of anions such as azide and fluoride (63). Susceptibility investigations (93, 104) indicate that the EPR-nondetectable copper cannot be paramagnetic, although the fraction of paramagnetic ions comes out to be 40 to 65 percent rather than exactly 50 percent. Because only four electron acceptors per molecule were found in early oxidation-reduction titrations (105), the EPR-nondetectable ions were generally considered to be univalent. Recent titrations indicate (106), however, that there are as many electron acceptors in ceruloplasmin as there are copper ions and that the optical absorption band at 330 nm, first observed by Holmberg and Laurell (61), is associated with the EPR-nondetectable electron acceptors. Thus ceruloplasmin seems analogous to the laccases, and again it was suggested that the EPR-nondetectable ions are involved in an electron-accepting unit (106). An interesting observation is that an anaerobic solution of ceruloplasmin with its blue color reduced to about 50 percent because of the addition of reductant is almost completely decolored on freezing to liquid-nitrogen temperatures (106). This is probably caused by a temperature-dependent electron shift and it illustrates the difficulties that might be encountered in comparing room-temperature optical absorption data and low-temperature EPR results.

The laccases and ceruloplasmin have in common that they catalyze the oxidation of diphenols and related substances by molecular oxygen. The reducing substances probably act as one-electron donors [ferrocyanide is quite a good substrate for fungal laccase (107)] and oxygen is reduced by four electrons to water without the release of hydrogen peroxide. The details of the mechanism are unknown, but the following suggestions, which are based mainly on work on fungal laccase, might apply to all laccases and to ceruloplasmin. Type 1 Cu^{2+} appears to be the acceptor to which the electrons go first, since the reduction of this ion is very fast and not affected by the presence of fluoride ions, although they do inhibit the enzyme activity (107). The next steps would involve the intramolecular transfer of electrons from Type 1 copper so that all four electron acceptors (eight in ceruloplasmin) are reduced and followed by a four-electron transfer to oxygen. It appears, however, that Type 2 Cu^{2+} is reduced slowly by the reducing substrate (56), and this observation makes the four-electron transfer unlikely. Recently an alternative function has been suggested (58) for Type 2 Cu^{2+}, based on the finding that hydrogen peroxide affects the Type 2 Cu^{2+} EPR signal of fungal laccase (Fig. 9-9*d*). This suggests that hydrogen peroxide or one of its ions binds to Type 2 Cu^{2+}. Thus in the catalytic reaction this copper ion could serve as a stabilizer of a peroxide intermediate, which would be formed by the reduction of oxygen by a pair of electrons coming from the two-electron acceptor discussed above. In a subsequent step the bound peroxide would be reduced to water by another two-electron transfer. It should be stressed that this mechanism is only a hypothesis and that several other models are possible (cf. Ref. 108). It would seem, though, that both types of Cu^{2+} and EPR-nondetectable copper are necessary for the catalysis of the reduction of oxygen to water by a one-electron reducing substrate. Proteins with only Type 1 copper cannot be readily reoxidized by oxygen, and oxidases with only Type 2 copper work on two-electron substrates, reducing oxygen only to the peroxide level (108).

Ascorbate oxidase, which is obtained from a variety of plants (109), also has a strong blue color. It contains 8 Cu/molecule and it has been reported (109) that six of them are EPR-detectable. It is clear from the results obtained by Beinert (see Ref. 109) and from EPR spectra published by Nakamura et al. (64) that there are two copper components in the protein, one with a narrow hyperfine splitting and one with a broader splitting (see Table 9-1). Thus it seems likely that this protein contains Types 1 and 2

Cu^{2+} also. In addition there is an optical absorption band at 330 nm (64), which makes the analogy with the laccases and ceruloplasmin even greater.

9.14 CYTOCHROME OXIDASE

The functional unit of this important enzyme is believed to contain two heme groups and two copper atoms. Since in principle, both heme and copper can be examined by EPR, this protein has been the subject of many such studies. In this chapter we restrict our discussion to some features particular to the copper component of the protein.

Cytochrome oxidase offers an interesting example of the use of EPR saturation for the discrimination between two copper components. This protein is often contaminated by extraneous copper with an EPR signal different from that of the native copper. If, however, the microwave power is high (about 100 mW at 100 K) the signal from the extraneous copper is saturated away (42, 110), whereas no saturation is observed for the relevant copper signal.

Only about 40 percent of the total copper in cytochrome oxidase is represented in the EPR signal (65) and the simplest explanation is that only one of the two copper atoms is detected. Alternatively, we might invoke a mechanism recently discussed by Leigh (111) in which a nearby rapidly relaxing paramagnetic ion could cause a decrease in an EPR signal without any appreciable change in its shape. However, a strong temperature dependence of the signal amplitude is predicted, but this is not observed for cytochrome oxidase. Therefore this mechanism is not considered to be the likely explanation for the low EPR intensity at temperatures below 100 K (112).

The copper EPR signal from cytochrome oxidase shows no deviation from axial symmetry and the hyperfine coupling constant $A_{\parallel}$ is very small. As discussed above, the protein has such a combination of $g_{\parallel}$ values and $A_{\parallel}$ values that it falls distinctly out of the range of Type 1 Cu^{2+} ions (see Fig. 9-5). On the other hand, kinetic studies (113) indicate that a rather strong optical absorption associated with copper may exist at about 600 nm, although it is masked by the very intense heme absorptions.

9.15 STUDIES ON COPPER INTERACTION WITH NONCOPPER PROTEINS

There are two main reasons for conducting experiments on the interaction of copper with proteins that *in vivo* do not contain copper. The first is that we hope to learn about the mode of copper binding to proteins in general and the second is that substitution of copper for another metal ion may provide useful information about the metal binding site itself.

The studies on copper binding to myoglobin and hemoglobin belong to the first category. These proteins were chosen because much is known about their structure. As might have been expected, their copper complexes are not good models for Type 1 Cu^{2+} but are more analogous to the simple copper-peptide complexes. With ferrimyoglobin X-ray data had revealed the presence of one preferred site for copper binding, and the EPR data were consistent with the binding to this site in solution also (66). When more than one copper ion is bound to the molecule (114), a reduction in the iron EPR signal is observed which is due to conformational changes induced by the copper ions. Hemoglobin preferentially binds two Cu^{2+}/molecule (67). Although ligand hyperfine structure indicates binding to nitrogen in both proteins, the EPR parameters have quite different values (see Table 9-1). Studies on the binding of copper to isolated chains of hemoglobin and to a tetramer of β chains (115) have led to the conclusion that in hemoglobin the copper ions bind to the β chains.

The EPR investigations by Brill and Venable (68) on Cu^{2+} bound to insulin provide interesting information on the metal-binding site in this protein. Insulin can be crystallized, but only in the presence of certain metal ions. As isolated, the protein normally contains Zn^{2+}. Brill and Venable replaced this ion with Cu^{2+} and performed the only single-crystal EPR study on a copper-protein complex yet reported. They suggested (68) that there were two binding sites per unit cell situated on a trigonal axis. From the Jahn-Teller theorem it follows that for Cu^{2+} such a symmetry is too high to be stable, and each site was distorted in one of three symmetry-related ways. This explains the presence of the six different orientations of the Cu^{2+} ions that were observed. The ligand hyperfine coupling indicated the interaction with two nitrogen atoms. From symmetry arguments, however, Brill and Venable concluded that a third nitrogen atom coordinates, although the above-mentioned distortions made it inequivalent to the other two nitrogen atoms.

The serum protein transferrin is *in vivo* an iron-containing protein which requires the presence of equimolar amounts of bicarbonate ions for the strong binding of iron. The iron protein has been extensively studied by EPR techniques (69). The apoprotein, however, can bind several other metal ions (116), one of which is Cu^{2+}. The EPR spectra of the copper complexes (69) are quite well resolved and ligand hyperfine coupling to nitrogen atoms can be observed on the low-field line also. The bicarbonate-free complex shows a coupling to four equivalent nitrogen atoms (69), whereas only one nitrogen atom is seen in the bicarbonate complex (see Fig. 9-11). The shifts in $g_{\parallel}$ and $A_{\parallel}$ on binding of bicarbonate are consistent

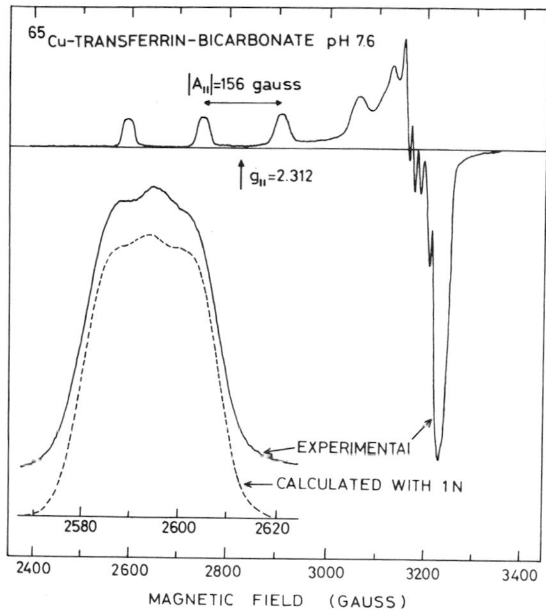

Fig. 9-11 EPR spectrum at 77 K and 9.151 GHz of ^{65}Cu-transferrinbicarbonate (69). The copper concentration was 0.9 m*M*. The dashed curve is a computer simulation which assumes a 9.5 G splitting due to interaction with one nitrogen only.

with a decrease in the number of coordinating nitrogen atoms. The relevance of this information for the binding of iron is of course uncertain, but at least the data show that nitrogen atoms must be seriously considered as ligand atoms for iron.

Several zinc-containing proteins in which the metal ion is replaced with Cu^{2+} have been studied by EPR. The amount of information is rather limited but the work on alkaline phosphatase (70a, b) may become useful in the characterization of the complexes between the protein and its substrates.

9.16 CONCLUDING REMARKS

EPR has been shown to be a valuable tool for the study of copper proteins. This is particularly true for the "blue" oxidases, from which has emerged a complex picture of the state and function of copper that could hardly have been obtained without the use of EPR. Although the EPR of Cu^{2+} in general is well understood, some features of Type 1 Cu^{2+} in proteins still lack an entirely satisfactory explanation. More direct structural information on the coordination of these ions would be most desirable.

ACKNOWLEDGMENTS

The cooperation of and discussions with a large number of people in this laboratory concerning work described in this chapter are gratefully acknowledged. I am deeply indebted to Mr. S.-O. Falkbring for his skilful preparation of the illustrations. The work was supported by the Swedish Natural Science Research Council.

REFERENCES

1. W. Blumberg, J. Eisinger, and S. Geschwind, *Phys. Rev.*, **130,** 900 (1963).
2. E. König in *Landolt-Börnstein,* K.-H. Hellwege, Ed., Vol. II: 2, p. 3–1.
3. H. Kuska and M. Rogers in *Radical Ions,* E. T. Kaiser and L. Kevan, Eds., Wiley-Interscience, New York, 1968, p. 579.
4. B. Malmström, R. Mosbach, and T. Vänngård, *Nature,* **183,** 321 (1959).
5. L. Broman, B. Malmström, R. Aasa, and T. Vänngård, *J. Mol. Biol.*, **5,** 301 (1962).
6. W. Blumberg, J. Eisinger, P. Aisen, A. Morell, and I. Scheinberg, *J. Biol. Chem.*, **238,** 1675 (1963).
7a. D. Gould and A. Ehrenberg in *Physiology and Biochemistry of Haemocyanins,* F. Ghiretti, Ed., Academic, New York, 1968, p. 95.
7b. R. Malkin and B. Malmström, *Advan. Enzymol.*, **33,** 177 (1970).
8a. B. Figgis, *Introduction to Ligand Fields,* Wiley-Interscience, New York, 1966.
8b. S. Kettle, *Coordination Compounds,* Nelson, London, 1969.
9. R. Coffman, *J. Chem. Phys.*, **48,** 609 (1968).
10. R. Pettersson and T. Vänngård, *Arkiv Kemi,* **17,** 249 (1961).
11. W. Blumberg in *The Biochemistry of Copper,* J. Peisach, P. Aisen, and W. Blumberg, Eds., Academic, New York, 1966, p. 49.
12. B. McGarvey in *Transition Metal Chemistry,* R. L. Carlin, Ed., Dekker, New York, 1966, Vol. 3, p. 90.
13. J. Ammeter, *Chimia,* **22,** 469 (1968).
14. K.-E. Falk, Thesis, University of Göteborg, 1970.
15. D. Schwarz, *Phys. Stat. Sol.*, **36,** 143 (1969).
16. A. Hausmann and P. Schreiber, *Solid-State Commun.*, **7,** 631 (1969).
17. G. Kokoszka, C. Reimann, and H. Allen, Jr., *J. Phys. Chem.*, **71,** 121 (1967).
18. A. Rockenbauer, *Acta Chim. Acad. Sci. Hung.*, **63,** 157 (1970).
19. A. Maki and B. McGarvey, *J. Chem. Phys.*, **29,** 31 (1958).
20. B. McGarvey, *J. Phys. Chem.*, **71,** 51 (1967).
21. L. Rollmann and S. Chan, *J. Chem. Phys.*, **50,** 3416 (1969).
22. D. Gould and H. Mason in *The Biochemistry of Copper,* J. Peisach, P. Aisen, and W. Blumberg, Eds., Academic, New York, 1966, p. 35.
23. K.-E. Falk, E. Ivanova, B. Roos, and T. Vänngård, *Inorg. Chem.*, **9,** 556 (1970).
24. G. Rist and J. Hyde, *J. Chem. Phys.*, **52,** 4633 (1970).
25a. G. Rist, J. Hyde, and T. Vänngård, *Proc. Natl. Acad. Sci.*, **67,** 79 (1970).

25b. A. Schoot Uiterkamp, *FEBS Letters*, **20,** 93 (1972).

26. J. Boas, J. Pilbrow, and T. Smith, *J. Chem. Soc.* (A), **1969,** 723.

27. C. Sigwart, P. Hemmerich, and J. Spence, *Inorg. Chem.*, **7,** 2545 (1968).

28. J. Boas, R. Dunhill, J. Pilbrow, R. Srivastava, and T. Smith, *J. Chem. Soc.*, (A) **1969,** 94.

29. A. Brill and J. Venable, Jr., in *Magnetic Resonance in Biological Systems*, A. Ehrenberg, B. Malmström, and T. Vänngård, Eds., Pergamon, Oxford, 1967, p. 365.

30. J. Venable, Jr., *ibid.*, p. 373.

31. J. Venable, Jr., Thesis, Yale University, New Haven, Connecticut.

32. T. Vänngård and R. Aasa in *Paramagnetic Resonance*, W. Low, Ed., Academic, New York, 1963, Vol. 2, p. 509.

33. R. Aasa, B. Malmström, P. Saltman, and T. Vänngård, *Biochim. Biophys. Acta*, **88,** 430 (1964).

34. H. Gersmann and J. Swalen, *J. Chem. Phys.*, **36,** 3221 (1962).

35. D. Getz and B. Silver, *J. Chem. Phys.*, **52,** 6449 (1970).

36. T. Vänngård in *Magnetic Resonance in Biological Systems*, A. Ehrenberg, B. Malmström, and T. Vänngård, Eds., Pergamon, Oxford, 1967, p. 213.

37. K.-E. Falk, H. Freeman, T. Jansson, B. Malmström, and T. Vänngård, *J. Am. Chem. Soc.*, **89,** 6071 (1967).

38. R. Ross, *J. Chem. Phys.*, **42,** 3919 (1965).

39. B. Malmström and T. Vänngård, *J. Mol. Biol.*, **2,** 118 (1960).

40. B. Malmström, B. Reinhammar, and T. Vänngård, *Biochim. Biophys. Acta*, **205,** 48 (1970).

41. R. Aasa and T. Vänngård, *J. Chem. Phys.*, **52,** 1612 (1970).

42. H. Beinert and G. Palmer in *Oxidases and Related Redox Systems*, T. King, H. Mason, and M. Morrison, Eds., Wiley, New York, 1965, Vol. 2, p. 567.

43. A. Brill, G. Bryce, and H. Maria, *Biochim. Biophys. Acta*, **154,** 342 (1968).

44a. L. Broman, B. Malmström, R. Aasa, and T. Vänngård, *ibid.*, **75,** 365 (1963).

44b. I. Sutherland and J. Wilkinson, *J. Gen. Microbiol.*, **30,** 105 (1963).

45. T. Stigbrand, B. Malmström, and T. Vänngård, *FEBS Letters*, **12,** 260 (1971).

46a. W. Blumberg and J. Peisach, *Biochim. Biophys. Acta*, **126,** 269 (1966).

46b. S. Katoh, I. Shiratori, and A. Takamiya, *J. Biochem.* (*Tokyo*), **51,** 32 (1962).

47. H. Yamada, K. Yasunobu, T. Yamano, and H. Mason, *Nature*, **198,** 1092 (1963).

48. H. Yamada, O. Adachi, and T. Yamano, *Biochim. Biophys. Acta*, **191,** 751 (1969).

49. B. Mondovì, G. Rotilio, M. Costa, A. Finazzi Agrò, E. Chiancone, R. Hansen, and H. Beinert, *J. Biol. Chem.*, **242,** 1160 (1967).

50. F. Buffoni, L. Della Corte, and P. Knowles, *Biochem. J.*, **106,** 575 (1968).

51. W. Blumberg, B. Horecker, F. Kelly-Falcoz, and J. Peisach, *Biochim. Biophys. Acta*, **96,** 336 (1965).

52. W. Blumberg, M. Goldstein, E. Lauber, and J. Peisach, *ibid.*, **99,** 187 (1965).

53. S. Friedman and S. Kaufman, *J. Biol. Chem.*, **241,** 2256 (1966).

54. M. Wishnick, M. Lane, M. Scrutton, and A. Mildvan, *ibid.*, **244,** 5761 (1969).

55a. G. Rotilio, A. Finazzi Agrò, L. Calabrese, F. Bossa, P. Guerrieri, and B. Mondovì, *Biochem.*, **10,** 616 (1971).

55b. J. Fee and B. Gaber, *Fed. Proc.*, **30,** 1294 (1971).

56. B. Malmström, B. Reinhammar, and T. Vänngård, *Biochim. Biophys. Acta*, **156**, 67 (1968).
57. R. Malkin, B. Malmström, and T. Vänngård, *FEBS Letters*, **1**, 50 (1968).
58. R. Brändén, B. Malmström, and T. Vänngård, *European J. Biochem.*, **18**, 238 (1971).
59. T. Nakamura and Y. Ogura in *The Biochemistry of Copper*, J. Peisach, P. Aisen, and W. Blumberg, Eds., Academic, New York, 1966, p. 389.
60. T. Omura, *J. Biochem.* (*Tokyo*), **50**, 264 (1961).
61. C. Holmberg and C.-B. Laurell, *Acta Chem. Scand.*, **2**, 550 (1948).
62. B. Magdoff-Fairchild, F. Lovell, and B. Low, *J. Biol. Chem.*, **244**, 3497 (1969).
63. L.-E. Andréasson and T. Vänngård, *Biochim. Biophys. Acta*, **200**, 247 (1970).
64. T. Nakamura, N. Makino, and Y. Ogura, *J. Biochem.* (*Tokyo*), **64**, 189 (1968).
65. H. Beinert, D. Griffiths, D. Wharton, and R. Sands, *J. Biol. Chem.*, **237**, 2337 (1962).
66. F. Gurd, K.-E. Falk, B. Malmström, and T. Vänngård, *ibid.*, **242**, 5724 (1967).
67. G. Bemski, T. Arends, and G. Blanc, *Biochem. Biophys. Res. Commun.*, **35**, 599 (1969).
68. A. Brill and J. Venable, Jr., *J. Mol. Biol.*, **36**, 343 (1968).
69. R. Aasa and P. Aisen, *J. Biol. Chem.*, **243**, 2399 (1968).
70a. H. Csopak and K.-E. Falk, *FEBS Letters*, **7**, 147 (1970).
70b. H. Csopak, K.-E. Falk, and H. Szajn, *Biochim. Biophys. Acta*, in press.
71. G. Bryce, *J. Phys. Chem.*, **70**, 3549 (1966).
72. D. Forster and V. Weiss, *ibid.*, **72**, 2669 (1968).
73. D. Gould and A. Ehrenberg, *European J. Biochem.*, **5**, 451 (1968).
74. A. Brill, R. Martin, and R. Williams in *Electronic Aspects of Biochemistry*, B. Pullman, Ed., Academic, New York, 1964, p. 519.
75. C. Bates, W. Moore, K. Standley, and K. Stevens, *Proc. Phys. Soc.*, **79**, 73 (1962).
76. M. Sharnoff, *J. Chem. Phys.*, **42**, 3383 (1965).
77. J. Peisach, W. Levine, and W. Blumberg, *J. Biol. Chem.*, **242**, 2847 (1967).
78. S.-P. Tang, J. Coleman, and Y. Myer, *ibid.*, **243**, 4286 (1968).
79. F. Bossa, G. Rotilio, P. Fasella, and B. Malmström, *European J. Biochem.*, **10**, 395 (1969).
80. K.-E. Falk and B. Reinhammar, to be published.
81. K. Wütrich, *Helv. Chim. Acta*, **49**, 1400 (1966).
82. A. Brill and G. Bryce, *J. Chem. Phys.*, **48**, 4398 (1968).
83. J. Harris and K. Ritchie, *Ann. N.Y. Acad. Sci.*, **153**, 706 (1969).
84. H. Mason, *Biochem. Biophys. Res. Commun.*, **10**, 11 (1963).
85. G. Strahs, *Science*, **165**, 60 (1969).
86. A. Finazzi Agrò, G. Rotilio, L. Avigliano, P. Guerrieri, V. Boffi, and B. Mondovì, *Biochem.*, **9**, 2009 (1970).
87. T. Nakamura and Y. Ogura, *J. Biochem.* (*Tokyo*), **64**, 267 (1968).
88. B. Mondovì, G. Rotilio, A. Finazzi Agrò, M. Vallogini, B. Malmström, and E. Antonini, *FEBS Letters*, **2**, 182 (1969).
89. D. Ballou, G. Palmer, and V. Massey, *Biochem. Biophys. Res. Commun.*, **36**, 898 (1969).
90. R. Malkin, B. Malmström, and T. Vänngård, *European J. Biochem.*, **7**, 253 (1969).
91. J. Fee, R. Malkin, B. Malmström, and T. Vänngård, *J. Biol. Chem.*, **244**, 4200 (1969).

92. R. Malkin, B. Malmström, and T. Vänngård, *European J. Biochem.*, **10,** 324 (1969).
93. A. Ehrenberg, B. Malmström, L. Broman, and R. Mosbach, *J. Mol. Biol.*, **5,** 450 (1962).
94. J. Fee and B. Malmström, *Biochim. Biophys. Acta*, **153,** 299 (1968).
95. T. Nakamura and H. Mason, *Biochem. Biophys. Res. Commun.*, **3,** 297 (1960).
96. J. Boas, J. Pilbrow, G. Troup, C. Moore, and T. Smith, *J. Chem. Soc.*, **(A) 1969,** 965.
97. K. Van Holde, *Biochem.*, **6,** 93 (1967).
98. B. Malmström, R. Aasa, and T. Vänngård, *Biochim. Biophys. Acta*, **110,** 431 (1965).
99. J. Fee, B. Malmström, and T. Vänngård, *ibid.*, **197,** 136 (1970).
100. J. Fee, B. Malmström, and T. Vänngård, 19. *Colloquium der Gesellschaft für Biologische Chemie, Mosbach/Baden* 1968, Springer-Verlag, Berlin 1968, p. 29.
101. T. Nakamura, A. Ikai, and Y. Ogura, *J. Biochem.* (*Tokyo*), **57,** 808 (1965).
102. W. Blumberg, W. Levine, S. Margolis, and J. Peisach, *Biochem. Biophys. Res. Commun.*, **15,** 277 (1964).
103. B. Reinhammar and T. Vänngård, *European J. Biochem.*, **18,** 463 (1971).
104. P. Aisen, S. Koenig, and H. Lilienthal, *J. Mol. Biol.*, **28,** 225 (1967).
105. B. Van Gelder and A. Veldsema, *Biochim. Biophys. Acta*, **130,** 267 (1966).
106. R. Carrico, B. Malmström, and T. Vänngård, *European J. Biochem.*, **20,** 518 (1971).
107. B. Malmström, A. Finazzi Agrò, and E. Antonini, *European J. Biochem.*, **9,** 383 (1969).
108. E. Frieden, S. Osaki, and H. Kobayashi, *J. Gen. Physiol.*, **49,** 213 (1965).
109. C. Dawson in *The Biochemistry of Copper*, J. Peisach, P. Aisen, and W. Blumberg, Eds., Academic, New York, 1966, p. 305.
110. H. Beinert and G. Palmer, *J. Biol. Chem.*, **239,** 1221 (1964).
111. J. Leigh, Jr., *J. Chem. Phys.*, **52,** 2608 (1970).
112. B. Van Gelder and H. Beinert, *Biochim. Biophys. Acta*, **189,** 1 (1969).
113. Q. Gibson and C. Greenwood, *J. Biol. Chem.*, **240,** 2694 (1965).
114. F. Gurd, K.-E. Falk, B. Malmström, and T. Vänngård, *ibid.*, **242,** 5731 (1967).
115. R. Nagel, G. Bemski, and P. Pincus, *Arch. Biochem. Biophys.*, **137,** 428 (1970).
116. P. Aisen, R. Aasa, and A. Redfield, *J. Biol. Chem.*, **244,** 4628 (1969).

CHAPTER TEN

Electron Spin Resonance Studies in Radiation Biology

EDMUND S. COPELAND

Walter Reed Army Institute of Research
Washington, D.C.

10.1 INTRODUCTION

Electron spin resonance spectroscopy has been one of the most useful, recently developed experimental techniques employed in molecular level radiation biology. As a result the literature on the subject is voluminous and somewhat confusing to a newcomer to the field. In this chapter an attempt has been made to clarify the various types of problems in radiation biology which can bc studied with ESR. The discussion is limited to the interaction of ionizing radiation with biological systems. No attempt has been made to review the literature exhaustively. A sufficient number of examples are cited, however, to point out experimental procedures found most useful and to demonstrate how certain experimental and theoretical pitfalls can be avoided.

10.1.1 The Place of ESR in Radiobiological Research: Defining the Problem

The cellular manifestations of ionizing radiation damage are temporally and chemically quite remote from the initial absorption of the energy from irradiation. An understanding of the mechanisms of the occurrence of cellular damage requires an understanding of the intervening physical, biophysical, and biochemical events. Theoretical and experimental analysis of these events indicates that free radical reactions play a key role in the transformation of radiant energy to cellular damage. ESR spectroscopy has therefore been of major importance in studies designed to elucidate these mechanisms.

10.1.1.1 Distortions of Existing Paramagnetic Signals

As discussed in the preceding chapters, many biological systems contain paramagnetic species. Since an excellent experimental groundwork has been laid for the nonirradiated state, analysis of radiation effects on naturally occurring paramagnetic species could be relatively straightforward. Little work has been done, however, in this area (26) and our discussion is limited to studies of radiation-induced ESR signals.

10.1.1.2 Radiation Induced Radicals

Irradiation of almost any substance, including biological materials, will produce free radicals. If the proper experimental conditions are applied, they can then be detected by ESR spectroscopy. The physics and chemistry underlying this transformation of the initial radiation energy into the formation and subsequent reactions of free radicals is beyond the scope of this book, but Table 10-1 outlines the time sequence of events preceding and following free radical formation.

Table 10-1 (9, 38)

Time (sec)	Events in solids at room temperature
10^{-16}	Excitation or ionization by a fast charged particle.
10^{-14}	Recapture of electrons by parent ions.
10^{-13}	Dissociation of chemical bonds.
10^{-12}	Relaxation of dielectric, reorientation of the lattice.
10^{-10}	Radical-radical reactions in a spur of ionizations.
10^{-8}	Reactions of kinetic or excited radicals.
10^{-5}	Reactions of small thermal radicals.
$\leq 10^{+2}$	Metastable situation.

Radiation-induced radicals are generally quite reactive and disappear too rapidly for observation by ordinary ESR methods. Therefore special techniques are required either to lengthen radical lifetimes or to shorten observation times (see Section 2.18). Radical lifetimes are lengthened by decreasing diffusion and/or lowering temperatures. Lyophilization or ordinary drying, with or without lowering temperature, has been employed in many studies to prevent diffusion. Such techniques have obvious limitations in radiobiological studies because of the important role of water in radiobiology. Many investigators have therefore turned to frozen aqueous solutions, usually at 77 K. Liquid nitrogen temperature (77 K) is low enough to stop many, but not all, diffusion-controlled reactions. Unless special steps are taken, hydrogen atoms will not be trapped at 77 K and will react further. If irradiation and observation are carried out at liquid helium temperature (4.2 K), most events can be stopped at about the 10^{-10} sec time frame (see Table 10-1). If one gradually raises the temperature after this initial observation, succeeding events listed in the table can be followed in a controlled way. (It should be kept in mind, however, that some quantitative variations in final products may occur when the reactions are allowed to proceed in discrete steps, compared with the continuous reactions that occur in the fully hydrated warm state.)

A more recent procedure is to observe early events directly with extremely rapid observation techniques. Pulsed ESR has been used to follow reactions occurring in intervals as short as 10^{-6} sec (4, 81). An ESR spectrometer was coupled with a linear accelerator so that a 15 MeV electron beam could be fired through the poles of the electromagnet to an aqueous sample cavity. With sufficiently fast electronic components and multichannel memory systems, the hydrated electron was observed in liquid water, and radical reactions involving radicals with 2 to 3 μsec lifetimes were followed. Whether similar techniques can be used to study macromolecules or bacterial systems remains to be seen. Because most ESR studies to date have employed low temperatures and/or drying to "freeze-in" certain stages of radical formation and reaction, only these conditions are discussed further (except for the flow work reviewed in Section 10.2.4.2).

10.1.2 Brief History of the Approach to Studying Radiobiological Problems with ESR

The work of Gordy and associates first reported in 1955 uncovered many phenomena observable when ESR was used to follow the free radicals induced by ionizing radiation in biological materials (33). These workers proposed structures for radicals formed in many of the amino acids. The cystinelike "sulfur resonance" dominated the ESR spectra of many proteins even when cystinyl residues made up but a small fraction of the amino acid population. An intramolecular transfer of electrons to form a radical cation at the disulfide bonds was suggested. A prominent glycylglycine type doublet was also noted and its preponderance was accounted for by assuming energy transfer to hydrogen bonded regions in which H nuclei would split the resonance of an unpaired electron stabilized on oxygen.

Numerous investigations followed to identify the molecular species that gave rise to these two resonance types in proteins and to attempt to provide an understanding of the mechanisms of the transfer of radiation energy which these first results indicated. Whether such transfer was intra- or intermolecular (15, 22, 34, 35, 40, 72, 73) or whether it was hydrogen bond-dependent (6, 7, 8, 41) and how it could be influenced (23, 36, 42,

79) have all been lively research topics. Also noted in the 1955 paper were the effect of oxygen on protein radicals and the postulation of the "peroxy" type radical. Since such results describe a molecular basis for the "oxygen effect" of radiation biology, it is understandable that such studies have been repeated and extended (43, 52, 53, 84).

One postulate of Gordy's early paper (33) seems neither to have been confirmed nor extensively studied. It was suggested that proteins, by virtue of their ability to stabilize radiation energy at their intermolecular links (disulfide and hydrogen bonds), were much more radioresistant than their constituent amino acids. Thus deamination and decarboxylation were avoided in proteins. It was suggested that this differential radiosensitivity allowed proteins to be evolutionarily favored during intense solar irradiation of the primordial soup.

It can be seen that the first paper that applied ESR to radiation biology uncovered many interesting theoretical problems, and most of them are still being actively investigated.

10.1.3 The Fundamental Experimental Problem: Physical versus Biological Relevance

Since the mid-1950's numerous investigators have examined various biological materials exposed to ionizing radiation and readily demonstrated free radical production whenever conditions were favorable to stabilize free radicals. The knowledge sought, however, is not whether free radicals are induced—because it is well known that they are—but rather what *roles* free radicals play in biologically important damage. It is quite clear that many detectable radiation-induced free radicals have little significant biological effect, and so one must be selective in what radical reactions are followed and how they are interpreted.

The major problem, then, in the application of ESR to biological systems is that although the greatest fundamental physical-chemical understanding of ESR results can be gleaned from experiments in which the chemical structure and orientation of the sample can be well defined, the most pertinent results for understanding mammalian radiobiology require whole cells or, preferably, live animals. However, as the system under study increases in complexity from amino acid or nucleic acid base to protein or nucleic acid and then to whole cells, the data that can be obtained by ESR become increasingly difficult to interpret in terms of specific molecular changes. Most ESR investigators have struggled with this problem and have settled on the most complex biological system that still gave results interpretable to them. The choices have varied from single crystals of amino acids to whole animals, with most workers settling on systems of intermediate complexity.

As more complicated systems such as whole cells are studied, one may have to give up studying radicals that can be rigorously identified in terms of hyperfine structure, etc. This does not necessarily mean that definitive identification of involved radical species in such systems is impossible, however. A variety of techniques is available that can be employed to identify tentatively the radical species of interest. These techniques include selective isotopic enrichment, power saturation properties, reactivity with added components, and cell fraction procedures. Such studies are likely to be quite difficult, however, and one must be prepared to deal with only partially characterized signals in many instances, just as has been the case in many of the biological and biochemical samples discussed in other chapters. Some of the results of studies of irradiated materials are considered in later sections.

10.2 EXPERIMENTAL PROBLEMS IN RADIOBIOLOGICAL ESR STUDIES

As suggested in the introduction, the nature of the problem leads to many experimental difficulties, some of which are dealt with explicity in this section.

10.2.1 Quantitative Studies

The desire to quantitate is prominent in most scientists and especially strong when physical scientists attack biological problems, perhaps because of their repulsion to the intrinsically less precise aspects of biological studies (due to specimen variability and so on). It is not surprising, therefore, that some of the earliest ESR radiobiological studies attempted to quantitate the yield of free radicals per unit energy absorbed (usually expressed as G values, molecules changed per 100 eV absorbed). Certainly it would be highly desirable to know accurately the yield of specific radical changes and to compare them with specific biological end points. With time, however, it has gradually become appreciated that quantitative ESR studies in radiation biology are quite difficult and any such study should be examined rigorously before its findings and implications are accepted.

Some of the difficulties in quantitation in this field are reflections of general problems of quantitative ESR discussed in detail in Chapter 3. Other aspects of the difficulties are particularly characteristic of radiation studies and are considered in more detail here. These additional aspects include saturation of radical concentrations (departures from linear dose-response relationships), changes in radical type with dose, power saturation (radiation-induced free radicals in frozen matrices may be exquisitely power saturable), and sample preparation techniques (yield is quite dependent on the ratio between amorphous and crystalline forms).

10.2.1.1 Saturation of Radical Concentration

Theoretically, initial radical production should be linearly related to dose, and although this certainly holds at low doses significant variations can occur at higher doses (Fig. 10-1). High doses have been used in many experiments, especially in earlier experiments which used spectrometers of relatively low sensitivity and in enzyme studies in which doses of 20 to 60 Mrads may be required to obtain inactivation in the solid state. There are several causes for this type of saturation, including the increased possibility of multiple hits at a single site, radiation-induced changes in substrates, and destruction of radicals by either radical-radical reactions (when two radicals are close to each other) or directly by radiation.

The appropriate technique to avoid these effects is to administer a series of doses and take quantitative data only from the linear portion of the curve. Present ESR spectrometers are sufficiently sensitive so that good resolution should be obtainable at the low dose levels required.

Closely related to the problem of saturation of radical production is the possibility that with increasing dose we may alter the type as well as the quantity of radicals, due to secondary reactions and/or the disproportionate buildup of a second species. Careful analysis of spectral shapes at different

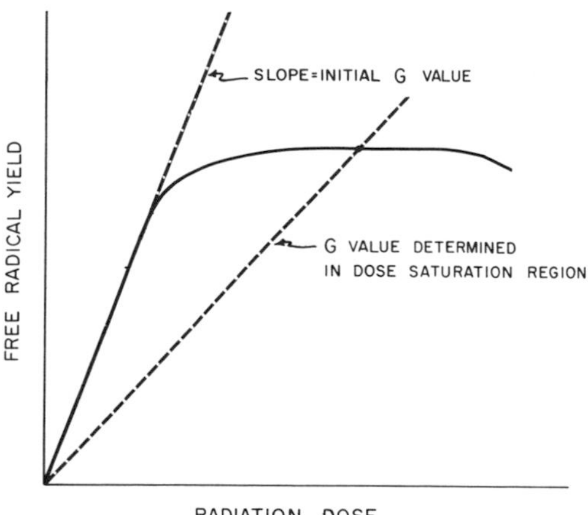

Fig. 10-1 Hypothetical radical yield versus radiation dose curve. The initial G value determination and a determination in the radical saturation region are shown.

dose levels should demonstrate whether this is an important problem in the particular system under investigation.

10.2.1.2 Saturation with Microwave Power

An equally difficult problem is that of power saturation. The area under an ESR absorption curve is only proportional to the number of free radicals present when the relaxation time of the radicals is sufficiently short at the microwave power levels employed (see Section 2.7 and Chapter 3). Thus, if an ESR spectrum of a radical were determined at a saturating microwave power, not all the radicals would be accounted for. This problem can be overcome by operating at progressively lower microwave powers until the signal height varies linearly with the square root of power. This is the region of no power saturation. When operating at very low temperatures (77 K or less), the region of no power saturation may be below 10 nW and this remains a persistent experimental problem. Accurate quantitative studies require that power saturation curves be determined experimentally before any conclusions are reached.

10.2.1.3 Sample Preparations

Even when saturation by radiation dose or microwave power is avoided, numerous other problems are encountered in quantitative ESR, some of which have been recently considered (9, 18) in detail and also reviewed in Chapter 3. A somewhat surprising source of variation occurring in irradiated samples reported independently by Henriksen (44) and ten Bosch (9) is that the radical yield in an irradiated solid organic material is dependent on the particle size and phase distribution (amorphous versus polycrystalline). Freeze-dried fluffs were found most capable of stabilizing and trapping radicals. As particle size increased, radical yield for the same radiation dose in the same material decreased (10, 11, 44). Thus sample preparation must be carefully described and considered.

10.2.1.4 General Considerations

Even when all the above factors are considered, interlaboratory variations remain disturbingly large.

In 1962 a number of workers (60) began an interlaboratory comparison of quantitative ESR techniques (see Table 10-2). Aliquots of stable free radicals, induced in sucrose by gamma irradiation, were measured on various spectrometers around the world using a variety of spin concentration standards. The results for this simple stable compound indicated variations as high as ± 50 percent. Such interlaboratory comparisons have been continued and the variations have been somewhat reduced, but the difficulty is a real one and must be considered in any radiation biological ESR work.

Table 10-2 Measured Radical Concentrations in Units of 10^{17} Spin Equivalents per Gram (59)

		Lignite BM3	Sucrose	DL-*a*-alanine
Braams, Casteleijn & ten Bosch Nijhuis	Utrecht	2.26	9.8	24.3
Depireux	Liege	2.0 ± 0.2	5.6 ± 0.2	41 ± 4
Ehrenberg Ehrenberg Löfroth	Stockholm	3.5	6.2	24
Hausser	Heidelberg	2.8 ± 0.3		
Henriksen	Oslo		6.3	
Hunt	Toronto		7.5	
Müller Köhnlein	Karlsruhe	2.4	9.5	24
Randolph Miller	Oak Ridge	2.45 ± 0.23 1.95 ± 0.26	4.3	23.5 ± 1.9 18.0 ± 2.5
Stratton	Boston	3.78 ± 0.08		27 ± 0.5
Vänngård Lund	Uppsala		6.8	
Weill	Strasbourg			15 ± 1.5

More complex and/or less stable samples probably lead to larger variations. It would be useful if national standard laboratories could provide calibrated spin concentration standard samples with various ESR shapes and g factors for ESR investigators. Such standards would help diminish interlaboratory variations. It also seems that readily saturating radicals with characterized hyperfine structure would be useful in determining saturation properties.

10.2.2 Model Systems

Although the ultimate goal of most research in radiation biology is to understand the response of intact mammals to ionizing radiation, there obviously must be frequent resort to model systems to obtain information. The general problem such compromises impose on ESR studies was considered in the introduction to this chapter in terms of physical versus biological relevance. It is considered here in additional detail, along with other problems associated with various model systems.

10.2.2.1 Restrictions Imposed by the Nature of Free Radicals

One of the principal experimental constraints encountered in this field is the need to stabilize the radiation-induced free radicals so that they may be observed in the ESR spectrometer (see Section 2.18). This essentially limits us to frozen and/or dried preparations, thus severely restricting the type of biological sample that can be used. These restrictions may be particularly bothersome if we conclude, as discussed below, that some type of biological correlation is an experimental prerequisite.

10.2.2.2 Biological Pertinence of Model

In view of the physical restrictions on sample state and the problems associated with interpreting spectra of irradiated complex materials, many investigators have turned to simple compounds for model studies, basing their choices on resemblance of the model to a particular biological property, such as appropriate chemical groupings, physical structure (e.g., membrane models), or chemical composition. Such systems can lead to precise data, but considerable caution and judgment must be used in applying these results to the living cell. With appropriate restrictions such models can lead to very valuable information, including information on energy transfer mechanisms and relative radiosensitivity of particular cell biochemicals. Use of more complex preparations does not automatically lead to biological pertinence. Whole cell preparations, after suitable manipulations, may lose all resemblance to living cells in regard to their response to ionizing radiation. Another example of this type is the use of impure, partly depolymerized, and/or crosslinked DNA as a model for studies of DNA response; such a preparation will probably show energy localization and delocalization quite uncharacteristic of DNA *in vivo*.

10.2.2.3 Relationship Between ESR and Biological Changes

One potential solution to many of the problems alluded to above is to choose a model system in which both biological and ESR parameters can be measured. Only a small number of such studies have been reported, however, because of their complexity. The Ehrenbergs studied the effect of oxygen and moisture content on ESR spectra and biological damage to the grass seed *Agrostis stolonifera* (30). Powers and his colleagues have investigated the effect of oxygen, heat, nitric oxide, and hydrogen sulfide on the survival and ESR spectra of spores of *Bacillus megaterium* (76). Conger has done analogous work with irradiated seeds (20). Swartz and Richardson found an inverse relation between the number of radiation induced radicals in frozen aqueous *E. coli* preparations and the log of their reproductive capability after rapid thawing and plating (86).

In each of these studies measurements of ESR and of biological parameters were made in parallel as different treatments were applied which modified the radiation response. The greater the number of variations employed and the closer the two sets of observations follow in parallel, the more likely that the two parameters are causally related. It must also be remembered, however, that such studies cannot *prove* cause and effect relationships. There may be a number of steps interposed between the two processes or both might result from a common cause. Such studies do, however, constitute one of the most direct and convincing approaches to demonstrating the biological role of free radical changes measured by ESR.

10.2.3 Limitations, Advantages, and Uses of Specific Classes of Model Systems

We shall now examine some of the types of model system or preparation that have been utilized in radiobiological ESR studies. A more complete discussion of the results obtained appears in Section 10.3 of this chapter. In this section, therefore, results are referred to primarily to indicate the type of information obtainable with these systems.

All types of preparation in which samples are irradiated share the common experimental problem that radiation will generate free radicals in virtually all materials. Therefore we must somehow handle the preparation so that only free radicals generated in the sample are studied. This means that the sample holder either must not be irradiated originally or must be changed after irradiation. The latter procedure is limited by the need to stabilize the radiation-induced radicals in the sample. However, a variety of procedures has been successfully worked out for each type of sample preparation, and the reader is referred to the literature for applications of his specific problem. It is most important, nevertheless, to be aware of this problem and to avoid the pitfall of studying radiation-induced signals in one's sample holder!

10.2.3.1 Single-Crystal Investigations

The most complete information about a free radical can be obtained in single-crystal studies because all the molecules are aligned in fixed positions to permit elucidation of anisotropic hyperfine splittings (see Chapter 1).

Single crystals of amino acids (or other biochemicals) are usually grown by slow evaporation from an aqueous solution. With the help of the crystallographic literature, by carrying out the requisite crystallographic measurements directly, or by working closely with a crystallography group the space group and number of molecules per unit cell are determined. The crystal axes are identified either optically or by X-ray diffraction, and the single crystal is mounted so that the relation between the molecular orientation and the crystal axes is known. The crystal is irradiated at the chosen temperature and placed in the ESR cavity, either on a fixed shaft around which the magnet can be rotated or on a rotating shaft fitted to a goniometer. By passing the external magnetic field through the molecules parallel or perpendicular to the crystallographic axes unique orientations can be found in which all unpaired electrons bear the same relation to the external magnetic field and in which well-resolved ESR spectra can be obtained. The theory involved in the determination of g tensors and splitting constants was outlined in Sections 1.4 and 1.6 and is discussed for radiation-induced radicals in many excellent reviews (e.g., 65).

By these procedures precise information on the structure of the radicals and the distribution of the unpaired electron can be obtained. Experimental techniques involved in such measurements have recently been summarized by Wyard (93), who outlined how the techniques of annealing, power saturation, measurement at two frequencies, and deuteration may be used to clarify ESR results.

Single-crystal studies provide the ultimate means by which a radical can be identified. Molecules, however, are randomly oriented in biological systems, and the anisotropic contributions to their ESR spectra are neither averaged out (as in liquids) nor coherent (as in single crystals), and analysis and identification may not be possible. Since single-crystal studies can provide much more information about these same radicals, the features of their ESR powder spectra may be identified by correlating studies of single crystals and polycrystalline samples.

One widely used result of single-crystal investigations has been that unpaired electrons stabilized on sulfur atoms show a marked g factor anisotropy in studies on irradiated cysteine and cystine. Such g-factor variations that are dependent on spin-orbit coupling result in broad ESR absorptions with characteristic components considerably removed from the free spin g factor. Studies of randomly oriented irradiated sulfur containing proteins show a peak at $g = 2.06$ in powdered samples. By using single crystal results such resonances in biological preparations can now be ascribed with confidence to unpaired electrons on cysteinyl sulfur.

Several recent reviews tabulate the qualitative ESR results found for a myriad of single organic crystals subjected to ionizing radiation at low temperatures followed by careful annealing and observation of the free radical transformations (12, 67, 93). The amino acids and certain dipeptides have been quite thoroughly analyzed. Single crystals of the nucleic acid bases have been fairly well examined (e.g., 45). When characteristic signals such as the low-field organosulfur radical absorption peak or the thymine octet are observed in protein or DNA, respectively, they can be identified with certainty because of the analytical groundwork done on single crystals.

Usually only very simple organic crystals can be thoroughly analyzed by ESR. At present several laboratories are engaged in examining irradiated protein-single crystals, and if the complex data can be unraveled it should be most enlightening. The only attempts reported to date to study oriented biological macromolecules have employed stretched strands of DNA (28).

10.2.3.2 Investigations with Lyophilized and Polycrystalline Materials

Because of the paucity of materials that can be obtained and analyzed as single crystals, many investigators have utilized randomly oriented dry solids. Virtually all materials can be obtained in this form, but we can no longer obtain the detailed information that is available from single crystals. However, mixtures as well as pure substances can be studied in the solid state, which permits investigation of the important problem of energy transfer. Materials ranging from mixtures of two amino acids to whole cells have been utilized to investigate the mechanisms of energy transfer with this type of preparation. The interpretation of such studies is somewhat limited because of the absence of most of the water normally present in functional biological materials.

Amorphous or polycrystalline dry solids are also of limited value in studies that attempt to obtain parallel biological results, although dried seeds and bacterial spores have been utilized with considerable success. Dry preparations do offer the opportunity to perform limited postirradiation radical scavenging and radical transformation experiments by introducing different gases after irradiation. The temperature dependence of these and other reactions can also be conveniently studied in dry preparations; gradual heating of the preparation within the ESR cavity is a particularly popular technique.

An excellent review of the use of ESR in studying radiation effects on solid biological materials has been written recently by Müller (67). He showed that the preponderance of research to date has been of two types: (a) the identification of intermediate radical products in irradiated biological compounds and (b) the correlation of radical yields with biological consequences of radical reactions; hence most of the work he reported dealt with radical identification and radiochemical yield determinations.

One paper that is particularly useful in ESR analysis of polycrystalline irradiated material is that by Kneubühl (58), who showed how the number of different g factors exhibited by the ESR spectrum of a free radical in a multioriented situation ("powder spectrum") can be deduced from the general spectral shape (see Fig. 10-2 and Figs. 1-3 and 1-4). A singlet suggests that no g-factor anisotropy exists. A first derivative ESR spectrum with five inflection points suggests two principal g factors: $g_{\|}$ and $g_{\perp}$, whereas a curve with seven inflection points represents a radical with all

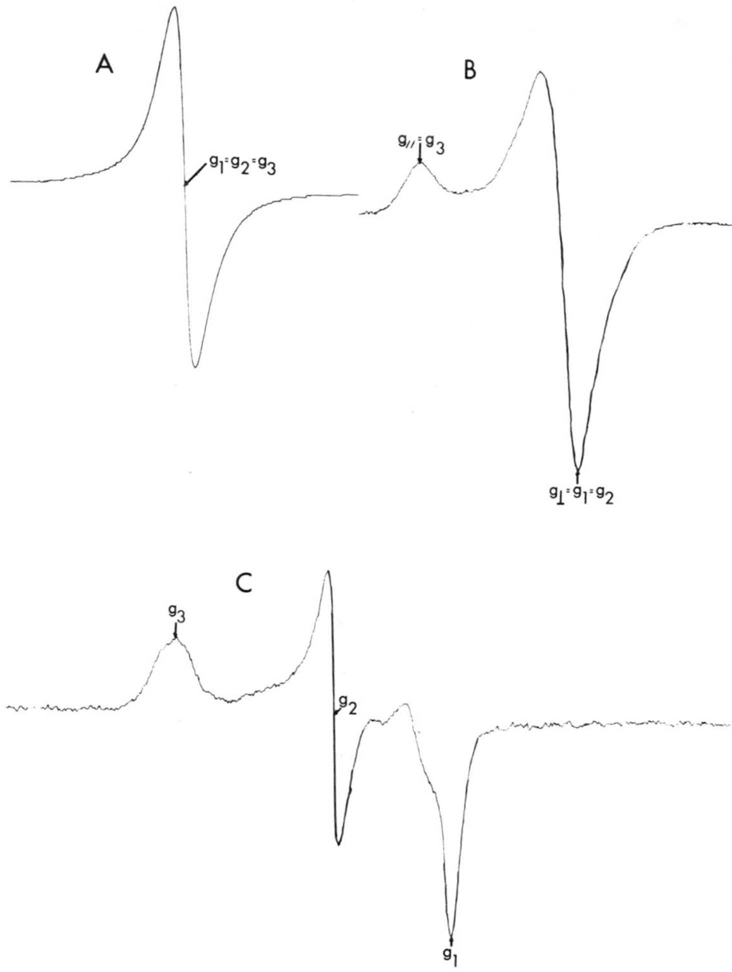

Fig. 10-2 Deduction of principal *g* factors from the general spectral shape. Three polycrystaline samples were chosen to illustrate the shapes found for radicals having one, two, or three unique principal *g* factors. A. a carbon standard, BM-3 (see Table 10-2), having three equal *g* factors. B. bacteria (*E. coli* B/r) γ-irradiated is an oxygen equilibrated frozen aqueous suspension. The radical, R00·, has two principal *g* factors. C. penicillamine hydrochloride γ-irradiated in a nitrogen equilibrated frozen aqueous solution. The sulfur radical, $RC(CH_3)_2S\cdot$, has three principal *g* factors.

three principal g factors unequal to one another. (Section 1.4 discusses conventions for assigning g factors.)

As mentioned above, the stable free radical in irradiated cystine, the organosulfur radical, has three principal g factors, and in polycrystalline systems it gives rise to ESR spectra resembling Fig. 10-2*c*. Such radicals have been identified in numerous solid-state biological preparations. Gordy's first reported work on irradiated biological materials showed sulfur radicals in hair, fingernails, and skin, as well as in proteins known to contain sulfhydryl or disulfide groups. An extensive analysis of this type of radical in many biochemicals can be found in work by Henriksen (46). The importance of this "organosulfur" radical is discussed in detail in Section 10.3.

10.2.3.3 Investigations with Frozen Aqueous Solutions

Because of the importance of water in biology and radiobiology, it is often desirable to perform ESR studies in materials that have not had the water removed. Such studies are usually performed by freezing the preparation to liquid nitrogen temperatures (77 K) or below, at which temperatures most, but not all (e.g., not H atoms), radiation-induced free radicals are indefinitely stabilized.

In such preparations radiation-induced radicals will be found in the water as well as the "solute." At 77 K the observed ESR spectrum of water is somewhat complex (Fig. 10-3). Single-crystal studies (13) indicate,

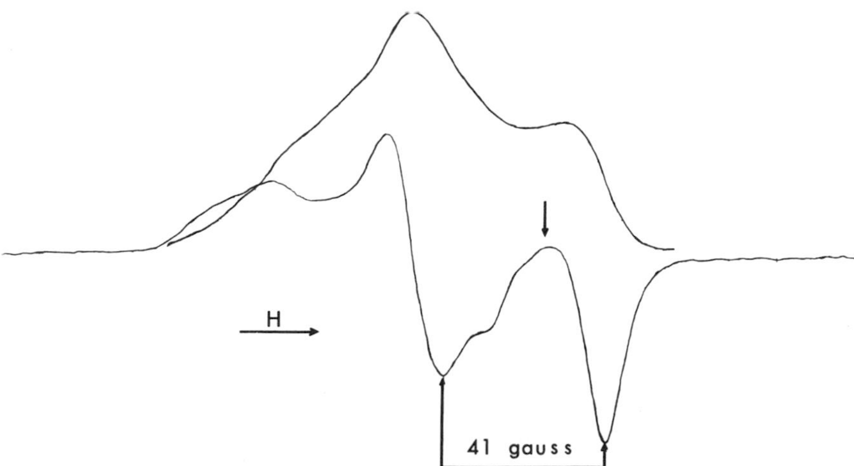

Fig. 10-3 The hydroxyl radical doublet shown as an absorption spectrum (*top*) and in first derivative form. The 41-G splitting can best be seen in the first derivative presentation. Distilled water was γ irradiated as a frozen cylinder at 77 K and the spectrum was observed at 77 K. The vertical arrow indicates $g = 2.0036$.

however, that the hydroxyl radical is the only stabilized free radical in neutral solutions, and its different orientations ($\sim$ 24) lead to the entire observable ESR spectrum. If the water is made strongly acid with an oxyanion acid (e.g., H_2SO_4), the hydrogen atom is also stabilized after irradiation at 77 K and can be recognized by its 507-G doublet. In oxygenated basic (pH = 12) preparations both O_2^- and e_{aq}^- are stable and can be recognized by their *g* factors, shape, and reaction behavior. Other water radicals, such as $HO_2^{\cdot}$ radicals, can also be observed under special conditions.

If we were interested primarily in those radicals induced directly or indirectly in the solute, several experimental techniques could be used. We could simply irradiate the preparation at a temperature at which all water radicals are unstable (e.g., 196 K, dry-ice temperature) or, to assess the interaction of solute with water radicals, irradiate at 77 K and then observe the ESR pattern after pulse annealing to increasing temperatures (see Sections 2.18.1 and 10.1.1.2). As indicated in Fig. 10-4, the water radicals disappear above 140 K. Most of the water radicals decay by recombination, but a small amount of the solute radical yield may be due to radiation energy transfer from radicals induced in a single molecular layer of bound water associated with macromolecules such as DNA and gelatin (77).

Henriksen and Snipes (47) have used the technique of acidification with an oxyanion acid to trap H atoms in frozen aqueous preparations of dihydrothymine. They were able to correlate a decrease in the amplitude of the

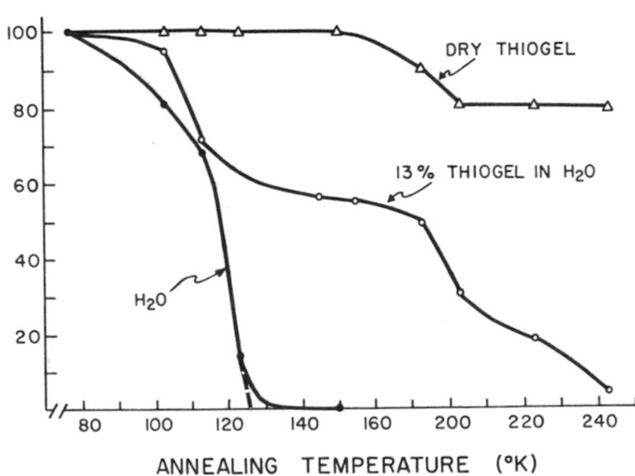

Fig. 10-4 Decay of hydroxyl radicals with annealing. Solutions of thiolated gelatin containing 0 percent (H_2O), 13 percent and 100 percent thiolgel by weight, were irradiated at 77 K and annealed for 3 min at the indicated temperatures with ESR observation at 77 K. All spectra were double integrated and the initial yield at 77 K set equal to 100 relative units. Note that the water radical yield reaches zero before 140 K.

507-G doublet with an increase in the 5-hydrothymine octet signal as the sample was gradually warmed. Thus they postulated a mechanism of radiation damage involving H atoms and furthermore suggested a greater indirect effect mediated by water radicals than is normally suspected.

Frozen solution studies may be used to obtain both ESR and biological results on the same samples if the biological preparation utilized can survive the freezing process. This approach has been useful in studying the mechanisms of action of radioprotective compounds in bacteria (86, 89, 90). Considerable caution must be attached to the interpretation of such studies, however. Most of the biological effects due to indirect damage (damage mediated by diffusable water free radicals, principally e_{aq}^-, $H^\cdot$ and $OH^\cdot$) are eliminated when frozen samples are irradiated, and therefore primarily direct effects are investigated with this technique. (It may, of course, be used to some advantage by permitting experimental separation of the two effects). Biological results may also be altered by damage due to the freezing process (see Section 2.18.1 and 4.2.5).

10.2.3.4 Unmodified Hydrated Preparations

The ultimate goal of most radiobiological studies is the understanding of what happens in the living, normally functioning cell. The various preparations described above are experimental compromises required because of the need to stabilize radicals and/or to obtain more interpretable ESR data. Some studies, however, can be profitably carried out on unmodified chemical and biological preparations.

Relatively long-lived free radicals can be studied by irradiating samples and then quickly transferring them to the ESR spectrometer for analysis. A variation of this technique, room-temperature irradiation followed by quick freezing, may also be employed (see Section 2.18.1). The latter allows a more leisurely ESR examination and provides an estimate of radical lifetimes (by employing variable periods between irradiation and freezing), but of course it prevents dynamic studies of radical decay and transformation. Another related technique is the use of continuous-flow procedures (see Section 2.18.2.2) in which the samples flow through an irradiator and then into the ESR cavity.

Using some of the above techniques, long-lived radicals (with lifetimes ranging from seconds to several days) have been found in preparations ranging from amino acids (56) to bacteria (87) and mammals (16, 88). The occurrence of such long-lived radiation-induced radicals is of considerable interest, both with respect to their capacity to cause damage after irradiation and their possible use in dosimetry. Such persistent radicals, of course, are a very small proportion of the total number of free radicals produced by irradiation.

Most recently techniques have been developed (4, 81) for the irradiation of aqueous materials in the ESR cavity with simultaneous ESR observations. These techniques have time resolutions as fast at 10^{-6} sec and therefore may be used to study a wide variety of radical reactions. Many technical problems had to be solved to allow such studies, and to date only a few laboratories have been able to perform them. Preliminary results have been reported for irradiated aqueous solutions and animal tissues (57). Although the broad bandwidth implied by a microsecond response time markedly reduces ESR sensitivity (see Section 2.11.1), this is obviously an area of great promise, and it may become one of the most productive ESR radiobiological techniques.

10.2.4 Use of Individual Components of Irradiated Water

Ionization and energy deposition in water causes much of the observed radiobiological effect. This seems quite reasonable, inasmuch as most cells are 50 to 90 percent water by weight. Most estimates of the role of these "indirect effects" range from 40 to 60 percent of the total observed biological damage. Many investigators have therefore attempted to determine the relative contribution of the various radiation products of water to this damage by experimental conditions that selectively produce individual components of irradiated water ($OH^{\cdot}$, $H^{\cdot}$, and e^-_{aq}, principally).

10.2.4.1 Hydrogen Atoms

Hydrogen atoms can be produced by excitation of hydrogen gas by radio-frequency radiation in a gas discharge tube (19, 39, 51, 54). The hydrogen atoms can then be allowed to flow over a sample (usually lyophilized), and the reaction products can be studied by ESR. The discharge also produces UV light (1216 Å), which can cause radical formation; and some early studies of hydrogen atom reactions were confounded by this effect. Jensen and Henriksen constructed T-shaped tubes (55) to obviate this difficulty.

Another approach to evaluate the effect of $H^{\cdot}$ is to modify its contribution in studies employing ionizing radiation. The yield of $H^{\cdot}$ from water is quite dependent on pH; at neutral and alkaline pH hydrated electrons replace hydrogen atoms as the predominent reducing species (47, 62), while at low pH, $H^{\cdot}$ predominates.

10.2.4.2 Hydroxyl Radicals

Hydroxyl radicals have been used extensively not only in the study of ionizing radiation effects but also as tools to produce free radicals in molecules of biochemical interest. They are usually produced by flow systems or by photolysis of hydrogen peroxide.

The rationale of the flow systems is quite straightforward (29) but the nature of the products remains open to some debate (27, 32). Generally, a solution containing the substrate for reaction plus a metal ion such as Ti^{3+} or Fe^{2+} is allowed to mix with a stream of hydrogen peroxide, and the products that result then flow through the ESR cavity (see Section 2.18.2.2). Because aqueous solutions are involved, a flat cell or capillary tube is generally used, which greatly reduces the sensitive volume for ESR study. Alternatively the reaction mixture may be quick-frozen and studied statically in the frozen state.

The area of controversy is over the nature of the oxidizing species produced. In principle $OH^{\cdot}$ is formed by reduction of hydrogen peroxide: $H_2O_2 + M^n \rightarrow OH^{\cdot} + OH^- + M^{n+1}$. However, depending on the systems and the rate of flow, convincing arguments have been made for the production of $HO_2^{\cdot}$ and various metal-$OH^{\cdot}$ and metal-$HO_2^{\cdot}$ complexes as well as $OH^{\cdot}$ as significant oxidizing species. It is neither appropriate nor possible to summarize the various arguments here, although it seems fair to conclude that either free $OH^{\cdot}$ radicals or weakly complexed forms with closely similar reactivity are produced by the Ti^{3+}/H_2O_2 system, whereas the oxidizing species from Fe^{2+}/H_2O_2 is different. The interested reader is urged to consult the literature thoroughly (32) before undertaking experiments with these systems if the nature of the oxidizing species is important in his experiments.

The photolysis of H_2O_2 may lead to $OH^{\cdot}$ and/or $HO_2^{\cdot}$, depending on the radiant energy utilized (64, 82) and the reader is again urged to examine his particular experimental procedure carefully in the light of the published literature.

The relative role of $OH^{\cdot}$ in irradiated water can also be modified by appropriate additions. Hydroxyl radical scavengers can be employed to reduce $OH^{\cdot}$ effects or nitric oxide may be added to convert hydrated electrons to $OH^{\cdot}$ (70). Details on the various scavengers and the conditions required can be obtained in standard radiation chemistry texts and/or review articles (2, 70).

10.2.4.3 Hydrated Electrons

Hydrated electrons have usually been studied by pulse radiolysis with optical detection methods, and relatively few ESR studies consider them in great detail (but see 83). As indicated above, their contribution to biological damage can be modified by appropriate additives. There is no widely used method that selectively produces hydrated electrons; however, electrons solvated in liquid ammonia have been used as reactants in some ESR flow experiments (17).

10.3 RESULTS OF SOME RADIOBIOLOGICAL ESR STUDIES

10.3.1 Early Radiation Products

Early radiation products are frequently free radicals which can be directly analyzed by ESR, whereas many ordinary chemical methods can provide only indirect evidence of their existence. The earlier the product in the radiation reaction sequence, the more reactive it is likely to be, and therefore data interpretation must include the consideration that the observed species may have been preceded by other more reactive chemical species. Hence species identified by ESR (or any other method) should usually be considered to be "early" rather than literally being the *initial* radiation products unless there is specific evidence that the observed products are indeed initial products.

As pointed out in Section 10.1.1.2, crystalline matrices at very low temperatures provide the best opportunities to trap and rigorously identify early radiation products, and a number of excellent studies have been carried out under these conditions (12, 37, 65). The interaction of electrons produced by ionizing radiation with a neutral diamagnetic organic molecule can result in the loss of an electron from the molecule and the formation of a paramagnetic radical cation. Another neutral diamagnetic molecule may capture the dissociated electron and become a paramagnetic radical anion. Both the anion and cation species so formed have been observed in single crystals of biologically interesting molecules (12).

Single-crystal studies with amino acids and simple organic molecules have shown that the first ESR-detectable species formed during this interaction are the cation and anion radical pair; for example, by irradiating and observing dithiodiglycolic acid single crystals at 4.2 K Box and coworkers have been able to identify both the anion radical at the site of a stabilized secondary electron and the cationic radical species at the site of ejection of this electron (12).

Similar studies have now been performed on a number of organic compounds, including amino acids, which provide important information on early radiation products of the constituents of more complicated molecules. Several investigators are attempting to obtain similar information directly from biological macromolecules, but obtaining and interpreting this information involves tremendous experimental difficulties.

10.3.2 Oxygen Effect

Although the radiation-sensitizing action of oxygen has been known for many years, ESR studies have now provided some of the best information on the molecular mechanisms of this effect (48). Because molecular oxygen contains two unpaired electrons, it reacts readily with free radicals but, unlike most radical-radical reactions, the product is also a free radical (only one of oxygen's unpaired electrons becomes paired in the reaction). The usual oxygen-addition radical is a peroxy-type radical, and because there is considerable spin-orbit coupling to an oxygen atom it has a fairly characteristic ESR spectrum (see Fig. 10-2*b*). The following equations, confirmed by ESR data, can therefore account for the oxygen effect (RH = any organic molecule).

(1)	RH + ionizing radiation	$\rightarrow R^{\cdot} + H^{\cdot}$	(initial damage)
(2)	$R^{\cdot} + O_2$	$\rightarrow ROO^{\cdot}$	(peroxy radical)
(3)	$R^{\cdot}$ + XH	$\rightarrow RH + X^{\cdot}$	(restoration)

Reaction 3 would restore the damaged molecule, whereas reaction 2 would fix the damage irreparably. Such reactions have now been demonstrated by ESR in a variety of systems ranging from simple organic molecules to whole bacteria (86). ESR has also provided a convenient way to follow processes that interfere with the effect of oxygen and to monitor reactions with certain related free radicals, such as nitroxides, which can also cause radiation sensitization. Most of the data supplied by ESR on the oxygen effect have confirmed and extended pre-existing theories rather than establishing new theories; this specific validation has been a highly valuable contribution.

10.3.3 Sulfur-Containing Compounds

Sulfur compounds are of special interest because of their roles in sensitizing to radiation damage and in radiation protection. Specific aspects are discussed in following sections, but first the basic information on radiation effects on sulfur containing compounds is considered.

Many ESR data have been obtained on early free radical products in crystals of sulfur-containing compounds; for example, both ionic species (cationic and anionic) have been identified in irradiated cystine crystals (12). In dithiodiglycolic acid and in cystine the cation radical is quite unstable thermally and decays rapidly when the temperature is raised to 77 K. At this temperature the anion radicals are fairly stable. The radical anion in cystine begins to transform when the temperature is raised above 77 K. Akasaka and colleagues have shown that the unpaired electron is first trapped on the disulfide bond. Then this bond breaks and the neutral sulfur radical forms as the temperature is raised above 77 K toward room temperature (1). The sulfur radical anion has its principal g factor at 2.01. Because this is somewhat above the main g factor of most protein ESR spectra (2.004 to 2.007), sulfur radical anions might be visible in spectra of sulfur-containing proteins irradiated at 77 K. In fact, Singh and Ormerod (80) and Stratton (85) noted that although nonsulfur proteins had rather symmetrical singlet ESR spectra, proteins containing disulfide bonds had asymmetric ESR spectra with good evidence of an underlying absorption at $g = 2.01$. They hypothesized that at 77 K electrons were stabilized on sulfur residues of proteins and designated such radicals "primary" sulfur radicals. This is another example of how fundamental processes clarified in single-crystal studies have been applied to more complex biological systems (see Section 10.2.3.1). An excellent source of information on sulfur radicals in polycrystalline systems is Henriksen's thesis (46).

10.3.4 Nucleic Acids and Components

Because it has been widely assumed that the ultimate radiobiological target molecule in cellular material is DNA, a great number of ESR investigations have been carried out on nucleic acids and their constituents (45, 68, 78). Some of the important findings and current areas of research are discussed here, and the reader is referred to some of the excellent recent review articles that are available (37, 69) for more detailed consideration of this subject.

Irradiation of dry preparations of DNA itself has produced a variety of results. Spectra reported include various "singlets," a doublet with 20-G splitting, a triplet with 20-G splitting, and some of their combinations with a "thymine octet" (69). The origin of the DNA, the physical preparation of the DNA, and the ESR observation conditions are all important factors in determining the shape of the ESR spectra that are observed. In addition, low molecular weight DNA appears to have a greater radical yield than higher molecular weight DNA, which is otherwise identical to it; the reason for this is not clear. As a result of these and perhaps other factors not considered here, literature values for G(DNA radicals) vary. One key question, however, has been satisfactorily answered by yield studies of DNA: it is quite clear that the radical yield greatly exceeds the biological inactivation yield (by about a factor of 100) so that radical formtion could be involved in inactivation (69). These data also imply that most of the radiation-induced free radicals in DNA are either repaired or are not biologically important. These yield figures hold for both 77 K and room-temperature experiments.

The relationship between modification of DNA and free radical formation and transformation has been studied by a number of workers. Studies of DNA in combination with other substances indicate that energy transfer can occur both to and from DNA. In nucleoproteins energy transfer has been shown to occur from protein to DNA (69). With radioprotective agents such as mercaptoethylamine (MEA) energy transfer from DNA to MEA has been demonstrated in dry preparations (66) and may play a role in biological protection, although there has been no direct evidence to indicate that it does. The mechanism of radiation sensitization caused by substitution of bromouracil in DNA has been studied, and energy transfer from residual thymine (DNA with 70 percent bromouracil substitution) to bromouracil has been demonstrated. The radicals appeared on the sugar moeity rather than the bromouracil (61). There appears to be some conflict in the literature whether the presence of bromouracil increases or decreases total radical yield (71) but the most important effect is probably redistribution of energy.

An area of current interest is the production of well-oriented complex preparations such as nucleoproteins, in which rigorous identifications of radicals similar to those obtained in single-crystal preparations of simple molecules could be made. If successful, these studies would be illuminating, but it has been difficult to produce such preparations. One partly successful approach has been to orient DNA fibers (31) to give a considerably more coherent preparation than in polycrystalline samples but still with less orientation than in a single crystal. Using such a preparation, the angular dependence of the thymine octet and an unresolved singlet were dramatically demonstrated.

Single-crystal and polycrystalline preparations of the various components of nucleic acids have been studied extensively and many radiation-induced radicals identified. Hydrogen addition appears to play a prominent role in radical formation in thymine, adenine, guanine, and cystosine (37). The radical induced in thymine has drawn particular interest because of its ESR prominence. It has been identified as the 5,6 dihydrothymin-5-yl radical with its unpaired electron largely localized on the C-5 atom of the thymine ring, where it interacts with the methyl protons of C-5; it also has some density on C-6 so that the spectrum is also affected by the C-6 methylene protons. The result is a characteristic eight-line spectrum (Fig. 10-5) frequently termed the "thymine octet." This spectrum extends over a broad region and so it can often be identified by its wings in the presence of other radicals. Thus the transformation of a portion of the nonspecific DNA spectrum into the thymine octet can be followed and some quantitative estimates made by using the wings to decompose the complex spectra (74). The mechanism of the formation of the thymine radical has been worked out; it is likely that similar mechanisms apply to the formation of radicals in other purine and pyrimidine bases. Hydrogen addition to the C-5—C-6 double bond appears to be the main pathway (69). This mechanism is based on the nature of the radical, the requirement of the hydrogen

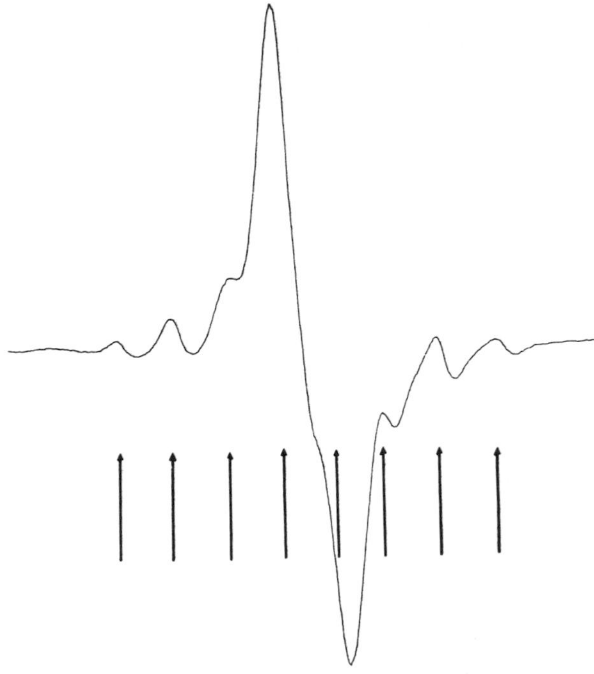

Fig. 10-5 γ-irradiated DNA showing the thymine octet. Solid calf thymus DNA was given 0.7 Mrads of ^{60}Co γ radiation at room temperature and observed at 77 K. At somewhat lower microwave power a doublet was observable in the center of the spectrum. The outer wings of the 5-thymyl radical, the octet, are clearly seen. The center lines are covered by the large singlet. The vertical arrows indicate the eight lines of the octet.

atom source for its formation, and observed incorporation of labeled hydrogen isotopes. Water appears to be the usual hydrogen source, although hydrogen gas or free hydrogen atoms can also serve. The detailed determination of the identity and mechanism of the formation of the thymine radical has been a great stimulus to ESR studies in radiation biology. The biological importance of the thymine radical, however, is not yet clear.

Free radical products of irradiated ribose and deoxyribose have also been determined and their ESR spectra are quite distinct from the bases. This has enabled the determination of the direction of energy migration in nucleosides and nucleotides. The radical yields *of the bases* are greatest in nucleotides, less in nucleosides, and least in the bases themselves, suggesting that radiation energy migrates from the phosphate and sugar to the bases (69). Consistent with this interpretation, the qualitative spectra of the nucleosides and nucleotides resemble those of the bases and not the sugars.

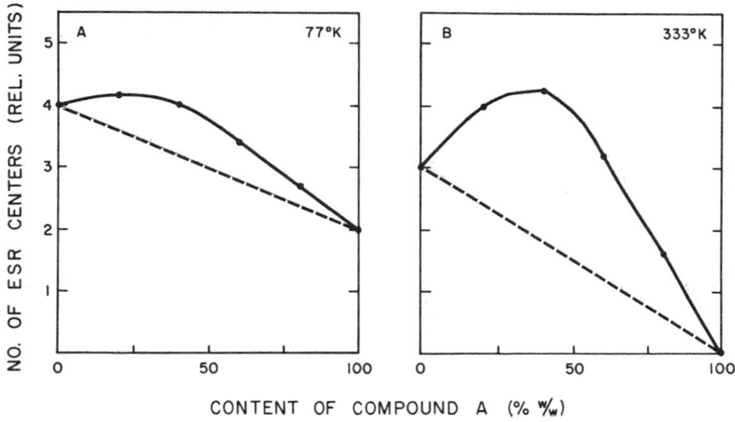

Fig. 10-6 Hypothetical quantitative ESR data from molecular mixtures of compounds A and B. The data at the left (A) was taken at 77 K and that at the right (B) after 10 min annealing at 333 K. The dotted lines indicate the yield expected if there were no interaction between the components and each behaved as when irradiated alone. Radical yield is plotted against the composition by weight of the molecular mixture.

10.3.5 Energy Transfer*

One of the most useful applications of ESR in radiation biology has been the study of energy transfer processes. Early experimental and theoretical considerations suggested that a large fraction of ionizing radiation damage occurs as a result of the migration of energy, both inter- and intramolecularly (15, 33, 34, 40). Energy transfer of this kind has now been shown to occur within proteins and nucleoproteins (63). It may be a fundamental aspect of radiation protection (36, 42). (We are not considering here another form of energy transfer, the "indirect effect," in which energy deposited initially in water migrates to other components via radiation products of water.)

Model systems have been especially useful in energy transfer studies. The general procedure is to lyophilize solutions or suspensions of two substances to produce a series of "molecular mixtures" in which the weight ratio of each material varies from zero to 100 percent (see Fig. 10-6). Examination of Fig. 10-6 suggests that compound *A* stabilizes radicals twice as effectively (on a weight basis) as compound *B* when irradiated and observed at 77 K. The dotted line represents the radical yield to be expected

* Energy transfer is used here in its broadest sense, including physical transfer of energy via migration of unpaired electrons and pure energy transfer by radiation processes.

with no interaction between components. The total radical yield is somewhat greater than expected. We might assume that there has been energy transfer from B to A, but qualitative spectra showing increased amounts of A are required to prove this interpretation.

If the samples are heat-treated for 10 min at 333 K, the curve at the right of Fig. 10.6 might be observed. Apparently pure compound B is of a nature such that it stabilizes no radicals, but at 333 K the total radical yield of the 1:2 and 1:1 $A:B$ mixtures is again greater than expected. Because of the instability of B-type radicals, it is reasonable to assume that energy initially deposited in B is transferred to A during heat treatment. If either substance has a characteristic ESR spectrum (e.g., sulfur radical, thymine octet), spectrum stripping can be employed to substantiate and quantitate the hypothetical energy transfer.

Henriksen, Sanner, and Pihl (40) reported in 1963 that for a variety of irradiated proteins the percentages of the total radical yield which could be attributed to sulfur-type radicals was related to the ratio of cysteine/(cysteine and glycine) in the protein. They suggested that "secondary radicals" were formed at stable trapping sites as a result of intermolecular diffusion-controlled radical reactions, due to a migration of unpaired spin species from their primary sites of formation. It was suggested that such radiation energy transfer was mediated by migrating small molecular entities such as hydrogen atoms. In an accompanying paper (42) they showed how nonconvalently bonded low molecular weight thiol compounds freeze-dried from a protein solution could prevent the formation of typical secondary radicals in the protein. Thus, when a 10 percent MEA (by weight) 90 percent bovine serum albumin molecular mixture was irradiated at room temperature, nearly 90 percent of the radicals found after room-temperature irradiation were located on MEA. In another example, using a mixed crystal of cysteine and butyric acid, the intermolecular transfer of a hydrogen atom from cysteine to butyric acid was unequivocally demonstrated, thus substantiating previous conclusions drawn from experiments with polycrystalline materials (14).

Numerous reports from these and other groups have shown that secondary radical reactions occur in irradiated proteins and in frozen aqueous systems. Such reactions appear to be mediated by diffusing radical species in that they depend on the degree of contact between components of a molecular mixture. Henriksen et al. (49) used the gel filtration material Sephadex as a component of molecular mixtures. By using penicillamine (PSH) solutions of various concentrations to swell the Sephadex beads and then lyophilizing, they produced molecular mixtures that had varying amounts of PSH bound within Sephadex pores, with the remainder of the PSH outside the Sephadex matrix. It was found that the transfer of ESR centers from Sephadex to PSH was maximal when the PSH was inside the pores and thus in close molecular contact with Sephadex.

Related studies (24) show a similar phenomenon of radiation energy transfer between Sephadex of various pore sizes and the macromolecule trypsin held within pores or adsorbed to the matrix surface. This type of model system indicates that there may be an increased radiosensitivity for macromolecules that are in intimate contact with a macromolecular matrix; perhaps a similar phenomenon occurs in cells; for example, in the enzyme complexes associated with mitochondrial membranes.

10.3.6 Modification of Radiation Damage—Radiation Protection and Radiation Sensitization

ESR techniques have played a major role in studies designed to elucidate the mechanisms of modification of radiation damage. These mechanisms usually involve the concepts of energy transfer, and the most frequently utilized protectors and sensitizers are compounds containing reactive thiol groups or are capable of binding to thiol groups. Hence the material covered in Sections 10.3.3 and 10.3.5 is quite pertinent to these studies.

Several theories of radiation protection have been offered which involve modification of free radical reactions (75). These include scavenging of water radicals by radioprotective agents, energy transfer to radioprotective compounds, and repair of radiation damage sites by radioprotective compounds. Experimental findings bearing on these and other mechanisms are discussed in some detail below; they represent some of the most useful results of radiobiological ESR studies.

Several workers have demonstrated by ESR that in lyophilized model systems a transfer of energy from irradiated proteins to radioprotective agents occurs (42). These studies have been aided by the fact that the high g factor of one component of the organosulfur radical permits accurate calculation of the number of spins localized on the sulfur atom. Irradiations of mixtures of protective agents (usually β-mercaptoethylamine, MEA) and proteins indicate that the yield of spins in the protective agents is much higher than would be expected if the energy were randomly deposited and not transferred (see Section 10.3.5). Similar results have been reported for mixtures of DNA and MEA (66). Such results have also been obtained in lyophilized bacteria and MEA, but only if the cell walls of the bacteria were first broken (5). The demonstration of energy transfer to MEA and/or repair by H atom donation by MEA fit in very well with intuitive concepts of how radioprotective agents work.

There are, however, several indications that the picture obtained in these studies, all of which utilized lyophilized preparations, may not reflect the events that lead to biological protection in viable cells. The time sequence of energy transfer to MEA can be studied in lyophilized preparations by controlled heating. The general picture has been that if the preparation is kept quite cold (77 K or lower) little transfer to sulfur is observed. The transfer occurs during warming (50). Careful analysis of the data, however, indicates that radicals in protein decay before radicals build up on the sulfur atom of MEA, suggesting that the ESR evidence does not outline the complete reaction sequence. Studies of frozen preparations of bacteria also suggest that stabilization of the unpaired spin on sulfur may not be a necessary step in protection (86, 89, 90). These studies indicate that in the presence of radioprotective agents the number of free radicals stabilized in bacteria is decreased *without* a corresponding rise in the number of radicals stabilized on the protective agent. This suggests that radioprotective compounds may play a catalytic role in which they accelerate decay of radiation-induced free radicals without themselves becoming radicals. Alternatively there may be energy transfer to the protective agent whose free radical forms may then decay rapidly. In recent studies (25) the organosulfur radical, typical of solid-state preparations, has been observed in frozen aqueous solutions but only at low pH. At higher pH an entirely different spectrum is observed. The only aminothiol that shows an organosulfur radical in physiological pH ranges is penicillamine, but this is a poor radioprotector (21).

The relationship between the structure of radioprotective compounds, their ability to provide biological protection, and their effect on radiation-induced free radicals has been investigated for aminothiol radioprotectants (86, 89, 90). These studies indicate that although there appears to be a correlation between biological protection and reduction of observable (by ESR) free radicals in irradiated bacteria for different concentrations of a single protective compound, no such general relationship exists between different compounds. Instead, it appears that protection by various aminothiols can be correlated with their ability to cause specific types of free radical modification. This suggests that radiation protection, at least under the conditions of these experiments, resulted from *specific* interactions of protective agents with cell components.

These studies (86, 89, 90) provide a good example of the complexities involved in attempting to use ESR to determine directly the mechanism of biological effects [see also (3)]. To be confident that the ESR changes observed are related to biological changes, we must perform both ESR measurements and bioassays on similar samples. This greatly restricts experimental options, but it may be the only alternative if we desire to ensure biological pertinence. A direct comparison of ESR with radiation damage *other* than mortality has been made by investigators (52, 53) using criteria of biological damage such as decreased enzyme activity in the case of irradiated enzymes.

10.3.7 Long-Lived Radiation-Induced Radicals

The preceding sections have considered experimental situations designed to trap radiation-induced radicals. However, several recent reports of relatively long-lived radiation-induced radicals (e.g., 16, 88), those that can be experimentally observed without special trapping procedures, have been made. These probably represent only a small percentage of the total yield of radiation-induced free radicals, but they are of interest for several reasons. Theoretically such radicals could lead to damage at later times and/or provide a means for damage to migrate large distances. Of more practical use is the potential of such long-lived radicals as dosimeters in radiation accidents because preliminary results indicate that the intensities of their ESR signals are proportional to dose over a wide range (16).

The radicals referred to here are to be distinguished from other long-lived radicals trapped in certain naturally occurring biological preparations, such as seeds and bacterial spores (30, 76, 91, 92). These systems, because they are naturally dehydrated, trap radicals in the same way as any other dried preparations, and the trapped radicals can cause considerable biological damage when the specimens are subsequently hydrated before growth initiation.

Long-lived radiation-induced radicals have now been found in several different animal tissues (teeth, bone, hair, muscle, and blood) and in bacteria, insect skeletons, and plants (16, 87, 88). Some pure biochemicals also show relatively long-lived free radicals that can be detected in flow systems in which the biochemical is irradiated in a gamma source and then circulated to an aqueous cell in an ESR spectrometer (56).

10.3.8 Free Radicals Observed in Tissues During Irradiation

Recently Kenny and Commoner (57) reported signals observed in tissues during irradiation. This experiment required the development of a spectrometer and a sample holder that permitted irradiation in the cavity without distortion of the ESR spectra of the tissue under study. Using a dose rate of about 3000 rad/sec, they were able to detect radiation-induced radicals in 100 mg of wet tissue at 15 C. All tissues studied showed radiation-induced signals. In tissues such as heart and liver the radiation-induced signals were qualitatively similar to, but more intense than, the signals seen in these tissues without radiation. The signal from testis was narrower and decayed faster than that seen in mature, differentiated tissues such as heart and liver. The authors concluded that there was a significant correlation between type of ESR response shown by a tissue and its radiosensitivity. They suggested that these correlations might be related to the mechanisms of radiosensitivity.

The noted empirical correlations are of great interest but their radiobiological significance is not yet clear. A limited number and type of tissue were investigated. The doses employed were very high (180,000 rad/min) and profound radiation-induced chemical alterations undoubtably took place before the first radiation-induced signals were recorded. Such doses induce a large number of radicals, but the observed signals were quite small, which indicates that the signals observed in this experiment were due to less than 1 percent of the radicals induced in the tissues. Experiments currently in progress at Commoner's laboratory should help eventually to determine the radiobiological significance of these preliminary results. (Further discussion of the problem of determining the biological significance of observed ESR changes is found in Sections 4.2, 7.1 and 10.2.2.3.)

10.4 THE FUTURE

As indicated in the preceding sections, ESR studies have made significant contributions to radiation biology in a number of areas, especially in regard to radical identification, spin transfer, and radiation protection. It is likely that ESR will have more to offer in these fields.

The recent development of ESR spectrometers capable of following relatively short-lived species (81) (lifetimes of milliseconds or less) has revealed exciting prospects that may become quite productive over the next few years. Related to this has been the development of spectrometers capable of following radicals in tissues irradiated within the ESR cavity (see Section 10.3.8).

As more and more radicals are characterized in biological materials by single-crystal ESR work there will be increased demand for biologists to assimilate this data and to look for ways to apply the information to more complex biological systems. Investigators involved in related analytical techniques, such as pulse radiolysis and radiation chemistry, will also continue to generate data, and it remains for more broadly based radiobiologists to couple these data meaningfully with ESR results. Such cross discipline extrapolation seems essential.

REFERENCES

1. K. Akasaka, S. Ohnishi, T. Suita, and I. Nitta, *J. Chem. Phys.*, **40,** 3110 (1964).
2. A. Allen, *The Radiation Chemistry of Water and Aqueous Solutions*, Van Nostrand, Princeton, New Jersey, 1961.
3. D. Aripova, Ye. Ganassi, L. Kayushin, M. Pulatova, and L. Eidus, *Biofizika*, **12,** 206 (1967).
4. E. Avery, J. Remko, and B. Smaller, *J. Chem. Phys.*, **49,** 951 (1968).
5. E. Baker, M. Ormerod, C. Dean, and P. Alexander, *Biochem. Biophys. Acta*, **114,** 169 (1966).
6. L. Bliumenfel'd and A. Kalmanson, *Biofizika*, **3,** 87 (1958).
7. L. Bliumenfel'd and A. Kalmanson, *Biofizika*, **2,** 546 (1957).
8. L. Bliumenfel'd and A. Kalmanson, *Proc. 2nd Intern. Conf. Peaceful Uses Atomic Energy*, Geneva, 1958, **22,** 524 (1958).
9. J. ten Bosch, "Radiation Effects in Collagen, A Quantitative Electron Spin Resonance Study," University of Utrecht, 1967.
10. J. ten Bosch and R. Braams, *Radiat. Res*, **36,** 544 (1968).
11. J. ten Bosch, *Intern. J. Rad. Biol.*, **13,** 93 (1967).
12. H. Box, H. Freund, K. Lilga, and E. Budzinski, *J. Phys. Chem.*, **74,** 40 (1970).
13. H. Box, K. Lilga, E. Budzinski, and R. Derr, *J. Chem. Phys.*, **50,** 5422 (1969).
14. H. Box, H. Freund, and E. Budzinski, *J. Chem. Phys.*, **45,** 2324 (1966).
15. R. Braams, *Nature*, **200,** 752 (1963).
16. J. Brady, N. Aarestad, and H. Swartz, *Health Phys.*, **15,** 43 (1968).
17. A. Buick, T. Kemp, and G. Neal, *J. Chem. Soc.*, **A,** 666 (1969).
18. G. Casteleijn and J. ten Bosch, *J. Appl. Phys.*, **39,** 4375 (1968).
19. T. Cole and H. Heller, *J. Chem. Phys.*, **42,** 1668 (1965).
20. A. Conger, *J. Cell. Comp. Physiol.*, **58,** Suppl. 1, 27 (1961).
21. E. Copeland and W. Earl, *Biophys. Soc. Abs. WPM-I-13* (1971).
22. E. Copeland, T. Sanner, and A. Pihl, *Rad. Res.*, **35,** 437 (1968).
23. E. Copeland, T. Sanner, and A. Pihl, *European J. Biochem.*, **1,** 312 (1967).
24. E. Copeland, T. Sanner, and A. Pihl, *Intern. J. Rad. Biol.*, **18,** 85 (1970).
25. E. Copeland and H. Swartz, *Intern. J. Rad. Biol.*, **16,** 293 (1969).
26. P. Cripper and A. Vecli, *Biophys. J.*, **10,** 269 (1970).
27. G. Czapski, H. Levanon, and A. Samuni, *Israel J. Chem.*, **7,** 375 (1969).
28. See, for example, A. Ehrenberg, A. Gräslund, A. Rupprecht, and G. Ström, *Book of Abstracts, 4th Intern. Congr. Rad. Res.*, Evian, 1970, Bellanger, Sarthe, 1970, p. 63.
29. W. Dixon and R. Norman, *J. Chem. Soc.*, 3119 (1963).
30. A. Ehrenberg and L. Ehrenberg, *Arch. Fysik*, **14,** 133 (1958).
31. A. Ehrenberg, A. Rupprecht, and G. Ström, *Science*, **157,** 1317 (1967).
32. R. Florin, F. Sicilio, and L. Wall, *J. Phys. Chem.*, **72,** 3154 (1968).
33. W. Gordy, W. Ard, and H. Shields, *Proc. Natl. Acad. Sci.*, **41,** 983 (1955).
34. W. Gordy and H. Shields, *Rad. Res.*, **9,** 611 (1958).

35. W. Gordy and H. Shields, *Proc. Natl. Acad. Sci.*, **46,** 1124 (1960).
36. W. Gordy and I. Miyagawa, *Rad. Res.*, **12,** 211 (1960).
37. W. Gordy, *Ann. N.Y. Acad. Sci.*, **158,** 100 (1969).
38. E. Hart and R. Platzman in *Mechanisms in Radiobiology*, Vol. I, M. Errera and A. Fossberg, Eds., Academic, New York, 1956, p. 93.
39. H. Heller, S. Schlick, and T. Cole, *J. Chem. Phys.*, Ithaca, **71,** 97 (1967).
40. T. Henriksen, T. Sanner, and A. Pihl, *Rad. Res.*, **18,** 147 (1963).
41. T. Henriksen, *Nucl. Sci. Ser.*, **43,** 81 (1966).
42. T. Henriksen, T. Sanner, and A. Pihl, *Rad. Res.*, **18,** 163 (1963).
43. T. Henriksen, *Solid State Biophysics*, S. Wyard, Ed., McGraw-Hill, New York, 1969, Chapter 6, p. 201.
44. T. Henriksen, *Acta. Chem. Scand.*, **20,** 2898 (1966).
45. T. Henriksen and W. Snipes, *Rad. Res.*, **42,** 255 (1970).
46. T. Henriksen, University Press, Oslo, 1963, and *J. Chem. Phys.*, **37,** 2189 (1962).
47. T. Henriksen and W. Snipes, *Rad Res.*, **41,** 439 (1970).
48. T. Henriksen, *Rad. Res.*, **32,** 892 (1967).
49. T. Henriksen and T. Sanner, *Rad. Res.*, **32,** 164 (1967).
50. T. Henriksen, *Scand. J. Clin. Lab. Invest.*, **22** (Suppl. 106), 7 (1968).
51. D. Holmes, L. Myers, and R. Ingalls, *Nature*, **209,** 1017 (1966).
52. J. Hunt, J. Till, and J. Williams, *Rad. Res.*, **17,** 703 (1962).
53. J. Hunt and J. Williams, *Rad. Res.*, **23,** 26 (1964).
54. R. Ingalls and L. Wall, *J. Chem. Phys.*, **35,** 370 (1961).
55. H. Jensen and T. Henriksen, *Acta. Chem. Scand.*, **22,** 2263 (1968).
56. D. Kalkwarf, *Book of Abstracts, 4th Intern. Congr. Rad. Res.*, Evian, 1970, Bellanger, Sarthe, 1970, p. 112. See also D. Kalkwarf, Batelle Northwest Laboratory Report BWNL-715, Part 2, p. 152, Batelle Northwest Laboratory, Richland, Washington, 1968.
57. P. Kenny and B. Commoner, *Nature*, **223,** 1229 (1969).
58. F. Kneubühl, *J. Chem. Phys.*, **33,** 1074 (1960).
59. W. Köhnlein, personal communication.
60. W. Köhnlein et al., *Abstract Papers 2nd Intern. Congr. Rad. Res.*, Harrogate, 1962, p. 22.
61. W. Köhnlein and F. Hutchinson, *Rad. Res.*, **39,** 745 (1969).
62. W. Köhnlein and D. Schulte-Frohlinde, *Rad. Res.*, **38,** 173 (1969).
63. I. Lenherr, A. Charlesby, and B. Singh, *Intern. J. Rad. Biol.*, **12,** 51 (1967).
64. R. Livingston and H. Zeldes, *J. Chem. Phys.*, **44,** 1245 (1966).
65. J. Morton, *Chem. Res.*, **64,** 453 (1964).
66. P. Milvy and I. Pullman, *Rad. Res.*, **34,** 265 (1968).
67. A. Müller, *Energetics and Mechanisms in Radiation Biology*, G. Phillips, Ed., Academic, New York, 1968.
68. A. Müller, *Abh. Math.-Naturw. Kl., Akad., Wiss.*, Mainz., **5,** 143 (1964) (privat dozent thesis).
69. A. Müller, *Prog. Biophys. Mol. Biol.*, **17,** 491 (1967).

70. K. Nakken, T. Brustad, and A. Karthum Hansen in "Radiation Chemistry," *Advan. Chem.*, R. Gould, Ed., **81,** 251 (1968).

71. M. Ormerod, *Progr. Biochem. Pharmacol.*, **1,** 137 (1965).

72. R. Patten and W. Gordy, *Rad. Res.*, **22,** 29 (1964).

73. R. Patten and W. Gordy, *Proc. Natl. Acad. Sci.*, **46,** 1137 (1960).

74. P. Pershan, R. Shulman, B. Wylunda and J. Eisinger, *Physics*, **I,** 163 (1964).

75. A. Pihl and T. Sanner in *Radiation Protection and Sensitization*, H. Moroson and M. Quintiliani, Eds., Taylor & Francis, London, 1970.

76. E. Powers, *Radiol. Clin. No. Amer.*, **3,** 197 (1965).

77. T. Sanner, *Rad. Res.*, **25,** 586 (1965).

78. H. Shields and W. Gordy, *Proc. Natl. Acad. Sci.*, **45,** 269 (1959).

79. B. Singh and M. Ormerod, *Biochem. Biophys. Acta*, **109,** 204 (1965).

80. B. Singh and M. Ormerod, *Nature*, **206,** 1314 (1965).

81. B. Smaller, J. Remko, and E. Avery, *J. Chem. Phys.*, **48,** 5174 (1968).

82. R. Smith and S. Wyard, *Nature*, **186,** 226 (1960).

83. V. Srinivasan, B. Singh, and A. Gopal-Ayengar, *Intern. J. Rad. Biol.*, **15,** 89 (1969).

84. K. Stratton, *Rad. Res. Suppl.*, **7,** 102 (1967).

85. K. Stratton, *Rad. Res.*, **35,** 182 (1968).

86. H. Swartz and E. Richardson, *Intern. J. Rad. Biol.*, **12,** 75 (1967).

87. H. Swartz, personal communication.

88. H. Swartz, *Rad. Res.*, **24,** 579 (1965).

89. H. Swartz, E. Copeland, and E. Richardson, *Rad. Res.*, **45,** 542, (1971).

90. H. Swartz, E. Richardson, E. Copeland, R. Lofberg, and R. Jandacek in *Radiation Protection and Sensitization*, H. Moroson and M. Quintilliani, Eds., Taylor & Francis, London, 1970, p. 21.

91. H. Tanooka, *Rad. Res.*, **27,** 570 (1966).

92. H. Tanooka and R. Hutchinson, *Biochem. Biophys. Acta*, **95,** 690 (1965).

93. S. Wyard, *Solid State Biophysics*, S. Wyard, Ed., McGraw-Hill, New York, 1969, Chapter 1.

CHAPTER ELEVEN

The Spin Label Method*

IAN C. P. SMITH

Biochemistry Laboratory,
National Research Council of Canada, Ottawa

* N.R.C.C. Number 12435.

11.1 INTRODUCTION TO THE METHOD

For many years labeling techniques have been used in biological investigations to probe the structure of biological systems and the mechanisms of biological reactions. As an example of the former type of application fluorescent labels on proteins have yielded significant information about the conformations of biological molecules. In the latter area labeling with ^{14}C has enabled the elucidation of the detailed mechanism of many biological reactions. Ideally we want a label that will report back on some function of the system without the label itself causing any disturbance of the system. This is fundamentally impossible; however, the question is to what degree does the label alter the system and is this disturbance subject to control and evaluation? The information that labels provide must be treated within the context of this limitation.

It is clear from the foregoing chapters that many biological systems naturally contain certain paramagnetic centers. These systems, however, are but a minute fraction of those in which the sensitivity of ESR spectroscopy could be useful. It would be most desirable if any biological system or molecule could be made paramagnetic in a specific way at will. It would seem a natural extension of the fluorescent label technique to develop "spin labels"—stable free radicals that could be attached to a specific site on a molecule in a complex system and whose ESR spectra would contain information about the environment of the label. Thus in 1964 Professor H. M. McConnell began a program to design and synthesize such spin labels and apply them to biological problems. From the pioneering papers in 1965 (1, 2) the spin label literature has grown to a prodigious size.

It is the aim of this chapter to demonstrate the manifold aspects of the method rather than to cover all applications intensively. Several articles discuss some particular applications up to mid-1968 (3, 4). A more up-to-date discussion of the physics and chemistry of spin labels has also appeared (5).

Before proceeding into the details of the spin label technique it would be well to outline briefly the kind of information that we might hope to obtain from an application of this technique:

1. The ESR spectra of spin labels are very sensitive to the *rate* at which the label is able to reorient. Thus a knowledge of this functional dependence will allow us to evaluate the degree of mobility allowed in the environment of the label. In particular, conformation changes brought about by some biochemical process are readily detected.
2. The g factor and hyperfine splitting of the spin label do vary slightly

with the polarity of the solvent. Thus we have a probe into the hydrophobic or hydrophilic nature of the environment around the label.

3. Biradical spin labels allow the study of certain intermolecular interactions, since the interaction of the two ends of the biradical is a strong function of the conformation of the biradical.

11.1.1 Requirements for Spin Labels

An essential property of a spin label is stability under conditions used in the study of biological molecules, such as aqueous solutions, pH 2–10, high and low salt concentrations, and temperatures from 20 to 70 C. It must be sensitive to its environment—preferably to polarity, acidity, spatial restrictions, and fluidity. The ESR spectra must be relatively simple and easy to interpret. To be generally useful it is necessary that the compounds used as spin labels have a well-understood chemistry that permits custom synthesis of functional groups for particular purposes. The first spin label was the cation radical of chloropromazine (1), but the most successful compounds used as spin labels to date are the nitroxides of general structural formula:

$$R_1-\underset{\underset{O^{\bullet}}{|}}{N}-R_2$$

Detailed accounts of the chemistry of nitroxides have been published (3, 6). The ESR spectra and parameters of many nitroxides are available in compendia of such data (7, 8).

11.1.2 Synthesis of Spin Labels

The most common synthesis of nitroxide spin labels has been by oxidation of the secondary amino group of a tetramethylpyrrolidine or tetramethylpiperidine derivative. Enormous contributions to nitroxide chemistry have been made by the groups of Rassat (Grenoble) and Rosantzev (Moscow). Unfortunately their publications are too numerous to document thoroughly. An excellent description of much of the recent nitroxide chemistry is given in the book by Rosantzev (18). In Fig. 11-1 we summarize many of the basic synthetic steps that may be taken. No attempt has been made to be comprehensive. The numbers in brackets indicate the literature sources for the reactions. Figure 11-1 includes a few general-purpose spin labels such as analogs of *N*-ethylmaleimide (12, 22), bromoacetamide (19), iodoacetamide (16, 19), diisopropylfluorophosphate (9), and the hapten trinitrobenzene (14). More detailed discussions of these and other labels appear in the following sections.

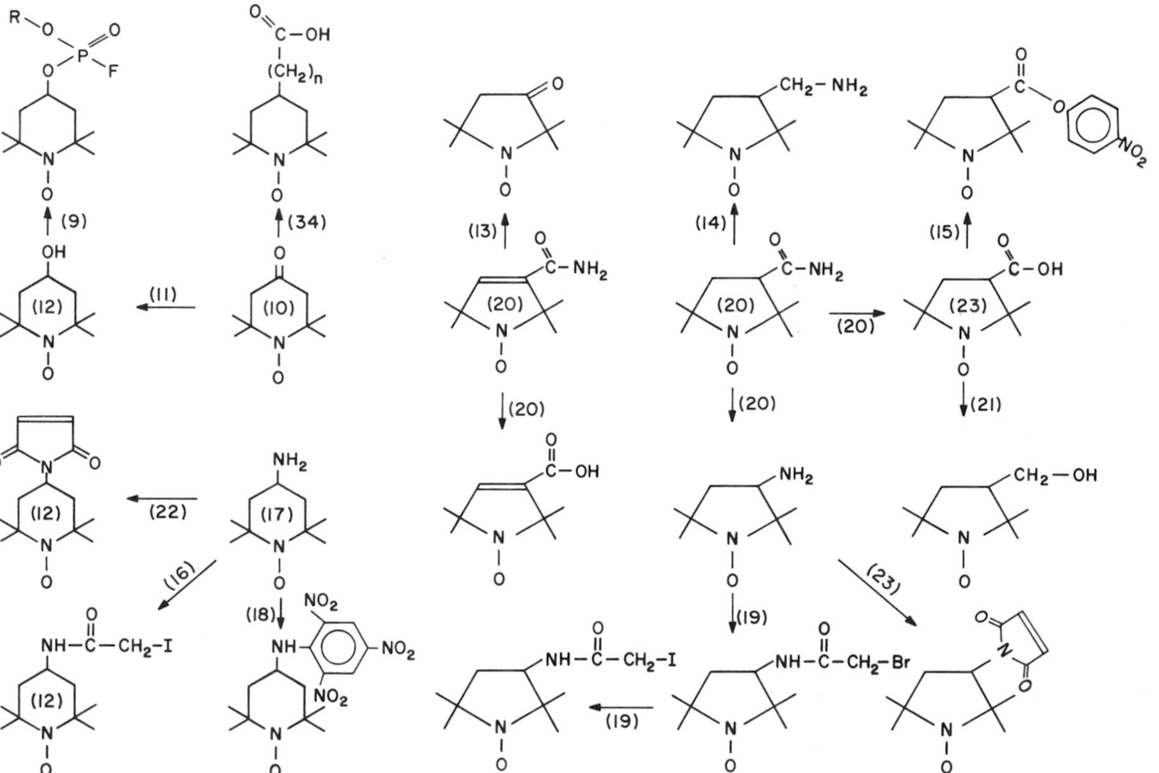

Fig. 11-1 Some representative spin labels and nitroxides. Reference numbers beside the arrows indicate the literature source for that synthetic route. Synthesis of starting nitroxides or alternative pathways to a given nitroxide are given by the reference numbers inside the molecular formulas.

Another approach to nitroxide synthesis, which has resulted in several useful spin labels, was suggested by Keana et al. (24). They demonstrated that a ketone could be converted to an oxazolidine and the corresponding nitroxide via the following reactions:

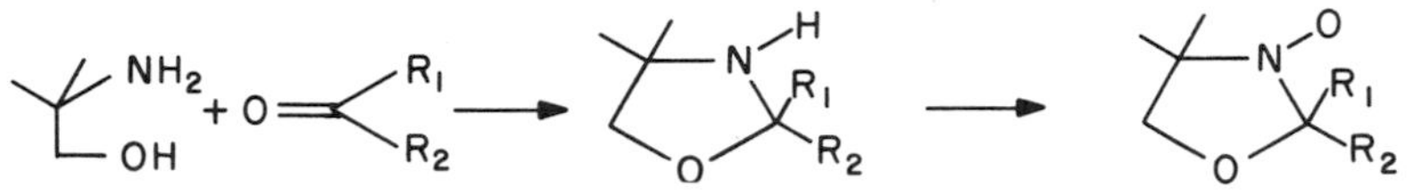

Two very useful compounds made by this method are spin labeled cholestane (24), I, and a spin labeled stearic acid (25), II. These radicals are fairly stable (several weeks) but less so than the tetramethyl nitroxides.

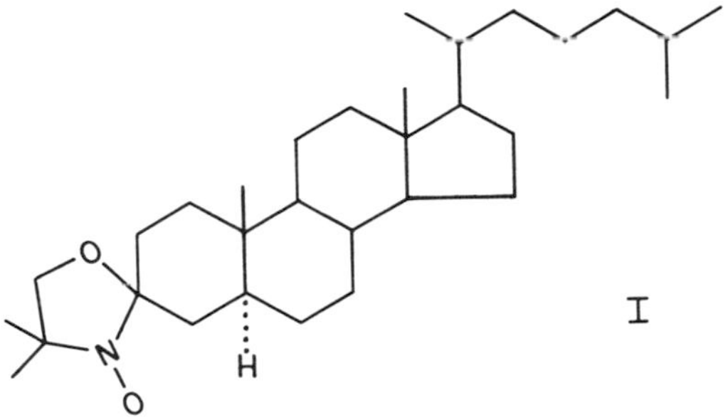

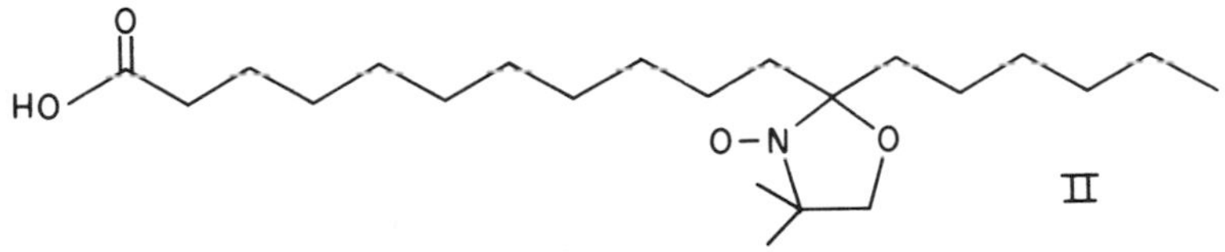

Another potentially useful series of nitroxides has been investigated by Ullman and co-workers (26, 27). The α-nitronylnitroxides are formed by the following reactions:

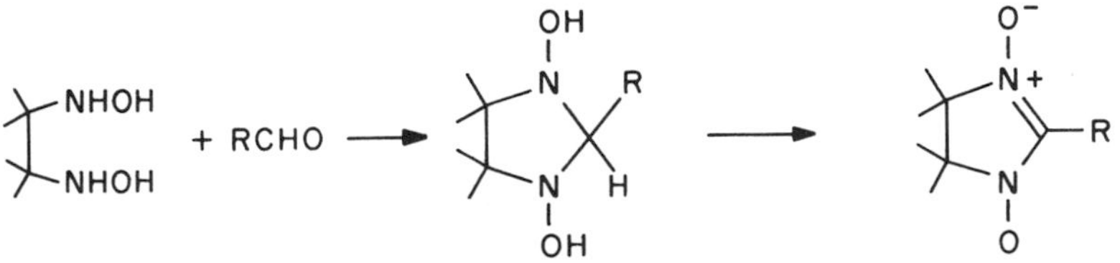

When R is aromatic, these radicals are reasonably stable in the dark but deteriorate over several weeks on exposure to light. If R is aliphatic, they deteriorate more rapidly. These compounds have not yet been applied as spin labels.

11.1.3 Information in a Nitroxide Spin Label Spectrum

Three classes of useful parameters are present in nitroxide spin label spectra—the g tensor, the nitrogen hyperfine coupling tensor, and the widths of the individual ESR lines. From their combinations information can be obtained about the orientation and mobility of the nitroxide.

11.1.3.1 The Hyperfine Coupling and g tensors

The first two parameters may be described in the formalism of Chapter 1 by the spin Hamiltonian (omitting the nuclear Zeeman term)

$$\hat{\mathscr{H}} = \beta \mathbf{H} \cdot \boldsymbol{g} \cdot \hat{\mathbf{S}} + h\hat{\mathbf{S}} \cdot \boldsymbol{A} \cdot \hat{\mathbf{I}}$$

where $\boldsymbol{g}$ and $\boldsymbol{A}$ are the g and hyperfine coupling tensors, respectively. (Other symbols are defined in Chapter 1.) The conventional axis system for nitroxides is defined below. The unpaired electron is considered to occupy a molecular orbital composed of the p_π orbitals of nitrogen and oxygen. The observed values for the components of the hyperfine tensor indicate that a substantial fraction of the unpaired electron is localized on the nitrogen atom and therefore suggest that the NO three-electron Π-bond has polar character, as represented here:

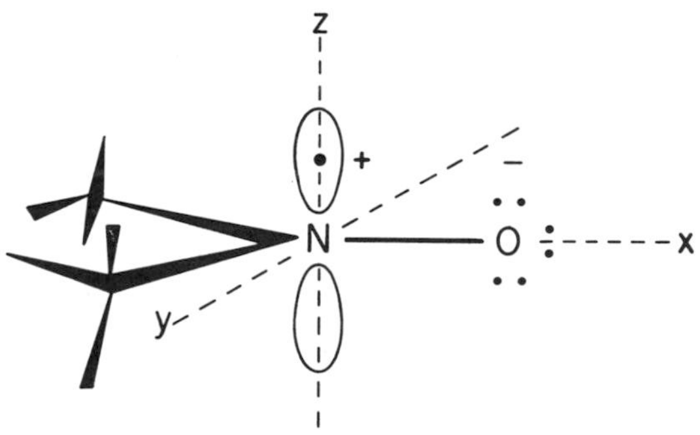

Because the molecular orbital containing the unpaired electron is made up in part of a degenerate oxygen p_π orbital, the g tensor for the nitroxide moiety is expected to be antistropic (28) ($g_{xx} \neq g_{yy} \neq g_{zz}$). The hyperfine coupling tensor is also anisotropic and is most often nearly axially symmetric ($A_{zz} \neq A_{xx} \simeq A_{yy}$) because of the occupation by the unpaired electron of a molecular orbital of Π-symmetry (29). Thus the magnetic field value at which the ESR spectrum of a nitroxide occurs, and the separations between the hyperfine lines, will depend very much on the orientation of the free radical with respect to the applied magnetic field.

To obtain the g tensor and hyperfine coupling tensor components accurately we must study the dependence of the nitroxide ESR spectrum on the angles between the applied magnetic field and the symmetry axes of the radical (Chapter 1). This is most conveniently achieved by doping a diamagnetic host crystal of known three-dimensional structure with the nitroxide of interest. This was done by Griffith et al. (30) for the nitroxides III to V in host crystals of tetramethyl-1,3-cyclobutanedione, VI. The principal axes of $\boldsymbol{g}$ and $\boldsymbol{A}$ were taken to be identical. The isotropic parameters $A_0 = \frac{1}{3}(A_{xx} + A_{yy} + A_{zz})$ and $g_0 = \frac{1}{3}(g_{xx} + g_{yy} + g_{zz})$ were measured in dilute solutions of di-*t*-butyl ketone.

Nitroxide

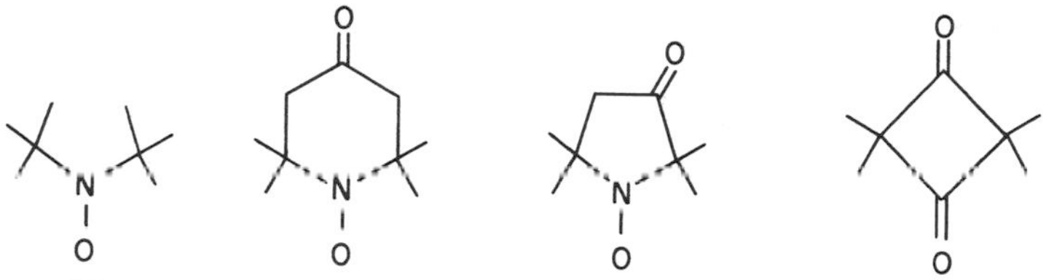

III IV V VI

	III	IV	V
A_{xx} (gauss)	7.1 ± 0.5	5.2	4.7
A_{yy}	5.6 ± 0.5	5.2	4.7
A_{zz}	32.0 ± 1.5	31	31
A_0	15.1 ± 0.5	14.3	14.0[a]
g_{xx}	2.0089 ± 0.0003	[b]	[b]
g_{yy}	2.0061 ± 0.0003	[b]	[b]
g_{zz}	2.0027 ± 0.0003	[b]	[b]
g_0	2.0060 ± 0.0002	2.0062	2.0060[a]

[a] Value for the corresponding amide.

[b] Not reported.

Despite numerous attempts, it has proved to be quite difficult to obtain dilute solid solutions of commonly used spin labels in appropriate hosts. Recently a study was presented of the cholestane spin label I which has the nitroxide moiety in a dimethyloxazolidine ring, in single crystals of cholesteryl chloride (31). The resultant parameters are $A_{xx} = 5.8$, $A_{yy} = 5.8$, and $A_{zz} = 30.8 \pm 0.5$ G; $g_{xx} = 2.0089$, $g_{yy} = 2.0058$, and $g_{zz} = 2.0021 \pm 0.0001$. Comparison with the data for III, IV, and V supports the following useful generalization: $32\text{ G} \simeq A_{zz} \gg A_{xx} \simeq A_{yy} \simeq 5\text{ G}$; $g_{xx} > g_{yy} > g_{zz}$.

Because of the ionic character of the nitroxide bond, the values of the g- and hyperfine-tensor components of a given spin label will vary with the polarity of the environment. In general, the isotropic hyperfine splitting constant will increase and the isotropic g factor will decrease as the polarity of the solvent increases (32); for example, the isotropic hyperfine splitting constant A_0 for the stearamide spin label VII varies from 15.8 G in aqueous

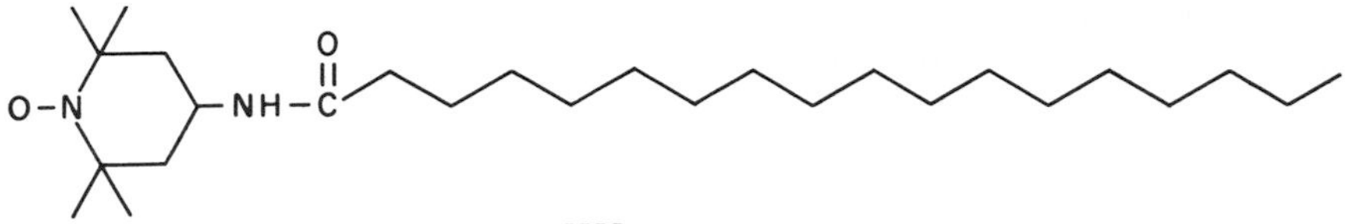

VII

solution to 14.0 G in mineral oil (33). Analysis of the lineshapes of the ESR spectrum of VII in phospholipid vesicles indicated that although A_0 was relatively unaffected g_0 was sensitive to asymmetric environment polarity (33). Thus arguments requiring detailed knowledge of the components of $\boldsymbol{A}$ and $\boldsymbol{g}$ should be made only when the values of the tensor components under comparable conditions are known. Good estimates of these components can often be made from the spectra of slowly tumbling or randomly immobilized nitroxides (see below, 4, 5). This sensitivity to environment polarity makes the spin labels extremely valuable as probes in situations in which perturbations are thought to cause rearrangement of the hydrophobic and hydrophilic components of a biological system.

It would be extremely useful if a spin label ESR spectrum were sensitive to the pH as well as to the polarity of the surrounding medium. The hyperfine splitting of the nitroxide VIII was found to increase by 0.5 G

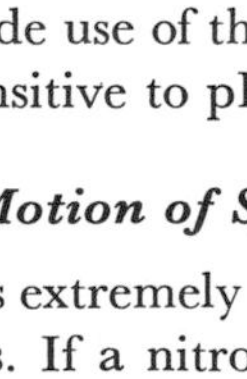

VIII

over the pH range 2–12 (35). No studies of the local acidities of a biological macromolecule have yet made use of this dependence. It is to be hoped that spin labels that are more sensitive to pH will be synthesized.

11.1.3.2 Isotropic Motion of Spin Labels

A spin label ESR spectrum is extremely sensitive to the nature and rate of the motions the label undergoes. If a nitroxide rotates symmetrically at a rate greater than the frequency corresponding to the largest differences between the principal components of the hyperfine coupling tensor ($\gg |A_{zz} - A_{xx}| \approx 73$ MHz) and g tensor ($\gg |g_{xx} - g_{zz}| \beta H h^{-1} \approx 29$ MHz for X-band spectrometers operating at fields of about 3.3 kG), the isotropic

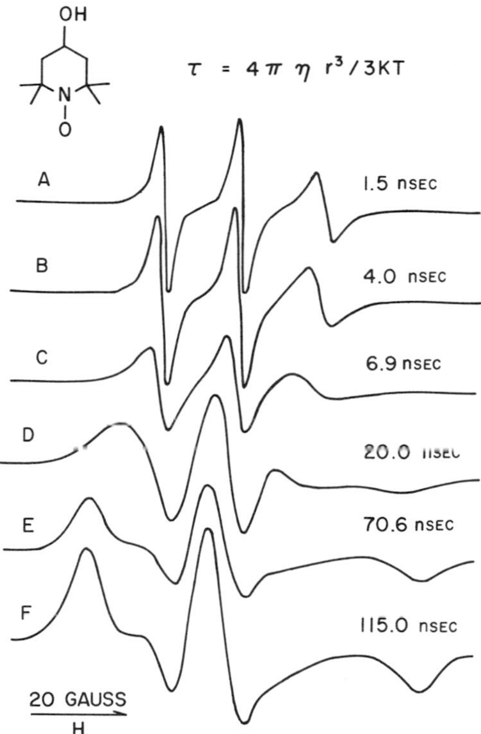

Fig. 11-2 ESR spectra of *N*-oxyl-2,2,6,6-tetramethyl-4-piperidinol in aqueous solutions of varying glycerol concentrations. Spectra were measured at the following viscosities and temperatures: A, 0.116 poise, 273 K; B, 0.367 poise, 293 K; C, 0.523 poise, 293 K; D, 1.58 poise, 283 K; E, 5.77 poise, 273 K; F, 9.4 poise, 273 K (14).

parameters A_0 and g_0 are observed and the ESR lines are narrow and of equal width. However, when the rate of rotation about any of the axes becomes comparable to these differences, changes in individual linewidths and positions occur. The simplest case, that of symmetrical rotation at gradually decreasing rates, is demonstrated by the spectra of Fig. 11-2, due to *N*-oxyl-2,2,6,6-tetramethyl-4-piperidinol (12) in aqueous solutions of varying glycerol content and viscosity (14). The times used to label each spectrum are rotational correlation times; they can be thought of as the times required for the molecules to forget what their previous spatial orientations were. In this case the correlation times were calculated from the Stokes law (assuming spherical symmetry)

$$\tau = \frac{4\pi\eta r^3}{3kT},$$

where τ is the correlation time, η, the viscosity, r, the effective radius of the molecule, k, the Boltzmann constant and T, the absolute temperature. Up to spectrum C we notice that the line positions change very little, but the relative widths change considerably with increasing τ. From spectrum D to spectrum F the high and low field lines move gradually to higher and lower fields, respectively. This is due to a manifestation of A_{zz}, the maximum component of the hyperfine coupling tensor. Spectrum F is often referred to as that of a "strongly immobilized nitroxide." It is approaching what is obtained for the ESR spectrum of a magnetically dilute powder, which is the envelope of the ESR spectra of nitroxide radicals with every possible orientation relative to the external magnetic field. Thus it is obvious that nitroxide ESR spectra are very sensitive to the rate of molecular rotation—covering a range of correlation times from 10^{-10} sec (spectrum of three narrow lines of almost equal width) to 10^{-7} sec (a strongly immobilized spin label spectrum). This range of correlation times includes those of most biological molecules, both large and small, and herein lies the very general applicability of the technique to conformational problems in molecular biology.

Theoretical treatment of the nitroxide motions leading to the spectra of Fig. 11-2 is complex and to a large extent undeveloped.* In the limit of rapid rotation, i.e., for correlation times shorter than approximately 5×10^{-9} sec (such as spectrum C of Fig. 11-2) the approximations made in the approaches of McConnell (37), Kivelson (38), and Freed and Fraenkel (39) are reasonable. The relative widths of the three nitroxide ESR lines can then be described by

$$\frac{\Delta H(\mathrm{m})}{\Delta H(0)} = 1 - \frac{\tau}{\sqrt{3}\,\pi\,\Delta\nu(0)}\,[c_1 m + c_2 m^2], \tag{11-1}$$

where $\Delta H(\mathrm{m})$ is the peak-to-peak linewidth (in gauss or Hertz) of the hyperfine line due to the nitrogen spin state of magnetic quantum number m ($m = +1$ for the low field line, zero for the center line, and -1 for the high field line), τ is the correlation time in seconds for the presumed isotropic rotation, $\Delta\nu(0)$ is the peak-to-peak width of the center line ($m = 0$) in Hertz [$\Delta\nu(0) = (g\beta/h)\,\Delta H(0)$], and c_1 and c_2 are constants determined by the magnetic properties of the free radical:

$$c_1 = \frac{-16\pi|\beta|H}{45h}\,[A_{zz} - A_{xx}][g_{zz} - \tfrac{1}{2}(g_{xx} + g_{yy})] \tag{11-2}$$

$$c_2 = \frac{2\pi^2}{9}\,[A_{zz} - A_{xx}]^2. \tag{11-3}$$

The A's are expressed in MHz. Assuming that the areas of the ESR lines are propor-

* An excellent discussion of the state of the art has been presented in Ref. 36.

tional to the products of their amplitudes (h) and their widths squared, we can rewrite (11-1) as

$$\left(\frac{h(\mathrm{o})}{h(\mathrm{m})}\right)^{1/2} = 1 - \frac{\tau}{\sqrt{3}\,\pi\,\Delta\nu(0)}\,[c_1 m + c_2 m^2] \tag{11-4}$$

which is the most convenient form for obtaining the correlation time from experimental spectra. By taking the sum and difference of $\sqrt{h(\mathrm{o})/h(-1)}$ and $\sqrt{h(\mathrm{o})/h(+1)}$ independent values for τ can be obtained from the terms of (11-4) in $c_1 m$ and $c_2 m^2$, respectively. In most cases these values are not identical (2, 40) and it has been found that the term in $c_1 m$ gives values of τ that are quite sensitive to the applied microwave power (40). It is therefore advisable to use the $c_2 m^2$ term for determination of τ unless a careful study of the microwave power dependence is done. Measurement of τ for attached spin labels as a function of strengths of perturbations such as pH and temperature has already proved useful in studying the structures of particular environments in polylysine (2), nucleic acids (40, 41, 42), and ribonuclease (43) (see 11.2.1.2).

Itzkowitz has developed a semiempirical approach to simulate nitroxide spectra over the entire range of correlation times (44, 45). This method involves solving an approximate spin Hamiltonian and use of the Monte Carlo method to perform ensemble averaging. Good agreement with the ESR spectrum of dansyl nitroxide (46) in viscous mixtures of water, glycerol, and ethanol was obtained (44, 45). Rotational correlation times were estimated; they agreed fairly well with those estimated by fluorescence depolarization (46). This approach requires the use of a high-speed digital computer.

11.1.3.3 The ESR Spectrum of a "Strongly Immobilized" Spin Label

In Fig. 11-3 we show the ESR spectrum of a nitroxide completely immobilized and randomly oriented in a rigid glass at −180 C (5). This is a powder spectrum, the envelope of the spectra of nitroxides in all possible orientations with respect to the applied magnetic field. The powder spectrum

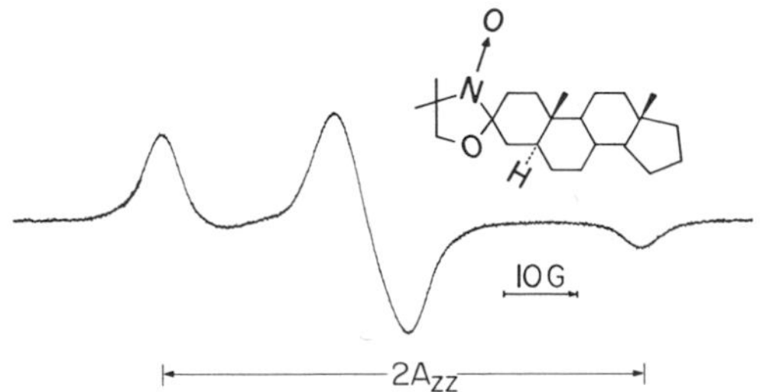

Fig. 11-3 ESR spectrum of the *N*-oxyl-4′,4′-dimethyloxazolidine derivative of 5α-androstan-3-one in a 1:1 isopentane-hexane glass at − 180 C (5).

is the limit approached by the spectra of spin labels which are totally constrained by a large molecule of very long correlation time; in this case, as far as the ESR spectrometer is concerned, all the spin labels are standing still with random orientations. (In practice this is seldom achieved because the spin label often has independent motion relative to that of the constraining macromolecule.) Because A_{zz} is considerably greater than A_{xx} or A_{yy} for a nitroxide, it is possible to obtain a reasonably accurate value for A_{zz} from such a powder spectrum, as demonstrated in Fig. 11-3. An upper limit for A_{xx} and A_{yy} can be obtained from the width of the central line. These approximate values are useful in ascertaining the influences of particular solvents on the components of the hyperfine coupling tensor, in particular because they are obtained so easily relative to single crystal measurements.

Recently Hyde et al. have shown that the saturation behavior of the ESR spectra of strongly immobilized radicals can be useful in estimating correlation times (47). Although the ESR spectra may all be identical, similar to Fig. 11-3, the saturation behavior will be determined by the correlation time, which can vary over a large range. This could be a valuable tool in the interpretation of spin-label spectra.

The ESR spectrum most often observed when the motion of a spin label is severely restricted by the structures of the macromolecule to which it is attached, resembles spectrum F of Fig. 11-2. This spectrum is often referred to as that of a strongly immobilized spin label. In this range it is difficult to estimate correlation times, particularly since the little motion the spin label has relative to the large molecule is undoubtedly anisotropic.* A useful experimental parameter in this situation is the separation between the two extreme components of the ESR spectrum. In the limit of complete immobilization of the spin label on a macromolecule of very long correlation time the separation corresponds to $2A_{zz}$. As the site of attachment expands, permitting only restricted rotation in relation to the macromolecule, the separation decreases (Fig. 11-2*D*, *E*). Thus, although theoretical treatments for extracting correlation times from this type of spectrum are lacking, this separation can be used as a qualitative estimate of the degree of immobilization of the spin label.

11.1.3.4 Complex Spin Label Spectra

With many of the general spin labels that have been commonly applied, such as analogs of bromoacetate (43), iodoacetamide (19), and *N*-ethylmaleimide (23), complex spectra containing at least two discernible sub-

* For a discussion on the effect of anisotropic motion on spin label spectra see the following sections on spin-labeled membranes (Section 11.2.2.4) and oriented films (Section 11.2.2.3), and Ref. 5.

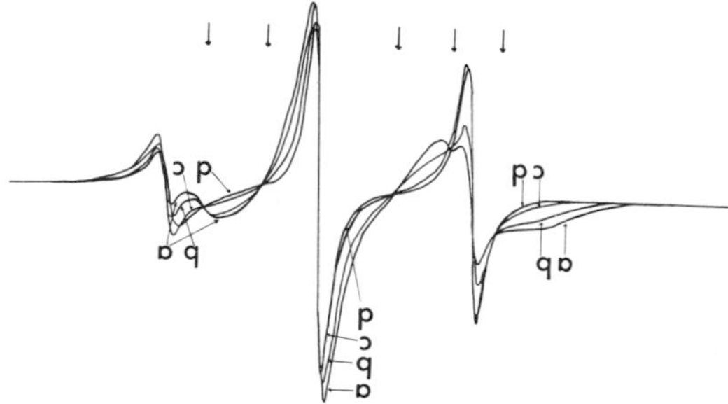

Fig. 11-4 Superposition of the ESR spectra of spin-labeled polyguanylic acid at different pH values (a) 10.45, (b) 10.95, (c) 11.60, (d) 11.80. The arrows at the bottom of the figure indicate isosbestic points (42).

spectra are observed; for example, in Fig. 11-4 we have the ESR spectra of polyguanylic acid labeled with an analog of bromoacetamide (42). Subspectra corresponding to highly constrained (strongly immobilized) and partly constrained (weakly immobilized) spin labels are evident. If these subspectra are due to two conformational states of the spin label attached to the same site on the macromolecule, it is often possible to observe isosbestic points in superpositions of spectra taken under variable conditions with the same total concentration of spin label (19, 42).* In Fig. 11-4 the pH was varied over the range of the ordered-disordered transition for poly *G*. Since the amplitude of the composite spectrum at any isosbestic point is proportional to the total concentration of spin label in both states, and since there are regions in the composite ESR spectra in which only one of the two types of spectrum makes a contribution to the amplitude (such as the broad low field line), the ratio of these amplitudes is related to the mole fraction of one component. This ratio serves as a useful qualitative monitor of conformational transitions (19, 42).

* Isosbestic points in ESR spectra are those points of equal amplitude at a given magnetic field that occur in superpositions of three or more spectra of a system under different conditions. Isosbestic points can be observed only for a system containing an equilibrium between *two* spectrally active states in which only the relative populations of the states have been changed. If a third state is introduced by varying the conditions, no isosbestic points will be observable. On the other hand, even if only two states of the system are involved, isosbestic points may not be observed. The other condition for their occurrence is that at the isosbestic point the spectral parameters for each state must not alter as conditions are changed. The intensity of an isosbestic point is directly related to the sum of the populations of the two states. An example of isosbesty is the superposition of optical spectra due to the tyrosine-tyrosinate equilibrium at various pH values.

In attempting to observe isosbestic points it is essential to keep all instrumental factors constant. The cavity *Q* can be monitored using the crystal leakage meter on the microwave bridge. To avoid errors all spectra should be run on the same piece of chart paper.

Quite often, particularly with the less specific spin labels, the complex spectra are due to labeling two or more sites in the molecule. It is still desirable to estimate the relative amounts of spin label contributing to the two general types of subspectra. One approach to this problem (48, 87) is to measure the area under the entire spectrum, as well as the area under the subspectrum due to the weakly immobilized component (one must assume a particular lineshape for the weakly immobilized component). The resultant areas for the subspectra are taken to be proportional to the concentrations of spin label in the two types of site. The total spin concentration can be estimated by totally denaturing the macromolecular components to yield ESR spectra of narrow lines whose amplitudes can be directly compared with those of a standard sample (48). Alternatively, a radioactive spin label can be used to estimate total spin concentration (49). A better approach is to use simulated spectra, synthesized by a computer from components of determined lineshape, to reproduce the observed spectrum (50). The relative intensities of the two principal subspectra can then be accurately calculated.

11.1.3.5 Stability of Spin Labels

Nitroxides may be oxidized or reduced quite readily. Polarographic measurements on di-*t*-butyl nitroxide in acetonitrile gave oxidation and reduction potentials of 0.55 and 1.65 V, respectively (51). Many common reducing agents react rapidly with nitroxides to form diamagnetic products; some of these agents are ascorbic acid, titanium (III), sodium dithionite, hydroxylamine, reduced glutathione, mercaptoethanol, cysteine, and phenylhydrazine. In some cases this reduction is reversed on exposure to air, particularly if the reduction product was a hydroxylamine (51, 52). This susceptibility of nitroxides to reduction by particular reagents (52, 53) has proved to be useful in estimating how deeply a spin label is buried in a macromolecular structure (see Section 11.2.2.4 on membranes).

Despite their sensitivity toward redox reagents, some nitroxides are surprisingly stable toward various strong reagents commonly used in synthetic organic chemistry; for example, Kosman and Piette showed that the keto group of nitroxide V could be reduced to the corresponding alcohol by lithium aluminium hydride without reduction of the nitroxide moiety; however, the six-membered nitroxide IV was reduced by this reagent (34). Hubbell and McConnell found that the alcohol of IV could be reacted with benzyl chloride, and the corresponding amine could be reacted with an acid chloride, without destruction of the nitroxide moiety (5).

11.2 APPLICATIONS OF THE SPIN LABEL TECHNIQUE

A spin label may be attached to the system of interest by a covalent bond, or by non-covalent forces such as those involved in enzyme-coenzyme,

enzyme-substrate, antibody-hapten, and membrane-steroid interactions. It is convenient to discuss the two types of attachment separately.

11.2.1 Covalent Spin Labels

11.2.1.1 Hemoglobin

One of the first and most fruitful applications of covalent attachment of spin labels to specific sites on a protein molecule is the study of hemoglobin conformations (16, 19, 22, 53–63, 71). Advantage was taken of the well-established reactivity of the sulfhydryl group of cysteine at position 93 in the sequence of the β chains toward alkylating agents such as *N*-ethylmaleimide, iodoacetamide, and *p*-chloromercuribenzoate. The spin labels used in the studies were analogs of these reagents (Fig. 11-5). Labels IX, X, XII, and XIII all reacted rapidly with cysteine β-93 in hemoglobin and in the case of oxyhemoglobin gave ESR spectra indicative of almost total constraint of spin-label motion relative to the protein as well as a weakly immobilized component (Fig. 11-6). Labels XI and XIV apparently reacted elsewhere in oxyhemoglobin, for their ESR spectra were indicative of considerable independent spin-label motion and were not sensitive to structural perturbations (53, 63). Label XI was very light-sensitive, making it inconvenient to work with.

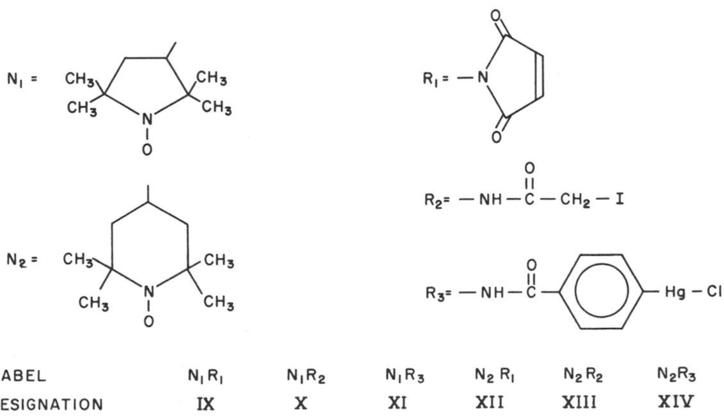

Fig. 11-5 Spin labels used to alkylate cysteine β-93 of hemoglobin. References to the use of these particular reagents are IX (23, 53), X (19, 57, 58, 59), XI (53), XII (22), XIII (56, 57, 58, 59), XIV (63).

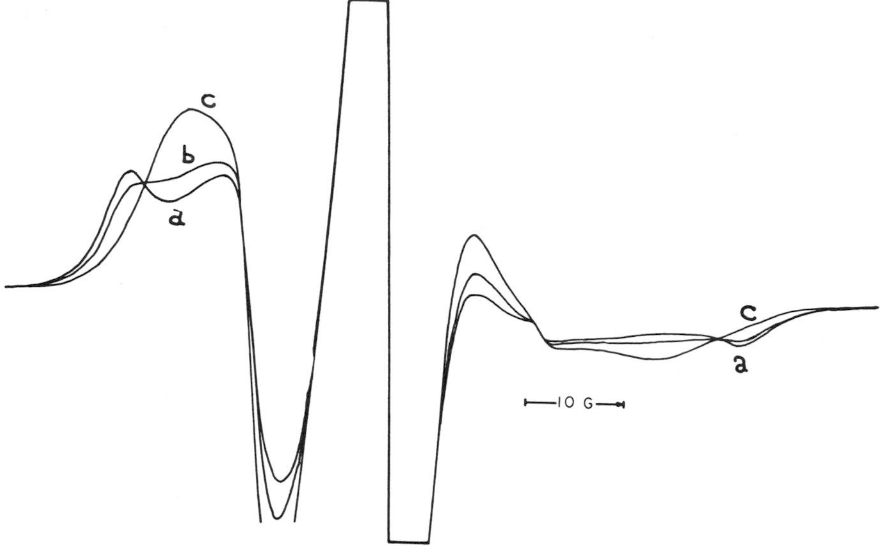

Fig. 11-6 ESR spectra of equine hemoglobin, spin-labeled with iodoacetamide nitroxide X, under varying degrees of oxygenation: (a) completely oxygenated, (b) partly oxygenated, (c) completely deoxygenated (19).

The complete immobilization of the spin labels bound to β-93 of hemoglobin in essentially its native conformation* turned out to be particularly advantageous. This is because a very small change in the protein structure in the region of the spin label will result in a significant change in the ESR spectrum. Thus, on deoxygenation of oxyhemoglobin, spin labeled with the five-membered nitroxyl-iodoacetamide X, the spectral changes shown in Fig. 11-6 were observed (19, 53). Of special significance are the isosbestic points in the low and high field regions of the superposition of spectra. They suggest that only one conformational change is associated with the oxygenation process and make possible quantitative measurement of the fraction of spin label in each of the two conformational states. Thus Ogawa and McConnell were able to compare the extent of oxygenation with the extent of conformational change at position β-93 (19). A linear relationship was observed; this is not what was expected on the basis of a symmetry-retaining model for cooperative oxygenation-induced conformational changes (64). In this model oxygenation of one β chain would result in corresponding conformational changes for both β chains. The data were consistent with the symmetry-breaking model for the allosteric phenomenon

* The effect of spin labels on macromolecular structure is discussed in Section 11.2.1.8.

(65). A crucial assumption here was that the conformational change observed via the spin label ESR spectra propagated to the α–β subunit contact region and was related to the cooperative subunit interaction and not merely to the presence of oxygen on the β chain (isolated spin-labeled β chains showed a somewhat similar change in ESR spectra on deoxygenation (19, 62). It appeared that the spin label on β-93 in the hemoglobin $\alpha_2\beta_2$ tetramer was sensitive to α–β subunit interactions, since the addition of unlabeled α chains to spin-labeled β chains resulted in a significant change in the ESR spectra. Conclusive evidence for the assertion that the spin labels on β-93 were monitoring a cooperative subunit interaction came with the studies of McConnell, Ogawa, and Horwitz, who used the six-membered nitroxyl-iodoacetamide XIII (57, 58). Deviations from isosbesty were observed in the superposition of ESR spectra due to human hemoglobin, labeled at β-93 with XIII, at various stages in the oxygenation-deoxygenation equilibrium. Thus, because of its different size and shape, label XIII sampled a slightly different region of space around β-93 and indicated the presence of conformational states other than those due merely to oxygenation or deoxygenation of β chains; the other state (or states) could obviously be dependent on the degree of oxygenation of the α chains. This was graphically demonstrated by comparison of the ESR spectra of reconstituted spin-labeled hemoglobins of compositions (cyanomet $\alpha)_2$-(spin labeled $\beta)_2$ and α_2(cyanomet spin labeled $\beta)_2$. In the cyanomet form neither the α nor the β chains can accept oxygen, and any observed conformational change is due to oxygenation of only the noncyanomet chains. With (cyanomet $\alpha)_2$(spin-labeled $\beta)_2$, oxygenation of the spin-labeled β chains produced a spectral change similar to that observed with normal ferrohemoglobin; with α_2(cyanomet spin labeled $\beta)_2$, oxygenation of the α chains produced a small but detectable change in the ESR spectra of the spin-labeled β chains. Thus the important points had been established, justifying the earlier speculation on the nature of subunit-subunit communication. It is unfortunate that the ESR spectral change observed in the latter case was so small that precise quantitative measurements were not possible. The search is now on for a spin label for β-93 that will show even greater deviations from isosbesty. It is interesting to note that a similar conclusion regarding the general nature of the conformational changes accompanying cooperative oxygen uptake by hemoglobin was reached independently by NMR studies, i.e., that the effect is essentially a protein conformational change transmitted via the subunit interfaces (66).

Recently Ho et al. have studied the uptake of carbon monoxide (145) and oxygen (146) by spin-labeled hemoglobin mutants with varying degrees of cooperativity. They concluded that subunit-subunit interaction detectable at β-93 was present only in hemoglobins exhibiting cooperative oxygen or carbon monoxide uptake, in support of the ideas of McConnell and co-workers.

The very detailed understanding of the spectral characteristics of spin-labeled hemoglobin derivatives has permitted many other valuable conclusions about the structure of the molecule (59, 63). We have mentioned the conformational differences between oxy- and deoxyhemoglobin; these had already been demonstrated by X-ray studies of single crystals (67–69). However, the solution ESR spectra of the carbon monoxy, met, met azide, and met fluoride derivatives were all slightly different (59). Apparently there are two distinct spatial orientations for a spin label attached to cysteine β-93 in these compounds, and the spectral differences could be interpreted in terms of slightly different populations of the two orientations in each compound. The spectra were all dependent on ionic strength and became more alike as the ionic strength increased. They were never identical, however, even in single crystal studies. The data were taken to indicate that very slight conformational differences exist among the derivatives and that they are so small as to be undetectable by X-ray techniques [it had been concluded from X-ray data that the met and met azide derivatives of hemoglobin have identical structures (67)]. These differences in conformation were shown to depend on the electronic state of the heme group (59, 63). It is interesting that the ESR spectra of polycrystalline suspensions or simple solutions of the various hemoglobin derivatives, in the same solvents, were virtually identical (59). This indicates that the structures around β-93 are identical in solution and in the crystalline state, a point of some satisfaction to the X-ray crystallographers.

Hemoglobin is known to form a very tight complex with an antibody-like group of proteins, known as the haptoglobins, which contain two light chains and two heavy chains per molecule (70). Recently the various complexes formed have been studied by means of spin labels at cysteine β-93 (71). The effect of complex formation on equine oxyhemoglobin labeled at β-93 with the five-membered nitroxyl-iodoacetamide, X, is shown in Fig. 11-7. Addition of haptolglobin results in an apparent depletion of the populations of the weakly and highly constrained spin labels in favor of a state of intermediate mobility. Viscosity effects on the system could be neglected, since addition of bovine serum albumin or γ-globulin in corresponding amounts had no influence on the ESR spectra. The ESR spectrum of the intermediate state is appreciably different from that of deoxyhemoglobin (Fig. 11-6). When the same experiments were performed with the six-membered nitroxyl-iodoacetamide XIII, a different result was obtained (71, 72); the ESR spectrum of the complex resembled closely that of deoxyhemoglobin labeled with XIII. Thus, in the absence of the data with label X, one might have concluded that the conformation around β-93 in

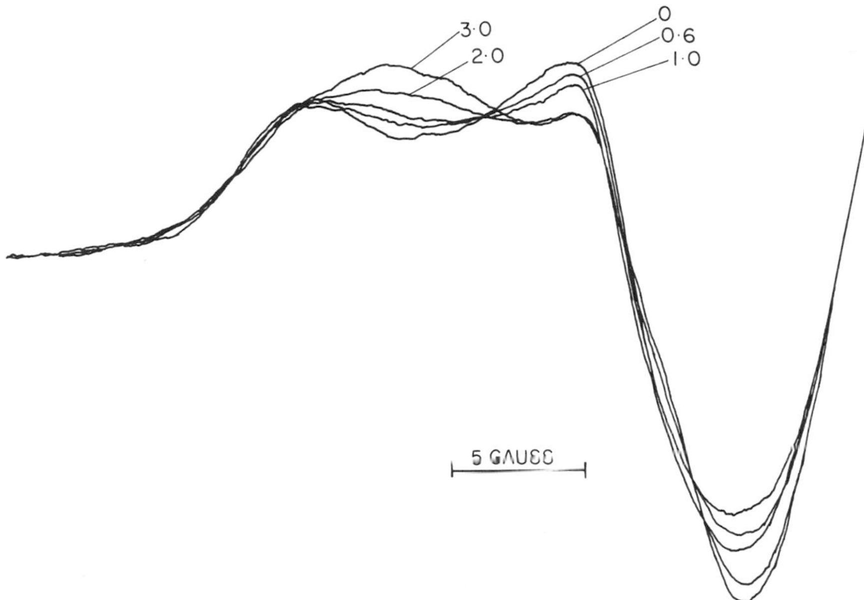

Fig. 11-7 ESR spectra of equine hemoglobin labeled at β-93 with the five-membered nitroxyl-iodoacetamide X in the presence of varying amounts of human haptoglobin 1-1 (71). The numbers above the spectra are the molar ratios of haptoglobin to hemoglobin. The apparent isosbestic point is an artifact due to the method of superposition of spectra and should be ignored.

the complex was the same as that in deoxyhemoglobin. This underlines the caution that must always be taken when applying the data from a labeled system to draw conclusions about the unlabeled system (see Section 11.2.1.8).

Malchy et al. also studied the binding of modified haptoglobins to hemoglobin labeled with X(71). Plasmin-digested and sialidase-digested haptoglobin produced the same ESR spectral change as modified haptoglobin. However, plasmin fragments P_1 or P_2 and reduced and alkylated haptoglobin produced no spectral change. The recombined P_1 and P_2 were as effective as unmodified haptoglobin. In this case, in which effects on the same labeled protein were studied, the comparisons and conclusions were justified.

The ESR spectral changes caused by haptoglobin of genetic types 1–1 and 2–1, which contain similar heavy chains but different light chains(73) were identical (71). This indicates that the nature of the binding is the same in both cases and suggests that the heavy chains are more involved in the binding process than are the light chains.

11.2.1.2 Ribonuclease A

The enzyme bovine pancreatic ribonuclease A has also been studied extensively by the spin label technique (43, 74, 75). It had been known for some time that bromoacetic acid and bromoacetamide reacted with the histidine residues at positions 12 and 119 in the RNase molecule, with concomitant inactivation of the enzyme. Alkylation of histidine-12 yielded the 3-substituted derivative, whereas reaction with histidine-119 gave the 1-substituted derivative. Analogs of these reagents were synthesized, XV

XV: $NH-\overset{O}{\overset{\|}{C}}-CH_2-\underset{Br}{\underset{|}{CH}}-COOH$ (on a 2,2,5,5-tetramethylpyrrolidine N–O ring)

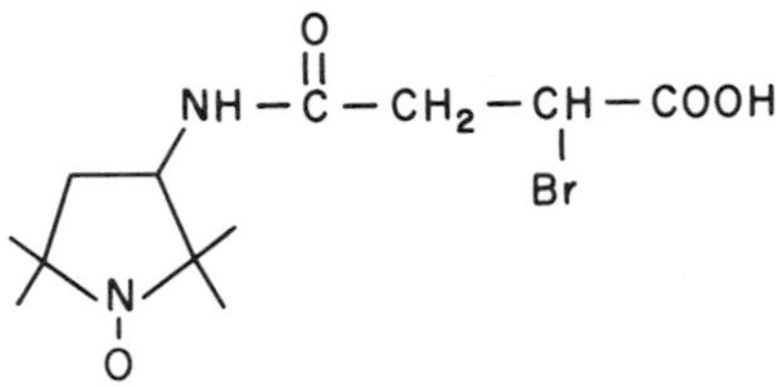

XVI: $NH-\overset{O}{\overset{\|}{C}}-CH_2-Br$ (on a 2,2,5,5-tetramethylpyrrolidine N–O ring)

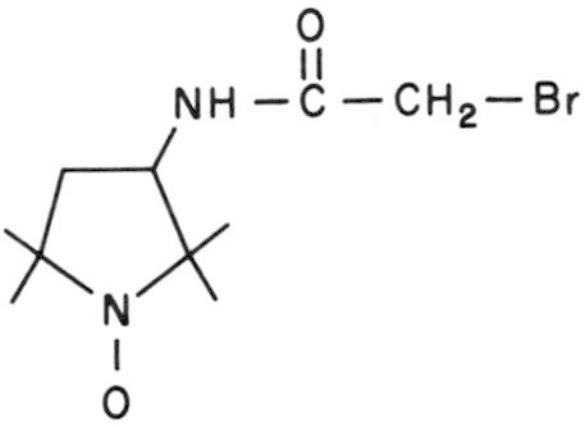

and XVI, and were found to react slowly with RNase A with a corresponding decrease in enzymic activity (43). Amino acid analysis of the products of reaction with XVI revealed the presence of 3-carboxymethylhistidine, the product expected if histidine-12 had been labeled (43). Thus it was concluded that XVI had reacted with histidine-12, although the ESR spectrum of the spin-labeled enzyme appeared to contain several sub-spectra which could have been due to enzyme molecules spin-labeled elsewhere. Amino acid analyses did not indicate the presence of any other labeled components. A detailed study was then pursued on the effects of pH, substrates, inhibitors, phosphate, and temperature on that region of the structure. One interesting observation was a structural change occurring in RNase A at a temperature of 45 C. This had been detected by optical measurements, which had demonstrated that a large disruption of structure occurred over the range 45 to 65 C (76). A quantitative study of the structural change was made by calculating spin label correlation times at various temperatures (Fig. 11-8). Because of the linearity of the data in Fig. 11-8, estimates could be made of energies of activation related to this structural change. It is interesting that the energies thus obtained for two derivatives, presumed to be labeled at different amino acids in the active center of RNase A (with label XVI, histidine-12; with label XII, lysine-41) were very similar; 5.4 and 9.6 kcal/mole with XVI, and 5.5 and 10.8 kcal/mole with XII. This suggested that the labels were monitoring the same region of the structure and that the information thus obtained did not depend strongly on the nature of the spin label. This, of course, will not always be the case, as demonstrated with hemoglobin in the preceding section.

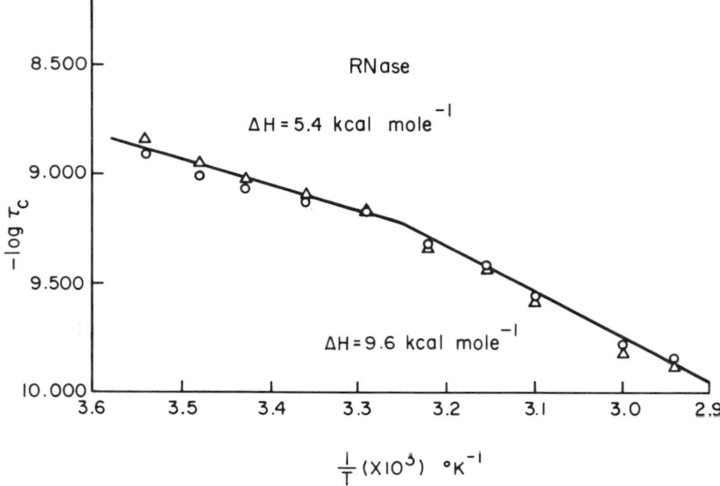

Fig. 11-8 Dependence of spin label correlation time on temperature for RNase A labeled with XII (43). The circles and triangles represent values calculated from the linear and quadratic terms respectively of Eq. 4.

More recently it has been possible to separate the products of reaction between RNase and label XVI by ion exchange chromatography (74, 75). Depending on conditions, a variety of products is obtained. Derivatives spin-labeled at methionine-29 (or 30), histidine-119, and histidine-105 have been characterized, and their ESR spectra under various conditions have been followed (74). An interesting feature of this study was the time dependence of the formation of enzyme-substrate complexes in urea solutions.

In studies such as those on RNase A, α-chymotrypsin (Section 11.2.1.3), and the antibody-hapten interaction (Section 11.2.2.1), in which only small quantities of pure derivatives were available, a simple device can be used to study the effects of increasing concentration of reagents. It is shown schematically in Fig. 11-9. Small volumes of concentrated solutions of the reagent (acid, base, urea, salt, etc.) are readily added when the sample is forced into the wide upper section of the cell by means of the syringe plunger. Manipulation of the plunger can be used to mix the sample and lower it back into the observed part of the cell. No disturbance of the position of the cell in the cavity, hence the tuning of the spectrometer, occurs. Thus spectra taken under identical instrument conditions can be obtained. Small intensity corrections to take account of dilution can be made accurately.

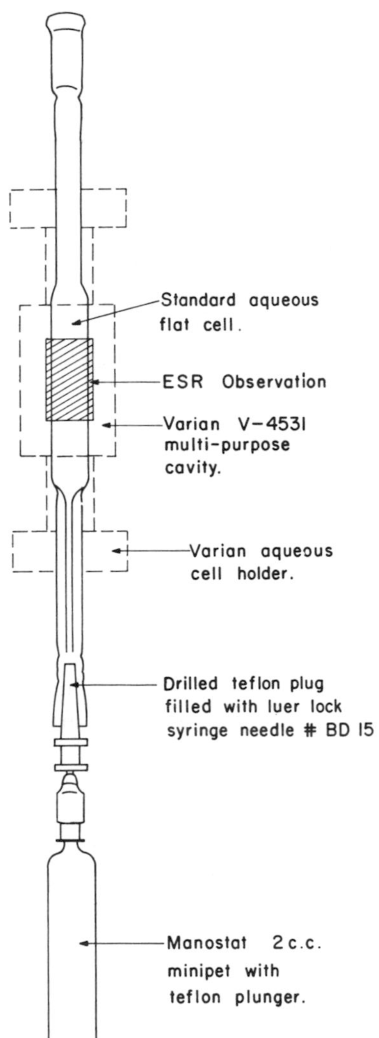

Fig. 11-9 Attachments for a standard flat cell to titrate small quantities of material without removing sample from the cell or disturbing the position of the cell in the cavity.

11.2.1.3 α-Chymotrypsin

A clever approach to labeling an enzyme at its active center was devised by Berliner and McConnell for α-chymotrypsin (15). It was known that in the hydrolysis of esters and amides by this enzyme an acylated enzyme intermediate was formed and later hydrolyzed. The liberated product of the first reaction was the alcohol or amine portion of the substrate; the product of the second reaction was the acid portion. They synthesized

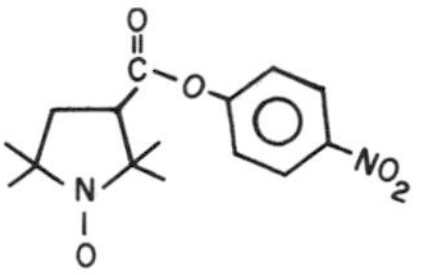

XVII

the substrate analog XVII, in which the acid portion was a nitroxide, and the alcohol portion a nitrophenol whose optical spectrum was sensitive to the state of esterification. Thus formation of the intermediate acyl enzyme resulted in attachment of the nitroxide label and release of nitrophenol. The kinetics of the acylation step could be monitored by the optical spectrum of the released phenolate ion and those of the second step by the ESR spectrum of the released nitroxide. By doing the reaction at low pH, at which the rate of deacylation was low, they were able to observe the ESR spectrum of the acyl enzyme. The spectrum was characteristic of a strongly immobilized spin label, indicating that the active center must be sufficiently flexible to admit the substrate but sufficiently rigid thereafter to immobilize the acyl component relative to the enzyme. Raising the pH to 6.8 resulted in rapid deacylation, for which the rate constant could be measured by the rate of appearance of the ESR spectrum of an unrestricted spin label. The latter step was shown to be rate-limiting for the overall hydrolysis. A large series of substrate spin labels has since been synthesized by Berliner (77). All became strongly immobilized on formation of the acyl-enzyme.

Berliner has also prepared a number of spin-labeled inhibitors for α-chymotrypsin, which are analogs of sulfonyl fluoride inhibitors (77).

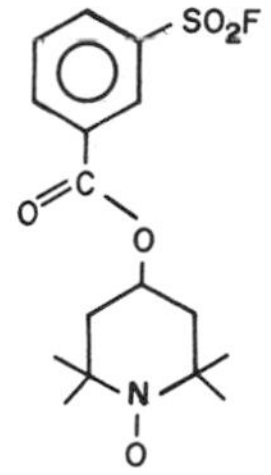

XVIII

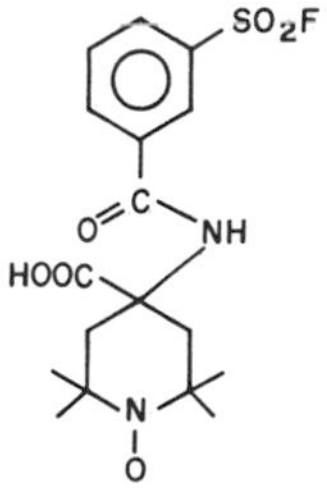

XIX

Inhibitor XVIII had the ESR spectrum of a weakly immobilized spin label when attached to the enzyme, whereas XIX was highly constrained. This was surprising in view of the similar distances between the point of attachment and the nitroxide in both cases. It was inferred that the active site region was only large enough to accommodate and immobilize the aromatic ring of the inhibitor (or the acyl portion of the substrate) and that immobilization of the nitroxide ring of the inhibitors was determined by interactions between it and other regions of the enzyme structure.

More recently Piette and co-workers have studied α-chymotrypsin in great detail by using substrate analogs XX-XXIII (78, 79), organophosphate spin labels XXIV, XXV (80) resembling diisopropylfluorophosphate (DFP), and a dinitroxide DFP analog (80) (Fig. 11-10). Changes in the ESR spectra of spin label-acylated α-chymotrypsin were correlated with the structures of the substrates, the presence or absence of indole, and structural modifications of the aryl binding region (methionine-192) and the amide binding region (methionine-180) of the enzyme. The data indicated a cooperative link between the aryl and amide binding regions. A model for the substrate binding site and the operational sequence of substrate hydrolysis was proposed (78, 79).

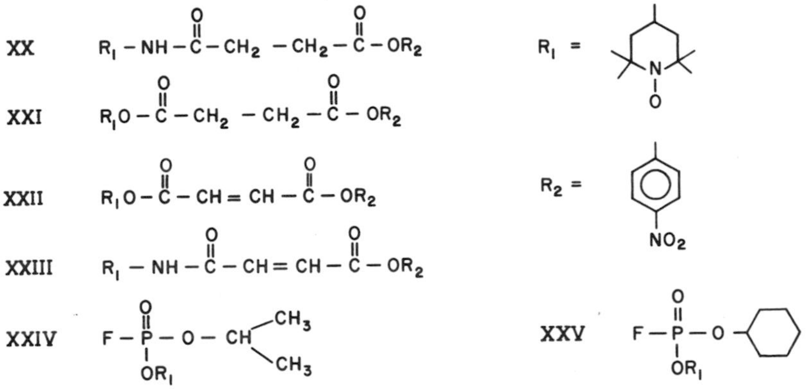

XX $R_1-NH-\overset{O}{\overset{\|}{C}}-CH_2-CH_2-\overset{O}{\overset{\|}{C}}-OR_2$

XXI $R_1O-\overset{O}{\overset{\|}{C}}-CH_2-CH_2-\overset{O}{\overset{\|}{C}}-OR_2$

XXII $R_1O-\overset{O}{\overset{\|}{C}}-CH=CH-\overset{O}{\overset{\|}{C}}-OR_2$

XXIII $R_1-NH-\overset{O}{\overset{\|}{C}}-CH=CH-\overset{O}{\overset{\|}{C}}-OR_2$

XXIV $F-\overset{O}{\overset{\|}{P}}(OR_1)-O-CH(CH_3)_2$

XXV $F-\overset{O}{\overset{\|}{P}}(OR_1)-O-$cyclohexyl

R_1 = 2,2,6,6-tetramethylpiperidine-N-oxyl (N–O)

R_2 = p-nitrophenyl (NO_2)

Fig. 11-10 Spin labels used by Piette and co-workers to study the active center of α-chymotryspin (78–80).

11.2.1.4 Other Proteins and Enzymes

The potential usefulness of DFP spin labels in studies of other enzymes containing essential serine residues, such as acetylcholinesterase, has been reported (80, 81). Interaction between a spin label on an essential sulfhydryl group in creatine kinase and paramagnetic metal ions has demonstrated a further possibility of the method—to determine the distance between two components in the active center of an enzyme (82). A similar approach was used to study the distance between a copper-containing paramagnetic dye and a nitroxide spin label, both attached to bovine serum albumin (83), and to hemoglobin (84).

11.2.1.5 Nonspecific Protein Labeling

A considerable amount of useful information on complex biological systems has been obtained by nonspecific labeling of sulfhydryl and amino groups with spin-labeled analogs of *N*-ethylmaleimide and iodoacetamide. Sandberg and Piette found that the maleimide-nitroxide XII reacted readily with membranes isolated from human red cells (erythrocyte ghosts) to yield a complex spectrum due to highly and weakly constrained spin labels (50). This indicated that at least two different types of site had been labeled. Blocking experiments have shown that the labeled sites were mainly sulfhydryl groups (85). Addition of psychotropic drugs such as chloropromazine caused further constraint of the more mobile labels, indicating that the drugs were able to produce conformational changes in membrane proteins. More recently, Holmes and Piette have done a similar study on erythrocyte ghosts, using the iodoacetamide spin label XIII (86). This label apparently reacted only with the sites that had evinced ESR spectra of less-constrained labels for XII. The absence of components due to strongly immobilized spin labels in the ESR spectra of ghosts labeled with XIII made possible the quantitative study of the drug effect, which is to convert weakly immobilized labels to strongly immobilized labels. It appeared that 50 percent of the sites labeled by XIII could be affected by interaction with phenothiazine-type drugs. A comparison was made of the effectiveness of various phenothiazine derivatives in inducing the conformational change.

Schneider and Smith have taken advantage of the sensitivity to protein conformational changes of the ESR spectra of erythrocyte ghosts spin-labeled with XII in a study of the various methods used to solubilize the membrane proteins (87). The aim was to determine the severity of protein structural perturbations caused by each method and the reversibility of the structural changes on removal of solubilizer. This is important because for many of the protein components there is no known function and therefore no assay of structural integrity after removal from the membrane. The data revealed that the solubilizers which disturbed protein conformations least, and which allowed isolation of spin-labeled proteins with ESR spectra equivalent to those they had while on the membrane, were agents acting mainly on the lipid components, e.g., n-butanol and sodium deoxycholate. Protein denaturants, such as pyridine and low or high pH, caused irreversible structural changes.

These authors have also shown that Mg^{2+} ions can induce a conformational change in spin-labeled ghosts, which can be largely reversed by adenosine triphosphate (ATP). This effect was attributed to binding of Mg^{2+} to the membrane; its subsequent reversal was proposed to be due to chelation by ATP rather than to an ATP effect related to transport or ATPase activities of the membrane. Justification for this view followed from similar reversal of the Mg^{2+} effect by nonsubstrate nucleoside triphosphates and by the chelating agent ethylenediamine tetracetic acid. At high ionic strengths in Tris Cl, NaCl, or KCl the Mg^{2+}-induced spectral change did not occur, which suggests that monovalent cations can compete for the Mg^{2+} binding sites but do not affect membrane protein structure in the same fashion (88).

Another demonstration of ATP-induced conformational changes was obtained by Landgraf and Inesi in a study of spin-labeled sarcoplasmic reticulum from rabbit skeletal muscle (89). The iodoacetamide nitroxide XIII reacted readily with the fragmented reticulum and gave an ESR spectrum due to strongly and weakly immobilized spin labels. Addition of ATP caused a conversion of some of the highly constrained labels to the more mobile state. This was taken to indicate a protein conformational change related to the ATPase system. Labeling the sarcoplasmic reticulum with an isothiocyanate spin label, XXVI, which is thought to react with

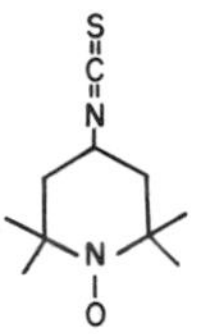

XXVI

amino or alcohol groups, yielded a spectrum similar to that obtained with XIII, but insensitive to ATP additions. Thus the ATP-induced conformational change observed with label XII must be small and localized in the region of the sulfhydryl groups.

Rabbit muscle fibers have been spin-labeled with the analogs of *N*-ethylmaleimide, XII, iodoacetamide, XIII, and isothiocyanate, XXVI (49). The ESR spectrum of label XII depended slightly on the angle between the fiber axis and the applied magnetic field, demonstrating a low but significant degree of orientation of the strongly immobilized spin label. When the fibers were shortened by the action of ATP, the ESR spectrum indicated a conversion of a small fraction of the spin labels from the weakly immobilized state to the strongly immobilized state. No spectral changes were observed with labels XIII or XXVI, however, underlining once again the different reactivities that the alkylating spin labels have toward sulfhydryl and amino groups in particular environments. Proteins were extracted from fibers labeled with XII and their ESR spectra were studied in solution. The spectra were insensitive to myosin-actin-ATP interactions but indicated a further immobilization of the spin label on actin polymerization. The sliding filament theory for muscle contraction could not account for these data without the introduction of some new interactions between the components. In a separate study Quinlivan et al. reported spin-labeling myosin with the five-membered nitroxyliodoacetamide X (90). Small spectral changes could be observed on activation of the ATPase system by *p*-mercuribenzoate.

Serum lipoproteins have been the object of several recent studies. Gotto and Kon reported labeling human high density and low density lipoproteins with XII and XXVI (91, 92). Removal of lipids from the mixture resulted in an increased mobility for the previously immobilized spin labels, suggesting that the lipids played a part in determining the conformations of the lipoproteins. More recently Martin et al. compared the environments around groups alkylated with XII in porcine serum lipoproteins (93). Besides the usual very low density (VLDL) and high density (HDL) lipoproteins (94), porcine serum contains two discrete and separable low density (LDL_1 and LDL_2) fractions (94). Strongly and weakly immobilized spin labels were observed in LDL_1, LDL_2, and HDL, with slightly different relative populations in each case. Variable temperature measurements (10 to 90 C) were performed; for all three types of lipoprotein increasing temperature resulted in conversion of strongly immobilized spin labels to weakly immobilized spin labels and increased mobility of the already mobile spin labels. Thus monitors of at least two regions of the structures were available. The area under the ESR spectrum of the strongly immobilized component was constant until 45 C for all three fractions and began to decrease thereafter. This indicated that no discernible change took place in that region of the structure until 45 C. Plots of the intensity of the low field line of the weakly immobilized spin label versus temperature, a measure of the increasing mobilization of the more mobile labels, gave two straight lines intersecting around 50 C. The estimated temperatures for these structural transitions were LDL_1, 51 C; LDL_2, 58 C; HDL, 58 C (all ± 2 C). Thus only slight structural differences between the proteins were detectable. The data indicated a trend to greater structural stability with increasing protein content. Such well-defined transitions had not been observed by other physical techniques. It is also noteworthy that the various structural changes observed all took place well below the thermal denaturation temperatures, 75 C (95, 96), of lipoproteins. This could be due to changes in lipid-protein interactions or in the helical content of the protein moieties.

Smith and Yamane have spin-labeled a protein component of *E. coli* ribosomes by using the bromoacetamide nitroxide XVI (42). The label was only weakly immobilized under conditions in which the ribosomes are thought to exist as separate 50S and 30S subunits and underwent no change in mobility on going to conditions in which the subunits are associated to form 70S ribosomes. Removal of the protein components from the ribosomes resulted in increased constraint of the spin label relative to the protein, indicating that solubilization caused a structural change in that region of the protein.

11.2.1.6 Single Crystal Studies

Measurement of the angular dependence of the g factor and hyperfine splitting in a single crystal of a spin-labeled biological macromolecule yields the orientation of the nitroxide moiety relative to the single crystal axes. Thus the measurements are sensitive to minute structural differences between crystals of one form of protein and another. The data can also indicate the presence of more than one labeled site per molecule, several isomeric states for labels in the same site, and the presence of noncrystallographic symmetry axes (symmetry axes related to the molecule itself and not simply to the symmetry of the crystals).

McConnell and co-workers have studied single crystals of hemoglobin labeled at β-93 (22, 54, 55, 59). They were able to separate the resonances for the two isomeric states of a spin label attached to β-93 (see Section 11.2.1.1). The orientations of the nitroxides in these states were shown to be identical in crystals of carbon-monoxyhemoglobin and methemoglobin; the spectra differed only in the relative populations of the two states. These data indicated that the crystal structures of the two derivatives were essentially the same, with a very small difference resulting in the population variation of the isomeric label states. This small difference was not detectable in the high resolution structures determined by X-ray diffraction (67).

Berliner has demonstrated that the spin label method can be used to locate noncrystallographic symmetry axes with relative ease. He studied single crystals of α-chymotrypsin spin-labeled by a substrate analog on the serine hydroxyl group of the active center (77, 158) (see Section 11.2.1.3).

11.2.1.7 Nucleic Acids

Smith and Yamane have demonstrated that the analogs of bromoacetic acid, XV, bromoacetamide, XVI, and *N*-ethylmaleimide, XII, labeled ribonucleic acid and deoxyribonucleic acid (41, 42). The labels reacted with the bases in the nucleic acids and had higher reactivities for the purines than for the pyrimidine bases. Studies of the order-disorder transitions for polyadenylic acid and polyguanylic acid were made (Fig. 11-4); the resultant pK values agreed with those obtained by optical spectroscopic methods. Isosbestic points in superpositions of ESR spectra indicated that each of these large polynucleotides existed in only two forms—one ordered and one disordered—and therefore that no intermediate forms were present. Spin label XVI on transfer RNA was located in a region with considerable secondary (or tertiary) structure, since RNase digestion resulted in greatly increased mobility for the label. Attempts to label the nucleic acid components of *E. coli* ribosomes resulted only in a preferential labeling of the proteins components (42).

Hoffman, Schofield, and Rich have reported a different and much more specific method for spin-labeling transfer RNA (97, 98). They synthesized

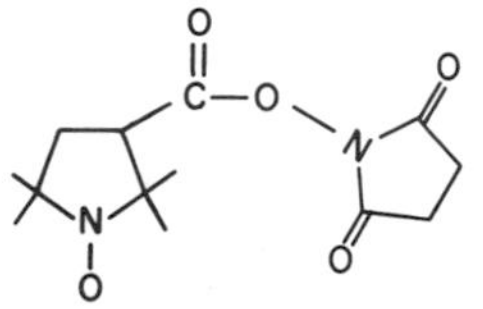

XXVII

a spin-labeled *N*-hydroxysuccinimide analog, XXVII, and reacted it with the aminoacyl residues on valyl-tRNA^{Val} (97, 98), and phenylalanyl-tRNA^{Phe} (98). The amino acids used were radioactive (^{14}C), and thus quantitative measurement of the extent of labeling could be readily made. Some nonspecific labeling of the RNA component occurred, but these products could be removed by chromatography (98). Graphs of log τ versus the reciprocal of absolute temperature for the spin-labeled tRNA showed discontinuous behavior, similar to that already discussed for RNase A (Section 11.2.1.2), Fig. 11-8). The temperature at which this discontinuity occurred was somewhat lower than the melting temperature obtained from the more conventional thermal-optical profiles and depended on the nature of the solvent and the ionic strength. The data were taken to indicate two molecular states of tRNA, in each of which constraint of the spin label differed.

The 4-thiouridine residue occurring in the tRNA of *E. coli* has been labeled with the nitroxylbromoacetamide, XVI (99). The amino acid accepting properties of tRNA^{Tyr}, tRNA^{fMet}, tRNA^{Val}, and tRNA^{Phe} were unaffected by this modification, whereas those of tRNA^{Glu} and tRNA^{Lys} were reduced. The ESR spectrum of the spin-labeled tRNA indicated only partial constraint of the spin label; the degree of constraint differed among the various types of tRNA. This application should prove to be exceedingly useful in studying conformational changes in tRNA during the various steps of protein synthesis.

11.2.1.8 Limitations of the Method

As with all approaches involving molecular modification, the onus is on the investigator to demonstrate that the data obtained are meaningful for the unmodified system. McConnell and McFarland have recently discussed this problem as it applies to the spin label method (5).

In cases such as α-chymotrypsin, in which the spin label is actually a substrate (15, 77–79), no justification need be made. The enzymic activity of ribonuclease modified at histidine-105 or methionine-29 (or 30) was only slightly reduced, and the optical absorption and rotatory dispersion characteristics were unchanged (74). Spin-labeled oxyhemoglobin took up oxygen more strongly than the unmodified protein (19) and bound haptoglobin normally (71), although Moffat has shown recently in an X-ray crystallographic study that there are some large conformational differences between native and spin-labeled hemoglobin (56). The results of the Malchy et al. (71) on the hemoglobin-haptoglobin complex (Section 11.2.1.1) demonstrate that it is advisable to use at least two spin labels of slightly different size when applying the results from the labeled system to draw conclusions about the unmodified system. In the studies of spin-labeled sarcoplasmic reticulum the overall activity of the membranes was only minimally altered (89). Spin-labeled erythrocyte ghosts retained a high ATPase activity (88). Keith et al. found that the bread mold *Neurospora crassa* was able to grow in media containing spin-labeled methyl stearate and that the spin label was incorporated into its lipid components (100). Some spin-labeled tRNA was capable of accepting amino acids, whereas some others had reduced capability (99). On the other hand, recombination of spin-labeled protohemin with apocytochrome *c* peroxidase yielded a synthetic enzyme with only 1 percent activity relative to the native enzyme (101; see Section 11.2.2.5). Thus each system behaves differently, and by careful choice of spin labels and labeling sites it should be possible to study almost any desired system without significant structural perturbation.

A further complication that may arise is the oxidation of sulfhydryl groups in proteins by the nitroxide spin labels. Morrisett and Drott have shown recently that large excesses of spin label (10:1) oxidize reduced glutathione to the corresponding cysteic acid (102). Significant oxidation of glutathione itself occurred only at high acid concentrations and high temperatures, indicating that disulfide bonds are relatively inert toward the nitroxides. Oxidation of sulfhydryl groups in a spin-labeled protein can be readily detected by amino acid analysis, and this check should always be made.

11.2.2 Noncovalent Spin Labels

The object with this type of spin label is to make it structurally as similar as possible to a natural component of a biological system or to a compound that interacts with the system. The spin label should then be bound to the system by the same noncovalent forces used to bind the natural or interacting species. The first reported spin label of this type was the chloropromazine radical cation, formed by oxidation of chloropromazine with persulfate

(1). Although it had the limitations of instability and a complicated ESR spectrum, valuable information relevant to the intercalation of chloropromazine into DNA was obtained. Since then a large number of nitroxides resembling biologically active compounds have been prepared and a great deal of biological information has been obtained.

11.2.2.1 Antibody-Hapten Interactions

Nitrophenyl derivatives have been used in a large number of antibody studies. Stryer and Griffith prepared the spin-labeled dinitrophenyl hapten,

O–N⟨ ⟩=N–NH–C$_6$H$_3$(NO$_2$)$_2$

XXVIII

XXVIII, and used it to study binding of the hapten to rabbit antidinitrophenyl antibody (103). Both the fluorescence of the dinitrophenyl group and the ESR spectrum of the nitroxide group were used to follow the binding. The presence of a nitroxide moiety apparently did not interfere with the specific, high affinity interaction of the dinitrophenyl group with the antibody. The ESR spectrum of the bound nitroxide-hapten was that of a strongly immobilized spin label (Fig. 11-11). The nitroxide moiety retained

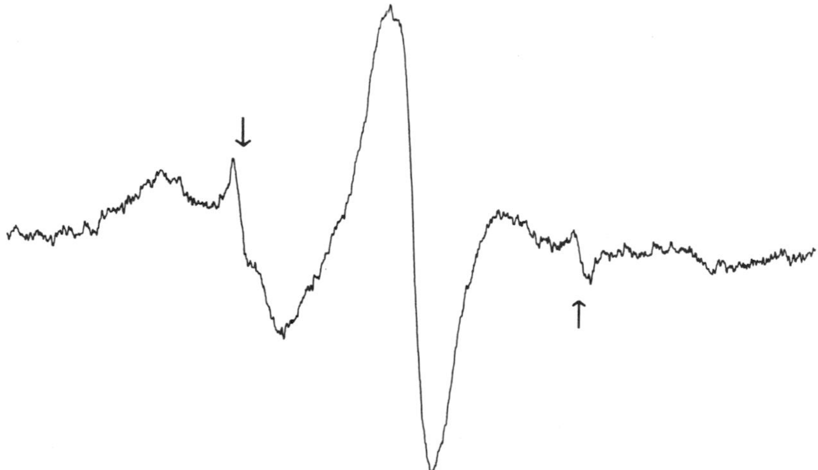

Fig. 11-11 ESR spectrum of the complex formed between rabbit antidinitrophenyl antibody and dinitrophenyl nitroxide XXVIII (103). The arrows indicate the observable narrow hyperfine lines due to unbound hapten.

some motion relative to the antibody, however, because the separation between the low field and center lines was less than that observed in a rigid glass containing the spin label. Because the ESR spectrum of the unbound hapten contained three narrow lines separated by only 15 G, the spectra of bound and unbound hapten could be readily distinguished, and the amount of unbound hapten could be measured by the intensity of its high field ESR line (indicated by the arrow at high field in Fig. 11-11). It was thus established that two moles of hapten were bound per mole of antibody, in agreement with results obtained by titration of fluorescence quenching. Measurement of the depolarization of fluorescence from the dansyl group of a dansyl nitroxide in viscous solution, whose ESR spectrum was the same as that of the antibody-hapten complex, yielded an approximate correlation time of 3.6×10^{-8} sec for the dinitrophenylnitroxide in the complex.

Hsia and Piette extended these studies by synthesizing dinitrophenylnitroxides in which the distance between the dinitrophenyl and nitroxide groups varied (104). As the distance increased, the nitroxide moiety of the hapten bound to antidinitrophenyl antibodies became more mobile. The mobility experienced a very rapid increase as the dinitrophenylnitroxide distance increased through 11 Å. An average depth of 10 Å was thus estimated for the antibody-hapten combining site. The same authors also compared the ESR spectra of nitrophenyl- and dinitrophenylnitroxides bound to rabbit antidinitrophenyl antibody (105). The cross-reacting nitrophenylnitroxide was less constrained in the antibody-hapten complex, as evinced by a smaller separation between the low and high field lines of its strongly immobilized spin label spectrum.

11.2.2.2 Liposomes and Detergent Micelles

One model for biological membranes is provided by the smectic mesophases (liposomes) formed by phospholipids when dispersed in aqueous solutions. These structures are thought to consist of concentric bimolecular layers of the phospholipids, separated by aqueous phase. Their hydrocarbon chains are thought to be perpendicular to the bilayer surface, whereas the ionic residues face the aqueous phase. This model is of interest because of the possibility that the phospholipids of membranes may be arranged in a closely similar structure (106, 107). Another model which has some feature of interest is the micellar phase formed by soaps or detergents. A study of the organization of the lipids in these structures is thus germane to the organization of the lipids of biological membranes.

Waggoner, Griffith, and Christensen have used the dinitrophenylnitroxide XXVIII, and the carboline derivative XXIX, to study micelles of sodium dodecyl sulfate by both ESR and optical spectroscopy (108). Since the nature of the solvent affects both ESR and optical properties

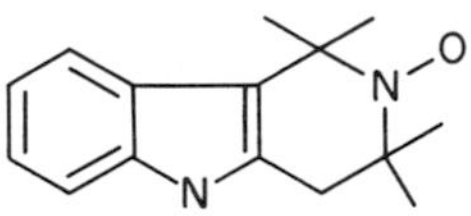

XXIX

of such compounds, it was hoped to determine the nature of the environment of the labels when associated with the micelles. It was demonstrated that XXVIII and XXIX do interact with the micelles such that their rotational correlation times are increased; the environment of the labels apparently was intermediate between that in pure hydrocarbon and that in water. A dynamic model for the label environment, in which the labels are moving rapidly from one type of environment to another, was proposed. Another study on micelles of sodium dodecyl sulfate, in which fatty acid esters of the form XXX were used, was reported by Waggoner, Keith, and Griffith (109). They concluded that the intercalated labels had a high degree of mobility relative to the micelles and that they experienced an average environment that was more like water than like hydrocarbon.

An analog of methyl stearate, XXXI, spin-labeled at position 12 of the hydrocarbon chain, has been used by Waggoner et al. to study liposomes of egg lecithin (110).

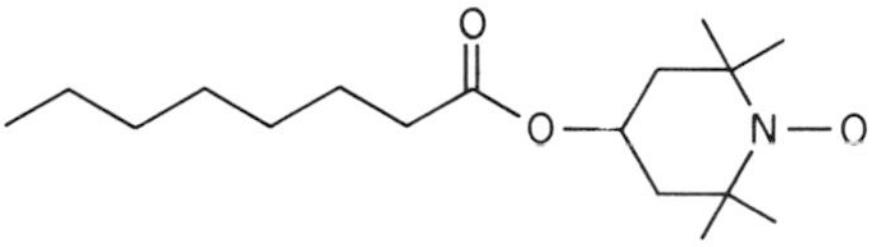

XXX

The nitroxide moiety had considerable motion in the lecithin liposomes but markedly less than that of the nitroxide groups of labels XXVIII to XXX in micelles of sodium dodecyl sulfate. This may be in part because the nitroxide moiety of this label is expected to sample the hydrocarbon region of the liposome and because the nitroxide moiety can undergo no single bond rotations relative to the rest of the spin label. Addition of cholesterol

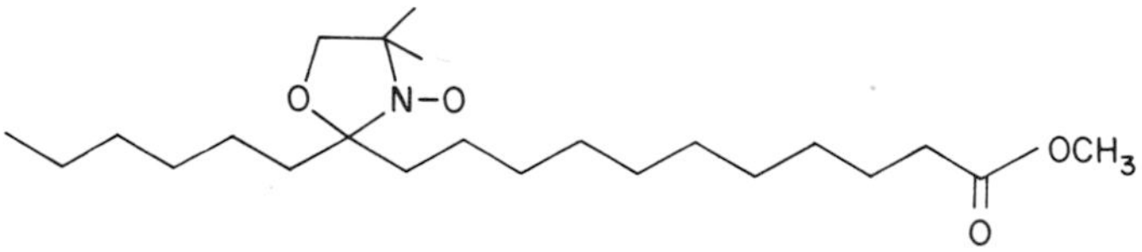

XXXI

to the liposomes resulted in decreased mobility of the nitroxide group of XXXI, demonstrating a decrease in the fluidity of the hydrocarbon region caused by cholesterol.

The influence of cholesterol on the organization of egg lecithin liposomes has also been studied by Hsia, Schneider, and Smith (33). They used a stearamide spin label, VII (see Section 11.1.3.1), in which the nitroxide group is located at the polar end of the long chain with the possibility of independent motion relative to the chain, and a cholestane nitroxide, I, in which the nitroxide group is locked onto a steroid backbone. Dramatically different effects of cholesterol were observed for the two labels. With the cholestane spin label the presence of cholesterol resulted in reduction in the mobility of the label (Fig. 11-12*a*). With the stearamide spin label, not

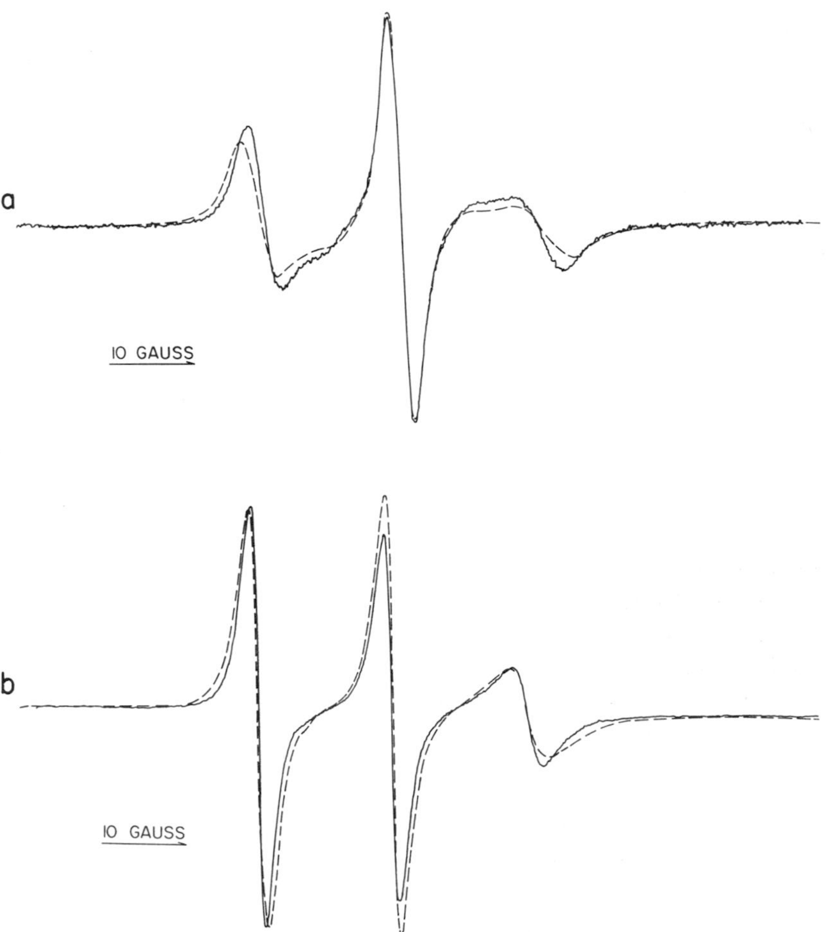

Fig. 11-12 ESR spectra due to (a) the cholestane spin label I and (b) the stearamide spin label VII in liposomes of egg lecithin. The dotted spectra show the effects of cholesterol. In (b) a higher gain was used for the dashed spectrum than for the solid spectrum (33).

only were the ESR lines broader in the presence of cholesterol but also the relative widths of the low field and center lines (Fig. 11-12*b*) were reversed. This latter effect could be due to a perturbation of the *g* or hyperfine tensor components as a consequence of a change in the spin label location. Since the observed hyperfine splitting was essentially the same in both cases, it appeared that on cholesterol addition the spin label moved to a region of asymmetric polarity, resulting in a change in the nitroxide *g* tensor with negligible effect on the hyperfine tensor. An explanation for the absence of this ESR spectral effect with the cholestane spin label probably lies in the inability of its nitroxide moiety to move independently of the lipid backbone. Thus the entire steroid must be moved if the nitroxide is to sample a region of different polarity. An alternate explanation of this behavior is that spin label VII undergoes anisotropic motion within a cone and that cholesterol addition results in a decrease in the volume of the cone (152). The spin label studies on lecithin liposomes have thus demonstrated that cholesterol plays an important role in the structure of phospholipid regions. This is in agreement with the results of other approaches (111, 112, 153, 159).

XXXII

As part of their study of rabbit vagus nerve, in which the incorporated spin label XXXII was used, Hubbell and McConnell investigated liposomes containing the label (113). Suspensions of soybean phosphatides (asolectin), phosphatidyl serine, phosphatidyl ethanolamine, and egg lecithin containing XXXII gave spectra similar to that shown in Fig. 11-13. This spectrum contains two subspectra of three lines with different average *g* values and hyperfine splittings. The two high field components of the subspectra due to spin label in hydrophobic (A in Fig. 11-13) and hydrophilic (B in Fig. 11-13) environments can be distinguished. A similar spectrum

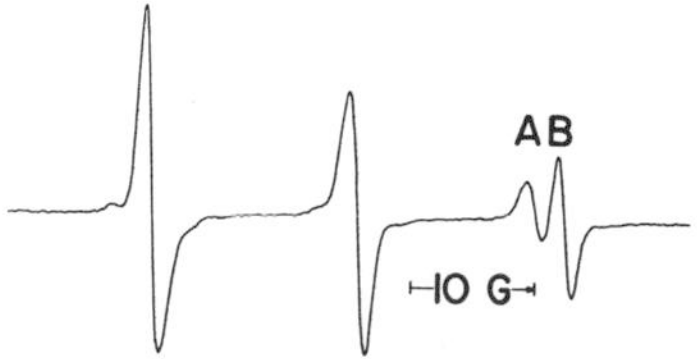

Fig. 11-13 ESR spectrum of spin label XXXII in rabbit vagus nerve (113). Hyperfine lines A and B are each part of the separate three-line spectra due to XXXII in the hydrophobic region of the nerve and the surrounding aqueous solution, respectively. The other two lines of the two types of spectrum occur at the same value of the magnetic field.

was obtained by superimposing the spectra of XXXII in dodecane and in water. Various agents were found to increase, or decrease, the solubility of XXXII in the hydrophobic region of the liposomes. Butanethiol, octylamine, and the anesthetic tetracaine increased ESR line A at the expense of B, indicating that they enhanced the solubility of XXXII in the hydrophobic region. Cholesterol in the liposomes, or calcium ion in the solution, caused an increase in line B at the expense of line A. It was proposed that the solubility changes were due to alterations in ordering of the liposome components caused by the added agents. Once again cholesterol was demonstrated to have an ordering effect on phospholipids in liposomes.

Hubbell and McConnell (114) also investigated the fluidity of the phospholipids in phosphatidyl serine liposomes by using steroid spin labels such as the oxazolidine derivative of 5α-androstan-3-one (formula shown in Fig. 11-3). The ESR spectra indicated that these rigid spin labels were able to tumble rapidly and isotropically, in contrast to their behavior in biological membranes (see Section 11.2.2.4).

The same authors have also prepared a series of amphiphilic spin labels [possessing two distinct molecular regions, one lipophilic (hydrophobic) and one hydrophilic] in which the position of the nitroxide along the fatty acid chain was varied (115). The labels may be described by the general formula XXXIII(*m*, *n*) in which *m* and *n* refer to the number of CH_2 groups between the nitroxide moiety and the lipophilic end and the hydrophilic end, respectively.

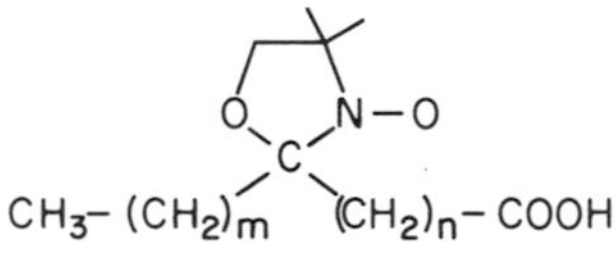

$CH_3-(CH_2)_m-C(-O-\ldots-N-O)-(CH_2)_n-COOH$

XXXIII (m,n)

In this family of spin labels the maximum component of the hyperfine tensor A_{zz} is approximately parallel to the long axis of the extended hydrocarbon chain, in contrast to the cholestane nitroxide I, in which A_{zz} is approximately perpendicular to the long molecular axis. Thus different spectra should be observed from oriented spin labels of types I and XXXIII, but they should provide self-consistent data on the orientation of the long molecular axes of the amphiphilic labels. Quite different spectra were obtained for labels XXXIII(*m*, *n*) in suspensions of soybean phosphatides, depending on the position of the nitroxide. With spin label XXXIII(17, 3), in which the nitroxide is near the polar head group, the spectrum shown in Fig. 11-14 was obtained. The well-defined hyperfine peaks in this spectrum indicate that the effective Hamiltonian for the spin label in this system is axially symmetric. This could come about only if

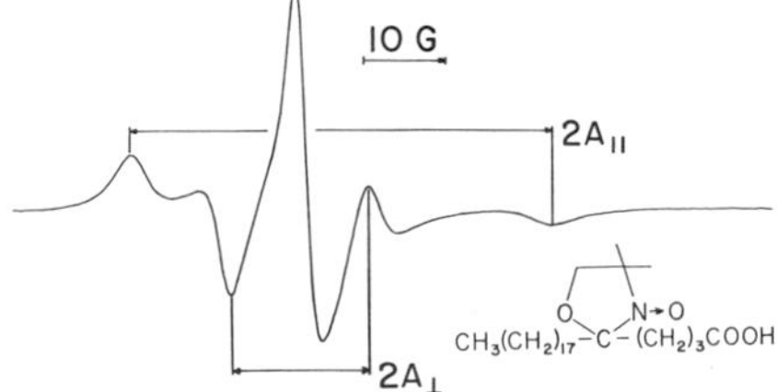

Fig. 11-14 ESR spectrum of spin label XXXIII (3, 17) in a dispersion of soybean phosphatides (115).

label XXXIII(17, 3) were undergoing anisotropic motion, with rapid rotation about the long axis of the extended hydrocarbon chain, but negligible motion about other possible axes. The separation between the outer hyperfine lines gives the effective $2A_{zz}$ resulting from this motion (labeled $2A_{\parallel}$ in Fig. 11-14); since it is very nearly equal to $2A_{zz}$ as measured for label I in crystals of cholesteryl chloride (115), motion about axes other than the long axis of the extended hydrocarbon chain must be slight. The sharpness of the spectrum in Fig. 11-14, compared with that of the usual strongly immobilized spin label, is due to averaging of g_{xx} and g_{yy} by the rapid motion about the long axis. This allows measurement of the effective axial hyperfine splitting ($A_{xx} = A_{yy}$, labeled $A_{\perp}$ in Fig. 11-14) and the effective g factors (from the center points of the effective hyperfine multiplets). As the distance between the nitroxide moiety and the polar head group of labels XXXIII(m, n) increased, the ESR spectra indicated that the motions of the spin labels were becoming more isotropic. This indicated that the phospholipid bilayers were more rigid near the polar head groups than they were in the pure lipid region.

Barratt et al. have used the ESR spectrum of the dinitrophenylnitroxide XXVIII to study the phase behavior of dipalmitoyl lecithin-water mixtures (116). This correlation time τ for the label provided an estimate of the fluidity of the dipalmitoyl lecithin region. A discontinuous change in τ occurred at the chain-melting temperature of the phospholipids, but its magnitude was much less than that expected if the label were present in a pure lipid environment. This led the authors to propose that the labels were located partly in the polar-head group region of the phospholipid layers and partly in the hydrocarbon region. Increasing the amount of water in the mixture up to 30 percent resulted in increased mobility for the spin labels; thereafter added water had no effect. This is consistent with the view that, up to about 40 percent water, all water is associated with phospholipid and therefore only above 40 percent does a free water phase appear (117). Addition of cholesterol to mixtures of dioleoyl lecithin containing XXVIII caused a reduction in spin label mobility (116).

11.2.2.3 Oriented Lipid Films

Another useful model membrane system consists of stacks of phospholipid bilayers deposited on a flat plate. This system is similar to liposomes in many ways but has the advantage of lamellar symmetry. Libertini et al. have reported that spin labels I and II (see Section 11.1.2) may be incorporated into films of egg lecithin deposited on glass slides (118). Hyperfine splitting patterns of three rather narrow lines were observed; the separations between the lines depended on the angle between the applied magnetic field and the plane of the lecithin film. The hyperfine splitting varied with this angle by as much as 12 G for label I and 10 G for label II (similar to the spectra in Fig. 11-15*b*). The degree of angular-dependence decreased as the temperature of the film increased, in a reversible fashion. The data indicated that the spin labels had preferred orientations with respect to the plane of the lipid films. Analysis of the angular variation of the observed splittings for both I and II indicated that they were located in the films with their long axes assembled roughly in a direction perpen-

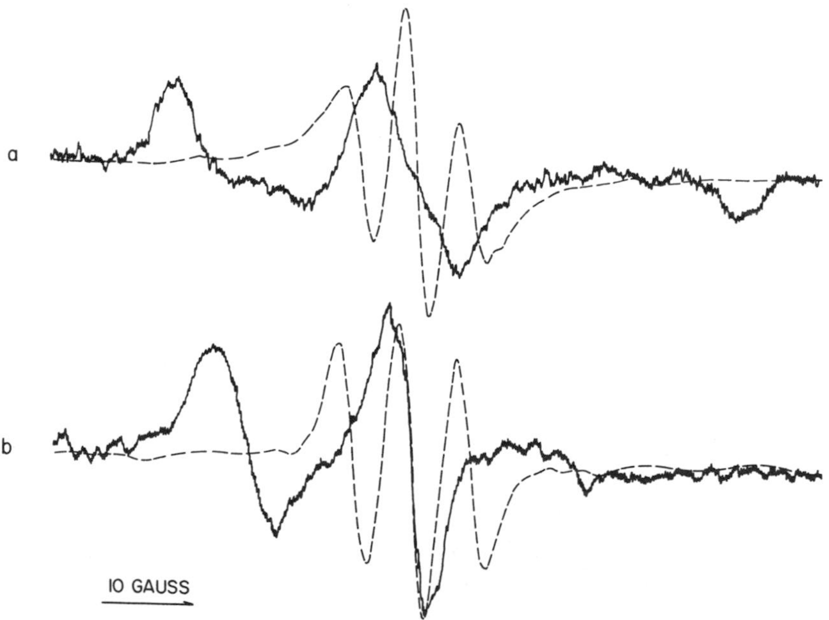

Fig. 11-15 ESR spectra of the cholestane spin label I in lipid films of cholesterol: lecithin ratio 2:1. The solid and dotted spectra were obtained with the magnetic field parallel and perpendicular to the plane of the film, respectively. (a) Dry film, (b) in the presence of an aqueous salt solution (119).

dicular to the plane of the film (see Fig. 11-16), suggesting that the phospholipids in the films were highly organized, with the long hydrocarbon chains perpendicular to the plane of the film. In no case was the maximum component of the hyperfine coupling tensor observed; the maximum detectable splittings were approximately 20 G. This suggested that the long axes of the spin labels were not completely fixed perpendicular to the plane and had some motion relative to this direction. In the case of the cholestane label I it appeared that the motion was rotation around the long axis of the steroid backbone.

Hsia, Schneider, and Smith have studied the influence of cholesterol and water on oriented egg lecithin layers containing label I (119). With perfectly dry lecithin films no preferred orientation of the spin label was observed; the ESR spectra were independent of the angle between the magnetic field and the plane of the film and were indicative of an isotropically tumbling spin label. Exposure of the films to an aqueous salt solution resulted in orientation of the spin label and angular-dependent

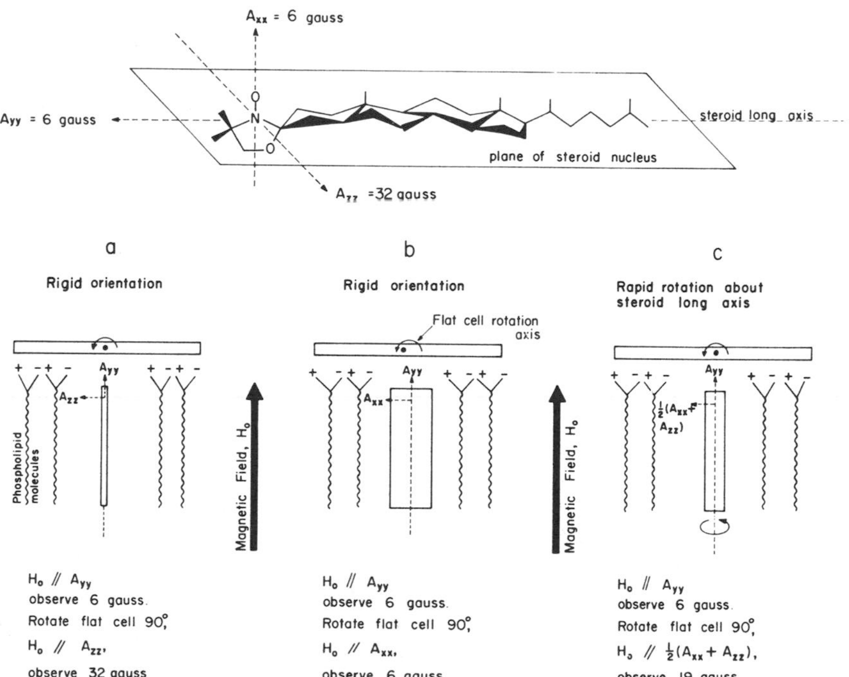

Fig. 11-16 Schematic representation of possible orientations and the corresponding ESR hyperfine splittings of the cholestane spin label I in films of egg lecithin. In (a), (b), and (c) the steroid backbone is represented as a plane (154).

spectra similar to those of Libertini et al. (118). The maximum and minimum hyperfine splittings observed were 16.5 G and 9.5 G, respectively. These deviate from the values of 32 and 6 G expected for complete immobilization and orientation of the label or 19 and 6 G expected for complete orientation of the long axis of the cholestane label, with rapid rotation about this axis to average A_{xx} and A_{zz} [$\frac{1}{2}(A_{xx} + A_{zz}) = 19$ G]. The deviations indicate that complete orientation of the long axis had not been achieved and/or more complicated types of motion were occurring. When the lecithin films contained cholesterol, however, the behavior was entirely different, (Fig. 11-15). For the perfectly dry film containing cholesterol at lecithin:cholesterol ratios of 1:2, maximum and minimum splittings of 32 and 6 G were observed, which indicated perfect orientation of the spin label and suggested a rigid and highly organized structure for the film. Exposing the cholesterol-containing film to aqueous salt solution resulted in maximum and minimum hyperfine splittings of 19 and 6.5 G, respectively. This demonstrated that in the presence of an aqueous phase the cholesterol-containing films are still highly organized, such that the long axis of the cholestane spin label is oriented perpendicular to the plane of the film, but sufficiently fluid that rotation about the long steroid axis of I can take place at a rate greater than the frequency difference between A_{zz} and A_{xx}, i.e., > 73 MHz. A schematic representation of the behavior of I in films of oriented lipids is given in Fig. 11-16. More recently the same authors have studied the effect of cholesterol in greater detail and found that it also occurs at much lower cholesterol:lecithin ratios (120). The ordering effect was analyzed in terms of the spin labels' being effectively oriented about a cone, the axis of which was perpendicular to the plane of the films. Increasing cholesterol concentration resulted in a decreased solid angle contained by the cone. The highest degree of orientation, corresponding to a deviation of the spin label long axis from perpendicularity by $10 \pm 3°$, was observed at 25 mole percent cholesterol. Between 25 and 50 mole percent the degree of order was constant. These results pointed very strongly to a possible role for cholesterol in membrane structure—to affect the order and fluidity of the phospholipids. More detailed analyses of the cholesterol effect for this (153) and other lipid systems (125, 154, 159) have appeared recently. A detailed theoretical treatment of these types of spectrum has been presented by Lapper et al. (153) and Jost et al. (155).

Further insight into the role of cholesterol comes from a study by Butler et al. on the nature of steroids which can effect order in spin-labeled multi-bilayers of the lipids from bovine brain (125). A planar steroid nucleus and an hydroxyl group in the 3β position were necessary for ordering; the hydrocarbon tail at position 17 was not essential but did increase the ordering effect. The degree of order induced by the various sterols paralleled their influence on membrane permeability and the growth of sterol-requiring organisms.

In a separate study Butler et al. have demonstrated that the concentration and nature of ions in the hydrating solution can have a profound effect on the degree of order of phospholipids in multibilayer films (121). The greater the charge of a cation, the greater the degree of order it induced in bovine brain lipids. These data are consistent with the view that ion-induced changes in membrane structure are crucial to some membrane processes (147).

Also in the bovine lipid system, it has been shown recently that although low concentrations of cholesterol ($<$ 50 percent) can induce ordering higher concentrations decrease the degree of order (148). The effects of antibiotics which increase the permeability of membranes to ions were studied. The data revealed complex behavior that depended on the nature of the antibiotic and on whether cholesterol was present. Local and general anesthetics were found to cause effects on ordering and motional freedom. These effects were correlated with the biological influence of the compounds.

Recently Verma et al. have shown that light-sensitive agents such as retinal and chlorophyll can cause changes in the organization of phospholipid films (149). On absorption of visible light a decrease in order was observed. The spin label also served as a detector of liberated electrons, its ESR signal decreasing steadily on prolonged irradiation in the presence of the light sensitive compounds. Similar effects were found in the rod outer segments from bovine retina (156).

Thus it appears that the oriented film technique will become increasingly important in studying the molecular mechanism of membrane processes associated with lipid organization. Combined with results from studies of spin-labeled liposomes, the data should provide a firm foundation for understanding the more complex spectra found in spin-labeled biological membranes.

11.2.2.4 Biological Membranes

The labeling of protein components of biological membranes such as red blood cell ghosts and sarcoplasmic reticulum was covered in Section 11.2.1.5. It is much more difficult to label covalently and specifically the lipid components of natural membranes. This difficulty can be circumvented by preparation of a spin label that resembles strongly the natural lipid components and introduction of the spin label into the membrane. The spin label would then be held in the membrane by the same noncovalent forces that bind together the natural lipids. Transfer of the spin label to the membrane has been accomplished in two ways: biosynthetically, by culturing an organism on media containing essential components which have already been spin-labeled; and physically by making use of the highest solubility of the lipidlike spin labels in environments most similar to themselves.

Keith, Waggoner, and Griffith (122) initiated the biosynthetic incorporation technique by growing the mold *Neurospora crassa* in media containing 10^{-4} *M* spin-labeled methyl stearate XXXI. No inhibition of growth by the spin label was detected. After 72 hr of growth less than 5 percent of the spin label was left in the medium. The mitochondria were isolated and their lipids separated into phospholipids, free fatty acids, and neutral lipids. Spin label XXXI was detected unchanged in the mitochondrial lipids by gas chromatography. The phospholipids contained approximately 2 percent spin-labeled hydrocarbon chains, presumed to have resulted from incorporation of XXXI into phospholipids such as the phosphatidyl ethanolamines. The ESR spectrum of the spin-labeled mitochondria contained at least two subspectra due to incorporated spin labels with different degrees of constraint; no subspectrum corresponding to a strongly immobilized spin label was present.

Tourtellotte, Branton, and Keith (127) have cultured *Mycoplasma laidlawii* on a medium containing spin-labeled stearic acid, XXXIII(6, 11). This organism is known to incorporate fatty acids from the medium into its phospholipids and glycolipids. Analysis of the lipids extracted from cells grown on media containing the spin label showed that XXXIII(6, 11) had been incorporated only into the polar lipid fraction. No unmodified spin label was detected. The ESR spectra of the spin-labeled cells were indicative of a high degree of isotropic spin label motion. The apparent frequency of the motion (determined from the correlation times, calculated as in Section 11.1.3.2) depended on the nature of the fatty acids in the growth medium; the spin label had a greater mobility in cells grown on oleate-rich media than it had in cells grown on stearate-rich media. The hyperfine coupling constant was approximately 14.2 G, indicating that the nitroxide moiety had a hydrophobic environment. Graphs of log τ versus $1/T$ gave straight lines over the temperature range 20 to 60 C, from which energies of activation could be calculated. The effects of temperature were completely reversible and apparently independent of the protein denaturation occurring at higher temperatures. This behavior and the slight difference between the ESR spectra of XXXIII(6, 11) in the intact membrane and in suspensions of extracted lipids, was taken as evidence for a weak protein-lipid interaction in the intact membranes.

Stanacev et al. have shown recently that spin label XXXIII(5, 10) can be incorporated biosynthetically into phosphatidic acid by the microsomal fraction of guinea pig liver (157), the first mammalian system to be studied by this technique.

The biosynthetic incorporation technique should prove to be even more valuable in the future as a probe of the membranes of living cells. The spectra of different spin labels, such as the various combinations for XXXIII(m, n), must be investigated to determine whether the conclusions are valid for large or small portions of the total membrane structure.

In attempting to incorporate spin-labeled compounds into membranes or liposomes by diffusion and preferential solubility, one is often hampered by the very low solubility of the lipidlike labels in the aqueous media surrounding the membranes. Hubbell and McConnell got around this difficulty by using a protein carrier for the spin label (114). For experiments with micelles or liposomes the label can usually be incorporated by agitation or sonication of the aqueous suspension (33, 110, 116).

Spin label XXXII has been introduced into the lipid regions of rabbit vagus nerve, the walking leg nerve of Maine lobster, and frog skeletal muscle (113). It could not be forced into membranes of human erythrocytes, glycerinated muscle fibers, or the mitochondrial membranes of *Neurospora crassa*. Failure in the latter cases was attributed to much stiffer lipid structures. When incorporation was successful, the ESR spectra were like Fig. 11-13. This type of spectrum and the effects of various agents thought to affect membranes, was discussed in Section 11.2.2.2. It was concluded that the low viscosity hydrophobic regions of the excitable membranes were very similar to those in liposomes and that agents such as tetracaine, cholesterol, and gramicidin S intercalated in the membranes to alter the ordering of the hydrophobic regions and thus change the volume available for incorporation of XXXII.

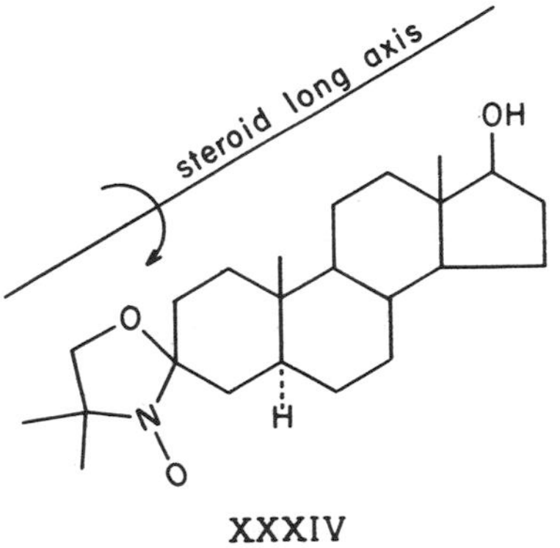

steroid long axis

OH

O

N

O

H

XXXIV

Steroid spin labels have been used to study the unmyelinated walking leg nerve fibers of the Maine lobster (114). One such label is the N-oxyl-4′,4′-dimethyloxazolidine derivative of 5α-androstan-3-one-17β-ol, XXXIV. In the nerve fiber label XXXIV had the ESR spectrum shown in Fig. 11-17a. The separation between the two outer hyperfine lines (indicated by the arrows) is 37 G. The shape and separation of the hyperfine lines

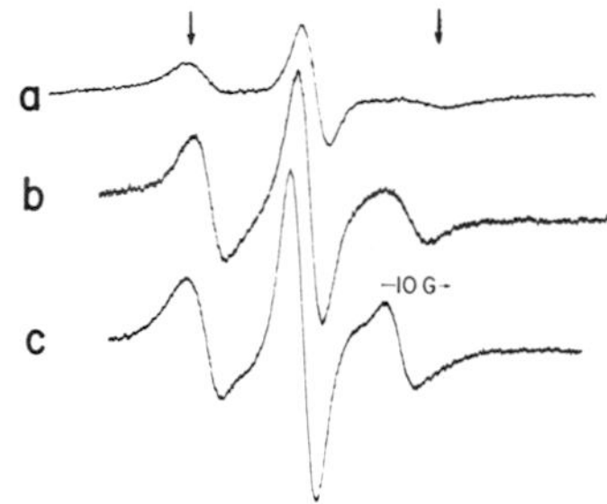

Fig. 11-17 ESR spectra of steroid spin labels in the walking-leg nerve of the Maine lobster (113). The spin labels were the *N*-oxyl-4′-4′-dimethyl-oxazolidine derivatives of (a) 5α-androstan-3-one-17β-ol, XXXIV, (b) 5β-androstan-3-one-17β-ol, and (c) 5α-androstan-3-one.

indicate rapid anisotropic motion about the long axis of the steroid backbone which results in rotational averaging of some tensor components and effective parameters for the spin Hamiltonian as follows: perpendicular to the steroid long axis $A'_{\perp} = \frac{1}{2}(A_{xx} + A_{zz}) = 18.5$ G, $g'_{\perp} = \frac{1}{2}(g_{xx} + g_{zz}) = 2.006$; parallel to the steroid long axis $A'_{\parallel} = A_{yy} = 6$ G, $g'_{\parallel} = g_{yy} = 2.006$. The effective axial symmetry of the g tensor thus causes the two extreme hyperfine lines of the pseudo-powder spectrum* to be symmetrically located about the center line, in contrast to the usual powder spectrum (Fig. 11-3), where g-tensor anisotropy produces an unsymmetrical displacement of the extreme lines. Such anisotropic motion was not detectable with the 5β isomer of XXXIV (Fig. 11-17*b*), which lacks the cylindrical shape of XXXIV, or with the spin label derived from 5α-androstan-3-one (Fig. 11-17*c*) which differs from XXXIV only in the absence of an hydroxyl group at position 17.† Hubbell and McConnell concluded that XXXIV could undergo anisotropic motion because (a) its cylindrical shape resulted in very little resistance to motion about the long steroid axis; (b) the presence of an hydroxyl group at position 17 resulted in that section of the steroid molecule being located in the polar head group region of the membrane, which they assumed formed a rigid "floor" to which the hydroxyl group was anchored. In contrast, the ESR spectra of phosphatidyl serine liposomes containing XXXIV showed no evidence of a high degree of rotational anisotropy; this was attributed to a lack of rigidity in the polar-head group region of the liposomes.

It is interesting to compare these data with those for the cholestane spin

* The nerve has cylindrical symmetry and the magnetic field is perpendicular to the cylinder axis. Thus, even if all spin labels had their long axes perpendicular to the cylinder surface, these long axes are still randomly oriented with respect to the applied magnetic field.

† McConnell has emphasized that rapid anisotropic spin label motion is most easily detected when the axis of the motion is perpendicular to the z axis (the p_{π} orbital), such as apparently occurs in this case (114). If the axis of rapid anisotropic motion made an angle of 54° with the z axis, a spectrum similar to that of an isotropically rotating spin label (Fig. 11-17*b*) would result.

label I in lecithin liposomes (Section 11.2.2.2) and in oriented films of lecithin (Section 11.2.2.3). In the liposomes the ESR spectra indicate some rotational anisotropy (Fig. 11-12*a*); in the films complete rotational anisotropy was observed (Fig. 11-15*b*). The cholestane spin label differs from the two androstane spin labels which did not rotate anisotropically by the presence of the hydrocarbon tail at position 17. This tail is apparently responsible in part for the higher degree of order achieved by the cholestane spin label. It also would appear that in the cholestane derivative the spin-labeled end is located in the polar regions of the liposomes and films in contrast to the androstane derivative XXXIV.

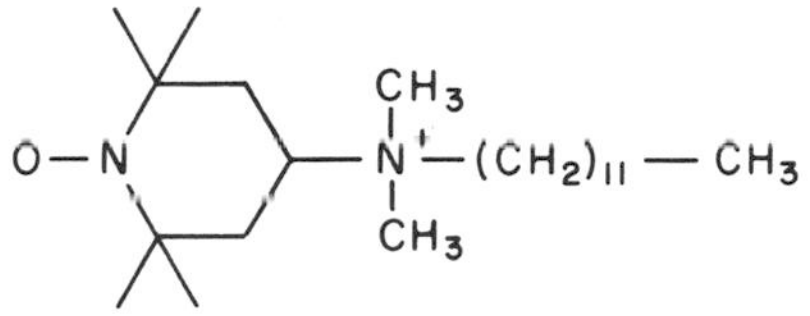

XXXV

Hubbell and McConnell demonstrated that the nitroxide moiety of label XXXIV was buried in the hydrocarbon regions of the nerve by measuring the rate of reduction of the nitroxide by sodium ascorbate in the bathing solution. With both minced and intact nerves, the rate of reduction was very slow compared with that of the label in the bathing solution. In contrast, spin label XXXV, whose nitroxide group is expected to lie in the polar region of the nerve, was rapidly reduced by ascorbate (114).

The amphiphilic spin labels XXXIII(m, n) have also been studied in the leg nerve fiber of the Maine lobster (115). The ESR spectrum of a suspension of minced nerve containing XXXIII(17, 3) is shown in Fig. 11-18*a*. It is much like the spectrum of XXXIII(17, 3) in liposomes of soybean phosphatides (Fig. 11-15), but with somewhat broader lines. This indicates that the label is undergoing anisotropic rotation of the type discussed in

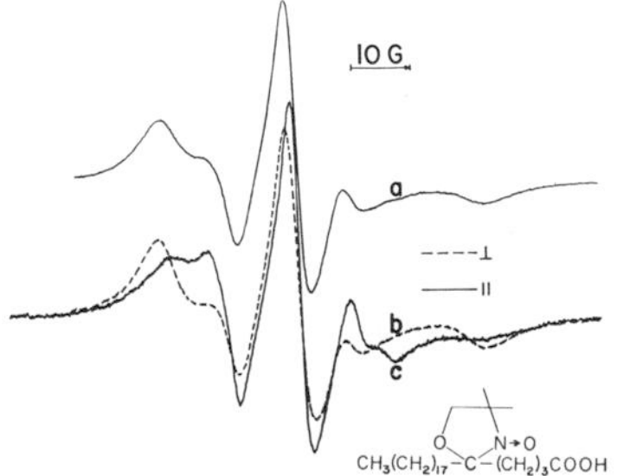

Fig. 11-18 ESR spectrum of spin label XXXIII (3, 17) in the walking-leg nerve fiber of the Maine lobster (115): (a) minced nerve, (b) magnetic field perpendicular to nerve cylindrical axis, (c) magnetic field parallel to nerve cylindrical axis.

Sections 11.2.2.2 and 11.2.2.3. When the intact nerve fibers were oriented with their fiber axes parallel and perpendicular to the applied magnetic field, the spectra of Fig. 11-18*b* and *c* resulted. It is possible in both cases to discern spectra due to spin labels experiencing the applied magnetic field parallel (outer hyperfine lines) and perpendicular (inner hyperfine lines) to the axis about which the rapid anisotropic motion is occurring. The relative intensities of these two subspectra depended on the orientation of the fiber axis relative to the applied magnetic field. Analysis of the relative intensities of the two subspectra indicated that the spin labels had a 5:1 preference for an orientation with the axis of the rapid anisotropic motion perpendicular to the nerve axis (i.e., the extended hydrocarbon chain of XXXIII(17, 3) perpendicular to the membrane surface) over an orientation in which the axis of motion was parallel to the membrane surface. For labels XXXIII(m, n) increasing the distance between the polar head group and the nitroxide moiety caused a decrease in the observable ESR spectral anisotropy: the nitroxide moiety became increasingly mobile, just as in the liposomes of soybean phosphatides. If the methyl esters of labels XXXIII(m, n) were used instead of the free acids, the mobility of the label was greater, demonstrating the importance of the charged head group in anchoring the label.

Spin label XXXIV in the lobster nerve fibers showed a relatively small ESR spectral anisotropy. Analysis of the angular dependence of the ESR spectra indicated that the preferred orientation of this label was with the long steroid axis perpendicular to the membrane surface (115).

Similar spectral anisotropy was detected in canine erythrocytes containing spin labels XXXIII(5, 10) or XXXIV, oriented by hydrodynamic shear (115). Although the observed degree of orientation of the labels in erythrocytes was not so high as that in nerve fibers, similar conclusions were reached regarding the orientations of the label relative to the membrane surface.

In summary, Hubbell and McConnell concluded that the phospholipid regions of both nerve and erythrocyte membranes strongly resembled lipid bilayers [postulated by Danielli and Davson (123) to be a general feature of membrane structure], with the phospholipids being more tightly packed in the erythrocytes than in the nerve fibers.

Koltover et al. (124) have reported reversible conformational changes in the electron transport particles of bovine heart mitochondria during the oxidation process, in which the intercalated spin label XXX was used. While the particles were oxidizing substrates, such as sodium succinate, the spin label had decreased mobility (a change in τ from 4×10^{-10} to 20×10^{-10} sec). The original mobility was regained on oxidizing the particles.

These data were taken as support for the postulate that conformational changes were involved in the respiratory cycle.

Hsia, Piette, and Noyes have shown that spin-labeled amides of fatty acids, such as VII, can intercalate in rabbit spermatozoa (126). There was no evidence of reduced sperm motility or specific activity due to labeling. It was hoped to use this method to detect and follow sperm in more complex situations.

Submitochondrial membranes have been studied by physical incorporation of spin-labeled cytochrome *c* and the androstan-3-one-17β-ol derivative XXXIV (128). Reversible changes in the mobility of the spin label attached to cytochrome *c* occurred when the metabolic state of the submitochondrial particles was altered.

11.2.2.5 Coenzymes and Inhibitors

A spin-labeled analog of the coenzyme nicotinamide adenine dinucleotide (NAD) has been synthesized and used to study complexes with liver alcohol dehydrogenase (129–131). The spin label XXXVI has a nitroxide moiety

XXXVI

coupled to the diphosphate group of adenosine-5′-diphosphate (ADP). Kinetic studies showed it to be a competitive inhibitor of both liver and yeast alcohol dehydrogenase (129). The ESR spectrum of XXXVI bound to liver alcohol dehydrogenase was indicative of a high degree of immobilization, and thus the spectra of free and bound labels could be distinguished. The decrease in intensity of the ESR spectrum due to free label, caused by addition of the enzyme, was used to determine the dissociation constant and number of binding sites involved in the complex. Evidence was found for both specific and nonspecific binding to the enzyme. Mildvan and Weiner studied the effect of the paramagnetic complex on the NMR relaxation times of water in the active site (130, 131; see Section 11.2.4).

Analogs of vitamin B_{12} have been synthesized by reaction of a bromoacetamide-nitroxide with cob(I)alamin, XXXVII, and by replacement of one coordinated water molecule of diaquocobinamide by a nitroxide alcohol, XXXVIII (132). It is hoped that these compounds will bind to proteins in a manner similar to vitamin B_{12} and thus help to elucidate the role of the vitamin as a coenzyme. A spin-labeled triphosphate XXXIX has been shown to act as a cofactor for the removal of oxygen from hemoglobin (5, 133) in a manner similar to that observed for 2,3-diphosphoglyceric acid. The monophosphate ester XXXX, an analog of the phosphate inhibitors of ribonuclease A, has been found to bind to the active site of the enzyme (134; see Section 11.2.4).

Protohemin has been labeled at porphyrin ring positions 6 and 7 by reaction with spin label VIII (101, 136). On combination with apocytochrome *c* peroxidase the spin labels on protohemin became highly constrained. The degree of constraint was sensitive to the nature of the heme

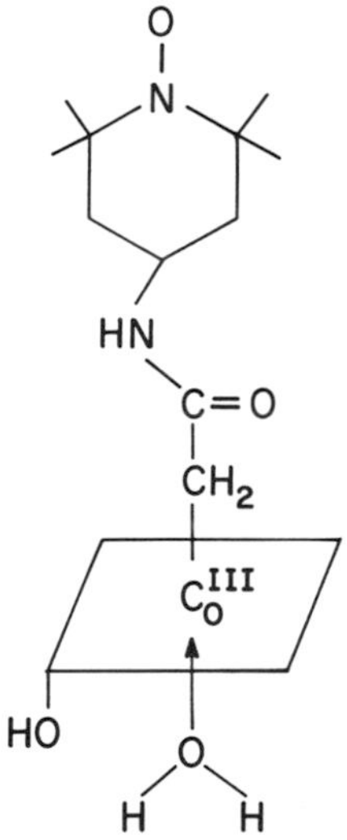

XXXVII

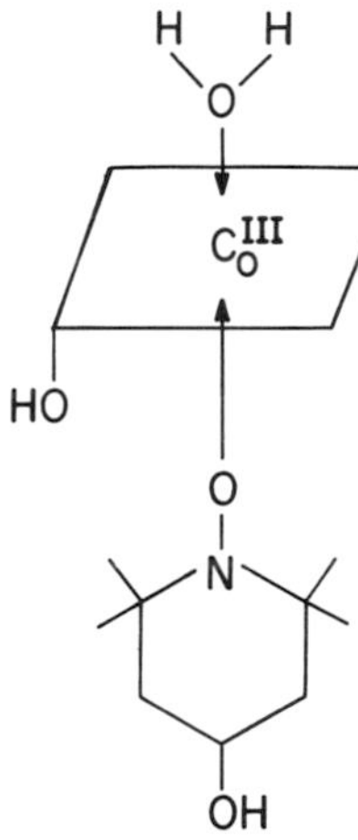

XXXVIII

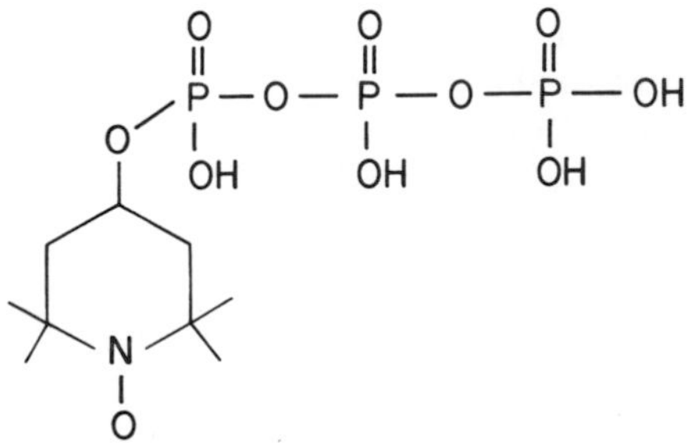

XXXIX

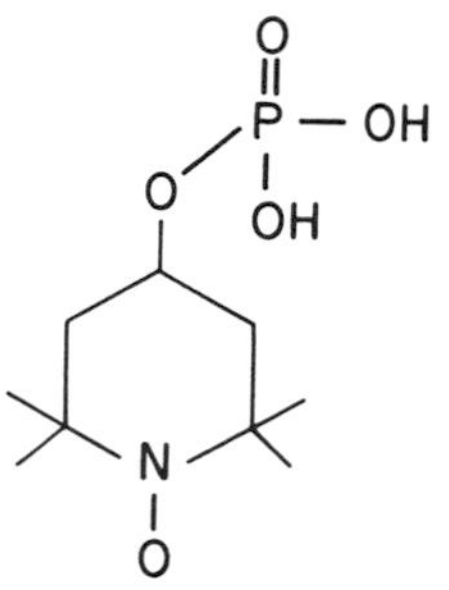

XXXX

ligands. It was inferred that the heme-protein interaction was altered by ligand binding. The synthetic enzyme had optical properties similar to those of the native enzyme, but only 1 percent of the enzymic activity. This is consistent with other work which had demonstrated the importance of unmodified side chains at positions 6 and 7 for retention of enzymic activity (135). In contrast, the ESR spectrum of the synthetic enzyme containing heme labeled at positions 2 and 4 of the porphyrin ring demonstrated a spin label mobility higher than in the other derivative (136). This led the authors to propose that the 6 and 7 positions of the porphyrin ring were directed inwards toward the protein binding site, whereas positions 2 and 4 were pointing outward (136).

11.2.3 Biradical Spin Labels

11.2.3.1 ESR Spectra of Biradical Spin Labels

Biradical spin labels are those containing two nitroxide groups. If the two nitroxides do not interact with one another, the ESR spectrum of the biradical will be simply a superposition of the two nitroxide spectra. If the two nitroxides are close enough, however, electron exchange between them can occur, and the spin states of the two unpaired electrons become correlated. In the limit of strong exchange the two nitroxide groups will behave as a triplet spin species (total electron spin = 1), and new hyperfine lines will be manifest in the composite ESR spectrum. If the two nitroxide moieties are identical and have isotropic hyperfine splittings A_0, the new lines will appear in the ESR spectrum at $\pm A_0/2$ G. In the limit of strong exchange the spectrum will contain five lines, separated by $A_0/2$ G, of relative intensities 1:2:3:2:1.

Two mechanisms for the exchange interaction between the two nitroxide moieties are possible: an indirect polarization mechanism through the bonds connecting the nitroxides or a direct coupling through space

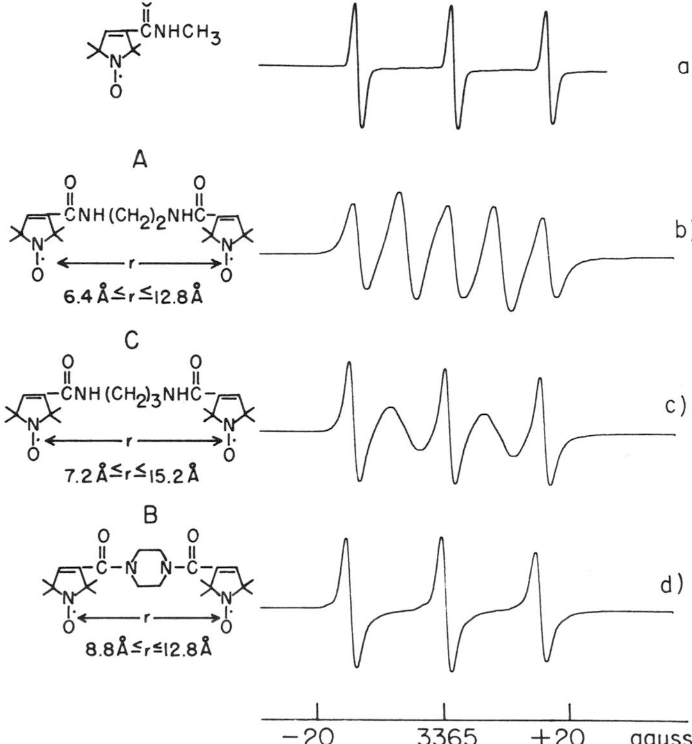

Fig. 11-19 ESR spectra of (a) a doublet nitroxide radical, (b-d) biradicals with increasingly large separation of the nitroxide moieties (142).

when the nitroxides are sufficiently close. The former mechanism undoubtedly operates if the nitroxides are separated by only a few bonds, but an increasing volume of evidence points to the latter mechanism being important in almost all cases (137–141). Figure 11-19 demonstrates the dependence of the electron exchange between nitroxide moieties on the distance separating them. Biradical A exhibits fairly strong exchange, since the spectrum approaches the intensity distribution 1:2:3:2:1; biradical C exhibits much weaker exchange, as shown by the decreased intensity of the second and fourth hyperfine lines; biradical B, with a minimum nitroxide separation of 8.8 Å, exhibits no electron exchange in its ESR spectrum. Thus, since the ESR spectra of biradicals depend strongly on the relative orientations and separations between the component nitroxides, they should be sensitive indicators of conformational changes in their immediate environment. The ESR spectra, of course, are also dependent on the rate of tumbling of the biradicals in solution, and thus the same line-broadening effects observed with doublet spin labels will be present. A further complication is that the spectral lineshape may depend also on the rate of modulation of the interaction between the two radical components. Thus Luckhurst and Pedulli have pointed out that spectra such as those in Fig. 11-19*b-d* could arise from a varying rate of modulation as well as from a decreased exchange interaction (150). A detailed description of linewidth effects arising from slow motions of biradicals, when modulation of the exchange interaction does not dominate the relaxation processes, is given in (151).

The foregoing demonstrates that interpretation of the ESR spectra of biradical spin labels is very difficult. A complete theoretical description of their relaxation behavior is lacking. For the present, at least, this makes them less desirable as spin labels. Nevertheless, several applications have already been reported (14, 80, 142).

11.2.3.2 Applications of Biradical Spin Labels

The isomeric biradical dinitrophenyl haptens XXXXI have been prepared (14). When bound to antidinitrophenyl antibodies, the ESR spectrum of XXXXI was a broad envelope, indicative of complete immobilization of the label. Calvin et al. have studied the ESR spectrum of biradical A (Fig. 11-19)

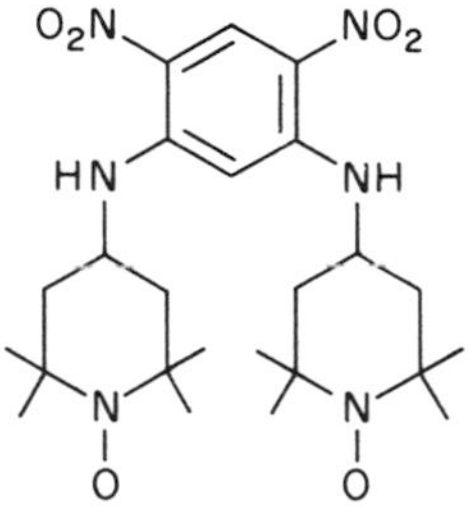

O_2N NO_2 HN NH N O N O

XXXXI

in lobster walking nerves (142). Surprisingly, the ESR spectrum in the nerve was almost that of a completely uncoupled biradical, in contrast to the spectrum in water at room temperature (Fig. 11-19). The ESR lines were very narrow, indicative of a rapid tumbling rate for the constituent nitroxides. Attempts to observe changes in the ESR spectrum during electrical excitation of the nerve were unsuccessful. Hsia, Kosman, and Piette have reported a fluorophosphate diester (similar to XXV; Section 11.2.1.3) in which both ester groups are nitroxides (80). The ESR spectrum of α-chymotrypsin inactivated by this label was composed of broad lines, but six individual components could be distinguished. Inactivation of cholinesterase by this label gave an ESR spectrum of narrow lines that exhibited intermediate coupling between the nitroxide moieties. These studies serve to demonstrate the versatility of the biradical spin-labeling technique, and it is likely that valuable applications of it will be made in the near future.

11.2.4 Nuclear Relaxation by Spin Labels

Because of the large magnetic moment associated with an unpaired electron, free radicals can cause enhanced relaxation of magnetic nuclei. The effect depends strongly on the separation between the unpaired electron and the nucleus. Thus a spin label attached to a biological molecule will in general broaden the magnetic resonances of all nuclei in proximity. This broadening can be useful in determining the distance between a spin label and various groups on the biological molecule or in assigning particular lines in complicated nuclear resonance spectra to molecular components in the vicinity of the attached spin label. First attempts at this were made by Sternlicht and Wheeler (143) and McConnell, Smith, and Bhacca (144), using nonspecific *N*-ethylmaleimide and bromoacetamide analogs. A general broadening of the proton resonances of lysozyme (143, 144). ribonuclease (144), bovine serum albumin (144), α-chymotrypsin (144), and hemoglobin (144) were observed, but no detailed analysis of the effects could be given. Roberts et al. have used the spin-labelled phosphate XXXX to perturb the NMR spectrum of ribonuclease A (134). Appreciable broadening of the proton resonances previously assigned to histidines −12 and −119 were observed, thus confirming that the phosphate was binding to the active site region of the enzyme. Broadening of the resonance assigned to histidine —12 was somewhat greater, implying that the nitroxide could approach this amino acid more closely than it could histidine —119.

Mildvan and Weiner have studied the influence of a spin-labeled analog of nicotinamide-adenine dinucleotide XXXVI (Section 11.2.2.5), bound to alcohol dehydrogenase, on the proton relaxation rate of water (130, 131). The data indicated two tight and six weak binding sites on the protein for the spin label; an interaction between the binding sites was detected (130). Studies of the ternary complexes formed between the spin label, the enzyme, and any one of ethanol, acetaldehyde, and isobutyramide resulted in models for the complexes (131).

This combination of NMR and ESR techniques appears to have a high potential for biological problems. The crucial requirements are that the spin label must resemble closely a natural component of the system, and the location of the spin label on the biological molecule must be known.

11.3 CONCLUSION

In conclusion it remains only to emphasize the extreme versatility of the spin label technique and the care which must be taken in interpreting the spectra and ensuring that the perturbations caused by the spin label are sufficiently small to produce relevancy of the results to the natural system. It is fitting to acknowledge here the manifold contributions of Professor Harden M. McConnell to this field. Without his efforts this chapter would have contained very little. It is a pleasure also to acknowledge the many authors who submitted preprints before publication and who permitted me to use their figures and diagrams. Doctors Shirley Mucillo, Hermann Dugas, Larry Berliner, and Hayes Griffith were very helpful in reading and criticizing the manuscript.

REFERENCES

1. S. Ohnishi and H. McConnell, *J. Am. Chem. Soc.*, **87**, 2293 (1965)
2. T. Stone, T. Buckman, P. Nordio and H. McConnell, *Proc. Natl. Acad. Sci.*, **54**, 1010 (1965).
3. C. Hamilton and H. McConnell in *Structural Chemistry and Molecular Biology*, A. Rich and N. Davidson, Eds., Freeman, San Francisco, 1968, p. 115.
4. O. Griffith and A. Waggoner, *Acc. Chem. Res.*, **2**, 17 (1969).
5. H. McConnell and B. McFarland, *Quart. Rev. Biophys.*, **3**, 91 (1970).
6. A. Forrester, J. Hay, and R. Thomson, *Organic Chemistry of Stable Free Radicals*, Academic London, 1968, p. 180.
7. H. Fisher, *Magnetic Properties of Free Radicals*, K. Hellwege and A. Hellwege, Eds., Springer, Berlin, 1967.
8. B. Bielski and J. Gebicki, *Atlas of Electron Spin Resonance Spectra*, Academic, New York, 1967.
9. J. Hsia, D. Kosman, and L. Piette, *Biochem. Biophys. Res. Commun.*, **36**, 75 (1969).
10. E. Rosantzev and M. Neimann, *Tetrahedron*, **20**, 131 (1964).
11. E. Rosantzev, *Izv. Akad. Nauk. SSSR, Ser. Khim.*, 2187 (1964).
12. This and other spin labels are commercially available from Syva, Palo Alto, California.
13. L. Krinitskaya, E. Rosantzev and M. Neimann, 1965, *ibid.*, 115.
14. J. Hsia and L. Piette, *Arch. Biochim. Biophys.*, **129**, 296 (1969).
15. L. Berliner and H. McConnell, *Proc. Natl. Acad. Sci.*, **55**, 708 (1966).
16. H. McConnell and C. Hamilton, *ibid.*, 776 (1968).
17. E. Rosantzev and Yu. Kokhanov, *Izv. Akad. Nauk. SSSR, Ser. Khim.*, **8**, 1477 (1966).
18. E. Rosantzev, *Free Nitroxyl Radicals*, Plenum, New York, 1970.
19. S. Ogawa and H. McConnell, *Proc. Natl. Acad. Sci.*, **58**, 19 (1967).
20. E. Rosantzev and L. Krinitzkaya, *Tetrahedron*, **21**, 491 (1965).
21. B. McFarland (unpublished).
22. S. Ohnishi, J. Boeyens, and H. McConnell, *Proc. Natl. Acad. Sci.*, **56**, 809 (1966).
23. O. Griffith and H. McConnell, *Proc. Natl. Acad. Sci.*, **55**, 8 (1966).
24. J. Keana, S. Keana, and D. Beetham, *J. Am. Chem. Soc.*, **89**, 3055 (1967).

25. A. Waggoner, T. Kingzett, S. Rottschaefer, O. Griffith, and A. Keith, *Chem. Phys. Lipids*, **3,** 245 (1969).
26. J. Osiecki and E. Ullman, *J. Am. Chem. Soc.*, **90,** 1078 (1968).
27. D. Boocock, R. Darcy, and E. Ullman, *J. Am. Chem. Soc.*, **90,** 5945 (1968).
28. A. Carrington and A. McLachlan, *Introduction to Magnetic Resonance,* Harper and Row, New York, 1967.
29. A. Carrington and H. Longuet-Higgins, *Mol. Phys.*, **5,** 447 (1962).
30. O. Griffith, D. Cornell, and H. McConnell, *J. Chem. Phys.*, **43,** 2909 (1965).
31. W. Hubbell and H. McConnell, *Proc. Natl. Acad. Sci.*, **64,** 20 (1969).
32. R. Briere, H. Lemaire, and A. Rassat, *Bull. Soc. Chim. France,* **11,** 3273 (1965).
33. J. Hsia, H. Schneider, and I. Smith, *Chem. Phys. Lipids*, **4,** 120 (1970).
34. D. Kosman and L. Piette, *Chem. Comm.*, 926 (1969).
35. H. McConnell, S. Ogawa, and I. Smith (unpublished results).
36. A. Hudson and G. Luckhurst, *Chem. Rev.*, **69,** 191 (1969).
37. H. McConnell, *J. Chem. Phys.*, **25,** 709 (1956).
38. D. Kivelson, *J. Chem. Phys.*, **33,** 1094 (1960).
39. J. Freed and G. Fraenkel, *J. Chem. Phys.*, **39,** 326 (1963).
40. B. Hoffman, P. Schofield, and A. Rich, *Proc. Natl. Acad. Sci.*, **62,** 1195 (1969).
41. I. Smith and T. Yamane, *Proc. Natl. Acad. Sci.*, **58,** 884 (1967).
42. I. Smith and T. Yamane in *Recent Developments of Magnetic Resonance in Biological Systems,* S. Fujiwara, Ed., Hirokawa. Tokyo, 1968, p. 95.
43. I. Smith, *Biochem.*, **7,** 745 (1968).
44. M. Itzkowitz, Ph.D. Thesis, California Institute of Technology (1967).
45. M. Itzkowitz, *J. Chem. Phys.*, **46,** 3048 (1967).
46. L. Stryer and O. Griffith, *Proc. Natl. Acad. Sci.*, **54,** 1785 (1965).
47. J. Hyde, L. Eriksson, and A. Ehrenberg, *Biochim. Biophys. Acta*, **222,** 688 (1970).
48. D. Stone, S. Provost, and J. Botts, *Biochem.*, **9,** 3937 (1970).
49. R. Cooke and M. Morales, *Biochem.*, **8,** 3188 (1969).
50. H. Sandberg and L. Piette, *Agressologie*, **9,** 59 (1968).
51. A. Hoffman and A. Henderson, *J. Amer. Chem. Soc.*, **83,** 4671 (1961).
52. E. Rozantzev, V. Golubev, and M. Neimann, *Izv. Akad. Nauk. SSSR, Ser. Khim.*, 379 (1965).
53. J. Boeyens and H. McConnell, *Proc. Natl. Acad. Sci.*, **56,** 22 (1966).
54. H. McConnell in *Magnetic Resonance in Biological Systems*, A. Ehrenberg, B. G. Malmström, and T. Vänngård, Eds., Pergamon, London, 1967, p. 313.
55. H. McConnell and J. Boeyens, *J. Phys. Chem.*, **71,** 12 (1967).
56. J. Moffat, *J. Mol. Biol.,* **55,** 135 (1971).
57. S. Ogawa, H. McConnell, and A. Horwitz, *Proc. Natl. Acad. Sci.*, **61,** 401 (1968).
58. H. McConnell, S. Ogawa, and A. Horwitz, *Nature*, **220,** 787 (1968).
59. H. McConnell, W. Deal, and R. Ogata, *Biochem.*, **8,** 2580 (1969).
60. S. Ogawa and H. McConnell in *Recent Developments of Magnetic Resonance in Biological Systems,* S. Fujiwara and L. Piette, Eds., Hirokawa, Tokyo, 1968, p. 88.
61. S. Ohnishi, T. Maeda, T. Ito, K. Hwang, and I. Tyuma, *ibid.*, p. 83.

62. S. Ohnishi, T. Maeda, T. Ito, K. Hwang, and I. Tyuma, *Biochem.*, **7,** 2662 (1968).
63. G. Likhtenshtein, P. Bobodzhanov, E. Rozantzev, and V. Suskina, *Molecular Biology* (USSR), **2,** 280 (1968).
64. J. Monod, J. Wyman, and J.-P. Changeux, *J. Mol. Biol.*, **12,** 88 (1965).
65. D. Koshland, G. Némethy, and D. Filmer, *Biochem.*, **5,** 365 (1966).
66. R. Shulman, S. Ogawa, K. Wüthrich, T. Yamane, J. Peisach, and W. Blumberg, *Science*, **165,** 251 (1969).
67. M. Perutz and F. Matthews, *J. Mol. Biol.*, **21,** 199 (1966).
68. W. Bolton, J. Cox, and M. Perutz, *ibid.*, **23,** 283.
69. H. Muirhead, J. Cox, L. Mazzarella, and M. Perutz, *ibid.*, **28,** 117 (1967).
70. H. Schultze and J. Heremans, *Molecular Biology of Human Proteins*, Vol. 1, Elsevier, Amsterdam, 1966.
71. B. Malchy, H. Dugas, F. Ofosu, and I. Smith, *Biochem.* (in press).
72. M. Makinen and H. Kon, *Biochem.* **10,** 43 (1971).
73. H. Hamaguchi, *Am. J. Human Genetics*, **21,** 440 (1969).
74. S. Paterson, H. Dugas, and I. Smith (manuscript in preparation, 1972).
75. J. Morrisett, Ph.D. Thesis, University of North Carolina, 1969.
76. J. Hermans, Jr., and H. Sheraga, *J. Am. Chem. Soc.*, **83,** 3283 (1961).
77. L. Berliner, Ph.D. Thesis, Stanford University, 1967.
78. D. Kosman, J. Hsia, and L. Piette, *Arch. Biochem. Biophys.*, **133,** 29 (1969).
79. D. Kosman and L. Piette in *Magnetic Resonances in Biological Research: An International Conference* (in press).
80. J. Hsia, D. Kosman, and L. Piette, *Biochem. Biophys. Res. Commun.*, **36,** 75 (1969).
81. J. Morrisett, C. Broomfield, and B. Hackley, Jr., *J. Biol. Chem.*, **244,** 5758 (1969).
82. J. Taylor, J. Leigh, Jr., and M. Cohn, *Proc. Natl. Acad. Sci.*, **64,** 219 (1969).
83. G. Likhtenshtein, *Molecular Biology* (*USSR*), **2,** 234 (1968).
84. G. Likhtenshtein and P. Bobodzhanov, *Biophysics* (*USSR*), **5,** 757 (1968).
85. H. Sandberg, R. Bryant, and L. Piette, *Arch. Biochem. Biophys.*, **133,** 144 (1969).
86. D. Holmes and L. Piette, *J. Pharmacol. Exp. Therap.*, **173,** 78 (1970).
87. H. Schneider and I. Smith, *Biochim. Biophys. Acta*, **219,** 73 (1970).
88. H. Schneider and I. Smith, unpublished results.
89. W. Landgraf and G. Inesi, *Arch. Biochem. Biophys.*, **130,** 111 (1969).
90. J. Quinlivan, H. McConnell, L. Stowring, R. Cooke, and M. Morales, *Biochem.*, **8,** 3644 (1969).
91. A. Gotto and H. Kon, *Biochem. Biophys. Res. Commun.*, **37,** 444 (1969).
92. A. Gotto, *Proc. Natl. Acad. Sci.*, **64,** 1119 (1969).
93. W. Martin, H. Dugas, and I. Smith, unpublished results.
94. M. Janado, W. Martin, and W. Cook, *Can. J. Biochem.*, **44,** 1201 (1962).
95. W. Martin (unpublished data).
96. *Structural and Functional Aspects of Lipoproteins in Living Systems*, E. Tria and A. Scanu, Eds., Academic, New York, 1969.
97. B. Hoffman, P. Schofield, and A. Rich, *Proc. Natl. Acad. Sci.*, **62,** 1195 (1969).
98. P. Schofield, B. Hoffman, and A. Rich, *Biochem.*, **9,** 2525 (1970).

99. H. Hara, T. Horiuchi, M. Saneyoshi, and S. Nishimura, *Biochem. Biophys. Res. Commun.*, **38,** 305 (1970).
100. A. Keith, A. Waggoner, and O. Griffith, *Proc. Natl. Acad. Sci.*, **61,** 819 (1968).
101. T. Asakura, H. Drott, and T. Yonetani, *J. Biol. Chem.*, **244,** 6626 (1969).
102. J. Morrisett and H. Drott, *J. Biol. Chem.*, **244,** 5083 (1969).
103. L. Stryer and O. Griffith, *Proc. Natl. Acad. Sci.*, **54,** 1785 (1965).
104. J. Hsia and L. Piette, *Arch. Biochem. Biophys.*, **129,** 296 (1969).
105. J. Hsia and L. Piette, *Arch. Biochem. Biophys.*, **132,** 466 (1969).
106. A. Bangham, *Progr. Biophys. Mol. Biol.*, **18,** 29 (1969).
107. *Biological Membranes*, D. Chapman, Ed., Academic, London, 1968.
108. A. Waggoner, O. Griffith, and C. Christensen, *Proc. Natl. Acad. Sci.*, **57,** 1198 (1967).
109. A. Waggoner, A. Keith, and O. Griffith, *J. Phys. Chem.*, **72,** 4129 (1968).
110. A. Waggoner, T. Kingzett, S. Rottschaefer, and O. Griffith, *Chem. Phys. Lipids*, **3,** 245 (1969).
111. E. Willmer, *Biol. Rev.*, **36,** 368 (1961).
112. D. Chapman and S. Penkett, *Nature*, **211,** 1304 (1966).
113. W. Hubbell and H. McConnell, *Proc. Natl. Acad. Sci.*, **61,** 12 (1968).
114. W. Hubbell and H. McConnell, *Proc. Natl. Acad. Sci.*, **63,** 16 (1969).
115. W. Hubbell and H. McConnell, *Proc. Natl. Acad. Sci.*, **64,** 20 (1969).
116. M. Barratt, D. Green, and D. Chapman, *Chem. Phys. Lipids*, **3,** 140 (1969).
117. D. Chapman, R. Williams, and B. Ladbrooke, *Chem. Phys. Lipids*, **1,** 445 (1967).
118. L. Libertini, A. Waggoner, P. Jost, and O. Griffith, *Proc. Natl. Acad. Sci.*, **64,** 13 (1969).
119. J. Hsia, H. Schneider, and I. Smith, *Biochim. Biophys. Acta*, **202,** 399 (1970).
120. H. Schneider, J. Hsia, and I. Smith, *Can. J. Biochem*, **49,** 614 (1971).
121. K. Butler, H. Dugas, H. Schneider, and I. Smith, *Biochem. Biophys. Res. Commun.*, **40,** 770 (1970).
122. A. Keith, A. Waggoner, and O. Griffith, *Proc. Natl. Acad. Sci.*, **61,** 819 (1968).
123. J. Danielli and H. Davson, *J. Cell. Comp. Physiol.*, **5,** 495 (1935).
124. V. Koltover, M. Goldfield, L. Hendel, and E. Rozantzev, *Biochem. Biophys. Res. Commun.*, **32,** 421 (1968).
125. K. Butler, I. Smith, and H. Schneider, *Biochim. Biophys. Acta*, **219,** 514 (1970).
126. J. Hsia, L. Piette, and R. Noyes, *J. Reprod. Fert.*, **20,** 147 (1969).
127. M. Tourtellotte, D. Branton, and A. Keith, *Proc. Natl. Acad. Sci.*, **66,** 909 (1970).
128. C. Lee, H. Drott, B. Johansson, T. Yonetani, and B. Chance in *Probes of Structure and Function of Macromolecules and Membranes*, B. Chance, C.-P. Lee, and T. Yonetani, Eds., Academic, New York (1971).
129. H. Weiner, *Biochem.*, **8,** 526 (1969).
130. A. Mildvan and H. Weiner, *Biochem.*, **8,** 552 (1969).
131. A. Mildvan and H. Weiner *J. Biol. Chem.*, **244,** 2465 (1969).
132. T. Buckman, F. Kennedy, and J. Wood, *Biochem.*, **8,** 4437 (1969).
133. R. Ogata and H. McConnell (unpublished).
134. G. Roberts, J. Hannah, and O. Jardetsky, *Science*, **165,** 504 (1969).

135. T. Asakura and T. Yonetani, *J. Biol. Chem.*, **244,** 537 (1969).

136. T. Asakura, H. Drott, and T. Yonetani in *Probes of Structure and Function of Macromolecules and Membranes*, B. Chance, C.-P. Lee, and T. Yonetani, Eds., Academic, New York (1971).

137. R. Dupeyre, H. Lemaire, and A. Rassat, *J. Am. Chem. Soc.*, **87,** 3771 (1969).

138. E. Rosantzev, M. Neimann, and V. Goubev, *Izv. Akad. Nauk. SSSR, Ser. Khim.*, **393,** 572, 718 (1965).

139. H. Lemaire, *J. Chim. Phys.*, **64,** 559 (1967).

140. R. Briere, R.-M. Dupeyre, H. Lemaire, C. Morat, A. Rassat, P. Rey, *Bull. Soc. Chim. (France)*, **11,** 3290 (1965).

141. P. Ferruti, D. Gill, M. Klein, and M. Calvin, *J. Am. Chem. Soc.*, **91,** 7765 (1969).

142. M. Calvin, H. Wang, G. Entine, D. Gill, P. Ferruti, M. Harpold, and M. Klein, *Proc. Natl. Acad. Sci.*, **63,** 1 (1969).

143. H. Sternlicht and E. Wheeler in *Magnetic Resonance in Biological Systems*, A. Ehrenberg, B. Malmström, and T. Vänngård, Eds., Pergamon, London, 1967, p. 325.

144. H. McConnell, I. Smith and N. Bhacca, *ibid.*, p. 335.

145. C. Ho, J. Baldassare, and S. Charache, *Proc. Natl. Acad. Sci.*, **66,** 722 (1970).

146. J. Baldassare, S. Charache, R. Jones, and C. Ho, *Biochem.*, **9,** 4707 (1970).

147. T. Hill, *Proc. Natl. Acad. Sci.*, **58,** 111 (1967).

148. K. Butler, P. Hwang, S. Paterson, H. Schneider, and I. Smith (submitted for publication).

149. S. Verma, I. Smith, and H. Schneider (unpublished results).

150. G. Luckhurst and G. Pedulli, *J. Am. Chem. Soc.*, **92,** 4738 (1970).

151. G. Luckhurst and G. Pedulli, *Mol. Phys.*, **20,** 1043 (1971).

152. D. Marsh, S. Schreier-Muccillo, K. McLaughlan, and I. Smith (unpublished).

153. R. Lapper, S. Paterson, and I. Smith, *Can. J. Biochem* (in press).

154. I. Smith, *Chimia*, **25,** 349 (1971).

155. P. Jost, L. Libertini, V. Hebert, and O. Griffith, *J. Mol. Biol.*, **59,** 77 (1971).

156. S. Verma and I. Smith (unpublished results).

157. N. Stanacev, L. Stuhne-Sekalec, S. Schreier-Muccillo, and I. Smith, *Biochem. Biophys. Res. Comm.*, **46,** 114 (1972).

158. L. Berliner and H. McConnell, *Biochem. Biophys. Res. Comm.*, **43,** 651 (1971).

159. S. Schreier-Muccillo, D. Marsh, H. Dugas, H. Schneider, and I. Smith, *Chem. Phys. Lipids* (in press).

Author Index

Numbers in parentheses are reference numbers and show that an author's work is referred to although his name is not mentioned in the text. Numbers in brackets indicate the pages on which the full references appear.

Subject Index

Numbers in parentheses indicate definitions or major coverage. Numbers in brackets indicate figure postscripts; *n* indicates footnote.

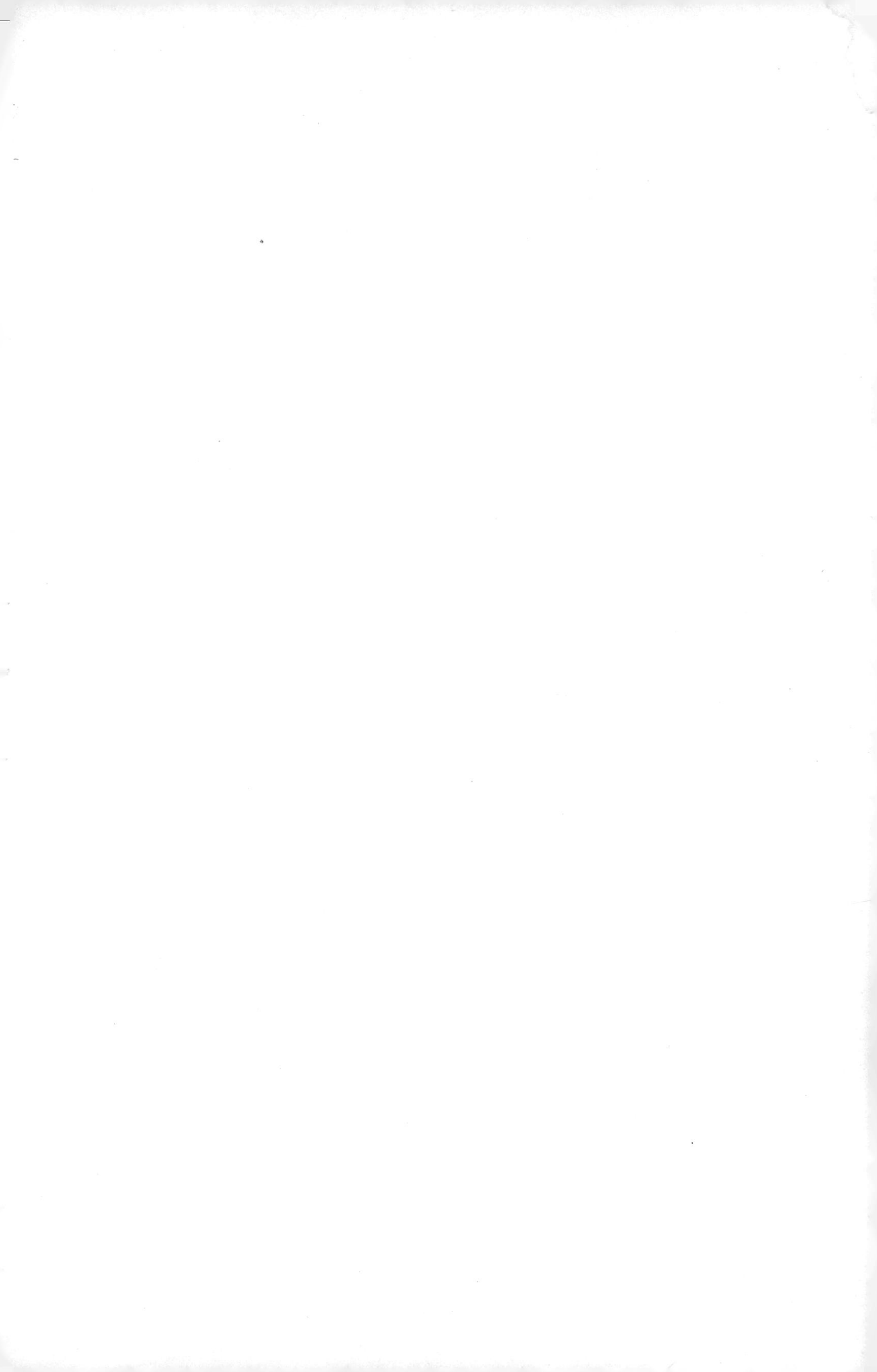